DIAGNOSTIC IMMUNOPATHOLOGY

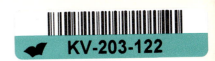

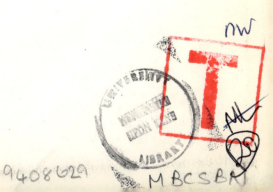

Diagnostic Immunopathology

Editors

Robert B. Colvin, M.D.   Atul K. Bhan, M.D.

Robert T. McCluskey, M.D.

Immunopathology Unit
Department of Pathology
Massachusetts General Hospital and
Harvard Medical School
Boston, Massachusetts

Raven Press New York

Raven Press, 1185 Avenue of the Americas, New York, New York 10036

Made in the United States of America

The material contained in this volume was submitted as previously unpublished material, except in the instances in which credit has been given to the source from which some of the illustrative material was derived.

Great care has been taken to maintain the accuracy of the information contained in the volume. However, neither Raven Press nor the editors can be held responsible for errors or for any consequences arising from the use of the information contained herein.

Materials appearing in this book prepared by individuals as part of their official duties as U.S. Government employees are not covered by the above-mentioned copyright.

9 8 7 6 5 4 3 2 1

Library of Congress Cataloging-in-Publication Data

Diagnostic immunopathology.

  Includes bibliographies and index.
  1. Diagnostic immunohistochemistry.   I. Colvin,
Robert B.   II. Bhan, Atul K.   III. McCluskey, Robert T.
[DNLM: 1. Immunohistochemistry.   2. Immunologic
Technics.   3. Immunologic Tests.   QY 250 D5365]
RB46.6.D53   1988   616.07'56   88-11640
ISBN 0-88167-452-4

Preface

The seed for this book was planted in Boston in 1976, the first year a course in diagnostic immunopathology was given by the editors and their colleagues at the annual meeting of the United States and Canadian Division of the International Academy of Pathology. The advances of the last decade are reflected in the topics added to the course over the subsequent years. In the beginning, there was immunofluorescence of the kidney and skin, with some discussion of E-rosettes and tissue autoantibodies. Soon immunoperoxidase techniques for the diagnosis of the lymphoid and endocrine tumors were discussed. By 1981 monoclonal antibodies had revolutionized the classification of lymphoid cells and automated flow cytometry had emerged as a clinical technique. In the years since, monoclonal antibodies to cell surface and cytoplasmic markers of differention have established immunohistochemistry as a major growth area in diagnostic immunopathology. Lately, molecular biologic techniques have been added to the diagnostic laboratory. The discovery that gene rearrangement is the basis of B and T cell clonal diversity led to the use of Southern blots to characterize B and T cell proliferative disorders. *In situ* DNA/RNA hybridization has demonstrated viral infection in the absence of protein products.

These remarkable advances rest on two pillars: dramatic insights into the molecular mechanisms of the immune system and dazzling technological innovations. Together, these will support a considerably larger edifice in the future. Here we attempt to capture the practicality of these newer diagnostic approaches without losing too much of the rigor or freshness of the underlying science. When choices of subject matter were necessary, we opted for the practical.

The primary purpose of this volume is to provide a practical and critical guide to the performance and interpretation of current immunologic tests performed in diagnostic pathology laboratories. The volume also gives a framework for the analysis of immunopathologic processes. The authors are experts in the diagnostic techniques they describe and were chosen for their contributions in the field. This volume will be of interest to practicing pathologists, clinical immunologists, and other physicians in practice or training with an interest in immunologic diseases and techniques.

Robert B. Colvin, M.D.
Atul K. Bhan, M.D.
Robert T. McCluskey, M.D.

Contents

Immunopathologic Mechanisms

Immunopathologic Diseases

Immunohistochemistry of Neoplasia

Immunopathologic Techniques

Contributors

Giuseppi A. Andres, M.D. *Department of Pathology and Biology, State University of New York at Buffalo, Buffalo, New York 14214*

Debra A. Bell, M.D. *Department of Pathology, Massachusetts General Hospital, Boston, Massachusetts 02114*

Atul K. Bhan, M.D. *Immunopathology Unit, Department of Pathology, Massachusetts General Hospital, Boston, Massachusetts 02114*

Jan R. Brentjens, M.D. *Department of Pathology and Biology, State University of New York at Buffalo, Buffalo, New York 14214*

C. Lynne Burek, M.D. *Department of Immunology and Infectious Disease, Johns Hopkins University, Baltimore, Maryland 21205*

A. Bernard Collins *Immunopathology Unit, Department of Pathology, Massachusetts General Hospital, Boston, Massachusetts 02114*

Robert B. Colvin, M.D. *Immunopathology Unit, Massachusetts General Hospital, Boston, Massachusetts 02114*

Ronald A. DeLellis, M.D. *Department of Pathology, New England Medical Center, Boston, Massachusetts 02111*

Harold F. Dvorak, M.D. *Department of Pathology, Beth Israel Hospital, Boston, Massachusetts 02115*

Thomas J. Flotte, M.D. *Dermatopathology Unit, Department of Pathology, Massachusetts General Hospital, Boston, Massachusetts 02114*

Arnold S. Freedman, M.D. *Division of Tumor Immunology, Dana Farber Cancer Institute, Boston, Massachusetts 02115*

James D. Griffin, M.D. *Division of Tumor Immunology, Dana Farber Cancer Institute, Boston, Massachusetts 02115*

Nancy L. Harris, M.D. *Department of Pathology, Massachusetts General Hospital, Boston, Massachusetts 02114*

James Linder, M.D. *Department of Pathology and Laboratory Medicine, University Nebraska Medical Center, Omaha, Nebraska 68105*

Randall J. Margolis, M.D.   *Dermatopathology Unit, Department of Pathology, Massachusetts General Hospital, Boston, Massachusetts 02114*

Robert T. McCluskey, M.D.   *Department of Pathology, Massachusetts General Hospital, Boston, Massachusetts 02114*

Martin C. Mihm, Jr., M.D.   *Dermatopathology Unit, Department of Pathology, Massachusetts General Hospital, Boston, Massachusetts 02114*

David Myerson, M.D.   *Pathology Section, Fred Hutchinson Cancer and Research Center, Seattle, Washington 98104*

Lee M. Nadler, M.D.   *Division of Tumor Immunology, Dana Farber Cancer Institute, Boston, Massachusetts 02115*

Frederic I. Preffer, Ph.D.   *Immunopathology Unit, Department of Pathology, Massachusetts General Hospital, Boston, Massachusetts 02114*

David T. Purtillo, M.D.   *Department of Pathology and Laboratory Medicine, University Nebraska Medical Center, Omaha, Nebraska 68105*

Noel R. Rose, M.D., Ph.D.   *Department of Immunology and Infectious Disease, Johns Hopkins University, Baltimore, Maryland 21205*

Robert E. Scully, M.D.   *Department of Pathology, Massachusetts General Hospital, Boston, Massachusetts 02114*

Thomas A. Seemayer, M.D.   *Department of Pathology, Montreal Childrens Hospital, Montreal Quebec H3M IP3 Canada*

Paul E. Swanson, M.D.   *Department of Laboratory Medicine and Pathology, University of Minnesota, Minneapolis, Minnesota 55455*

John Q. Trojanowski, M.D.   *Department of Pathology and Laboratory Medicine, University of Pennsylvania School of Medicine, Philadelphia, Pennsylvania 19104*

Mark R. Wick, M.D.   *Department of Laboratory Medicine and Pathology, University of Minnesota, Minneapolis, Minnesota 55455*

Robert H. Young, M.D.   *Department of Pathology, Massachusetts General Hospital, Boston, Massachusetts 02114*

Introduction

This volume is divided into four parts: immunopathologic mechanisms, immunopathologic diseases, immunohistochemistry of neoplasia, and immunopathologic techniques. The subjects and interrelationships are outlined below to indicate the conceptual organization in more detail.

IMMUNOPATHOLOGIC MECHANISMS

The two primary mediators of the immune system are T cells and antibodies. These have immunologic specificity and recruit, arm, and activate the secondary mediators, such as macrophages, mast cells, and the complement system. Some years ago Gell and Coombs proposed a simple classification of immunologic mechanisms that became widely accepted. In Table 1 we give our proposed modification of the Gell-Coombs schema, that incorporates further knowledge of the primary and secondary mechanisms. The principal changes are the addition of another type of cell mediated reaction (cytotoxicity), the division of circulating and *in situ* immune complex mechanisms, and the clearer distinction of reactions to cell and basement membranes. Few diseases are pure examples of these mechanisms. The individual types of reactions can be regarded as "elements" that are combined in various proportions to form the "compounds" typical of actual diseases.

This volume begins with T cells, as most immune responses are under their ultimate control. Chapter 1 by Bhan and McCluskey deals with the current status of the classification and function of human T cells in cell mediated reactions, particularly as revealed by the application of monoclonal antibodies to surface differentiation markers. Chapter 7 (transplantation) extends and applies this information. A table of the current "cluster designations" (CD) of the anti-leukocyte monoclonal antibodies is given in Chapter 18 (flow cytometry). We have adhered to the CD terminology (with common synonyms indicated), because it provides a useful *lingua franca* until the specific functions of the molecules are known.

The mechanisms by which antibodies cause tissue injury is addressed in Chapter 2 by Brentjens and Andres. Particular emphasis is placed on animal models that reveal recently recognized mechanisms of *in situ* immune complex formation, and reaction of antibodies with surface antigens of tissue cells. Autoantibodies to surface molecules are now known to underlie certain autoimmune diseases (Chapters 4,5,6).

IMMUNOPATHOLOGIC DISEASES

Classification of renal disease became the first widely accepted diagnostic application of the immunofluorescence technique developed in the 1940s by Albert Coons at Harvard Medical School. Immunofluorescence has extended knowledge of pathogenesis and is essential in the practice of diagnostic nephropathology. In Chapter 3 McCluskey critically

TABLE 1. *Classification of immunopathologic reactions*

	Reaction	Primary mechanism	Secondary mechanisms	Consequences	Prototype disease or reaction	Gell and Coombs classification[a]
Antibody Mediated						
I	Anaphylactic	Combination of antigen with IgE antibody on mast cells and basophils	Release of mediators: histamine, leukotrienes, PAF, ECF-A	Smooth muscle contraction, vasopermeability, mucus secretion	Asthma Anaphylaxis	Type I (Anaphylactic, reagin dependent)
II	Cell surface	Reaction of antibodies with cell surface antigens	Activation of the complement system; opsonization, antibody dependent cellular cytotoxicity (Fc receptors); activation, blocking, or modulation of antigen	(A) Cytolysis (B) Stimulation of receptor function (C) Loss of receptor function	(A) Hemolytic disease of newborn (B) Graves' disease (C) Myasthenia gravis	Type II (cytotoxic or cell stimulating)
III	Immune complex	Extracellular accumulation of immune complexes formed (A) in the circulation or (B) *in situ*	Activation of the complement system; leukocyte chemotaxis and activation; release of enzymes and toxic O_2 products	Necrosis of nearby cells; damage to matrix; vascular injury; increased permeability	(A) Lupus glomerulonephritis (B) Anti-GBM disease	Type III (immune complex)
T Lymphocyte Mediated						
IV	Delayed-type hypersensitivity (lymphokine)	MHC restricted[b] interaction of T cells with antigen on antigen presenting cell	Liberation of lymphokines; recruitment and activation of other leukocytes (macrophages, NK cells, LAK cells) and modulation of parenchymal cells, fibroblasts, endothelium	Induration; vasopermeability; fibrin deposition; vascular injury; necrosis; granuloma formation; fibrosis	Tuberculin reaction Tuberculoid leprosy	Type IV (delayed hypersensitivity)
V	Cytotoxic	MHC restricted[b] interaction of T cells with antigen on target cell	Contact triggered release of membrane damaging molecules	Cytolysis of target cell	Viral hepatitis (HBV) Graft-vs-host disease	

[a]Coombs, R.R.A., and Gell, P.G.H. (1975): Classification of allergic reactions responsible for clinical hypersensitivity and disease. In *Clinical Aspects of Immunology*, 3rd ed., edited by P.G.H. Gell, R.R.A. Coombs, and P.J. Lachmann, pp. 761–781. Blackwell Scientific Publications, Oxford.
[b]CD4[+] T cells are usually restricted by class II, and CD8[+] T cells by class I MHC molecules.

reviews the current interpretation of renal biopsies using immunofluorescence and related tests.

The recognition in the early 1960s that a variety of inflammatory skin diseases were mediated by antibodies stimulated the diagnostic application of immunofluorescence to skin biopsies and tests for serum autoantibodies reactive to skin components. In Chapter 3, Flotte, Margolis, and Mihm review the state-of-the-art in diagnostic immunodermatopathology and provide useful algorithms for diagnostic interpretation. The related characterization of the cellular inflammatory component in skin diseases is discussed in Chapter 1.

A thorough, succinct review of tests for autoantibodies and their disease correlations is given in Chapter 5 by Burek and Rose. Emphasis is on the classification and interpretation of the complex and prevalent antinuclear antibodies. Assays for antireceptor antibodies that cause Graves' disease and myasthenia gravis are described, as well as those for more traditional autoantibodies. Renal and skin specific autoantibodies are discussed in Chapters 3 and 4, respectively.

The inherited and acquired immunodeficiencies are devastating diseases, which show with dramatic clarity the consequences of specific defects in the immune system. The most common disease in this category, of course, is the acquired immunodeficiency syndrome (AIDS). The diagnosis of these diseases is largely the province of the immunopathologist and clinical immunologist. In Chapter 6 Purtillo, Linder, and Seemayer discuss the immunologic consequences, the immunopathogenesis, and the key diagnostic tests for the diagnosis of the major immunodeficiencies.

Transplantation of kidneys and other organs has advanced substantially over the last decade with the introduction of more effective immunosuppressive agents. During the same period, patient management has become more complex and the pathologist is confronted with more biopsies for interpretation. Chapter 7 by Colvin is a comprehensive guide to the diagnostic evaluation of renal allograft biopsies, which continue to be the most definitive way to diagnose and classify graft rejection. The alternative diagnostic techniques that are discussed include fine needle biopsy, flow cytometry of leukocytes, and assay of interleukin 2 receptor in the serum.

IMMUNOHISTOCHEMISTRY OF NEOPLASMS

The diagnosis of neoplasia was one of the early beneficiaries of the marriage of immunoperoxidase techniques with monoclonal antibodies. Their union has spawned thousands of articles describing applications in tumor pathology. This literature has been culled with considerable effort by the authors of this section to yield those markers with the most practical and durable value in solving problems beyond the ken of dye-based light microscopy. The authors stress the limits of the interpretation of the technique with the view that tumors can be fickle and heterogeneous.

In Chapter 8, Bhan provides an orientation of the most useful markers which are cross-referenced to the other chapters in this section. The key properties and distribution of individual antigens, including the cytokeratins, are summarized. The strategies that have proved useful in solving specific recurrent pathologic differential diagnoses are emphasized. General principles are discussed to provide a framework for future developments.

The cytoskeletal proteins, especially the intermediate filaments, are discussed further in Chapter 9 by Trojanowski with reference to neural tumors. The extreme complexity of this family of proteins is revealed by the author's detailed investigation of the features in medulloblastomas. An important point developed in this chapter is the possibility that immunochemical techniques can detect chemical modifications of proteins that can be used to detect cellular activity (e.g., phosphorylation).

Most of the known molecules related to leukocyte differentiation were discovered by the analysis of the reactivity of monoclonal antibodies; over 45 molecules have been identified. In Chapter 10, Freedman, Griffin, and Nadler define the ontogeny of leukocytes by means of such antibodies (several of which were discovered in their laboratories). This information is then applied to classify leukemias and to predict their behavior.

Monoclonal antibodies have similarly extended the classifications of lymphomas, and are a necessary adjunct to their diagnosis. Chapter 11 by Harris emphasizes the practical approach to an immunochemical lymphoma workup, with the intent of providing standardized, manageable panels that address the important pathologic distinctions. The most reliable criteria for classification are presented from the author's experience in running a busy diagnostic service.

Endocrine tumors have long been defined by the hormone produced, in addition to the cell of origin. Immunohistochemistry provides the most incisive tool to demonstrate the peptide hormones (and certain others) in tissue, and has become an important technique to delineate the normal components of the endocrine system and their pathologic counterparts. DeLellis in Chapter 12 describes the most commonly detected hormones and the diagnostic implications of their presence in a neoplasm. The normal cells and their corresponding neoplasms are compared, and the critical issue of neoplasms with ectopic synthesis is addressed.

The immunohistochemical techniques that have been applied to gynecologic and genitourinary tumors are assessed in Chapter 13 by Bell, Young, and Scully. These experienced diagnosticians look with critical eyes for those instances in which antibodies can yield useful information beyond that appreciable with standard light microscopy. Several antibodies currently meet this test, e.g., prostatic acid phosphatase, prostate specific antigen, and human chorionic growth hormone. No doubt many more will be proposed in the future, but these must pass the stringent criteria implicit in this chapter to achieve widespread clinical acceptance.

Soft tissue tumors and spindle cell tumors in general are among the most frustrating for pathologists, because of the difficulties in appreciating specific lines of differentiation. Chapter 14 by Wick and Swanson describes with clarity the considerable advances afforded by the immunochemical analysis of such tumors and their differential diagnosis. The authors give their strategies in the choice of diagnostically useful panels of antibodies and their interpretation.

Careful analysis of the tumor stroma reveals many similarities with a healing wound, or, more precisely, a wound that does not heal. These aspects of the host-tumor relationship are discussed in Chapter 15 by Dvorak. The pathologic features that indicate the behavior of tumors, such as basement membrane transgression and lymphatic invasion, are more closely related to prognosis than appearance of individual cells. The analysis of normal stromal elements and growth factors (e.g., oncogene products) in tumors may lead to diagnostically and therapeutically useful information in the future.

IMMUNOPATHOLOGIC TECHNIQUES

The last section of the book deals with the implementation of four important techniques, immunofluorescence (Chapter 16, Collins), immunoperoxidase (Chapter 17, Bhan), flow cytometry (Chapter 18, Preffer), and *in situ* hybridization (Chapter 19, Myerson). The emphasis in each chapter is on specific step-by-step descriptions of techniques in use in the author's laboratory. Problems and pitfalls are discussed in detail. These chapters are intended for neophytes who wish to initiate these techniques and for more experienced users looking for refinements and solutions to specific problems.

Diagnostic Immunopathology,
edited by R.B. Colvin,
A.K. Bhan, and R.T. McCluskey.
Raven Press, New York © 1988.

1 / *T Cell Mediated Reactions*

Atul K. Bhan and Robert T. McCluskey

*Department of Pathology, Massachusetts General Hospital, Harvard Medical School,
Boston, Massachusetts 02114*

The purpose of this chapter is to provide a background for the characterization of T cell mediated reactions in man, through analysis of mononuclear cells in inflammatory infiltrates, principally by using monoclonal antibodies and immunohistochemical techniques. The main emphasis will be on how evidence can be obtained concerning the nature of the inflammatory reaction and the role of various types of T cells within infiltrates.

CLASSIFICATION OF CELL MEDIATED REACTIONS

Before discussing how mononuclear cell inflammatory infiltrates in human diseases can be analyzed, categories of cell mediated reactions will be reviewed. Two prototypic local T cell mediated reactions are recognized: delayed type hypersensitivity (DTH or lymphokine mediated reactions) and cytotoxic T cell mediated reactions (see the Introduction).

DTH Reactions

The development of DTH depends on proliferation of sensitized T cells in lymphoid tissue following exposure to certain antigens. The sensitized cells enter the circulation, making it possible for them to interact with antigen virtually anywhere in the host; however, DTH reactions are usually elicited in the skin. Reactions are triggered by interaction of a few sensitized T cells that traverse the vascular barrier and encounter antigen presented on accessory cells—such as macrophages or dendritic cells—in association with major histocompatibility complex (MHC) products. Most of the T cells that initiate DTH reactions have the CD4$^+$ (T4) phenotype; however, since CD8$^+$ (T8) cells can also sometimes trigger DTH reactions (56,108), and since it appears that not all of the heterogeneous class of CD4$^+$ T cells mediate DTH reactions (1,45,86) the functional designation Tdh is useful. Following contact with antigen, the Tdh cells are stimulated to produce and release lymphokines, which result in a slowly developing inflammatory reaction, with recruitment of various leucocytes (23). Prominent among the cells that emigrate at sites of DTH reactions are monocytes and recently formed lymphocytes, with various antigen specificities and phenotypes (64,66,105). The DTH reaction generally peaks at about 2 days in man.

The infiltrates in DTH reactions elicited under various conditions are quite diverse. Species differences are notable. In most species, including man, lymphocytes or mononuclear phagocytes predominate. Lymphocytes tend to concentrate around small vessels (perivascular cuffs) (30). The macrophages in DTH infiltrates become activated, providing a major mechanism for resistance to certain intracellular pathogens, such as *Mycobacterium*. Neutrophils are also seen in many DTH reactions in man, but usually in small numbers. In mice, however, neutrophils predominate in most DTH reactions (100). Even within a given species, the composition of the infiltrate in T cell mediated reactions varies considerably, depending on the tissue involved, the time at which the reaction is studied, the method of immunization, and the physical state of the eliciting antigen. For example, the injection of an insoluble antigen may result in a granulomatous lesion, with nodular accumulation of epithelioid mononuclear phagocytes and predominantly peripherally arranged lymphocytes, whereas another reaction in the same host elicited by a soluble form of the antigen may be characterized by a diffuse infiltrate of lymphocytes and macrophages.

A type of reaction in man and guinea pigs that has generally been considered to be T cell mediated and a variant of DTH is characterized by basophil rich infiltrates [cutaneous basophil hypersensitivity (CBH)]; however, several observations indicate that CBH reactions are heterogeneous and that some may depend not only on T cells but also on antibodies (6,95,97). Cutaneous basophil hypersensitivity reactions lack interstitial fibrin deposition and severe endothelial cell injury, which are characteristic features of classical DTH reactions (30).

Another type of reaction that is generally classified as a form of DTH is contact sensitivity, in which the immunogens consist of conjugates of small molecular weight substances with autologous proteins, formed after application of the sensitizer to the skin. Many contact reactions contain numerous basophils and therefore can be considered as a form of CBH. It is also possible that contact reactions involve the effects of cytolytic T cells directed against neoantigens on epidermal cells (99,101). In contact reactions infiltrates are more intense in the epidermis and upper dermis than in DTH reactions elicited by intradermal injection. This difference in distribution reflects the sites of maximal antigen concentrations.

In most DTH reactions, eosinophils are inconspicuous. In certain situations, however, such as with the retest reaction (elicited by antigen injection at sites of earlier reactions) or schistosome granulomas, numerous eosinophils are found; their accumulation may result either from associated antibody reactions or from lymphokines (23,24).

It seems likely that the diversity of DTH reactions results in part because various reactions are initiated by different subsets of T cells. There is evidence that different subsets of murine CD4$^+$ T cells produce distinctive kinds of lymphokines (1,45,72,86), but evidence that the known subsets of human CD4$^+$ T cells (70,71) produce different lymphokines is lacking.

Reactions also vary because of the concomitant effects of other causes of tissue injury, including antibody-mediated mechanisms, which will be discussed later. In any case, histologic features clearly do not provide a reliable guide to the identification of DTH reactions.

Cytolytic T Cell Reactions

The second major prototypic T cell reaction, T cell mediated cytolysis has been studied mainly *in vitro*; however, evidence for cytolytic T cell killing *in vivo* has also been obtained, especially in experimental viral infections (107), in allografts undergoing rejection, and possibly in tumors. The killing of a target cell by a cytolytic T cell requires close contact between the two cells. The binding of a cytolytic T cell to its target (an MHC restricted event) stimulates the cell's cytolytic activity. Although the mechanism of lysis has not been fully elucidated, there is evidence that the cytolytic cells secrete factors that damage cell membranes (48,106). Most human T cells that exert cytolytic effects belong to the CD8$^+$ subset and recognize target cells bearing class I MHC antigens (67). However, CD4$^+$ T cells can also function as cytolytic T cells, against targets bearing class II MHC antigens (49).

Although it is likely that the predominant role of cytotoxic T cells is direct cell killing, there is evidence, as noted earlier, that T cells with the CD8$^+$ phenotype may also produce effects through release of lymphokines. Furthermore, in most, if not all reactions in which cytolytic T cells play a major role, CD4$^+$ T cells as well as CD8$^+$ lymphocytes are found among the infiltrating cells. Based on this finding and certain experimental observations (52) it seems likely that most, if not all, cytolytic T cell reactions occur in combination with DTH reactions. The DTH component may facilitate the emigration of cytolytic T cells and also may contribute directly to injury through direct effects of lymphokines and changes in the microvasculature (30).

Natural Killer (NK) and Lymphokine Activated Killer Cells (LAK)

In addition to MHC restricted cytolytic T cells, other cells with the morphologic appearance of lymphocytes may exert cytolytic effects in some T cell mediated reactions. These include two groups of lymphocytes that have been designated NK and LAK cells. These populations of cells (which probably overlap to some extent) have the capacity to kill a broad range of target cells *in vitro*, particularly malignant or viral infected cells. However, LAK cells react with a broader range of targets than NK cells. By definition, NK cells are cells with the ability to lyse target cells without prior sensitization to target antigens (88). LAK cells are defined as lymphocytes that have been stimulated to become cytolytic by interleukin-2 (IL-2) (36). The recognition of target cells by both groups of lymphocytes is not MHC restricted. The products recognized on target cells have not been identified. Lysis requires contact between target and effector cells, but the mechanisms responsible for killing are unknown. Most cells with NK activity are described as large granular lymphocytes. Both LAK cells and NK cells are phenotypically heterogeneous. Most NK cells are said to be CD3$^-$, CD16$^+$, Leu 19$^+$, Leu 7$^+$, and NKH-1$^+$ (N901$^+$) (35,54,103); these cells fail to show gene rearrangements of the T cell antigen receptors. Clones of CD3$^+$ cells with NK activity, however, have been identified. Such clones also exhibit MHC restricted cytolytic activity against targets bearing Class I antigens (98). Populations of LAK cells apparently consist mainly of CD3$^+$ cells; however, it has been reported that precursors of LAK cells do not express CD3 (36).

There is evidence that NK cells participate in certain reactions *in vivo*, particularly those occurring in response to viral infected cells (4), tumors or allografts (58), as well as in certain autoimmune diseases (7,28). The finding of the relatively distinctive markers Leu 7 or NKH-1 on infiltrating cells is suggestive of NK activity, but is not entirely specific.

Since IL-2 is released at sites of cell mediated reactions, it is reasonable to assume that LAK cells are induced in such reactions and are represented among the activated T cells in the infiltrates. There are, however, no unique markers that can be used to identify LAK cells. And even when the administration of LAK cells to tumor-bearing patients is followed by tumor regression, it is unknown to what extent the administered LAK cells contribute to mononuclear infiltrates at tumor sites; indeed, it appears likely that most of the cells are secondarily recruited.

Cell Mediated Reactions Combined with Antibody or Other Mechanisms

Reactions involving T cells may take place in association with antibody mediated mechanisms. Antibodies may produce immune complex injury or effects on cell surfaces (see Introduction and Chapter 2). Small numbers of B cells and plasma cells are found in some cell mediated mechanisms. B cells may function not only in antibody production, but also as antigen presenting cells (1). In some longstanding lesions that appear to have been initiated by T cells, ectopic lymphoid tissue develops with follicle and germinal center formation. This provides a setting for the local generation of lymphocytes involved in the reaction. Antigen reactive cells are also generated in infiltrates lacking lymphoid architecture, although probably less efficiently.

Combinations of cell and antibody mediated components probably take place in most naturally occurring immunological reactions. However, not all components are of equal importance. For example, T cells generally account for allograft rejection, even when some B cells and plasma cells are found in the infiltrate. And many immunogens elicit either a predominantly cellular or a humoral response.

Some of the inflammation in cell mediated reactions is secondary to destruction of tissue. For example, during the final stages of allograft rejection, when necrosis becomes widespread, numerous neutrophils usually appear.

ANALYSIS OF CELL MEDIATED REACTIONS IN EXPERIMENTAL STUDIES AND HUMAN DISEASE

In view of the diversity and complexity of cell mediated reactions, the question may be asked: how can the role of individual types of mononuclear cells be analyzed? In experimental models, this question can be studied in transfer experiments. The demonstration that the transfer of T cells, but not of serum, from an affected donor to normal syngeneic recipients results in lesions within a few days at sites where antigen is present provides the most reliable evidence for a primary role of T cells. Similarly, the importance of suppressor cells can best be shown through transfer experiments. For two major reasons, however, there are limitations in the interpretation of transfer studies, even when pure subsets or clones of cells are used: (1) the transferred cells almost never act entirely on their own, but rather lead to the participation of recipient cells in the reaction (and in some instances the recruited cells may be the principal effector cells) (90); and (2) the cells used for transfer, maintained or propagated *in vitro*, may not migrate normally *in vivo* and may therefore fail to induce a reaction.

Obviously, transfer studies cannot be performed in man. Four approaches that have been taken to obtain evidence of a role of T cells in human beings are: (1) demonstration of *in vitro* correlates of cell mediated immunity (for example, lymphokine production) following interaction of the patient's lymphocytes with putative pathogenic antigens (89); (2) analysis of the phenotype of infiltrating cells in tissue sections by immunohistochemical techniques with monoclonal antibodies; (3) studies *in vitro* of functional properties of cells obtained from lesions; and (4) the effect of ablation of T cells by administration of monoclonal antibodies. For example, it has been shown that anti-CD3 monoclonal antibodies (OKT3) can reverse cellular renal graft rejection (see Chapter 7).

ANALYSIS OF THE ROLE OF INFILTRATING CELLS BY IMMUNOHISTOCHEMICAL TECHNIQUES

Immunohistochemical studies of tissue sections make it possible to identify various cell types within infiltrates. The methods also make it possible to obtain information concerning the topographical relationships of inflammatory cells to one another and to resident tissue components, which cannot be obtained by analysis of cells isolated from tissue. Moreover, immunohistochemical studies allow recognition of alterations in resident cells, such as expression of activation markers on endothelial cells (52) or inappropriate or increased expression of major histocompatibility complex (MHC) antigens on parenchymal cells, which may be of pathogenetic importance in certain lesions, as will be discussed.

Both immunofluorescence and immunoenzyme techniques have been used to stain mononuclear cells in tissue sections (see Chapters 16 and 17). Immunoperoxidase methods allow a high level of amplification, which is needed for detection of many cell surface antigens. Analogous immunoelectron microscopic techniques can be used for further characterization and localization of infiltrating cells.

Most lymphocyte cell surface antigens are altered by the methods of fixation and processing used in routine diagnostic studies. Therefore, staining of cell surface antigens is usually performed on frozen tissue sections, in which preservation of morphological details is suboptimal. Recently, a few monoclonal antibodies have been described that recognize lymphocyte surface antigenic determinants in sections prepared from formalin-fixed and paraffin-embedded tissue. Antigens that are heavily glycosylated are apparently especially likely to be preserved after fixation (57).

There are several problems with interpreting immunohistochemical studies of infiltrating mononuclear cells. High background staining, in particular for immunoglobulins, can create difficulties in lesions with serum protein accumulations, such as sites of inflammation or necrosis. Moreover, cells with endogenous peroxidase activity (see Chapter 17), such as granulocytes, may result in false positive staining. This problem may be minimized by blocking endogenous peroxidase activity. In addition, precise enumeration of individual subsets of mononuclear cells in tissue sections is difficult at best. Often it is only possible to obtain a rough estimate of the proportions of positively stained cell subsets. One problem stems from the fact that antigen negative cells may appear stained due to diffusion of reaction product from adjacent positive cells; this is especially likely to occur in dense aggregates. Enumeration of dendritic cells whose processes are stained can be difficult, because multiple processes of a single cell may appear in a given section. Additional problems stem from the fact that many of the monoclonal antibodies commonly used to characterize mononuclear cells are not specific for a particular cell type, and phenotypes do not directly correspond to function, as will be discussed later.

Despite these problems, there is reason to believe that characterization of subsets of mononuclear cells in inflammatory infiltrates can provide evidence for certain cellular mechanisms. Thus, the finding of large numbers of T cells in a lesion, especially cells with activation markers (IL-2 receptors) (9), transferrin receptors (85), class II MHC antigens (21), especially HLA-DR (22,74), or very late activation antigen complex (92) indicates that T cells are playing an active role, probably in response to an antigen present at the site. In addition, the proportions and distribution of T cell subsets may give further insight into the nature of the reaction. As noted earlier, most DTH reactions are mediated by CD4$^+$ T cells, whereas most cytolytic T cells have the CD8$^+$ phenotype. Therefore, a preponderance of CD4$^+$ T cells (especially in association with mononuclear phagocytes) is indicative of DTH reaction. Indeed, as discussed below, studies of classical DTH reactions have shown that CD4$^+$ cells are the predominant type of T cell. Furthermore, since most nucleated cells bear class I MHC antigens and are targets for CD8$^+$ cell cytolysis, lesions with CD8$^+$ cells in juxtaposition to parenchymal cells undergoing necrosis may be interpreted as cytolytic T cell reactions. Studies of human viral infections (79), autoimmune diseases (10), and allografts undergoing rejection support this view, as discussed below.

Although these interpretations are probably valid in general, they are not definitive and do not provide a complete picture of cellular events in an inflammatory reaction, largely because of the following considerations. Individual available monoclonal antibodies do not recognize unique subsets of mononuclear cells. For example, antibodies against CD4 antigens react not only with a major subset of T cells, but also with some mononuclear phagocytes (13). Furthermore, the early interpretation that CD4$^+$ T cells and CD8$^+$ cells comprise subsets with distinct functions is now known to be invalid. Rather, CD4$^+$ T cells and CD8$^+$ cells are characterized by their ability to identify antigens associated either with Class II or Class I MHC products respectively (49,67) (Fig. 1). Although probably most CD4$^+$ T cells function as helper or inducer cells, this category of functions is in itself quite broad. Thus, helper/inducer CD4$^+$ T cells can function to initiate DTH reactions, to induce suppressor or cytotoxic cells, and to provide help in antibody production. Furthermore, CD4$^+$ cells can exhibit effector functions, including cytotoxic activity against cells bearing certain antigens in association with class II MHC products and probably even effector suppressor function. Similarly, CD8$^+$ cells are capable of several functions, including cytolytic effects, suppression and initiation of DTH reactions.

Recently, monoclonal antibodies have been described that are capable of reacting with T cell subsets with functions more limited than those possessed by whole populations of CD4$^+$ or CD8$^+$ T cells. It has been reported that the monoclonal antibody 9.3 reacts with CD8$^+$ cells with cytotoxic function, but not with CD8$^+$ cells with antigen-specific suppressor functions (27). CD11 (Leu 15) is said to be on CD8$^+$ suppressor cells but not cytotoxic CD8$^+$ cells (53). Similarly, CD4$^+$ cells allegedly can be divided into two groups with a monoclonal antibody anti-Leu-8: CD4 cells that activate suppressor cells are Leu 8$^+$, whereas CD4$^+$ cells with helper function do not express Leu-8 antigen (33). Schlossman and his associates have described a monoclonal antibody (anti 2H4) (CD45R) that identifies the inducer of suppressor cells among human CD4 T cells, and another (anti-4B4) CDw29 that identifies the helper/inducer population (70,71).

A major problem with the antibodies that subdivide functional subsets of CD4$^+$ T cells or CD8$^+$ cells is that they are not restricted to either major set of T cells, or even to T cells. It is therefore necessary to perform double-staining studies to identify the subsets just described. Unfortunately, with most antibodies, double staining of two closely associated cell membrane antigens has not been successfully performed in tissue sections (see Chapter 17 for further details). Even without double staining, however, inferences about the function of subsets may sometimes be drawn. For example, it has been reported that the lymphocytes in rheumatoid synovial tissue, which include both CD4 and CD8 sets, are almost entirely 2H4 negative (80). Thus, it can be concluded that most of the T lymphocytes in the infiltrates are not inducers of suppressor cells and may well be inducers of helper cells.

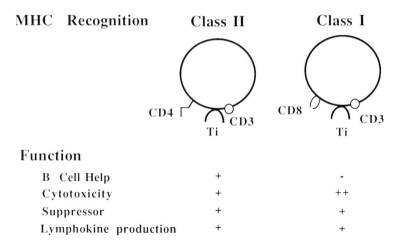

FIG. 1. Reactivities and functions of CD4⁺ and CD8⁺ T cells.

Another major problem with the use of present monoclonal antibodies to characterize lymphocytes is that no information is obtained about their antigen reactivity. Methods for detection of antigen reactivity of T cells recovered from infiltrates are discussed later.

STUDIES OF INFLAMMATORY INFILTRATES IN SELECTED HUMAN DISEASE

Infiltrating lymphocytic subsets have been analyzed in a wide variety of inflammatory conditions in which immunological mechanisms are known or thought to play an important pathogenetic role (12,13). These include inflammatory lesions in the skin (5,17,44,55, 61,75,76), kidney (20,22,26,65), brain (9,39,102), heart (59,84), liver (31,69), conjunctiva (16), thyroid (3,10,41,60), joints (21,29), and salivary glands (2,32). In addition, inflammatory infiltrates in allografts (14,38,46,58,81) (Chapter 7) and tumors (8,15,43,91) have been extensively investigated. Since it is beyond the scope of this chapter to discuss all of these conditions, selected studies will be reviewed, especially those that help explain the role of lymphocyte subsets.

Studies of skin lesions have been particularly informative. It is relatively easy to obtain punch biopsies of the skin and to sample lesions in different stages of development. Furthermore, it has been possible to study prototypic cell mediated reactions elicited in the skin of patients and volunteers.

A finding that has been recognized in lymphocytic infiltrates in various tissues is the tendency of CD4⁺ T cells to accumulate in aggregates, often in perivascular locations, and of CD8⁺ lymphocytes to be more widely scattered, often among parenchymal cells (Figs. 2A and B).

Skin Allografts

There is abundant experimental evidence that both cytolytic T cells and DTH reactions participate in the rejection of solid allografts (52) (see Chapter 7). The findings obtained in immunohistochemical studies of rejecting human allografts also provide evidence for

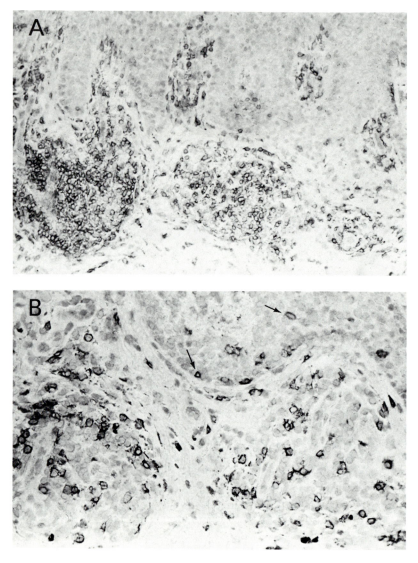

FIG. 2. Frozen sections of an inflammatory skin lesion (chronic eczematous dermatitis) stained for CD4 (**A**) and CD8 (**B**). Most of the lymphocytes in perivascular regions in the dermis are CD4 +. Scattered CD8 + cells are present in the dermis and epidermis (*arrows*). (A × 125, B ×200).

this conclusion. This in turn supports the general validity of interpretations concerning the role of infiltrating cells based on immunohistochemical studies. Bhan et al. (18) performed a study on skin allografts in nonimmunosuppressed adult volunteers. Both CD8 + and CD4 + cells were abundant. The CD8 + cells were more numerous than the CD4 + cells in the epidermis and hair follicles, which is consistent with direct killing of epithelial cells by CD8 + cytotoxic cells. In contrast, CD4 + cells predominated in perivascular infiltrates, both within the graft and in the graft bed, which is consistent with a DTH component.

Studies of GVH reactions have shown that the infiltrates in the epidermis contain predominantly CD8 + cells, which may be responsible for cytolytic effects (40).

DTH Reactions

The CD4$^+$ cells have been found to be the predominant T cell in the infiltrates of the classical DTH tuberculin reaction, especially in perivascular cuffs (82). Of interest is that test sites in tuberculin negative individuals have also shown a lymphocyte-rich infiltrate in which CD4$^+$ cells predominate (82). (Of course many more cells were seen at positive sites as the DTH reaction developed.) As seen in one study (82), the CD4/CD8 ratio in the positive test site was greater than in the blood at 6 hours, but at 15 to 18 hours the ratio was the same in the blood and in the tissue. In control sites, the CD4/CD8 ratio was the same in the blood and tissue at both times (82). In another study perivascular cuffs were found to show a higher CD4/CD8 ratio than did infiltrates throughout the dermis (34); the factors responsible for this difference are unknown. Langerhans cells (CD1$^+$) have been found in the dermal infiltrates as early as 6 hours, which suggests that these cells play a role in the early phase of DTH reactions (47).

In studies of contact reactions, it has been shown that both CD4$^+$ and CD8$^+$ T cells are abundant; of interest is that early infiltrates in contact and toxic reactions have been found to be similar (87,93).

There is experimental evidence that activation of T cells occurs in DTH reactions and is crucial for their development. Evidence of T cell activation in human DTH reaction sites has been obtained by the demonstration on T cells of IL-2 receptors, T9 (transferrin receptor), and CD38 (T10) (82). The proportion of T cells showing activation markers has been observed to increase during the course of DTH reactions, but not in negative control sites.

Granulomatous Reactions

As mentioned earlier, DTH reactions elicited by certain insoluble antigens have granulomatous features. In two conditions with granulomatous lesions, sarcoidosis (11) and tuberculoid leprosy (77,104), that have been studied, CD4$^+$ T cells have been found to be more numerous than CD8$^+$ cells. In addition, distinctive topographic relationships between the T cell subsets have been observed (77). The CD4$^+$ T cells have been described to be diffusely distributed among the macrophages in the granuloma, whereas the CD8$^+$ cells are concentrated among the lymphoid cells at the periphery of the granulomas. It is unclear how the microanatomical distribution of T cell subsets and macrophages relates to the granulomatous reaction. It is possible that the CD8$^+$ cells at the periphery are in large part suppressor cells, which serve to restrict the inflammatory response (68).

Lepromatous Leprosy

The presence of suppressor cells within inflammatory infiltrates has been well documented in studies of lepromatous leprosy. In this condition, T cell reactivity to lepra bacilli is deficient or absent, and there is a lack of granuloma formation. Numerous bacilli-laden macrophages are found in the dermal infiltrates, which reflects the inability of macrophages that have not been activated by T cell products to kill intracellular pathogens. Relatively few T cells are found and most of these are CD8$^+$ (104). It has been shown that CD8$^+$ clones derived from skin lesions of lepromatous leprosy suppress CD4$^+$ T cells responsive to *M. leprae* (68,78). It is reasonable to assume that this type of suppressor function contributes to the paucity of CD4$^+$ T cells in lepromatous infiltrates, possibly through interference with proliferation of CD4$^+$ T cells or through their destruction.

T Cells in Human Viral Infections

Based on numerous experimental studies, it can be concluded that the principal *in vivo* role of cytolytic T cells is to defend against viral infections, which is accomplished mainly by destruction of viral infected cells. Investigations of the phenotype of T cells in human viral infections have also provided evidence for T cell cytolytic destruction of infected cells. Thus, studies of infiltrates in the liver in patients with chronic active hepatitis resulting from hepatitis B infection have revealed that CD8[+] cells predominate in areas of piecemeal necrosis and in lobular parenchyma (79). Moreover, *in vitro* studies have shown that T cells are able to lyse autologous hepatocytes that express HBcAg. It has not been clearly demonstrated, however, that the CD8[+] T cells in the parenchyma are located in juxtaposition to viral infected hepatocytes. Investigation of this issue is difficult, in part because double staining for lymphocyte phenotypes and viral antigens in hepatocytes is required, and because it is unknown exactly what form of viral antigen expressed on the surface of hepatocytes provides the target for cytolytic T cells.

Obviously, the CD8[+] cells are not completely successful in eliminating viral infection in chronic hepatitis and indeed may serve principally to produce hepatic cell injury. An injurious role of cytolytic T cells has been clearly established in models of lymphocytic choriomeningitis (LCM) virus infection in mice. The LCM virus (like the hepatitis B virus) is not cytopathic and in the absence of cytolytic T cells produces no damage.

In other human viral infections that have been studied, roughly equal numbers of CD4[+] T cells and CD8[+] cells have been found in infiltrates, without any distinctive pattern (94).

Many of the CD4[+] T cells and even some of the CD8[+] cells found in infiltrates of virus-induced lesions may function as Tdh cells. As noted earlier, there is evidence that a DTH component may play a role in viral infections, although the final effector mechanism is generally cytolytic destruction of virus-infected cells (56,108).

Antigen Specificities of T Cells in Infiltrates

Interaction between specifically sensitized T cells and antigen initiate cell mediated reactions. The results of numerous experimental studies have shown that lymphocytes of multiple specificities migrate at sites of cell mediated reactions and that there is no preferential migration of specifically sensitized cells in the site containing the corresponding antigen (64,66,83,105). Thus, small numbers of lymphocytes can initiate reactions. It appears, however, that in longstanding reactions there is preferential proliferation of cells with specificity toward antigens present at the site (52,62,63). Regardless of their numbers, antigen-reactive T cells are of crucial importance, since they initiate and drive the reaction.

At present, the only way the antigen specificity of T cells in infiltrates can be examined is by studies of cells isolated or propagated from the affected tissue. Generally large specimens are required to prepare suspensions with adequate numbers of cells directly from tissue. An approach that has made it possible to propagate T cells from small specimens has been developed by Kurnick and his associates, using IL-2 containing media (50). The lymphokine, IL-2, reacts preferentially with activated T cells that express high affinity receptors for it. With specimens that contain intense infiltrates, as many as 10 million T cells can be propagated from a cubic millimeter of tissue within 7 to 10 days. The cells can be expanded further by addition of antigen (when this is known) or of polyclonal activators. The availability of large numbers of T cells makes it possible to detect specific antigen reactivity, through assays that measure proliferation, cytotoxic effects or lympho-kine production. Using this approach, Kurnick and associates have demonstrated donor reactive T cells derived from renal allografts (62,63,98) and T cells with cytolytic activity toward autologous neoplastic cells derived from tumor infiltrates (51).

Similar methods have been used to demonstrate alloreactive cells derived from liver and heart allografts, as well as antigen-specific suppressor cells in cells propagated from lep-romatous skin lesions (68).

Increased Expression of Class II Antigens on Parenchymal Cells in Cell Mediated Reactions

Increased expression of MHC antigens (especially Class II antigens) by resident cells is a common feature of inflammatory reactions, including cell mediated reactions. Some ex-amples of conditions in which this phenomenon has been described are: thyroiditis (3,41, 73), salivary glands in Sjögren's syndrome (32,42), acute interstitial nephritis (25) and renal allografts (37). Interferon-γ is probably of major importance in the induction of Class II antigen in cell mediated reactions (see Chapter 7).

It has been suggested that enhanced expression of MHC Class II antigens plays a role in the pathogenesis of cell mediated autoimmune and other reactions, by causing parenchymal cells to function as antigen-presenting cells (19). This hypothesis requires that some event initiate MHC antigen expression. It has been suggested that a viral infection of an organ, such as the thyroid, might bring about an influx of T lymphocytes, including activated T cells, whose products induce Class II MHC expression on thyrocytes. The thyroid cells might then trigger an autoimmune response. There is, however, no direct evidence that this sequence of events takes place. Even if a viral infection initiates inflammation, thyroid antigens might be released from damaged cells and be processed by "conventional" antigen presenting cells to initiate an autoimmune response. Nevertheless, increased expression of MHC antigens on parenchymal cells may render these cells more susceptible to cytotoxic injury, and thus potentiate certain autoimmune diseases or rejection of allografts.

CONCLUSION

We have discussed how Immunohistochemical studies with monoclonal antibodies have been used to analyze human inflammatory infiltrates, and the limitations of these methods have been reviewed. To date such studies have not revealed diagnostically useful patterns, although certain findings are often of value in distinguishing between inflammatory pro-cesses and lymphoproliferative disorders (see Chapter 11). The major information gained so far relates to the nature of cell mediated reactions and the role of individual cell types. In addition, certain studies have led to the recognition of expression of MHC products by parenchymal cells, which may become targets of the immune response.

Further progress should come with the development of additional monoclonal antibodies that recognize subsets with restricted or unique functional properties and with the develop-ment of techniques that permit staining of individual cells with multiple monoclonal anti-bodies. Other approaches will certainly be useful: analysis of T cell antigen gene rearrange-ment as a way of detecting dominant clones (96); and identification of lymphokines in tissue through the use of monoclonal antibodies or of mRNA for particular lymphokines. Studies in which *in situ* hybridization is combined with immunohistochemistry may shed light on the identity of viral infected cells and on the relationship between these cells and the nature of the juxtaposed cells. Finally, new information obtained from research in basic immunology, as well as from studies of experimental models on the role and interaction of various cell types and lymphokines in cell mediated reactions, should help in the interpretation of human lesions.

REFERENCES

1. Abbas, A. K. (1987): Cellular interactions in the immune response. The roles of B lymphocytes and Interleukin-4. *Am. J. Pathol.*, 129:26–33.
2. Adamson, T. C., 3rd., Fox, R. I., Frisman, D. M., and Howell, F. V. (1983): Immunohistologic analysis of lymphoid infiltrates in primary Sjögren's syndrome using monoclonal antibodies. *J. Immunol.*, 130:203–208.
3. Aichinger, G., Fill, H., and Wick. G. (1985): *In situ* immune complexes, lymphocyte subpopulations, and HLA-DR positive epithelial cells in Hashimoto thyroiditis. *Lab. Invest.*, 52:132–140.
4. Allen, J. E., and Doherty, P. C. (1986): Natural killer cells contribute to inflammation but do not appear to be essential for the induction of clinical lymphocytic choriomeningitis. *Scand. J. Immunol.*, 24:153–162.
5. Andrews, B. S., Schenk, A., Barr, R., Friou, G., Mirick, G., and Ross, P. (1986): Immunopathology of cutaneous human lupus erythematosus defined by murine monoclonal antibodies. *J. Am. Acad. Dermatol.*, 15:474–481.
6. Askenase, P. W. (1973): Cutaneous basophil hypersensitivity in contact-sensitized guinea pigs. I. Transfer with immune serum. *J. Exp. Med.*, 138:1144–1155.
7. Bagnasco, M., Ferrini, S., Venuti, D., Prigione, I., Torre, G., Biassoni, R., and Canonica, G. W. (1987): Clonal analysis of T lymphocytes infiltrating the thyroid gland in Hashimoto's thyroiditis. *Int. Arch. Allergy Appl. Immunol.*, 82:141–146.
8. Bell, D. A., Flotte, T. J., and Bhan, A. K. (1987): Immunohistochemical characterization of seminoma and its inflammatory cell infiltrate. *Hum. Pathol.*, 18:511–520.
9. Bellamy, A. S., Calder, V. L., Feldmann, M., and Davison, A. N. (1985): The distribution of interleukin-2 receptor bearing lymphocytes in multiple sclerosis: evidence for a key role of activated lymphocytes. *Clin. Exp. Immunol.*, 61:248–256.
10. Bene, M. C., Derennes, V., Faure, G., Thomas, J. L., Duheille, J., and Leclere, J. (1983): Graves's disease: *In situ* localization of lymphoid T cell subpopulations. *Clin. Exp. Immunol.*, 52:311–316.
11. Beuchner, S. A., Winkelmann, R. K. and Banks, P. M. (1983): T-cell subsets in cutaneous sarcoidosis. *Arch. Dermatol.*, 119:728–732.
12. Bhan, A. K. (1985): Detection and enumeration of T cells in tissues. In: *Investigation of Cell-Mediated Immunity*, edited by T. Yoshida, pp. 37–48, Churchill Livingstone, London.
13. Bhan, A. K. (1984): Application of monoclonal antibodies to tissue diagnosis. In: *Advances in Immunohistochemistry*, edited by R.A. DeLellis, pp. 1–39, Masson Publishing Inc., New York.
14. Bhan, A. K., Colvin, R. B., Cosimi, A. B., and McCluskey, R. T. (1982): Nature of cellular infiltrate in renal allograft rejection. *Kidney Int.* (abstract), 21:293.
15. Bhan, A. K., and Desmarais, C. L. (1983): Immunohistologic characterization of major histocompatibility antigens and inflammatory cellular infiltrate in human breast cancer. *JNCI*, 71:507–516.
16. Bhan, A. K., Fujikawa, L., and Foster, C. S. (1982): T cell subsets and Langerhans cells in normal and diseased conjunctiva. *Am. J. Ophthalmol.*, 94:205–212.
17. Bhan, A. K., Harrist, T. J., Murphy, G. F., and Mihm, M. C., Jr. (1981): T cell subsets and Langerhans cells in lichen planus: *In situ* characterization using monoclonal antibodies. *Br. J. Dermatol.*, 105:617–622.
18. Bhan, A. K., Mihm, M. C., Jr., and Dvorak, H. F. (1982): T cell subsets in allograft rejection: *In situ* characterization of T cell subsets in human skin allografts by the use of monoclonal antibodies. *J. Immunol.*, 129:1579–1583.
19. Bottazzo, G. F., Pujol-Borrell, R., Hanafusa, T., and Feldmann, M. (1983): Role of aberrant HLA-DR expression and antigen presentation in induction of endocrine autoimmunity. *Lancet*, 2:1115–1119.
20. Boucher, A., Droz, D., Adafer, E., and Noel, L. H. (1986): Characterization of mononuclear cell subsets in renal cellular interstitial infiltrates. *Kidney Int.*, 29:1043–1049.
21. Burmester, G. R., Yu, D. T., Irani, A. M., Kunkel, H. G., and Winchester, R. J. (1981): Ia⁺ T cells in synovial fluid and tissues of patients with rheumatoid arthritis. *Arthritis Rheum.*, 24:1370–1376.
22. Caligaris-Cappio, F., Bergui, L., Tesio, L., Ziano, R., and Camussi, G. (1980): HLA-Dr⁺ T cells of the Leu 3 (helper) type infiltrate the kidneys of patients with systemic lupus erythematosus. *Clin. Exp. Immunol.*, 59:185–189.
23. Cohen, S. (1986): Physiologic and pathologic manifestations of lymphokine action. *Hum. Pathol.*, 17:112–121.

24. Cohen, S., and Ward, P. A. (1971): *In vitro* and *in vivo* activity of a lymphocyte and immune complex-dependent chemotactic factor for eosinophils. *J. Exp. Med.*, 133:133–146.

25. Colvin, R. B. (1986): Pathogenesis of interstitial nephritis: Role of Ia expression. In: *Drugs and the Kidney*, edited by, T. Bertani, G. Remuzzi, and S. Garattini, vol. 33, pp. 175–183, Raven Press, New York.

26. DAgati, V. D., Appel, G. B., Estes, D., Knowles, D. M., 2nd., and Pirani, C. L. (1986): Monoclonal antibody identification of infiltrating mononuclear leukocytes in lupus nephritis. *Kidney Int.*, 30:575–581.

27. Damale, N. K., Mohagheghpour, N., Hansen, J. A., and Engleman, E. G. (1983): Alloantigen-specific cytotoxic and suppressor T lymphocytes are derived from phenotypically distinct precursors. *J. Immunol.*, 131: 2296–2300.

28. Del Prete, G. F., Vercelli, D., Tiri, A., Maggi, E., Mariotti, S., Pinchera, A., Ricci, M., and Romagnani, S. (1986): *In vivo* activated cytotoxic T cells in the thyroid infiltrate of patients with Hashimoto's thyroiditis. *Clin. Exp. Immunol.*, 65:140–147.

29. Duke, O., Panayi, G. S., Janossy, G., and Poulter, L. W. (1982): An immunohistological analysis of lymphocyte subpopulations and their microenvironment in the synovial membranes of patients with rheumatoid arthritis using monoclonal antibodies. *Clin. Exp. Immunol.*, 49:22–30.

30. Dvorak, H. F., Galli, S. J., and Dvorak, A. M. (1986): Cellular and vascular manifestation of cell-mediated immunity. *Hum. Pathol.*, 17:122–137.

31. Eggink, H. F., Houthoff, H. J., Huitema, S., Gips, C. H., and Poppema, S. (1982): Cellular and humoral immune reactions in chronic active liver disease. I. Lymphocyte subsets in liver biopsies of patients with untreated idiopathic autoimmune hepatitis, chronic active hepatitis B and primary biliary cirrhosis. *Clin. Exp. Immunol.*, 50:17–24.

32. Fox, R. I., Bumol, T., Fantozzi, R., Bone, R., and Schreiber, R. (1986): Expression of histocompatibility antigen HLA-DR by salivary gland epithelial cells in Sjögren's syndrome. *Arthritis Rheum.*, 29:1105–1111.

33. Gatenby, R. A., Kansas, G. S., Xian, C. Y., Evans, R. L., and Engleman, E. G. (1982): Dissection of immunoregulatory subpopulations of T lymphocytes within the helper and suppressor sublineages in man. *J. Immunol.*, 129:1997–2000.

34. Gibbs, J. H., Ferguson, J., Brown, R. A., Kenicer, K. J., Potts, R. C., Coghill, G., and Swanson-Beck, J. (1984): Histometric study of localization of lymphocyte subsets and accessory cells in human Mantoux reactions. *J. Clin. Pathol.*, 37:1227–1234.

35. Griffin, J. D., Herscend, T., Beveridge, R., and Schlossman, S. F. (1983): Characterization of an antigen expressed by human natural killer cells. *J. Immunol.*, 130:2947–2951.

36. Grimm, E. A., Ramsey, K. M., Mazumder, A., Wilson, D. J., Djeu, J. Y., and Rosenberg, S. A. (1983): Lymphokine-activated killer cell phenomenon. II. The precursor is serologically distinct from peripheral T-lymphocytes, memory, CTL and NK cells. *J. Exp. Med.*, 157:884–897.

37. Hall, B. M., Bishop, G. A., Duggin, G. G., Horvath, J. S., Phillips, J., and Tiller, D. J. (1984): Increased expression of HLA-DR antigens on renal tubular cells in renal transplants: relevance to the rejection response. *Lancet*, 2:247–251.

38. Hancock, W. W., Thomson, N. M., and Atkins, R. C. (1983): Composition of interstitial cellular infiltrate identified by monoclonal antibodies in renal biopsies of rejecting human renal allografts. *Transplantation*, 35:458–463.

39. Hauser, S. L., Bhan, A. K., Giles, F., Kemp, M., Kerr, C. K., and Weiner, H. L. (1986): Immunohistochemical analysis of the cellular infiltrate in multiple sclerosis lesions. *Ann. Neurol.*, 19:578–587.

40. Janossy, G., Montano, L., Selby, W. S., Duke, O., Panayi, G., Lampert, I., Thomas, J. A., Granger, S., Bofill, M., Tidman, N., Thomas, H. C., and Goldstein, G. (1982): T cell subsets abnormalities in tissue lesions developing during autoimmune disorders, viral infection and graft-vs-host disease. *J. Clin. Immunol.*, 2:42s–56s.

41. Jonsson, R., Karlsson, A., and Forsum, U. (1984): Intrathyroidal HLA-DR expression and T lymphocyte phenotypes in Graves' thyrotoxicosis, Hashimoto's thyroiditis and nodular colloid goiter. *Clin. Exp. Immunol.*, 58:264–272.

42. Jonsson, R., Klareskog, L., Backman, K., and Tarkowski, A. (1987): Expression of HLA-D-Locus (DP, DQ, DR)-coded antigens, β_2-microglobulin and interleukin 2 receptor in Sjögren's syndrome. *Clin. Immunol. Immunopathol.*, 45:235–243.

43. Kabawat, S. E., Bast, R. C., Welch, W. R., Knapp, R. C., and Bhan, A. K. (1983): Expression of major histocompatibility antigens and nature of inflammatory cellular infiltrate in ovarian neoplasms. *Int. J. Cancer*, 32:547–554.

44. Kanerva, L., Ranki, A., and Lauharanta, J. (1984): Lymphocytes and Langerhans cells in patch tests. An immunohistochemical and electron microscopic study. *Contact Dermatitis*, 11:150–155.

45. Killar, L., MacDonald, G., West, J., Woods, A., and Bottomly, K. (1987): Cloned, Ia-restricted T cells that do not produce interleukin 4(IL4)/B cell stimulatory factor 1(BSF-1) fail to help antigen-specific B cells. *J. Immunol.*, 138:1674–1679.

46. Kolbeck, P. C., Tatum, A. H., and Sanfilippo, F. (1984): Relationships among the histologic pattern, intensity, and phenotypes of T cells infiltrating renal allografts. *Transplantation*, 38:709–713.

47. Konttinen, Y. T., Bergroth, V., Visa-Tolvanen, K., Reitamo, S., and Forstrom, L. (1983): Cellular infiltrate

in situ and response kinetics of human intradermal and epicutaneous tuberculin reactions. *Clin. Immunol. Immunopathol.*, 28:441–449.

48. Kranz, D. M., Pasternack, M. S., and Eisen, H. N. (1987): Recognition and lysis of target cells by cytotoxic T lymphocytes. *Fed. Proc.*, 46:309–312.

49. Krensky, A. M., Clayberger, C., Reiss, C. S., Strominger, J. L., and Burakoff, S. J. (1982): Specificity of OKT4$^+$ cytotoxic T lymphocyte clones. *J. Immunol.*, 129:2001–2003.

50. Kurnick, J. T., Gronvik, K. O., Kimura, A. K., Lindblom, J. B., Skoog, V. T., Sjoberg, O., and Wigzell, H. (1978): Long term growth *in vitro* of human T cell blasts with maintenance of specificity and function. *J. Immunol.*, 122:1255–1260.

51. Kurnick, J. T., Kradin, R. L., Blumberg, R., Schneeberger, E. E., and Boyle, L. A. (1986): Functional characterization of T lymphocytes propagated from human lung carcinomas. *Clin. Immunol. Immunopathol.*, 38:367–380.

52. Kurnick, J. T., and McCluskey, R. T. (1988): Perspective on cell mediated immunity *in vivo*. In: *The Role of Lymphokines in The Immune Response*, edited by S. Cohen, CRC Press Inc., Boca Raton, Florida.

53. Landay, A., Gartland, G. L., and Clement, L. T. (1983): Characterization of a phenotypically distinct subpopulation of Leu-2$^+$ cells that suppresses T cell proliferative responses. *J. Immunol.*, 131:2757–2761.

54. Lanier, L. L., Le, A. M., Cwirla, S., Federspiel, N., and Phillips, J. H. (1986): Antigenic, functional, and molecular genetic studies of human natural killer cells and cytotoxic T lymphocytes not restricted by the major histocompatibility complex. *Fed. Proc.*, 45:2823–2828.

55. Leung, D. Y. M., Bhan, A. K., Schneeberger, E. E., and Geha, R. S. (1983): Characterization of the mononuclear cell infiltrate in atopic dermatitis using monoclonal antibodies. *J. Allergy Clin. Immunol.*, 71:47–56.

56. Lin, Y. L., and Askonas, B. A. (1981): Biological properties of an influenza A virus-specific killer T cell clone. Inhibition of virus replication *in vivo* and induction of delayed-type hypersensitivity reactions. *J. Exp. Med.*, 154:225–234.

57. Linder, J., Ye, Y., Harrington, D. S., Armitage, J. O., and Weisenburger, D. D. (1987): Rapid Communication. Monoclonal Antibodies marking T lymphocytes in paraffin-embedded tissue. *Am. J. Pathol.*, 127:1–8.

58. Marboe, C. C., Knowles, D. M., II, Chess, L., Raetsma, K., and Fenoglio, J. J. (1983): The immunologic and ultrastructural characterization of the cellular infiltrate in acute cardiac allograft rejection. Prevalence of cells with the natural killer (NK) phenotype. *Clin. Immunopathol.*, 27:141–151.

59. Marboe, C. C., Knowles, D. M., II, Weiss, M. B., and Fenoglio, J. J., Jr. (1985): Monoclonal antibody identification of mononuclear cells in endomyocardial biopsy specimens from a patient with rheumatic carditis. *Hum. Pathol.*, 16:332–338.

60. Margolick, J. B., Hsu, S. M., Volkman, D. J., Burman, K. D., and Fauci, A. S. (1984): Immunohistochemical characterization of intrathyroid lymphocytes in Graves' disease. Interstitial and intraepithelial populations. *Am. J. Med.*, 76:815–821.

61. Margolis, R., Tonnesen, M. C., Harrist, T. J., Bhan, A. K., Wintroub, B. U., Mihm, M. C., Jr., and Soter, N. A. (1983): Lymphocyte subsets and Langerhans/indeterminate cells in erythema multiforme. *J. Invest. Dermatol.*, 81:403–406.

62. Mayer, T. G., Fuller, A. A., Lazarovits, A. I., Boyle, L. A., and Kurnick, J. T. (1985): Characterization of *in vivo*-activated allospecific T lymphocytes propagated from human renal allograft biopsies undergoing rejection. *J. Immunol.*, 134:258–264.

63. Mayer, T. G., Lazarovits, A. I., Boyle, E. R., Sullivan, E. R., Leary, C. P., Fuller, A. A., Fuller, T. C., Cosimi, A. B., Bhan, A. K., Colvin, R. B., Collins, A. B., and Kurnick, J. T. (1985): Functional allospecific T lymphocytes isolated from human renal allograft biopsy. *Transplant. Proc.*, 17:816–818.

64. McCluskey, R. T., Benacerraf, B., and McCluskey, J. W. (1963): Studies on the specificity of the cellular infiltrate in delayed hypersensitivity reactions. *J. Immunol.*, 90:466–477.

65. McCluskey, R. T., and Bhan, A. K. (1986): Cell-mediated immunity in renal diseases. *Hum. Pathol.*, 17:146–153.

66. McCluskey, R. T., and Bhan, A. K. (1977): Cell-mediated reactions *in vivo*. In: *Mechanisms of Tumor Immunity*, edited by I. Green, S. Cohen, and R.T. McCluskey, pp. 1–25. John Wiley and Sons, New York.

67. Meuer, S. C., Hussey, R. E., Hodgdon, J. C., Hercend, T., Schlossman, S. F., and Reinherz, E. L. (1982): Surface structures involved in target recognition by human cytotoxic T-lymphocytes. *Science*, 218:471–473.

68. Modlin, R. L., Kato, H., Mehra, V., Nelson, E. E., Fan, X. D., Rea, T. H., Pattengale, P. K., and Bloom, B. R. (1986): Genetically restricted suppressor T cell clones derived from lepromatous leprosy lesions. *Nature*, 322:459–461.

69. Montano, L., Aranguibel, F., Boffill, M., Goodall, A. H., Janossy, G., and Thomas, H. C. (1983): An analysis of the composition of the inflammatory infiltrate in autoimmune and hepatitis B virus-induced chronic liver disease. *Hepatology*, 3:292–296.

70. Morimoto, C., Letvin, N. L., Distaso, J. A., Aldrich, W. R., and Schlossman, S. F. (1985): The isolation and characterization of the human suppressor inducer T cell subset. *J. Immunol.*, 134:1508–1515.

71. Morimoto, C., Letvin, N. L., Boyd, A. W., Hagan, M., Brown, H. M., Kornacki, M. M., and Schlossman, S. F. (1985): The isolation and characterization of the human helper inducer T cell subset. *J. Immunol.*, 134:3762–3769.

72. Mosmann, T. R., Cherwinski, H., Bond, M. W., Giedlin, M. A., and Coffman, R. L. (1986): Two types of murine helper T cell clone. I. Definition according to profiles of lymphokine activities and secreted proteins. *J. Immunol.*, 136:2348–2357.

73. Most, J., Knapp, W., and Wick, G. (1986): Class II antigens in Hashimoto thyroiditis. I. Synthesis and expression of HLA-DR and HLA-DQ by thyroid epithelial cells. *Clin. Immunol. Immunopathol.*, 41:165–174.

74. Most, J., Wick, G. (1986): Class II antigens in Hashimoto thyroiditis. II. Expression of HLA-DR on infiltrating mononuclear cells in peripolesis. *Clin. Immunol. Immunopathol.*, 41:175–183.

75. Muhlbauer, J. E., Bhan, A. K., Harrist, T. J., Bernhard, J. D., and Mihm, M. C., Jr. (1983): Papular polymorphus light eruption: An immunoperoxidase study employing monoclonal antibodies. *Br. J. Dermatol.*, 108:153–162.

76. Muhlbauer, J. E., Bhan, A. K., Harrist, T. J., Moscicki, R. A., Rand, R., Caughman, W., Loss, B., and Mihm, M. C., Jr. (1984): Immunopathology of pityriasis lichneoides acuta. *J. Am. Acad. Dermatol.*, 10:783–795.

77. Narayanan, R. B., Ramu, G., Malaviya, G. N., Sengupta, U., and Desikan, K. V. (1985): *In situ* characterization of cells in the dermal infiltrates of lepromin reaction using monoclonal antibodies. *Indian J. Lepr.*, 57:265–272.

78. Ottenhoff, T. H. M., Elferink, D. G., Klatser, P. R., and deVries, R. R. P. (1986): Cloned suppressor T cells from a lepromatous leprosy patient suppress Mycobacterium leprae reactive helper T cells. *Nature*, 322:462–464.

79. Paronetto, F. (1986): Cell-mediated immunity in liver disease. *Hum. Pathol.*, 17:168–178.

80. Pitzalis, C., Kingsley, G., Murphy, J., and Panayi, G. (1987): Abnormal distribution of the helper-inducer and suppressor-inducer T-lymphocyte subsets in rheumatoid joint. *Clin. Immunol. Immunopathol.*, 45:252–258.

81. Platt, J. L., LeBien, T. W., and Michael, A. F. (1981): Interstitial mononuclear cell populations in renal allograft reflection: Identification by monoclonal antibodies in tissue sections. *J. Exp. Med.*, 155:17–30.

82. Platt, J. L., Grant, B. W., Eddy, A. A., and Michael, A. F. (1983): Immune cell populations in cutaneous delayed type hypersensitivity. *J. Exp. Med.*, 158:1227–1242.

83. Prendergast, R. A. (1964): Cellular immunity in the homograft reaction. *J. Exp. Med.*, 119:377–387.

84. Raizada, V., Williams, R. C., Jr., Chopra, P., Gopinath, N., Prakash, K., Sharma, K. B., Cherian, K. M., Panday, S., Arora, R., Nigam, M., Zabriskie, J. B., and Husby, G. (1983): Tissue distribution of lymphocytes in rheumatic heart valves as defined by monoclonal anti-T cell antibodies. *Am. J. Med.*, 74:90–96.

85. Ralfkiaer, E., and Lange-Wantzin, G. (1984): *In situ* immunological characterization of the infiltrating cells in positive patch tests. *Br. J. Dermatol.*, 111:13–22.

86. Reinherz, E. L., Morimoto, C., Fitzgerald, K. A., Hussey, R. E., Daley, J. F., and Schlossman, S. F. (1982): Heterogeneity of human T4$^+$ inducer T-cells defined by a monoclonal antibody that delineates two functional subpopulations. *J. Immunol.*, 128:463–468.

87. Reitamo, S., Tolvanen, E., Konttinen, Y. T., Kayhko, K., Forstrom, L., and Salo, O. P. (1981): Allergic and toxic contact dermatitis: Inflammatory cell subtypes in epicutaneous test reactions. *Br. J. Dermatol.*, 105:521–527.

88. Reynolds, C. W., and Ortaldo, J. R. (1987): Natural killer activity: The definition of a function rather than a cell type. *Immunol. Today*, 8:172–174.

89. Rocklin, R. E., Lewis, E. J., and David, J. R. (1970): *In vitro* evidence for cellular hypersensitivity to glomerular basement membrane antigens in human glomerulonephritis. *N. Engl. J. Med.*, 283:497–501.

90. Rosenberg, A. S., Mizuochi, T., Sharrow, S., and Singer, A. (1987): Phenotype, specificity and function of T cell subsets and T cell interactions involved in skin allograft rejection. *J. Exp. Med.*, 165:1296–1315.

91. Ruiter, D. J., Bhan, A. K., Harrist, T. J., Sober, A. J., and Mihm, M. C., Jr., (1982): Major histocompatibility antigens and mononuclear inflammatory infiltrates in benign nevomelanocytic proliferations and malignant melanoma. *J. Immunol.*, 129:2808–2815.

92. Saltini, C., Hemler, M. E., and Crystal, R. G. (1988): T lymphocytes compartmentalized on the epithelial surface of the lower respiratory tract express the very late activation antigen complex VLA-1. *Clin. Immunol. Immunopathol.*, 46:221–223.

93. Scheynius, A., Fischer, T., Forsum, U., and Klareskog, L. (1984): Phenotypic characterization *in situ* of inflammatory cells in allergic and irritant contact dermatitis in man. *Clin. Exp. Immunol.*, 55:81–90.

94. Sobel, R. A., Collins, A. B., Colvin, R. B., and Bhan, A. K. (1986): The *in situ* cellular immune response in acute herpes simplex encephalitis. *Am. J. Pathol.*, 125:332–338.

95. Sobel, R. A., Hanzakos, J. L., Blanchette, B. W., Williams, A. M., Dellapelle, P., and Colvin, R. B. (1987): Anti-T cell monoclonal antibodies *in vivo*. I. Inhibition of delayed hypersensitivity but not cutaneous basophil hypersensitivity reactions. *J. Immunol.*, 138:2500–2506.

96. Stamenkovic, I., Stegagno, M., Wright, K. A., Krane, S. M., Amento, E. P., Colvin, R. B., Duquesnoy, R. J., and Kurnick, J. T. (1988): Clonal dominance among T lymphocyte infiltrates in arthritis. *Proc. Natl. Acad. Sci.* (in press).

97. Stashenko, P. P., Bhan, A. K., Schlossman, S. F., and McCluskey, R. T. (1977): Local transfer of delayed hypersensitivity and cutaneous basophil hypersensitivity. *J. Immunol.*, 119:1987–1993.

98. Stegagno, M., Boyle, L. A., Preffer, F. I., Leary, C. P., Colvin, R. B., Cosimi, A. B., and Kurnick, J. T. (1987): Functional analysis of T cell subsets and clones in human renal allograft rejection. *Transplant. Proc.*, 19:394–397.

99. Sunday, M. E., and Dorf, M. E. (1981): Hapten-specific T cell response to 4-hydroxy-3-nitrophenyl acetyl. X. Characterization of distinct T cell subsets mediating cutaneous sensitivity responses. *J. Immunol.*, 127: 766–768.

100. Sy, M. S., Schneeberger, E., McCluskey, R., Greene, M. I., Rosenbert, R. D., and Benacerraf, B. (1983): Inhibition of delayed-type hypersensitivity by heparin depleted of anti-coagulant activity. *Cellular Immunol.*, 82:23–32.

101. Tamaki, K., Fujiwara, H., Levy, R. B., Shearer, G. M., and Katz, S. I. (1981): Hapten specific TNP-reactive cytotoxic effector cells using epidermal cells as targets. *J. Invest. Dermatol.*, 77:225–229.

102. Traugott, U., and Raine, C. S. (1984): Further lymphocyte characterization in the central nervous system in multiple sclerosis. *Ann. N.Y. Acad. Sci.*, 436:163–180.

103. Trinchieri, G. (1986): Surface phenotype of natural killer cells and macrophages. *Fed. Proc.*, 45:2821–2822.

104. van Vorrhis, W. C., Kaplan, G., Sanno, E. N., Horwitz, M. A., Steinman, R. M., Levis, W. R., Nogueira, N., Hair, L. S., Gattas, C. R., Arrick, B. A., and Cohn, Z. A. (1982): The cutaneous infiltrate of leprosy: Cellular characterization and predominant T cell phenotype. *N. Engl. J. Med.*, 307:1593–1597.

105. Werdelin, O., and McCluskey, R. T. (1971): The nature of the specificity of mononuclear cells in experimental autoimmune inflammation and mechanisms leading to their accumulation. *J. Exp. Med.*, 133:1242–1263.

106. Young, J. D. E., Damiano, A., DiNome, M. A., Leong, L. G., and Cohn, Z. A. (1987): Disassociation of membrane binding and lytic activities of the lymphocyte pore-forming protein (perforin). *J. Exp. Med.*, 165:1371–1382.

107. Zinkernagal, R. M., Haenseler, E., Leist, T., Cerny, A., Hengartner, H., and Althage, A. (1986): T cell-mediated hepatitis in mice infected with lymphocytic choriomeningitis virus. *J. Exp. Med.*, 164:1075–1092.

108. Zinkernagel, R. M., Leist, T., Hengartner, H., and Althage, A. (1985): Susceptibility to lymphocytic choriomeningitis virus isolates correlates directly with early and high cytotoxic T cell activity, as well as with foot pad swelling reaction, and all three are regulated by H-20. *J. Exp. Med.*, 162:2125–2141.

Diagnostic Immunopathology,
edited by R.B. Colvin,
A.K. Bhan, and R.T. McCluskey.
Raven Press, New York © 1988.

2 / *Antibody-Mediated Reactions*

Jan R. Brentjens and Giuseppe A. Andres

Departments of Pathology, Microbiology, and Medicine, School of Medicine, State University of New York, Buffalo, New York 14214; and the Renal Research Laboratory, Buffalo General Hospital, Buffalo, New York 14203

According to the modified classification of Gell and Coombs (see Preface), there are three different mechanisms by which antibodies may induce tissue injury (126). In type I or anaphylactic hypersensitivity, the antigen reacts with antibody (IgE in man), bound through its Fc piece to mast cells or circulating basophils. This leads to degranulation of these cells and release of various mediators of inflammation. In type II hypersensitivity, antibodies bind to antigens present on the surface of cells. In type III or immune complex-mediated hypersensitivity, antigen-antibody complexes deposited from the circulation (IIIA), or formed *in situ* (IIIB), cause inflammatory lesions. This chapter will discuss tissue injury caused by type II or type III hypersensitivity reactions.

Most of our insight into antibody-mediated immunopathology has been derived from the study of experimentally induced or spontaneously developing tissue lesions in laboratory animals. The organs most extensively studied, namely the kidney and lung, will feature prominently in this chapter. The establishment of an animal model can result in the recognition of the occurrence of a similar immunopathologic process in man. An effort will be made to discuss our more limited knowledge of human antibody-mediated tissue lesions in light of data generated by animal experimentation.

The organ that has received the most attention from immunopathologists is the kidney (7,8,42,119,156). In the 1960s, pioneering work by Germuth and Dixon and their associates led to the widely accepted hypothesis that granular immune deposits in the kidney were indicative of a nephropathy caused by circulating immune complexes (type IIIA hypersensitivity), whereas the presence of immune reactants in a linear pattern pointed to anti-basement membrane antibody-mediated nephritis (type IIIB hypersensitivity). Since the end of the 1970s, however, it has become increasingly evident that granular immune deposits may also arise from the local interaction of antibody with tissue-bound antigens (8,44, 147). The possibility of local or *in situ* immune deposit formation had already been proposed earlier to explain experimental lesions in tissues other than the kidney (8).

Examples of type II and III hypersensitivity reactions will be discussed under interactions of antibodies with intrinsic plasma membrane antigens; with endogenous antigens "leaking" from or secreted by cells; with intrinsic antigens present in basement membranes or intercellular matrix; or with antigens planted in tissue. Next the validity of the concept of tissue damage caused by deposition of circulating immune complexes will be assessed.

Finally, the current thinking on humoral and cellular mediation of antibody-induced tissue pathology will be summarized.

INTERACTION OF ANTIBODIES WITH INTRINSIC PLASMA MEMBRANE ANTIGENS (TYPE II)

Animal Models

Antibodies to Endothelial Cells

Angiotensin converting enzyme (ACE) is one of many proteins expressed on the plasma membrane of endothelial cells. Although ACE is found on the surface of endothelial cells in all vascular districts, a major site of ACE activity appears to be the lung. Rabbits or rats given a large intravenous dose of anti-ACE antibodies develop increased vascular permeability and frequently die from pulmonary edema. In one study (13), rabbits received relatively small doses of goat anti-rabbit ACE antibodies for 1 to 4 days. Due to pulmonary edema, many animals did not survive the first day of injection. Immunofluorescence microscopy revealed distinctly granular deposits of goat IgG, rabbit C3, and ACE along the alveolar capillary endothelium (Fig. 1). The granular distribution of ACE antigen after interaction *in vivo* with antibody is contrasted with the even, linear expression of the antigen on the surface of the alveolar endothelium observed in normal lung *in vitro* (Fig. 2). Rabbits surviving the 1st day tolerated subsequent administration of anti-ACE anti-

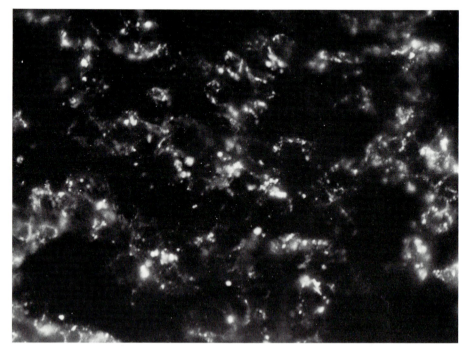

FIG. 1. Lung of a rabbit that received an intravenous injection of anti-ACE antibodies. The immunofluorescence micrograph shows a granular distribution of ACE along the alveolar capillary walls. ($\times$ 600)

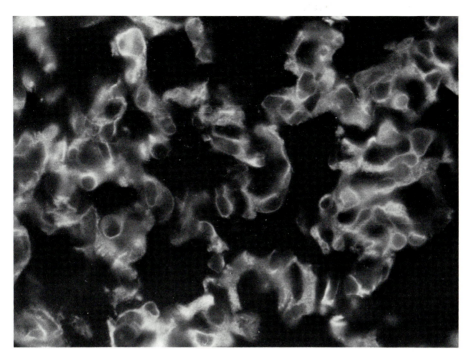

FIG. 2. Lung of an untreated rabbit. The immunofluorescence micrograph shows the normal, linear distribution of ACE along the alveolar capillary endothelium. (× 600)

bodies without apparent ill effects. This dramatic change in the response to antibody injection could be explained by the disappearance of ACE from the lung after continued *in vivo* interaction with specific antibody. In lungs of rabbits killed on the 4th day of injection, deposits of goat IgG and rabbit C3 were not present and ACE itself could no longer be demonstrated. Thus, in animals that did not die during the 1st day of anti-ACE antibody injection, a precipitous decrease in antigen availability protected the alveolar endothelium from further antibody-mediated injury. Within 24 hours of discontinuing antibody administration, ACE was again detectable in the lung.

The *in vivo* "immunological enzymectomy" of ACE from the lung is an example of antigenic modulation (17,66,132) due to the fluidity of the plasma membrane. Proteins present in this structure tend to have a random distribution; however, a rearrangement of plasma membrane proteins occurs when they are cross-linked by antibodies or other appropriate ligands. This phenomenon has been documented in detail *in vitro*. When antibodies react with plasma membrane antigens, such as immunoglobulins on B-lymphocytes or viral antigens on virus-infected cultured cells, successive changes take place in the plasma membrane. After an initial clustering of the immune complexes on the cell surface, the small patches form larger aggregates or caps. The redistribution of the plasma membrane proteins is followed by endocytosis and/or shedding of the immune complexes, leaving the surface of the cell temporarily free of antigenic sites. The ligand-mediated redistribution of plasma membrane proteins is optimal at 37°C, requires cross-linking, and is dependent on energy and a functionally intact cytoskeletal system.

The interpretation that similar events occur in the lungs of rabbits treated with anti-ACE antibodies is further supported by two observations. First, *in vivo* injected monovalent Fab fragments of anti-ACE IgG do not induce a redistribution of ACE in the lung; instead, they bind in a linear pattern along the alveolar endothelium (13). Second, chlorpromazine, a calmodulin antagonist that displaces calcium ions from binding sites linking the plasma membrane to the cytoskeleton and that blocks the redistribution of Ig on the surface of B-lymphocytes exposed to anti-Ig antibodies, prevents the redistribution *in vivo* of ACE by anti-ACE antibodies (unpublished observations).

Lungs of rabbits killed after 4 days of injections with anti-ACE antibodies show acute interstitial pneumonitis. In animals kept alive this lung disease appears completely reversible (13). In an attempt to induce chronic lung lesions, rabbits rendered immunologically tolerant to goat IgG were treated every other day for 6 weeks with goat anti-ACE IgG (29). Each time the animals received the immune IgG, they became dyspneic as a consequence of the interaction between ACE and specific antibody. When the rabbits were killed after the last antibody administration, granular deposits composed of goat IgG, rabbit C3, and ACE were found along alveolar capillary walls. Light and electron microscopy revealed acute inflammatory lesions and degenerative changes of endothelial and epithelial cells. Within a few days after suspension of the antibody injections, these lesions disappeared and the lung structure was restored to normal; goat IgG and rabbit C3 were no longer detected, and ACE was expressed again in a linear pattern along the alveolar capillary endothelium. Thus, there is a remarkable absence of chronic progressive lung lesions in animals chronically subjected to antibody-mediated alveolar endothelial injury, suggesting resistance to injury and rapid recovery of endothelial cells.

Because the monovalent Fab fragments of goat anti-ACE IgG would not be removed by patching and shedding, investigators became interested in the effect on lung structure of prolonged binding *in vivo* of these fragments to the surface of alveolar endothelium (29). In contast to the response to intact anti-ACE IgG, no clinically adverse effects were noted on the first 2 days of administration of Fab fragments. On the 3rd day, however, the animals appeared sick and dyspneic, and none of them survived the 4th day of injection. By immunofluorescence microscopy, the Fab fragments, as well as C3 and fibrinogen, were localized in a linear pattern along the alveolar endothelium. Histologically, a severe, acute interstitial pneumonitis was found. The explanation for the pathogenicity of Fab fragments is unclear. Fab fragments covering the plasma membrane may have altered the normal function of alveolar endothelial cells, thereby initiating an inflammatory response.

The observation that ACE is expressed on the plasma membrane of rabbit oocytes provided an opportunity to study the fate of immune complexes shed into a basement membrane-like structure, the zona pellucida, which surrounds oocytes in the ovary (107). *In vivo* binding of divalent anti-ACE antibodies to ACE on the oolemma resulted in the formation in the zona pellucida of granular immune deposits, recognizable ultrastructurally as electron dense deposits. The zona pellucida offers an ideal substrate for immune complex aggregation because soluble immune complexes preferentially precipitate in a polysaccharide milieu as a consequence of "steric exclusion" (98). With time the immune deposits migrated toward the outer part of the zona pellucida. This centrifugal movement of the immune deposits represents passive transport following the turnover rate of the zona pellucida, which is mainly synthesized by the oocyte.

Although weakly, ACE is expressed on the plasma membrane of glomerular capillary endothelial cells in the kidney. Immune complexes formed after *in vivo* interaction with antibody are shed from the endothelium and appear to relocate at the epithelial side of the glomerular basement membrane (108). These findings suggest that hydrodynamic forces exert an influence on the ultimate location of immune deposits formed in capillary beds specialized in filtration.

Heymann Nephritis

Another example of an experimental immunopathologic process involving antibodies reacting with plasma membrane antigens is Heymann nephritis in the rat. The nephropathy is considered to be the animal counterpart of idiopathic human membranous glomerulonephritis (see Chapter 3). The disease is characterized by the presence of immune deposits exclusively at the epithelial side of the glomerular basement membrane (GBM). Heymann nephritis may be produced either by active immunization of rats with antigens from the brush border of rat renal proximal tubules or by the passive administration of heterologous anti-rat brush border antibodies. The subepithelial immune deposits result from the *in situ* interaction of antibodies with a glycoprotein (gp330) expressed not only on the brush border of proximal tubules, but also on the plasma membrane of glomerular visceral epithelial cells (94).

Recent evidence supports the concept that antibody-mediated shedding of gp330 from the surface of visceral epithelial cells plays a pivotal role in the formation of subepithelial immune deposits in Heymann nephritis. Exposure of cultured rat glomerular visceral epithelial cells to anti-gp330 antibodies induces rapid clustering, patching, capping, and then shedding of gp330-antibody complexes (28). This process does not occur if monovalent antibodies are used, if incubation with antibodies is performed at 4°C instead of at 37°C, or if energy production or the cytoskeletal system is incapacitated (28). Thus, the rearrangement of gp330 by antibodies is governed by the same requirements as in other examples of ligand-induced redistribution of plasma membrane antigens (17,132). Furthermore, passive Heymann nephritis fails to develop after injection of monovalent Fab fragments of anti-brush border antibodies (28). Finally, inactivation of the cytoskeletal system by chlorpromazine prevents the induction of passive Heymann nephritis (30).

Morphologic Consequences

All these studies illustrate that the morphological and immunohistological features of the lesions produced by circulating divalent antibodies reacting with cell surface antigens depend upon the anatomical and physiological properties of the organ or structure in which the interaction takes place. When the antigen is expressed on the surface of cells facing the bloodstream in vascular structures not specifically involved in filtration, immune complexes are shed into the circulation, and immune deposits are not formed in tissue. By contrast, when the antigen is expressed on the surface of cells surrounded by a basement membrane or by a collagen matrix, shedding of immune complexes from the cell membrane results in the local formation of immune deposits. Thus, the distinction between a cell surface reaction (type II) and extracellular *in situ* deposition (type IIIB) is not always clear in tissue studies.

Human Pathology

At present, the list of human diseases in which there is evidence that antibody-mediated redistribution of cell surface antigens occurs is short, but will surely be extended in the future (see Chapter 5) (76). Once identified, it is not always clear whether and how antibody-cell surface interaction contributes to the pathogenesis of the disease. In fact, by inducing antigenic modulation, antibody-mediated antigen redistribution may, under certain conditions, even have a protective, beneficial effect. Furthermore, this or any other antibody-mediated pathogenic event should be viewed in context, because it is becoming increasingly apparent that in most immunological diseases several effector mechanisms cooperate, linking together antibody and T-cell-mediated mechanisms (114).

Antibody-mediated antigen redistribution may take place on cells in the circulation. For instance, in certain forms of autoimmune neutropenia, anti-neutrophil antibodies provoke patching and endocytosis of neutrophil antigens, a modulation that may protect the target cells from the effect of cytolytic antibodies or T-cells (152). Similar events could be relevant to our understanding of chronic viral infections, in which removal of viral antigens from the surface of infected cells may promote viral persistence (66).

Autoantibodies against plasma membrane receptors have been reported in Graves' disease (thyroid-stimulating hormone receptor), myasthenia gravis (acetylcholine receptor), insulin-resistant diabetes (insulin receptor), and in certain allergic conditions (beta-adrenergic receptor) (76). The pathophysiologic significance of these antibodies is discussed in Chapter 5.

Patients with pemphigus vulgaris, a skin disease characterized by intraepidermal bulla formation, have circulating and tissue-bound autoantibodies against antigenic determinants present on the surface of differentiating keratinocytes (see Chapter 4). The pathogenicity of these autoantibodies has been firmly established (50). Based on *in vitro* experiments involving cultured epidermal cells, it has been proposed that in patients with pemphigus vulgaris, antibody-mediated disappearance of epidermal surface antigens, caused by cross-linkage with subsequent redistribution and endocytosis, leads to epidermal cell to cell detachment.

Transplantation antigens expressed on the surface of endothelial cells are likely candidates for topographical redistribution and antigenic modulation. Indeed, it has been suggested that prolonged survival of renal allografts in the presence of transplantation antibodies is due to disappearance of transplantation antigens (60). However, this theory has yet to be confirmed (77) (see Chapter 7).

Because glomerular damage in Heymann nephritis has been shown to result from autoantibodies directed against a plasma membrane antigen of visceral epithelial cells, most, if not all, cases of idiopathic membranous glomerulonephritis in humans may have a similar immunopathogenesis (42) (see Chapter 3). Antigens of the brush border of proximal tubules similar to those responsible for Heymann nephritis have been identified in glomerular immune deposits in a few patients (52,113). However, most attempts to demonstrate that particular antigen-antibody system in the pathogenesis of human membranous nephropathy have been met with failure (8). More elaborate and sophisticated studies have to be conducted to settle the question of whether circulating antibodies binding to plasma membrane antigens of visceral epithelial cells produce membranous glomerulonephritis in man (8). Similarly, the possibility that this nephropathy is not a homogeneous disease entity, but is instead composed of various subgroups each with a different pathogenesis, should not be neglected. Therefore, aside from redistribution of intrinsic plasma membrane antigens, mechanisms involving circulating immune complexes, antibodies binding to secreted antigens, or antibodies binding to foreign antigens planted in the glomerular capillary wall, all deserve consideration in studies on the pathogenesis of human membranous glomerulonephritis.

INTERACTION OF ANTIBODIES WITH ENDOGENOUS ANTIGENS "LEAKING" FROM OR SECRETED BY CELLS (TYPE IIIB)

Animal Models

Rabbits immunized with glomeruli-free rabbit kidney cortex or given repeated renal allografts develop tubulointerstitial nephritis associated with granular deposits of IgG and C3 along the basement membrane of proximal tubules (95,96). The serum and kidney eluates of these animals contain autoantibodies that bind *in vitro* to cells of proximal tubules of normal kidneys. In addition, these antibodies react with antigens present in the granular, tubular basement membrane (TBM) deposits in diseased kidneys. Passive transfer of serum from rabbits with tubulointerstitial nephritis to normal rabbits results in focal deposition of immunoglobulin along TBM, in a pattern identical to that seen in the donors. These observations led to the original formulation of the hypothesis that granular immune deposits in tissues may form by the local reaction of circulating antibodies with antigens leaking from cells surrounded by basement membrane. A similar mechanism may be operative in various other experimental conditions. Tamm-Horsfall protein, the most abundant protein in normal urine, is produced by the cells of the thick ascending limb of the loop of Henle. An infiltration of inflammatory cells around the thick ascending limb can be found in rats that have been actively or passively immunized with Tamm-Horsfall protein (80,134). In these animals, Tamm-Horsfall protein, together with IgG and C3, is located in granular deposits at the base of the epithelium of the thick ascending limb. The immune deposits are believed to arise by the *in situ* reaction of antibodies with Tamm-Horsfall protein present as a secretion product on the surface of the tubular cells. Binding of circulating antibodies to thyroglobulin leaking from thyroid cells might be the mechanism responsible for the thyroiditis seen in guinea pigs injected with heterologous anti-guinea pig thyroglobulin serum or in mice actively immunized with heterologous thyroglobulin (35, 91). Comparable injury occurs in the testes of bilaterally vasectomized rabbits. These animals develop high levels of antibodies to sperm antigens and a "membranous orchitis" characterized by granular immune deposits along the basement membrane of seminiferous tubules (15). The antibodies eluted from the testes react with the acrosome of spermatozoa. Thus, the immune deposits are probably formed when circulating autoantibodies react with sperm antigens, as they diffuse out of the seminiferous tubules (15).

Local interaction of antibodies with secreted antigens may be involved in the granular immune deposit formation in $HgCl_2$ nephropathy. Regular, frequent injections of small doses of $HgCl_2$ induce, in conjunction with polyclonal B-cell activation, a biphasic autoimmune disease in rabbits and in Brown-Norway rats (3,127,131). In the early weeks after starting injections of $HgCl_2$, deposition of IgG in a linear pattern can be seen along the GBM. Later in the course of the disease, the distribution of immunoglobulin assumes a discrete granular pattern and electron dense deposits are found at the epithelial side of the GBM. Studies of sera of diseased rats reveal antibodies to laminin, type IV collagen, heparan sulfate proteoglycan, and entactin, the major components of the GBM. Antibodies with the same specificities can be eluted from kidneys with linear as well as granular deposits of immunoglobulin along the GBM. The eluates from nephritic kidneys react with antigens synthesized and secreted by cultured rat glomerular visceral epithelial cells (67). These data are consistent with the hypothesis that prolonged, continuous interaction of antibodies with basement membrane antigens secreted by visceral epithelial cells may contribute to the formation of granular immune deposits in the subepithelial part of the GBM

(67). In this concept, both phases of $HgCl_2$ nephropathy are different expressions of the same underlying process. One of the several possible alternative explanations is that the granular glomerular immune deposits in $HgCl_2$ nephropathy are derived from circulating immune complexes (79). However, against such an event and in favor of *in situ* immune complex formation is the finding, in rabbits and rats treated with $HgCl_2$, of granular immune deposits in organs and structures not especially involved in filtration and generally not affected by injury resulting from entrapment of circulating immune complexes (3,18).

In the experimental diseases reviewed above, the *in situ* immune deposit formation is regarded as a passive process governed merely by physicochemical forces. However, if the responsible antigens are at some time present on the surface of the secreting or leaking cells and connected to the cytoskeletal system, antibody-mediated antigen redistribution could represent a contributory pathogenic mechanism.

Human Pathology

Based on experimental immunopathological conditions in animals, one can only speculate in which human diseases an interaction of circulating antibodies with antigens leaking from or secreted by tissue cells is of pathogenic significance. The examples are few and the participating antigens have not been identified.

In long-functioning renal allografts, granular deposits of immunoglobulin and C3 are sometimes found along TBM in a pattern similar to that seen in rabbits receiving multiple renal allografts (6). Antigens coming from follicular cells may combine with autoantibodies to form immune deposits along the follicular basement membrane in certain forms of thyroiditis (90). Another human condition in which leaking antigens may feature is the orchitis of infertile males. About 30% of these patients have granular deposits of IgG and C3 along the basement membrane of seminiferous tubules (137). Lastly, one may entertain the possibility that a mechanism similar to that postulated to explain the biphasic course of experimental $HgCl_2$ glomerulonephritis, is occasionally relevant in patients in which a transition of anti-GBM nephritis into membranous glomerulonephritis is observed (122).

INTERACTION OF ANTIBODIES WITH INTRINSIC ANTIGENS PRESENT IN BASEMENT MEMBRANES OR INTERCELLULAR MATRIX (TYPE IIIB)

Animal Models

Anti-GBM nephritis has been produced in several animal species by the administration of heterologous anti-GBM antibodies or by active immunization with a GBM preparation (7,119,156). Autoimmune anti-GBM nephritis following immunization with xenogeneic or allogeneic GBM was first described in sheep (138,139). Antibodies elicited against the foreign GBM cross-react with autologous antigens to induce nephritis. The kidneys of immunized animals show a proliferative, exudative and crescentic glomerulonephritis; crescent formation is so dominating that it has become the histological hallmark of the disease. By immunohistochemical analysis, IgG and complement are found in a linear pattern along the GBM. Autoantibodies against GBM are found in serum as well as in eluates of diseased kidneys. The course of autoimmune nephritis in sheep is rapidly progressive, leading to renal failure and death. The importance of circulating anti-GBM antibodies has been convincingly demonstrated by passive transfer experiments. Normal recipients of anti-GBM antibodies develop a glomerulonephritis that is indistinguishable from the disease of the actively immunized donor. The nephritogenic antigens implicated in experimental as well as human autoimmune anti-GBM nephritis have molecular weights in the range of 50K and 26K and reside in the noncollagenous, nonhelical carboxy terminal domain (NCl) of collagen type IV. Studies of amino acid composition suggest that the 50K is a dimer of the 26K component (154).

Sheep antibodies that bind to GBM, react *in vitro* with alveolar basement membrane (ABM). Furthermore, immunization of sheep with ABM induces anti-GBM nephritis (139). As anti-basement membrane antibodies in kidney eluates can be removed by absorption with either GBM or ABM, it appears that the autoantibodies recognize antigens common to GBM and ABM. However, despite the presence of circulating antibodies that react with ABM *in vitro*, sheep immunized with basememt membrane antigens do not exhibit signs of lung disease. Other factors in addition to the presence of autoantibodies in the circulation are probably essential for the expression of autoimmune lung disease.

The possibility that increased permeability of the alveolar capillary is needed to give antibodies access to the ABM has been tested in animals exposed to toxic doses of oxygen (20,53,84). In contrast to what is observed in normal animals, in oxygen-treated animals intravenously administered anti-ABM antibodies do bind to the ABM and induce inflammatory lung lesions. The interpretation of these findings is that under normal physiologic conditions the endothelium prevents the binding of antibodies to the ABM. In contrast to glomerular capillaries, alveolar capillaries have a continuous, nonfenestrated endothelial lining. Indeed, physiologic and ultrastructural tracer studies show that such a continuous endothelial layer forms a barrier for macromolecules the size of IgG. Oxygen toxicity increases alveolar capillary wall permeability and thereby serves as a nonimmunologic factor, allowing the development of anti-ABM antibody-mediated lung lesions.

Mice, rats, guinea pigs, rabbits, monkeys and chickens have also been used for the study of autoimmune anti-GBM nephritis (16a,156). In rabbits the disease may be induced by immunization with GBM antigens present in normal allogeneic or autologous urine (100). One may speculate that the granular immune deposits sometimes observed along the GBM of these animals result from the interaction of autoantibodies with corresponding, secreted basement membrane antigens. The finding that bursectomized chickens develop severe glomerular lesions following immunization with bovine GBM antigens, despite an absence of anti-GBM antibodies, suggests that cell mediated mechanisms may play a role in other forms of anti-GBM disease (16a).

That formation of autoantibodies against GBM invariably leads to proliferative glomerular lesions, is illustrated in mice. Swiss-Webster mice immunized with human GBM do not develop a proliferative, crescentic glomerulonephritis but instead show conspicuous subepithelial extensions or "spikes" of the GBM, which are not separated from each other by immune deposits (16). Of interest is the finding that these spikes contain laminin, but not collagen type IV (106). This may be the consequence of excessive production by visceral epithelial cells of laminin, a basement membrane component involved in the attachment of epithelial cells to the basal lamina (143). Thus, while laminin and collagen type IV are normally co-distributed, this is not necessarily the case in pathologic conditions.

Sera of mice, rats, guinea pigs, or goats actively immunized with heterologous renal TBM contain autoantibodies that bind *in vitro* and *in vivo* in a linear pattern to the basement membrane of proximal tubules of the kidney. The *in vivo* binding may be associated with the development of a severe tubulointerstitial nephritis (anti-TBM nephritis) (21,156). Histologic examination of kidneys at the height of the disease reveals tubular lesions and the presence of numerous mononuclear leukocytes, mostly of the monocyte-macrophage series in the cortical interstitium. Macrophage derived multinucleated giant cells, particularly prominent in the guinea pig, appear actively involved in the destruction of tubules (10). Conclusive evidence of the pathogenic role of the autoantibodies is provided by the successful passive transfer of tubulointerstitial nephritis to normal animals by sera or kidney eluates from animals actively immunized with TBM (12,21). The phenomenon of autoimmune amplification may be relevant for the understanding of the progressive course of anti-TBM nephritis. Active immunization of guinea pigs with rabbit TBM elicits production of anti-TBM antibodies of both IgG_1 and IgG_2 isotypes. The separate transfer of either isotype induces nephritis, but also stimulates the synthesis of anti-TBM antibodies of both immunoglobulin subclasses by the recipient (75). The significance of antibodies in the initiation of anti-TBM nephritis is further illustrated by studies in which partial inhibition of the disease was achieved by utilizing anti-idiotype antibody (25,116,158). The concept that antibodies initiate the tubulointerstitial nephritis does, of course, not exclude the participation of cellular immunity in the expression of the disease. In fact, the model of anti-TBM nephritis has provided an opportunity to analyze the interaction between humoral and cellular immunity in detail (114,117). It has been proposed that an antibody-dependent, cell-mediated immune reaction, involving macrophages as effector cells, is an important mode of tissue damage in this model of tubulointerstitial nephritis (10,115). Furthermore, T-cells appear to modulate and amplify the expression of the disease. Lastly, it has been reported that in mice the disease can be passively transferred with T-lymphocytes (159). The nephritogenic TBM antigen isolated from rabbit kidney has been characterized as a 48K glycoprotein (36); this antigen shows similarity with the human nephritogenic TBM antigen (37,61). In the rat, the nephritogenic TBM antigen is an alloantigen. Transplantation of a TBM antigen positive kidney into an alloantigen negative rat results in the production by the recipient of anti-TBM antibodies that bind in vivo to the graft but not to the recipient's kidney (21). Surprisingly, the alloimmune response is not accompanied by damage of the graft.

The nephritogenic potential of monospecific xenogeneic antibodies against GBM components such as laminin, collagen type IV, and the core protein of heparan sulfate proteoglycans has been studied in rats and mice (1,58,104,112,153,157). The histologic or functional damage observed in the xenospecific (heterologous) phase of disease induction is mild or absent and does not compare in severity with that found in the xenospecific phase of anti-GBM nephritis (for the autologous phase of these models, see next section) (156). However, the xenospecific phase is of short duration (4 to 5 days), and it may be argued that a more sustained, chronic interaction of antibodies with individual GBM components, in animals rendered tolerant to the xenogeneic immunoglobulins or actively immunized with GBM components, could lead to more significant glomerular pathology.

Formation of mesangial, electron dense immune deposits has been reported in mice following intravenous administration of monoclonal antibodies against an antigen that is exclusively present in the glomerular mesangial matrix (111). The antigen is collagenase resistant and trypsin sensitive and has a molecular weight of 81K. A more precise characterization of this unique mesangial component awaits further biochemical studies. Functional or light microscopic abnormalities were not noted in this model.

Another example of a condition mediated by antibodies against a matrix substance is collagen-induced arthritis. Rats or mice actively immunized with collagen type II, a collagen whose distribution is primarily limited to cartilage, develop a polyarthritis that morphologically resembles that of human rheumatoid arthritis (40,146). This experimental arthritis is associated with humoral as well as cellular immunity to collagen. Successful passive transfer experiments attest to the importance of antibodies in the pathogenesis of this disease (141,142).

Human Pathology

The formation of autoantibodies against GBM is an infrequent cause of rapidly progressive, crescentic glomerulonephritis in man (7,119,156) (see Chapter 3). In Goodpasture's disease, autoantibodies reactive with GBM as well as ABM are assumed to induce both glomerulonephritis and a hemorrhagic pneumonitis (20,156). From animal experiments it may be inferred that a focal or diffuse increase in alveolar capillary wall permeability is required for autoantibodies to bind to the ABM in man (53,84). This view is consistent with the observation that in patients with anti-GBM nephritis lung disease may be absent, despite the presence in the circulation of antibodies cross-reacting *in vitro* with ABM, and with the demonstration that the titer of circulating antibodies does not correlate with the severity of lung pathology in patients with Goodpasture's syndrome. Factors that may enhance alveolar capillary wall permeability include pulmonary or systemic infection, fluid overload, and exposure to smoke or certain chemicals.

Circulating anti-TBM antibodies and linear deposits of IgG along the basement membrane of kidney tubules may occasionally be found in different nephropathies, but are common in patients with anti-GBM nephritis (9,21). Idiopathic anti-TBM nephritis is extremely rare. The demonstration in the latter disease that the membrane attack complex of the complement system co-locates with IgG along the TBM, supports the notion of a pathogenic role of anti-TBM antibodies *(unpublished observations)*. However, efforts to passively transfer anti-TBM nephritis with serum of patients to laboratory animals have been unsuccessful (21) *(unpublished data)*. The reason may be that the number of relevant, biologically active anti-TBM antibodies in the circulation of patients is relatively small, as most of these antibodies have bound to the diseased kidneys (12).

Antibodies against one or more of the following basement membrane components— collagen type IV, laminin and heparan sulfate proteoglycans—have been identified in sera of patients with rheumatic diseases including rheumatoid arthritis and systemic lupus erythematosus, with poststreptococcal glomerulonephritis, or with preeclampsia (57,59,62, 93,123). Furthermore, antibodies of the IgA class reacting with structures common to collagen type I, II, and IV have been found in the circulation of patients with IgA nephropathy (34). The pathogenic significance of these antibodies has yet to be established.

In patients with bullous pemphigoid, a blistering skin disease, autoantibodies against the epidermal basement membrane zone are present in the circulation and are localized together with complement in a linear pattern along this structure. There is evidence to implicate these autoantibodies in the development of this skin disorder (49) (see Chapter 4).

INTERACTION OF ANTIBODIES WITH ANTIGENS PLANTED IN TISSUE (TYPE IIIB)

Animal Models

Antibodies may bind to antigens that are present in tissue for a fortuitous reason. When exogenous, soluble antigens that have diffused into a vessel wall meet their corresponding antibodies coming from the circulation, the ensuing *in situ* immune complex formation initiates an inflammatory reaction resulting in vasculitis. In the classical Arthus reaction, the antigen is injected intradermally in an animal with high levels of antibody in the circulation (39). The subsequent dermal vasculitis affects primarily the postcapillary venules. The reaction peaks after 6 to 8 hours and is morphologically characterized by exudative, necrotizing, and hemorrhagic lesions. The locally formed immune deposits are phagocytized by neutrophils and quickly become undetectable by immunohistochemistry. In most experiments, the reversed passive Arthus reaction is used because this condition is easier to quantitate by injecting varying, known quantities of antibody intradermally and a fixed amount of antigen intravenously (45). A mechanism similar to that of the Arthus reaction appears responsible for severe pneumonitis in animals that first have antibodies of the IgG or IgA class instilled in the alveolar space and then receive an intravenous injection of corresponding antigens (87-89). Immunofluorescence studies suggest that antigens and antibodies diffuse toward each other and form complexes in the vessel walls or in the alveolar septa.

Antibodies may combine with exogenous antigens bound to tissue because of an immunological reaction. This is the case in Masugi or nephrotoxic nephritis (156). In the xenospecific (heterologous) phase of this disease, xenogeneic antibodies bind to the GBM. In the autologous phase, specific antibodies generated by the recipient react with the planted xenogeneic immunoglobulin. In both phases of the nephritis immune reactants are found in a linear pattern along the GBM. The histological and functional lesions in the autologous phase are more severe than those in the xenospecific phase (156). Similar observations have been made in laboratory animals that received xenogeneic antibodies against individual components of the GBM (1,58,104,112). However, in contrast to nephrotoxic nephritis, the glomerular damage in the autologous phase of the latter models is less conspicuous or more complicated to produce (58). The autologous phase of pneumotoxic pneumonitis has been reported in the rat, with rat IgG present in the same linear pattern along the ABM as the xenogeneic anti-ABM IgG (53).

Antibodies may react with exogenous antigens bound to tissue because of electrical charge. The glomerular capillary wall has fixed negative charges and cationic antigens, such as cationized ferritin or cationized serum proteins will preferentially localize in this structure especially in the GBM. Once implanted, exposure of the antigens to autologous or xenogeneic antibodies leads to a glomerulonephritis characterized by the formation of granular, electron dense deposits at the epithelial side of the GBM (2,42,121,148). Thus, the consequence of this antigen-antibody interaction at the level of the GBM is different from that encountered in the autologous phase of nephrotoxic nephritis and other related models in which linear immune deposits are found. The difference may be explained by the fact that the immune complexes need to undergo aggregation and condensation for identifiable immune deposits to form (105). Immune complexes formed with cationic antigens or with certain plasma membrane antigens (8) are capable of such rearrangements, whereas those formed with antigens firmly anchored in a basement membrane are not.

Antibodies may form a complex with antigens present in tissue because of a chemical reaction. Certain lectins bind to glucose or mannose of structural glycoproteins (101). In one study the glycoprotein-binding of concanavalin A was utilized to plant this antigen in glomeruli of rats. The subsequent reaction with anti-concanavalin antibody, either administered systemically or actively induced, resulted in an exudative and proliferative glomerulonephritis (73). Of relevance to the possible occurrence of *in situ* immune deposit formation in human systemic lupus erythematosus glomerulonephritis are studies on the affinity of DNA for various components of the extracellular matrix. Present data indicate that DNA does not preferentially bind to collagen type IV and laminin of the GBM (81,82) but instead reacts with collagen type V of the mesangial matrix (70). The basis for the binding of DNA to collagen type V molecules appears to be provided by ionic interactions as well as by the unique spatial arrangement of amino acid side chains in native collagen molecules.

Lastly, antibodies may bind to antigens contained within tissue because of a physical property, such as size. Aggregated protein molecules injected intravenously into animals tend to accumulate in the glomerular mesangium. Passively transferred antibodies to the planted proteins may then provoke a proliferative mesangial glomerulonephritis (109).

Human Pathology

It has been proposed that some forms of vasculitis are produced by an Arthus-like reaction. This notion is not supported by rigorous evidence (19).

Hypersensitivity pneumonitis, also referred to as extrinsic allergic alveolitis, seems like a condition in which an Arthus-like reaction might play an important role. However, it has become apparent that the pathogenesis of this disease is more complicated and probably involves not only antibody- but also T-cell-mediated mechanisms (26).

The precise pathogenesis of acute poststreptococcal glomerulonephritis is still unknown. However, the disease is generally assumed to be caused by immune complexes (156). It has been hypothesized that the nephritis is initiated by *in situ* immune deposit formation involving extracellular, cationic, streptococcal antigens (149). This concept is inconsistent with the findings of a recent study in which a unique, anionic (pI 4.75), 46K streptokinase was tentatively identified as the responsible nephritogenic antigen (85).

TISSUE DAMAGE CAUSED BY DEPOSITION OF CIRCULATING IMMUNE COMPLEXES (TYPE IIIA)

Animal Models

The hypothesis that circulating immune complexes cause damage to tissues in which they localize was first formulated to explain the pathogenesis of serum sickness in rabbits (39,51,71). The acute form of serum sickness is induced by a single intravenous injection of a foreign protein, usually bovine serum albumin (BSA). From 9 to 15 days after the injection, rabbits with an immune response against BSA develop an actue glomerulonephritis and inflammatory lesions of the joints and the cardiovascular system. The manifestations of acute serum sickness coincide with the immune elimination of BSA from the circulation, the appearance of circulating immune complexes, and the presence in affected tissues of immune deposits containing BSA and specific antibody. In the kidney, the immune deposits are found in the glomerular capillary wall at the epithelial side of the GBM. From these observations, it was concluded that serum sickness results from the trapping in tissue of phlogogenic immune complexes formed in the circulation.

Numerous studies have addressed the conditions necessary for the formation and tissue localization of biologically active, circulating immune complexes (156). It appears that quality as well as quantity of the immune complexes are important. In addition, increase in vascular permeability by an IgE-dependent mechanism is a prerequisite for deposition in tissues of circulating immune complexes (39).

It seems that immune complexes that are intermediate in size, soluble, and able to activate mediators of inflammation are biologically the most potent, inflicting damage especially to filtering structures, such as renal glomeruli (39,156). The size of immune complexes depends on the molar ratio of antigen to antibody and on the nature of the antigen (size, valency) and antibody (isotype, avidity) involved. Because of phagocytosis by the macrophage-phagocyte system, only a small fraction of the immune complexes formed in the circulation will localize in tissue (156). Overloading of the macrophage-phagocyte system may enhance the severity of tissue injury (63,74).

Another important qualitative determinant of tissue-localizing immune complexes concerns electrical charge. As mentioned earlier, the glomerular capillary wall is endowed with negatively charged sites, making its permeability to macromolecules not only a function of size and shape but also of electrical charge (92,124). *In vitro* prepared, positively charged immune complexes accumulate upon injection into animals at the epithelial side of the GBM (33,68,69). In contrast, immune complexes with a negative net charge deposit in mesangial areas but not in the glomerular capillary wall. The role of electrical charge is also illustrated by the observation that when the anionic sites of the glomerular capillary wall are neutralized by polyethyleneimine—a synthetic polycation—circulating immune complexes localize in the glomerular capillary wall, regardless of their isoelectric point (14).

The formation of large amounts of circulating immune complexes may be responsible for the manifestations of chronic serum sickness, a condition that has been produced in several animal species by daily injections of foreign protein for a long period of time (118,156). Animals thus treated develop a systemic immune complex disease (18). The glomerulonephritis of these animals is associated with extensive subepithelial, subendothelial, and mesangial glomerular immune deposits; immune deposits are also observed at extraglomerular sites in the kidney. In addition to the kidney, vascular immune deposits are found in other organs, including lung, gastrointestinal tract, spleen, endocrine and exocrine glands, choroid plexus, and eye (4,18,22). Immune deposits are notably absent from the liver and the basement membrane zone of the skin. Remarkably, the inflammatory response varies from organ to organ (18). Physiological as well as anatomical factors may account for this phenomenon. For example, their precise location within tissue may determine the interaction between immune deposits and humoral and cellular mediators of inflammation; the degree and extent of this interaction will in turn influence the expression of the immune injury (129).

Once formed in tissue, immune deposits are subject to changes in size and composition. These changes are brought about by the interaction of immune deposits with free antibodies, free antigens, complement components, rheumatoid factors, and anti-idiotypic antibodies (110).

Despite its conceptual attraction and considerable experimental support, the hypothesis that circulating immune complexes may cause tissue damage has recently been challenged (41,42,44). *In vitro* prepared immune complexes injected into animals usually do not form subepithelial glomerular immune deposits, which are typical of active serum sickness. Instead, they become transiently trapped at mesangial and subendothelial sites and do not induce significant damage. Preformed immune complexes with a positive electrical charge or complexes made with low avidity antibodies, however, do deposit at the epithelial side of the GBM (68,72). It has been argued that these immune complexes pass the GBM in dissociated form to then recombine in the subepithelial space. However, covalently linked immune complexes that cannot dissociate, form subepithelial immune deposits, provided they are appropriately cationized (33).

The alternative to tissue localization of circulating immune complexes is *in situ* formation of immune complexes. To explain how anionic antigens, such as native BSA, might form *in situ* immune deposits, two charge-related mechanisms have been proposed (42). Anionic antigens may preferentially elicit cationic antibodies (135). These cationic antibodies become planted in the negatively charged glomerular capillary wall and then bind their corresponding anionic antigens. The second mechanism would involve the binding of nonimmune cationic proteins derived from inflammatory cells or platelets to the anionic sites of the glomerular capillary wall (32,42). Anionic antigens may combine with the planted cationic proteins, an event that may be followed by local immune complex formation.

While serum sickness has been most extensively studied in this respect, circulating immune complexes have been implicated in a great number of experimental or spontaneous diseases in laboratory animals. Important examples are murine lupus-like syndromes, graft versus host and host versus graft disease, some models of IgA nephropathy, and glomerulonephritis seen in association with chronic viral infections (7,55,103,119,145,156).

Human Pathology

Circulating immune complexes have been described in many human diseases. In most of them, however, there is little or no indication that they play a pathogenic role. It is only in a few conditions that there is circumstantial evidence of their active participation in the disease process. One obvious example is acute serum sickness, following the administration to patients of xenogeneic anti-thymocyte globulin (46,99). In acute poststreptococcal glomerulonephritis, a nephropathy that immunopathologically resembles experimental acute serum sickness, circulating immune complexes containing streptococcal antigens and specific antibodies, have been detected at the time of the development of the glomerular lesions (65). Systemic lupus erythematosus, like chronic serum sickness in laboratory animals, is a systemic immune complex disorder (18,23,97). In patients with active disease, nuclear antigen-antibody complexes have been shown to be present in the circulation as well as in glomerular and pulmonary immune deposits (23,24,97). Additional antigen-antibody systems may also be important in the pathogenesis of vascular lupus lesions (97). Of great theoretical interest is the finding that anti-DNA antibodies, which are so characteristic of lupus, are polyspecific and react with a whole variety of targets, including IgG, basement membrane components, T and B cells, red blood cells, platelets, glomerular cells, and neuronal tissue (57,83,123,133). The implication is that in lupus all of the antibody-mediated pathogenic mechanisms reviewed above, may cooperate to induce tissue lesions. Circulating IgA-containing immune complexes, at least in part representing IgA rheumatoid factor-IgG complexes, have been demonstrated in patients with idiopathic IgA nephropathy (47,55,136). It is conceivable that these complexes localize and aggregate in glomerular mesangial areas and initiate the functional and morphological abnormalities of this common type of nephropathy. The systemic vasculitis of essential mixed cryoglobulinemia may be due to the deposition in the wall of vessels of circulating IgM rheumatoid factor-IgG complexes (19,64). In most other human systemic vasculitic syndromes evidence for an immune complex pathogenesis is less compelling or lacking (19). Finally, there are diseases presumably mediated by antibodies, in which the responsible mechanism has not yet been definitely established, e.g., membranous glomerulonephritis and certain other forms of immune complex nephritis, idiopathic interstitial pneumonia, and connective tissue diseases other than systemic lupus erythematosus (48,54,88,156). There is the possibility that circulating immune complexes may take part in the development of these conditions.

MEDIATION OF ANTIBODY-INDUCED TISSUE INJURY

Antibody alone causes tissue damage only exceptionally. Mediators of inflammation are almost always required to bring antibody-mediated injury to its full expression (42,43, 56,156). Cellular as well as many humoral mediators have been recognized. The extent of involvement of an individual mediator in an immunopathological reaction may be tested in experiments in which this mediator is either depleted or pharmacologically inhibited. It should be realized, however, that a negative test does not exclude a role for the mediator under study. The mediators are known to interact and collaborate with each other, and the abolition of a mediator that normally partakes in a pathologic process may not be noticed because other effector systems may compensate for its absence. On the other hand, a positive result provides a strong indication for the pathogenic significance of a mediator system.

The complement system (generating biologically active C3a, C5a, $\overline{C3b5b67}$, and the membrane attack complex), neutrophils, and monocytes/macrophages have been extensively studied as possible mediators of lesions observed in such models as the Arthus reaction, nephrotoxic nephritis (xenospecific as well as autologous phase), serum sickness, glomerulonephritides initiated by implantation of cationic antigens, Heymann nephritis, and forms of antibody-mediated pneumonitis (13,42,45,86,88,144,151,156). The results are rather bewildering and can only be touched on in the most general terms. It appears that the significant mediators vary widely from model to model and depend on the animal species used. One or more of the three mediator systems mentioned may be essential for disease expression; they may act independently of each other, or they may cooperate together. As an example of injury involving a single mediator, one should consider passive Heymann nephritis, a disease in which proteinuria is initiated exclusively by activation of the complement system (130). As an example of cooperation of mediators in other settings, activation of the complement system is frequently required to bring neutrophils and monocytes into play; at the same time accumulation and activation of inflammatory cells seem to be separate processes (144). Less well defined than that of the complement system, is the role of other cascading systems in immunologic inflammation, i.e., the coagulation, fibrinolytic, and kinin systems (78,155).

In recent years much attention has been given to oxygen radicals, to products of arachidonic acid, and to platelet activating factor (PAF) as mediators of antibody-induced tissue injury. Activated neutrophil and monocytes/macrophages release a variety of proteases that mainly affect noncellular targets (e.g., matrix components, basement membranes). In addition, these inflammatory cells generate reactive oxygen species including hydrogen peroxide, superoxide anion, hydroxyl radical, and singlet oxygen. Evidence coming from pharmacological inhibition experiments directly implicates oxygen radials in inflicting cell damage in experimental antibody-induced diseases (86,151).

Prostaglandins, lipids derived from arachidonic acid via the cyclooxygenase pathway, influence hemodynamic processes, salt and water metabolism, and the immune system. Administration of prostaglandins or inhibition of their synthesis has been shown to modulate some forms of immunological renal disease (140,150). Inhibition of thromboxane, a potent vasoconstrictor, may be of benefit in renal transplant rejection (38). Leukotrienes, metabolites of arachidonic acid produced by the lipoxygenase pathway, are functionally linked to the prostaglandins (120,140).

Another potent lipid mediator of inflammation is PAF. PAF is a long chain alkyl ether with a glyceryl core also containing an acetyl and a phosphocholine group (27). PAF acts on vessels, recruits and activates platelets, neutrophils, and monocytes, and may be released not only from inflammatory cells, including basophils and mast cells, but also from integral tissue cells such as endothelial cells (27). The synthesis of PAF is triggered by immunological as well as nonimmunological stimuli, as the activation of the coagulation or kinin system. PAF also causes the generation of other mediators (e.g., other autacoids, certain enzymes, and oxygen radicals). The availability of an increasing number of synthetic or natural competitive inhibitors of PAF offers the opportunity to clarify the place of PAF in the maze of mediators of immunological inflammation (31). Several biologically active substances (interleukin 1, growth factors, heparin-like substances) are not discussed here, but certainly contribute to cellular events of the inflammatory response (102).

Nonimmunological factors determining the progression of antibody-induced diseases have become the focus of intense investigation (11). One such factor in kidney diseases is glomerular hyperfiltration, an event that promotes the development of sclerosis. Dietary (low protein intake) or pharmacological measures, by lowering glomerular hyperfiltration, show promise in slowing the deterioration of function in diseased kidneys (5,128). The mode of action of dietary fish oil in reducing progression of renal desease has not yet been determined (125).

CONCLUSION

This review focuses on the mechanisms of experimental and human type II and III hypersensitivity diseases. Not addressed are etiologic factors, genetics and therapeutic modalities. It is clear that the repertoire of available animal models has greatly expanded in recent years; however, our knowledge of human immunological diseases is still fragmentary. Therefore, the search for experimental diseases that faithfully mimic human conditions should continue. Progress made in the analysis and pharmacological modulation of the inflammatory response provides reason for optimism. It is conceivable that, even in the absence of complete understanding of all the pathogenic mechanisms, inhibitors of mediators of inflammation will find their therapeutic application in human pathology.

ACKNOWLEDGMENTS

This work was supported by Grant AM-36807 of the National Institutes of Health, United States Public Health Service. The authors thank Mrs. Marilyn Fitzsimmons for typing the manuscript.

REFERENCES

1. Abrahamson, D. R., and Caulfield, J. P. (1982): Proteinuria and structural alterations in rat glomerular basement membranes induced by intravenously injected anti-laminin immunoglobulin G. *J. Exp. Med.*, 156: 128–145.
2. Adler, S. G., Wang, H. J., Cohen, A. H., and Border, W. A. (1983): Electric charge. Its role in the pathogenesis and prevention of experimental membranous nephropathy in the rabbit. *J. Clin. Invest.*, 71:487–499.
3. Albini, B., and Andres, G. (1983): Autoimmune disease induced in rabbits by administration of mercuric chloride: Evidence suggesting a role for antigens of the connective tissue matrix. In: *Immune Mechanisms in Renal Disease*, edited by N. B. Cummings, A. F. Michael, and C. B. Wilson, pp. 249–260. Plenum Medical Book Co., New York.

4. Albini, B., Ito, S., Brentjens, J. R., and Andres, G. A. (1983): Splenomegaly and immune complex splenitis in rabbits with experimentally-induced chronic serum sickness. Immunopathological findings. *J. Reticuloendoth. Soc.*, 34:485–500.

5. Anderson, S., Rennke, H. G., and Brenner, B. M. (1986): Therapeutic advantage of converting enzyme inhibitors in arresting progressive renal disease associated with systemic hypertension in the rat. *J. Clin. Invest.*, 77:1993–2000.

6. Andres, G. A., Accinni, L., Hsu, K. C., Penn, I., Porter, K. A., Randall, J. M., Seegal, B. C., and Starzl, T. E. (1970): Human renal transplants. III. Immunopathologic studies. *Lab. Invest.*, 22:588–604.

7. Andres, G. A., and Brentjens, J. R. (1984): Autoimmune diseases of the kidney. *Proc. Soc. Exp. Biol. Med.*, 176:226–237.

8. Andres, G., Brentjens, J. R., Caldwell, P. R. B., Camussi, G., and Matsuo, S. (1986): Formation of immune deposits and disease. *Lab. Invest.*, 55:510–520.

9. Andres, G. A., Brentjens, J., Kohli, R., Anthone, R., Anthone, S., Baliah, T., Montes, M., Mookerjee, B., Prezyna, A., Sepulveda, M., Venuto, R., and Elwood, C. (1978): Histology of human tubulo-interstitial nephritis associated with antibodies to renal basement membranes. *Kidney Int.*, 13:480–491.

10. Andres, G. A., Szymanski, C., Albini, B., Brentjens, J. R., Milgrom, M., Noble, B., Ossi, E., and Steblay, R. (1979): Structural observations on epithelioid cells in experimental autoimmune tubulointerstitial nephritis in guinea pigs. *Am. J. Pathol.*, 96:21–29.

11. Baldwin, D. S. (1982): Chronic glomerulonephritis: Non-immunologic mechanisms of progressive glomerular damage. *Kidney Int.*, 21:109–120.

12. Bannister, K. M., and Wilson, C. B. (1985): Transfer of tubulointerstitial nephritis in the Brown Norway rat with anti-tubular basement membrane antibody: Quantitation and kinetics of binding and effect of decomplementation. *J. Immunol.*, 135:3911–3917.

13. Barba, L. M., Caldwell, P. R. B., Downie, G. H., Camussi, G., Brentjens, J. R., and Andres, G. (1983): Lung injury mediated by antibodies to endothelium. I. In the rabbit a repeated interaction of heterologous anti-angiotensin-converting enzyme antibodies with alveolar endothelium results in resistance to immune injury through antigenic modulation. *J. Exp. Med.*, 158:2141–2158.

14. Barnes, J., and Venkatachalam, M. A. (1984): Enhancement of glomerular immune complex deposition by a circulating polycation. *J. Exp. Med.*, 160:286–293.

15. Bigazzi, P. L., Kosuda, L. L., Hsu, K. C., and Andres, G. A. (1976): Immune complex orchitis in vasectomized rabbits. *J. Exp. Med.*, 143:382–404.

16. Bolton, W. K., Benton, F. R., and Sturgill, B. C. (1978): Autoimmune glomerulotubular nephropathy in mice. *Clin. Exp. Immunol.*, 33:463–473.

16a. Bolton, W. K., Tucker, F. L., Sturgill, B. L. (1984): New avian model of experimental glomerulonephritis consistent with mediation by cellular immunity. *J. Clin. Invest.*, 73:1263–1276.

17. Braun, J., and Unanue, E. R. (1980): B lymphocyte biology studied with anti-IgG antibodies. *Immunol. Rev.*, 52:3–28.

18. Brentjens, J. R., and Andres, G. A. (1982): The pathogenesis of extra-renal lesions in systemic lupus erythematosus. *Arthritis Rheum.*, 25:880–886.

19. Brentjens, J. R., and Andres, G. (1985): Immunopathogenesis of renal vasculitis. *Semin. Nephrol.*, 5:3–14.

20. Brentjens, J. R., Camussi, G., Andres, G. A., and Caldwell, P. R. B. (1986): Experimental antibody-mediated lung disease. In: *Physiology of Oxygen Radicals*, edited by A.E. Taylor, S. Matalon, and P.A. Ward, pp. 109–118. Am. Physiol. Soc., Bethesda, Maryland.

21. Brentjens, J. R., Noble, B., and Andres, G. A. (1982): Immunologically mediated lesions of kidney tubules and interstitium in laboratory animals and in man. *Springer Semin. Immunopathol.*, 5:357–378.

22. Brentjens, J. R., O'Connell, D. W., Pawlowski, I. B., Hsu, K. C., and Andres, G. A. (1974): Experimental immune complex disease of the lung. The pathogenesis of a laboratory model resembling certain human interstitial lung diseases. *J. Exp. Med.*, 140:105–125.

23. Brentjens, J., Ossi, E., Albini, B., Sepulveda, M., Kano. K., Sheffer, J., Vasilion, P., Marine, E., Baliah, T., Jocklin, H., and Andres, G. A. (1977): Disseminated immune deposits in systemic lupus erythematosus. *Arthritis Rheum.*, 20:962–968.

24. Brentjens, J. R., Sepulveda, M., Baliah, T., Bentzel, C., Erlanger, B. F., Elwood, C., Montes, M., Hsu, K. C., and Andres, G. A. (1975): Interstitial immune complex nephritis in patients with systemic lupus erythematosus. *Kidney Int.*, 7:342–350.

25. Brown, A. C., Carey, K., and Colvin, R. B. (1979): Inhibition of autoimmune tubulointerstitial nephritis in guinea pigs by heterologous antisera containing anti-idiotype antibodies. *J. Immunol.*, 123:2102–2107.

26. Calvanico, N. J., Fink, J. N., and Keller, R. H. (1984): Hypersensitivity pneumonitis. In: *Immunology of the Lung and Upper Respiratory Tract*, edited by J. Bienenstock, pp. 365–385. McGraw-Hill Book Company, New York.

27. Camussi, G., Brentjens, J., Bussolino, F., and Tetta, C. (1986): Role of platelet activating factor in immunopathological reactions. *Adv. Inflamm. Res.*, 11:97–109.

28. Camussi, G., Brentjens, J. R., Noble, B., Kerjaschki, D., Malavasi, F., Roholt, O. A., Farquhar, M. G., and Andres, G. (1985): Antibody-induced redistribution of Heymann antigen on the surface of cultured glomer-

ular visceral epithelial cells: Possible role in the pathogenesis of Heymann glomerulonephritis. *J. Immunol.*, 135:2409–2416.

29. Camussi, G., Caldwell, P. R. B., Andres, G., and Brentjens, J. R. (1987): Lung injury mediated by antibodies to endothelium. II. Studies of the effect of repeated antigen-antibody interactions in rabbits tolerant to heterologous antibody. *Am. J. Path.*, 127:216–228.

30. Camussi, G., Noble, B. Van Liew, J., Brentjens, J. R., and Andres, G. (1986): Pathogenesis of passive Heymann glomerulonephritis: Chlorpromazine inhibits antibody-mediated redistribution of cell surface antigens and prevents development of the disease. *J. Immunol.*, 136:2127–2135.

31. Camussi, G., Pawlowski, I., Saunders, R., Brentjens, J., and Andres, G. (1987): Receptor antagonist of platelet activating factor inhibits inflammatory injury induced by *in situ* formation of immune complexes in renal glomeruli and in the skin. *J. Lab. Clin. Med.*, 110:196–206.

32. Camussi, G., Tetta, C. Mazzucco, G., Monga, G., Roffinello, C., Alberton, M., Dellabona, P., Malavasi, F., and Vercellone, A. (1986): Platelet cationic proteins are present in glomeruli of lupus nephritis patients. *Kidney Int.*, 30:555–565.

33. Caulin-Glasser, T., Gallo, G. R., and Lamm, M. E. (1983): Nondissociating cationic immune complexes can deposit in glomerular basement membrane. *J. Exp. Med.*, 158:1561–1572.

34. Cederholm, G., Wieslander, J., Bygren, P., and Heinegård, D. (1986): Patients with IgA nephropathy have circulating anti-basement membrane antibodies reacting with structures common to collagen I, II, and IV. *Proc. Natl. Acad. Sci.*, 83:6151–6155.

35. Clagett, J. A., Wilson, C. B., and Weigle, W. O. (1974): Interstitial immune complex thyroiditis in mice. The role of autoantibody to thyroglobulin. *J. Exp. Med.*, 140:1439–1456.

36. Clayman, M. D., Martinez-Hernandez, A., Michaud, L., Alper, R., Mann, R., Kefalides, N. A., and Neilson, E. G. (1985): Isolation and characterization of the nephitogenic antigen producing anti-tubular basement membrane disease. *J. Exp. Med.*, 161:290–305.

37. Clayman, M. D., Michaud, L., Brentjens, J., Andres, G. A., Kefalides, N. A., and Neilson, E. G. (1986): Isolation of the target antigen of human anti-tubular basement membrane antibody-associated interstitial nephritis. *J. Clin. Invest.*, 77:1143–1147.

38. Coffman, T. M., Yarger, W. E., and Klotman, P. E. (1985): Functional role of thromboxane production by acutely rejecting renal allografts in rats. *J. Clin. Invest.*, 75:1242–1248.

39. Cochrane, C. G., and Koffler, D. (1973): Immune complex disease in experimental animals and man. *Adv. Immunol.*, 16:185–264.

40. Courtenay, J. S., Dallman, M. J., Dayan, A. D., Martin, A., and Mosedale, B. (1980): Immunization against heterologous type II collagen induces arthritis in mice. *Nature* (Lond), 283:666–668.

41. Couser, W. G. (1981): What are circulating immune complexes doing in glomerulonephritis? *N. Engl. J. Med.*, 304:1230–1232.

42. Couser, W. (1985): Mechanisms of glomerular injury in immune-complex disease. *Kidney Int.*, 28:569–583.

43. Couser, W. G., Darby, C., Salant, D. J., Adler, S., Stilmant, M. M., and Lowenstein, L. M. (1985): Effect of antibody to glomerular basement membrane on protein excretion in the isolated perfused rat kidney. *Am. J. Physiol.*, 249:F241–F250.

44. Couser, W. G., and Salant, D. J. (1980): *In situ* immune complex formation and glomerular injury. *Kidney Int.*, 17:1–13.

45. Crawford, J. P., Movat, H. Z., Ranadive, N. S., and Hay, J. B. (1982): Pathways to inflammation induced by immune complexes: Development of the Arthus reaction. *Fed. Proc.*, 41:2583–2587.

46. Cunningham, E., Chi, Y., Brentjens, J., and Venuto, R. (1987): Acute serum sickness with glomerulonephritis induced by anti-thymocyte globulin. *Transplantation*, 43:309–312.

47. Czerkinsky, C., Koopman, W. J., Jackson, S., Collins, J. E., Crago, S. S., Schrohenloher, R. E., Julian, B. A., Galla, J. H., and Mestecky, J. (1986): Circulating immune complexes and immunoglobulin A rheumatoid factor in patients with mesangial immunoglobulin A nephropathies. *J. Clin. Invest.*, 77:1931–1938.

48. Dales, S., and Wallace, C. A. (1985): Nuclear pore complexes deposited in the glomerular basement membrane are associated with autoantibodies in a case of membranous nephritis. *J. Immunol.*, 134:1558–1593.

49. Diaz, L. A., Anhalt, G. J., Patel, H. P., Provost, T. T. (1985): Autoimmune cutaneous diseases. In: *The Autoimmune Diseases*, edited by N.R. Rose, and R. Mackay, pp. 443–467. Academic Press, New York.

50. Diaz, L. A., Roscoe, J. T., Eaglstein, N. F., Labib, R. S., Patel, H. P., Mutasim, D. F., and Anhalt, G. J. (1985): Human pemphigus autoantibodies are pathogenic to squamous epithelium. *Ann. N.Y. Acad. Sci.*, 475:181–190.

51. Dixon, F. J., Feldman, J. D., and Vasquez, J. J. (1961): Experimental glomerulonephritis. The pathogenesis of a laboratory model resembling the spectrum of human glomerulonephritis. *J. Exp. Med.*, 113:899–920.

52. Douglas, M. F. S., Rabideau, D. P., Schwartz, M. M., and Lewis, E. J. (1981): Evvidence of autologous immune-complex nephritis. *N. Engl. J. Med.*, 305:1326–1329.

53. Downie, G. H., Roholt, O. A., Jennings, L., Blau, M., Brentjens, J. R., and Andres, G. A. (1982): Experimental anti-alveolar basement membrane antibody-mediated pneumonitis. II. Role of endothelial injury and repair, induction of autologous phase, and kinetics of antibody deposition. *J. Immunol.*, 129:2677–2682.

54. Dreisin, R. D. (1981): Diseases of the lung associated with immune complexes. *Am. Rev. Resp. Dis.*, 124:748–752.

55. Emancipator, E. N., Gallo, G. R., and Lamm, M. E. (1985): IgA nephropathy: Perspectives on pathogenesis and classification. *Clin. Nephrol.*, 24:161–179.

56. Emancipator, S. N., and Lamm, M. E. (1986): Pathways of tissue injury initiated by humoral immune mechanisms. *Lab. Invest.*, 54:475–478.

57. Faaber, P., Ryke, T. P. M., Van de Putte, L. B. A., Capel, P. J. A., and Berden, J. H. M. (1986): Cross-reactivity of human and murine anti-DNA antibodies with heparan sulfate, the major glycosaminoglycan in glomerular basement membranes. *J. Clin. Invest.*, 77:1824–1830.

58. Feintzeig, I. D., Abrahamson, D. R., Cybulski, A. V., Dittmer, J. E., and Salant, D. J. (1986): Nephritogenic potential of sheep antibodies against glomerular basement membrane laminin in the rat. *Lab. Invest.*, 54:531–542.

59. Fillit, H. S., Damle, S. P., Gregory, J. D., Volin, C., Poon-King, T., and Zabriskie, J. (1985): Sera from patients with poststreptococcal glomerulonephritis contain antibodies to glomerular heparan sulfate proteoglycan. *J. Exp. Med.*, 161:277–289.

60. Fine, R. N., Batchelor, J. R., French, M. E., and Shumak, K. H. (1973): The uptake of ^{125}I-labeled rat alloantibody and its loss after combination with antigen. *Transplantation*, 16:641–654.

61. Fliger, F. D., Wieslander, J., Brentjens, J. R., Andres, G. A., and Butkowski, R. J. (1987): Identification of a target antigen in human anti-tubular basement membrane nephritis. *Kidney Int.*, 31:800–807.

62. Foidart, J-M., Hunt, J., Lapiere, C-M., Nusgens, B., De Rycker, C., Bruwier, M., Lambotte, R., Bernard, A., and Mahieu, P. (1985): Antibodies to laminin in preeclampsia. *Kidney Int.*, 29:1050–1057.

63. Ford, P. M. (1975): The effect of manipulation of reticuloendothelial system activity on glomerular deposition of aggregated protein and immune complexes in two different strains of mice. *J. Exp. Pathol.*, 56:523–529.

64. Franklin, E. C. (1980): The role of cryoglobulins and immune complexes in vasculitis. *J. Allerg. Clin. Immunol.*, 66:269–273.

65. Friedman, J., van de Rijn, I., Ohkuni, H., Fischetti, V. A., and Zabriskie, J. B. (1984): Immunological studies of post-streptococcal sequelae. Evidence for presence of streptococcal antigens in circulating immune complexes. *J. Clin. Invest.*, 74:1017–1034.

66. Fujinami, R. S., and Oldstone, M. B. A. (1983): Antigenic modulation: A mechanism of viral persistence. *Prog. Brain Res.*, 59:105–111.

67. Fukatsu, A., Brentjens, J. R., Killen, P. D., Kleinman, K. D., Martin, G. R., and Andres, G. A. (1987): Studies on the formation of glomerular immune deposits in Brown Norway rats injected with mercuric chloride. *Clin. Immunol. Immunopathol.*, 45:35–47.

68. Gallo, G. R., Caulin-Glaser, R. T., and Lamm, M. E. (1981): Charge of circulating immune complexes as a factor in glomerular basement membrane localization in mice. *J. Clin. Invest.*, 67:1305–1313.

69. Gauthier, V. J., Mannik, M., and Striker, G. E. (1982): Effect of cationized antibodies in preformed immune complex on deposition and persistence in renal glomeruli. *J. Exp. Med.*, 156:766–777.

70. Gay, S., Losman, M. J., Koopman, W. J., and Miller, E. J. (1985): Interaction of DNA with connective tissue matrix proteins reveals preferential binding to type V collagen. *J. Immunol.*, 135:1097–1100.

71. Germuth, F. G. (1953): A comparative histologic and immunologic study in rabbits of induced hypersensitivity of the serum sickness type. *J. Exp. Med.*, 97:257–282.

72. Germuth, F. G., Jr., Rodriguez, E., Lorelle, C. A., Trump, E. I., Milano, L., and Wise, O'L. (1979): Passive immune complex glomerulonephritis in mice: Models for various lesions found in human disease. II. Low avidity complexes and diffuse proliferative glomerulonephritis with subepithelial deposits. *Lab. Invest.*, 41:366–371.

73. Globus, S. M., and Wilson, C. B. (1979): Experimental glomerulonephritis induced by "*in situ*" formation of immune complexes in glomerular capillary wall. *Kidney Int.*, 16:148–157.

74. Haakenstad, A. O., and Mannik, M. (1974): Saturation of the reticuloendothelial system with soluble immune complexes. *J. Immunol.*, 112:1939–1948.

75. Hall, C. H., Colvin, R. B., Carey, K., and McCluskey, R. T. (1977): Passive transfer of autoimmune disease with isologous IgG_1 and IgG_2 antibodies to the tubular basement membrane in Strain XIII guinea pigs. *J. Exp. Med.*, 146:1246–1260.

76. Harrison, L. C. (1985): Antireceptor antibodies. In: *The Autoimmune Diseases*, edited by N.R. Rose, and R. MacKay, pp. 617–668. Academic Press, New York.

77. Hart, D. N. J., Wineorls, C. G., and Fabre, J. W. (1980): Graft adaptation: Studies on possible mechanisms in long-term surviving rat renal allografts. *Transplantation*, 30:73–80.

78. Holdsworth, S. R., and Tipping, P. G. (1985): Macrophage-induced glomerular fibrin deposition in experimental glomerulonephritis in the rabbit. *J. Clin. Invest.*, 76:1367–1374.

79. Houssin, D., Druet, E., Hinglais, N., Verroust, P., Grossetete, J., Bariety, J., and Druet, P. (1983): Glomerular and vascular IgG deposits in $HgCl_2$ nephritis: Role of circulating antibodies and immune complexes. *Clin. Immunol. Immunopathol.*, 29:167–180.

80. Hoyer, J. R. (1980): Tubulo-interstitial immune complex nephritis in rats immunized with Tamm-Horsfall protein. *Kidney Int.*, 17:284–292.

81. Izui, S., Lambert, P-H., Fournié, G. J., Türler, H., and Miescher, P. A. (1977): Features of systemic lupus erythematosus in mice injected with bacterial lipopolysaccharides. Identification of circulating DNA and renal localization of DNA-anti-DNA complexes. *J. Exp. Med.*, 145:1115–1136.

82. Izui, S., Lambert, P-H., and Miescher, P. A. (1976): *In vitro* demonstration of a particular affinity of glomerular basement membrane and collagen for DNA. A possible basis for a local formation of DNA-anti-DNA complexes in systemic lupus erythematosus. *J. Exp. Med.*, 144:428–443.

83. Jacob, L., Lety, M-A., Louvard, D., and Bach, J-F. (1985): Binding of a monoclonal anti-DNA auto-antibody to identical protein(s) present at the surface of several human cell types involved in lupus pathogenesis. *J. Clin. Invest.*, 75:315–317.

84. Jennings, L., Roholt, O. A., Pressman, D., Blau, M., Andres, G. A., and Brentjens, J. R. (1981): Experimental anti-alveolar basement membrane antibody-mediated pneumonitis. I. The role of increased permeability of the alveolar capillary wall induced by oxygen. *J. Immunol.*, 127:129–134.

85. Johnston, K. H., and Zabriskie, J. B. (1986): Purification and partial characterization of the nepthritis strain-associated protein from *Streptococcus pyogenes*, group A. *J. Exp. Med.*, 163:697–712.

86. Johnson, K. J. (1986): Neutrophil-independent oxygen radical-mediated tissue injury. In: *Physiology of Oxygen Radicals*, edited by A.E. Taylor, S. Matalon, and P.A. Ward, pp. 151–162. American Physiological Society, Bethesda, Maryland.

87. Johnson, K. J., and Ward, P. A. (1974): Acute immunologic pulmonary alveolitis. *J. Clin. Invest.*, 54:349–357.

88. Johnson, K. J., and Ward, P. A. (1984): Immune complexes. In: *Immunology of the Lung and Upper Respiratory Tract*, edited by J. Bienenstock, pp. 232–241. McGraw-Hill Book Company, New York.

89. Johnson, K. J., Ward, P. A., Kunkel, R. G., and Wilson, B. S. (1986): Mediation of IgA induced lung injury in the rat. Role of macrophages and reactive oxygen products. *Lab. Invest.*, 54:499–506.

90. Kalderon, A. E., Bogaars, H. A., and Diamond, I. (1975): Immune complex deposition in thyroid carcinoma associated with chronic thyroiditis. *Clin. Immunol. Immunopathol.*, 4:101–107.

91. Kåresen, R., and Godal, T. (1969): Induction of thyroiditis in guinea pigs by intravenous injection of rabbit anti-guinea pig thyroglobulin serum. *Immunology*, 17:863–874.

92. Kaysen, G. A., Myers, B. D., Couser, W. G., Rabkin, R., and Felts, J. M. (1986): Mechanisms and consequences of proteinuria. *Lab. Invest.*, 54:479–498.

93. Kefalides, N. A., Pegg, M. T., Ohno, N., Poon-King, T., Zabriskie, J., and Fillit, H. (1986): Antibodies to basement membrane collagen and to laminin are present in sera from patients with poststreptococcal glomerulonephritis. *J. Exp. Med.*, 163:588–602.

94. Kerjaschki, D., and Farquhar, M. G. (1983): Immunocytochemical localization of the Heymann nephritis antigen (gp330) in glomerular epithelial cells of normal Lewis rats. *J. Exp. Med.*, 157:667–685.

95. Klassen, J., and Milgrom, F. (1969): Autoimmune concomitants of renal allografts. *Transplant. Proc.*, 1:605–608.

96. Klassen, J., Milgrom, F., and McCluskey, R. T. (1977): Studies of the antigens involved in an immunologic renal tubular lesion in rabbits. *Am. J. Pathol.*, 88:135–144.

97. Kunkel, H. G. (1980): The immunopathology of SLE. *Hosp. Pract.*, 4:47–56.

98. Laurent, T. C. (1968): On the solubility of antigen-antibody complexes in the presence of dextran and some glycosaminoglycans from connective tissue. *Acta Univ. Ups. Abstr. Uppsala Diss. Sci.*, 58:7–16.

99. Lawley, T. J., Bielory, L., Gascon, P., Yancey, K. B., Young, N. S., and Frank, M. M. (1984): A prospective clinical and immunologic analysis of patients with serum sickness. *N. Engl. J. Med.*, 311:1407–1435.

100. Lerner, R. A., and Dixon, F. J. (1968): The induction of acute glomerulonephritis in rabbits with soluble antigens isolated from normal homologous and autologous urine. *J. Immunol.*, 100:1277–1287.

101. Lis, H., and Sharon, N. (1973): The biochemistry of plant lectins (phytohemagglutinins). *Am. Rev. Biochem.*, 45:541–574.

102. Lovett, D. H., and Sterzel, R. B. (1986): Cell culture approaches to the analysis of glomerular inflammation. *Kidney Int.*, 30:246–254.

103. Luzuy, S., Merino, J., Engers, H., Izui, S., and Lambert, P. H. (1986): Autoimmunity after induction of neonatal tolerance to alloantigens: Role of B cell chimerism and Fl donor B cell activation. *J. Immunol.*, 136:4420–4426.

104. Makino, H., Gibbons, J. T., Reddy, M. K., and Kanwar, Y. S. (1986): Nephritogenicity of antibody to proteoglycans of the glomerular basement membrane—I. *J. Clin. Invest.*, 77:142–156.

105. Mannik, M., Agodoa, L. Y. C., and David, K. A. (1983): Rearrangement of immune complexes leads to persistence and development of electron dense deposits. *J. Exp. Med.*, 157:1516–1528.

106. Matsuo, S., Brentjens, J. R., Andres, G., Foidart, J-M., Martin, G. R., and Martinez-Hernandez, A. (1986): Distribution of basement membrane antigens in glomeruli of mice with autoimmune glomerulonephritis. *Am. J. Pathol.*, 122:36–49.

107. Matsuo, S., Caldwell, P. R. B., Brentjens, J. R., and Andres, G. (1985): *In vivo* interaction of antibodies with cell surface antigens. A mechanism responsible for *in situ* formation of immune deposits in the zona pellucida of rabbit oocytes. *J. Clin. Invest.*, 75:1369–1380.

108. Matsuo, S., Fukatsu, A., Taub, M. L., Caldwell, P. R. B., Brentjens, J. R., and Andres, G. (1987): Glomerulonephritis induced in the rabbit by anti-endothelial antibodies. *J. Clin. Invest.*, 79:1798–1811.

109. Mauer, S. M., Sutherland, D. E. R., Howard, R. J., Fish, A. J., Najarian, J. S., and Michael, A. F. (1973): The glomerular mesangium: III. Acute mesangial injury. A new model of glomerulonephritis. *J. Exp. Med.*, 137:553–570.

110. McCluskey, R. T. (1983): Modification of glomerular immune complex deposits. *Lab. Invest.*, 48:241–244.

111. Mendrick, D. L., and Rennke, H. G. (1986): Immune deposits formed *in situ* by a monoclonal antibody recognizing a new intrinsic rat mesangial matrix antigen. *J. Immunol.*, 137:1517–1526.

112. Miettinen, A., Stow, J. L., Mentone, S., and Farquhar, M. G. (1986): Antibodies to basement membrane heparan sulfate proteoglycans bind to the laminae rarae of glomerular basement membrane (GBM) and induce subepithelial GBM thickening. *J. Exp. Med.*, 163:1064–1084.

113. Naruse, T., Kitamura, D., Miykawa, Y., and Shibata, S. (1973): Deposition of renal tubular epithelial antigen along the glomerular capillary walls of patients with membranous glomerulonephritis. *J. Immunol.*, 110:1163–1166.

114. Neilson, E. G., Clayman, M. D., Haverty, T., Kelly, C. J., and Mann, R. (1986): Experimental strategies for the study of cellular immunity in renal disease. *Kidney Int.*, 30:264–279.

115. Neilson, E. G., and Phillips, S. M. (1981): Cell-mediated immunity in interstitial nephritis. IV. Anti-tubular basement membrane antibodies can function in antibody-dependent cellular cytotoxicity reactions: Observation on a nephritogenic effector mechanism acting as an informational bridge between the humoral and cellular immune response. *J. Immunol.*, 126:1990–1993.

116. Neilson, E. G., and Phillips, S. M. (1982): Suppression of interstitial nephritis by auto-anti-idiotypic immunity. *J. Exp. Med.*, 155:179–189.

117. Neilson, E. G., and Zakheim, B. (1983): T cell regulation, anti-idiotypic immunity, and the nephritogenic immune response. *Kidney Int.*, 24:289–302.

118. Noble, B., and Brentjens, J. R. (1987): Experimental serum sickness. *Methods Enzymol.*, 162:484–501.

119. Noble, B., Brentjens, J. R., and Andres, G. A. (1985): Autoimmune kidney diseases. In: *The Autoimmune Diseases*, edited by N.R. Rose, and R. MacKay, pp. 339–370. Academic Press, New York.

120. O'Flaherty, J. T. (1982): Lipid mediators of inflammation and allergy. *Lab. Invest.*, 47:314–329.

121. Oite, T., Batsford, S. R., Mihatsch, M. J., Takamiya, H., and Vogt, A. (1982): Quantitative studies of *in situ* immune complex glomerulonephritis in the rat induced by planted, cationized antigen. *J. Exp. Med.*, 155:460–474.

122. Pettersson, E., Törnroth, T., and Miettinen, A. (1984): Simultaneous antiglomerular basement membrane and membranous glomerulonephritis: Case report and literature review. *Clin. Immunol. Immunopathol.*, 31:171–180.

123. Petty, R. E., Hunt, D. W. C., and Rosenberg, A. M. (1986): Antibodies to type IV collagen in rheumatic diseases. *J. Rheum.*, 13:246–253.

124. Rennke, H. G., Cotran, R. S., and Venkatachalam, M. A. (1975): Role of molecular charge in glomerular permeability: Tracer studies with cationized ferritins. *J. Cell. Biol.*, 67:638–646.

125. Robinson, D. R., Prickett, J. D., Makoul, G. T., Steinberg, A. D., and Colvin, R. B. (1986): Dietary fish oil reduces progression of established renal disease in (NZBxNZW) F_1 mice and delays renal disease in BxSB and MRL/1 strains. *Arthritis Rheum.*, 29:539–546.

126. Roitt, I. (1984): *Essential Immunology.* 5th Edition, pp. 233–267. Blackwell Scientific Publications, Oxford.

127. Roman-Franco, A. A., Turiello, M., Albini, B., Ossi, E., and Andres, G. A. (1976): Anti-basement membrane antibody (A-BM Ab) and immune complexes (IC) in rabbits injected with mercuric chloride ($HgCl_2$). *Kidney Int.* (Abstract), 10:549.

128. Rosman, J. B., Meijer, S., Sluiter, W. J., ter Wee, P. M., Piers-Brecht, T. P., and Donker, A. J. M. (1984): Prospective randomized trial of early dietary protein restriction in chronic renal failure. *Lancet*, 2:1291–1295.

129. Salant, D. J., Adler, S., Darby, C., Capparell, N. J., Groggel, G. C., Feintzeig, I. D., Rennke, H. G., and Dittmer, J. (1985): Influence of antigen distribution on the mediation of immunological glomerular injury. *Kidney Int.*, 27:938–950.

130. Salant, D. J., Belok, S., Madaio, M. P., and Couser, W. G. (1980): A new role for complement in experimental nephropathy in rats. *J. Clin. Invest.*, 66:1339–1350.

131. Sapin, C., Druet, E., and Druet, P. (1977): Induction of anti-glomerular basement membrane antibodies in the Brown-Norway rat by mercuric chloride. *Clin. Exp. Immunol.*, 28:173–179.

132. Schreiner, G. F., and Unanue, E. R. (1976): Membrane and cytoplasmic changes in B-lymphocytes induced by ligand-surface immunoglobulin interaction. *Adv. Immunol.*, 24:37–165.

133. Schwartz, R. S. (1986): Anti-DNA antibodies and the problem of autoimmunity. *Cellul. Immunol.*, 99:38–43.

134. Seiler, M. W., and Hoyer, J. R. (1981): Ultrastructural studies of tubulo-interstitial immune complex nephritis in rats immunized with Tamm-Horsfall protein. *Lab. Invest.*, 45:321–327.

135. Sela, M., and Mozes, E. (1966): Dependence of the chemical nature of antibodies on the net electrical charge of antigens. *Proc. Natl. Acad. Sci. USA*, 55:445–452.

136. Sinico, R. A., Fornasieri, A., Oreni, N., Benuzzi, S., and D'Amico, G. (1986): Polymeric IgA rheumatoid factor in idiopathic IgA mesangial nephropathy (Berger's disease). *J. Immunol.*, 137:536–541.

137. Solomon, F., Saremaslani, P., Jo-Kob, M., and Hedinger, C. E. (1982): Immune complex orchitis in infertile man. *Lab. Invest.*, 47:555–567.

138. Steblay, R. W. (1962): Glomerulonephritis induced in sheep by injections of heterologous glomerular basement membrane and Freund's complete adjuvant. *J. Exp. Med.*, 116:253–272.

139. Steblay, R. W. (1979): Anti-glomerular basement membrane glomerulonephritis. *Am. J. Pathol.*, 96:875–878.

140. Stork, J. E., Rahman, M. A., and Dunn, M. J. (1986): Eicosanoids in experimental and human renal disease. *Am. J. Med.*, 80 (Suppl. 1A):34–45.

141. Stuart, J. M., Cremer, M. A., Townes, A. S., and Kang, A. H. (1982): Type II collagen-induced arthritis in rats: Passive transfer with serum and evidence that IgG anticollagen antibodies can cause arthritis. *J. Exp. Med.*, 155:1–16.

142. Stuart, J. M., and Dixon, F. J. (1983): Serum transfer of collagen-induced arthritis in mice. *J. Exp. Med.*, 158:378–392.

143. Terranova, V. P., Rohrbach, D. H., and Martin, G. R. (1980): Role of laminin in the attachment of PAM212 (epithelial) cells to basement membrane collagen. *Cell*, 22:719–726.

144. Thaiss, F., Batsford, S., Mihatsch, M. J., Heitz, P. U., Bitter-Suermann, D., and Vogt, A. (1986): Mediator systems in a passive model of *in situ* immune complex glomerulonephritis. Role for complement, polymorphonuclear granulocytes, and monocytes. *Lab. Invest.*, 54:624–635.

145. Theofilopoulos, A. N., and Dixon, F. J. (1985): Murine models of SLE. *Adv. Immunol.*, 37:269–358.

146. Trentham, D. E., Townes, A. S., and Kang, A. H. (1977): Autoimmunity to type II collagen: An experimental model of arthritis. *J. Exp. Med.*, 146:857–869.

147. Van Damme, B. J. C., Fleuren, G. J., Bakker, W. W., Vernier, R. L., and Hoedemaeker, Ph. J. (1978): Experimental glomerulonephritis in the rat induced by antibodies against tubular antigens. IV. Fixed glomerular antigens in the pathogenesis of heterologous immune complex glomerulonephritis. *Lab. Invest.*, 38: 502–509.

148. Vogt, A. (1984): New Aspects of the pathogenesis of immune complex glomerulonephritis: Formation of subepithelial deposits. *Clin. Nephrol.*, 21:15–20.

149. Vogt, A., Batsford, S., Rodriguez-Iturbe, B., and Garcia, P. (1983): Cationic antigens in post-streptococcal glomerulonephritis. *Clin. Nephrol.*, 20:271–279.

150. Vriesendorp, R., Donker, A. J. M., de Zeeuw, D., De Jong, P. E., van der Hem, G. K., and Brentjens, J. R. H. (1986): Effects of nonsteroidal anti-inflammatory drugs on proteinuria. *Am. J. Med.*, 81 [Suppl. 2B]:84–94.

151. Ward, P. A., Johnson, K. J., and Till, G. O. (1986): Oxygen radicals, neutrophils, and acute tissue injury. In: *Physiology of Oxygen Radicals*, edited by A. E. Taylor, S. Matalon, and P. A. Ward, pp. 145–150. American Physiological Society, Bethesda, Maryland.

152. Weitzman, S. A., Desmond, M. D., and Stossel, T. P. (1979): Antigenic modulation and turnover in human neutrophils. *J. Clin. Invest.*, 64:321–325.

153. Wick, G., Muller, P. U., and Timpl, R. (1982): *In vivo* localization and pathological effects of passively transferred antibodies to type IV collagen and laminin in mice. *Clin. Immunol. Immunopathol.*, 23:656–666.

154. Wieslander, J., Langeveld, J., Butkowski, R., Jodlowski, M., Noelken, M., and Hudson, B. G. (1985): Physical and immunochemical studies of the globular domain of type IV collagen: Cryptic properties of the Goodpasture antigen. *J. Biol. Chem.*, 260:8564–8570.

155. Wiggins, R. C. (1985): Hageman factor in experimental nephrotoxic nephritis in the rabbit. *Lab. Invest.*, 53:335–348.

156. Wilson, C. B., and Dixon, F. J. (1985): The renal response to immunological injury. In: *The Kidney*, 3rd Edition, edited by B. M. Brenner, and F. C. Rector, Jr., pp. 800–889. Saunders, Philadelphia.

157. Yaar, M., Foidart, J-M., Brown, K. S., Rennard, S. I., Martin, G. R., and Liotta, L. (1982): The Goodpasture-like syndrome in mice induced by intravenous injections of anti-type IV collagen and anti-laminin antibody. *Am. J. Pathol.*, 107:79–91.

158. Zanetti, M., Mampaso, F., and Wilson, C. B. (1983): Anti-idiotype as a probe in the analysis of autoimmune tubulointerstitial nephritis in the Brown Norway rat. *J. Immunol.*, 131:1268–1273.

159. Zakheim, B., McCafferty, E., Michael-Phillips, S., Clayman, M., and Neilson, E. G. (1984): Murine interstitial nephritis. II. The adoptive transfer of disease with immune T lymphocytes produces phenotypically complex interstitial lesions. *J. Immunol.*, 133:234–239.

Diagnostic Immunopathology,
edited by R.B. Colvin,
A.K. Bhan, and R.T. McCluskey.
Raven Press, New York © 1988.

3 / *Renal Diseases*

Robert T. McCluskey

*Department of Pathology, Massachusetts General Hospital, Harvard Medical School,
Boston, Massachusetts 02114*

The main purpose of this chapter is to review the most important diagnostic uses of immunofluorescence in renal diseases. Comments will also be made about certain recent insights into immunopathogenetic mechanisms.

Direct immunofluorescence studies of human renal biopsy specimens were first performed in the 1950s. It soon became apparent that in addition to providing evidence concerning pathogenic mechanisms, the findings were helpful in classifying and diagnosing glomerular diseases. By the early 1970s, general agreement had been reached on the classification of the major forms of glomerulonephritis, and the main immunofluorescence findings in these diseases had been delineated (66); additional useful observations continue to be made, however. The reason immunofluorescence has proven to be so useful is, of course, that most of the major forms of glomerulonephritis are characterized by conspicuous glomerular accumulation of immunoglobulins, complement components, or both, often in distinctive patterns or with predominance of a particular immunoglobulin class. In most cases, the reactants are found as irregular, granular deposits, and by electron microscopy, corresponding extracellular accumulation of electron dense material is usually seen. It is assumed that such deposits generally represent antigen-antibody complexes, and the diseases are therefore generally classified as forms of immune complex glomerulonephritis (Table 1). However, proving that deposits are immune complexes requires demonstration of specific antibodies and/or corresponding antigens in the deposits. This type of evidence has been obtained only rarely, notably in some cases of lupus nephritis and of hepatitis B associated glomerulonephritis. For diagnostic purposes, there is no need to search for antigens. It is likely that certain immunoglobulin containing glomerular deposits are not immune complexes, but rather nonspecifically trapped or aggregated immunoglobulins; this interpretation is especially plausible when the only immunoglobulin class is IgM, as for example in focal glomerular sclerosis or when only small irregular deposits are seen in sites of necrosis. Despite these problems with interpretation, immunofluorescence studies provide compelling evidence that immune complexes are involved in the pathogenesis of major forms of human glomerulonephritis, in large part because of the resemblance of findings to those of established experimental models.

Immune complex glomerulonephritis was first thought to result only from deposition of circulating complexes. Attempts to obtain evidence for this mechanism through the use of assays designed to detect circulating immune complexes have been inconclusive. For one

TABLE 1. *Usual immunofluorescence findings in major glomerular diseases*

Disease category	Pattern of staining for IgG, C3, IgM, and IgA
I. Presumed or known immune complex glomerulonephritis	
Acute poststreptococcal glomerulonephritis	Scattered granular deposits of C3, alone or with IgG, and sometimes with IgM along the GBM, and/or in mesangial regions
Lupus nephritis*	
Mesangial (minimal)	Mesangial IgG, C3, and usually IgM and IgA
Mild (focal) proliferative	Mesangial IgG, C3, and usually IgG and IgA; focal peripheral loop deposits
Severe (diffuse) proliferative	Irregular, broad deposits along the GBM and in mesangial regions of IgG C3 and usually of IgM and IgA
Membranous	Granular deposits of IgG, C3, and often of IgA and IgM along the GBM
*Tubular or interstitial deposits may be seen in any form of lupus nephritis, especially severe forms.	
Henoch-Schönlein purpura Nephritis	
Mild	Mesangial IgA, IgG, C3, and IgM
Severe	As above, usually plus irregular, granular staining along the GBM
Nephritis in idiopathic mixed cryoglobulinemia	Granular staining for IgG, IgM, and usually C3 along the GBM and in intraluminal masses ("thrombi")
Idiopathic membranous glomerulonephritis	Granular deposits of IgG and C3 all along the GBM; fainter or irregular deposits of IgA or IgM also often found
Membranoproliferative glomerulonephritis, type I	Broad, irregular deposits of C3, and usually of IgG and IgM along the GBM and often in mesangial regions
IgA nephropathy (Berger's disease)	Mesangial deposits of IgA, and often of IgG, C3, and IgM; deposits less often seen along the GBM.
Idiopathic crescentic glomerulonephritis: type II	Irregular, granular, often scanty deposits of IgG, C3, and sometimes of IgM along the GBM or in mesangial regions
Chronic infections (Endocarditis, shunt nephritis, visceral abscess, parasitic diseases	Granular mesangial and GBM deposits, of IgG, IgM, and C3 (resembling type I MPGN)
II. Anti-GBM nephritis (Idiopathic crescentic glomerulonephritis, type I)	Linear accumulation of IgG, infrequently with associated IgA or IgM; C3 found about 75%, usually in irregular or interrupted linear deposits; linear staining for IgG along the TBM in many cases
III. Diseases with Obscure or Atypical Immunologic Mechanisms	
Dense deposit disease (MPGN type II)	Large granular deposits (globules) of C3 in mesangial regions; often ribbon-like deposits of C3 along the GBM and TBM. IgG usually absent; IgM occasionally present along the GBM
Light chain nephropathy	Broad, linear deposits of one type of light chain (usually kappa) along the TBM and GBM, in blood vessels and interstitium
IV. Diseases Without Impressive Evidence of Immunologic Mechanisms	
Idiopathic nephrotic syndrome minimal change disease	Often no immunoglobulins or C3; occasionally mesangial deposits of IgM and C3
Focal glomerular sclerosis	IgM and C3 commonly found in sclerotic lesions
Most case of chronic sclerosing glomerulonephritis	Often no IgG or C3; sometimes irregular, sparse deposits
Idiopathic crescentic glomerulonephritis type III	No Ig or C3
Glomerulonephritis in Wegener's granulomatous or periarteritis nodosa	Scanty or no Ig and C3
Benign recurrent hematuria	No immunoglobulins or C3
Hereditary nephritis	No immunoglobulins or C3 (Absent GBM Ag)
Diabetes mellitus	Diffuse linear BM accumulation of IgG and albumin

thing, the tests are generally negative in certain forms of glomerulonephritis with glomerular deposits (notably membranous glomerulonephritis). And although positive results are generally obtained in certain categories of immune complex glomerulonephritis, the tests are also often positive in patients without evidence of renal diseases (67). Furthermore, experimental evidence obtained in the past decade clearly shows that glomerular immune complex deposits may form *in situ*, as discussed in Chapter 2. The term immune complex glomerulonephritis is now generally applied to any glomerular disease in which extracellular immune deposits are found, without consideration of the mechanism of their formation. Anti-glomerular basement membrane (GBM) nephritis, which is characterized by continuous (linear) deposition of IgG in the GBM, resulting from combination of autoantibodies with GBM antigens, is usually classified separately because of the absence of discrete deposits and for historical reasons.

Immunofluorescence studies of renal biopsy specimens have also revealed tubulointerstitial deposits or accumulation of immunoglobulins along tubular basement membranes in some renal diseases. These findings are helpful in the diagnosis of certain uncommon forms of tubulointerstitial nephritis, as will be discussed.

Although immunoglobulins and complement components have been demonstrated in vessels in some cases of arteritis, these observations have been essentially valueless in diagnosis or classification (68).

The immunofluorescence procedures routinely used in our laboratory are reviewed in Chapter 16. Despite the development of more sensitive immunohistochemical techniques, immunofluorescence has remained the method of choice for the study of renal biopsies. Immunoperoxidase techniques are useful, however, when no frozen tissue is available and have been used with monoclonal antibodies to study infiltrating mononuclear cells, as discussed in Chapter 1.

MAJOR DIAGNOSTIC USES OF IMMUNOFLUORESCENCE

Demonstration of distinctive patterns of deposition of immunoglobulins, light chains, or complement components is generally required for the diagnosis of the following diseases: membranous glomerulonephritides; IgA nephropathies; anti-glomerular basement membrane (GBM) nephritis; light chain nephropathy, and the poorly defined or controversial conditions, IgM and Clq nephropathies (16,51). In addition, immunofluorescence studies are generally helpful in the diagnosis and subclassification of lupus nephritis and in the differential diagnosis of several conditions that may present clinically with the acute nephritic syndrome and exhibit diffuse endocapillary hypercellularity, namely, postinfectious glomerulonephritis, membranoproliferative glomerulonephritis (types I and II), and the glomerulonephritis of mixed cryoglobulinemia. Absence of immunoglobulins or complement components from glomeruli may support certain diagnoses, in particular minimal change disease, idiopathic crescentic glomerulonephritis (type III), periarteritis nodosa and Wegener's granulomatosis. In addition, recent studies have shown that immunofluorescence can be used to detect alteration or absence of native glomerular basement components. Such findings are helpful in diagnosing hereditary nephritis, as discussed later.

Although immunofluorescence findings are of great value in interpreting renal biopsies, a final diagnosis should be made only after consideration of clinical, histological, and laboratory findings. Electron microscopy is useful in about half of the biopsies with glomerular lesions. Even after all information has been considered, some cases will remain unclassified.

MEMBRANOUS GLOMERULONEPHRITIDES

Membranous glomerulonephritis is a descriptive diagnosis, which includes the following forms: idiopathic (the most common); membranous lupus nephritis; iatrogenic; membranous glomerulonephritis associated with hepatitis B infections or malignant tumors; and recurrent or *de novo* membranous glomerulonephritis in renal allografts. In all forms of membranous glomerulonephritis, the immunofluorescence findings are essentially the same, with granular deposits of IgG all along the glomerular basement membrane (Fig. 1). In rare cases the deposits are so confluent as to give a pseudolinear appearance, but at high magnification the granular nature of the deposits can be seen. Only in cases with extensive glomerular sclerosis is the pattern sometimes nondiagnostic, since the staining for IgG may be scanty and irregular.

Patients with membranous glomerulonephritis usually present with the nephrotic syndrome, and on clinical grounds the condition cannot be distinguished from most other diseases associated with heavy proteinuria, in particular minimal change disease and focal glomerulosclerosis. Immunofluorescence is the most reliable and efficient method for diagnosing membranous glomerulonephritis; although histologic findings are generally characteristic, cases with small deposits may be missed and erroneously diagnosed as minimal change disease. Electron-microscopic findings are generally diagnostic, but this technique is costly and time-consuming. However, electron microscopy provides the best means for detecting mesangial deposits, whose presence points toward lupus or hepatitis B associated disease. Electron microscopy can also be used to stage membranous glomerulonephritis, but this has only limited, if any prognostic value (87). When membranous

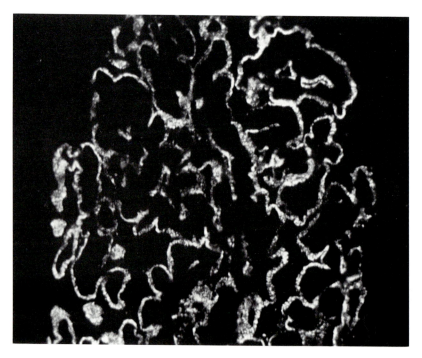

FIG. 1. Membranous glomerulonephritis. IgG is seen in granular form along the glomerular capillary walls.

glomerulonephritis is diagnosed, attempts should be made to identify known causes or associated conditions, before the disease is labeled idiopathic.

Membranous Lupus Nephritis

Membranous lupus nephritis should be suspected if the patient is young and female or if there are mesangial deposits (86), appreciable mesangial hypercellularity, or tubulointerstitial deposits of IgG. A definite diagnosis depends on serological and clinical findings of systemic lupus erythematosus. In rare cases, however, membranous nephritis may be the first manifestation of systemic lupus erythematosus, with other features appearing only months or years later (95,96).

Iatrogenic Membranous Glomerulonephritis

Iatrogenic membranous glomerulonephritis has been reported in patients given gold, penicillamine, captopril, or mercury (42,46). Although it is difficult to be certain that the agents were responsible for the associated nephritis in all cases, it is obviously prudent to discontinue these drugs in patients who develop evidence of membranous nephritis. In some patients, the renal disease has apparently disappeared following cessation of therapy.

Hepatitis B Associated Membranous Glomerulonephritis

Hepatitis B associated membranous glomerulonephritis has been reported principally from areas where there is a high incidence of chronic hepatitis B infection, notably Poland, Hungary, and Asia (12,48,101,121). In the United States the association is uncommon, but probably every patient with membranous glomerulonephritis should be studied for circulating hepatitis B surface antigen (HBsAg). Hepatitis antigens have been demonstrated in glomerular deposits in some cases; this argues for a causal role of the infection. In early studies HBsAg was thought to be the antigen present in epimembranous deposits; more recent studies indicate that HBe is probably the antigen involved (19,49,121), although in at least one recent study evidence for the presence of HBsAg was reported (48). Hepatitis B surface antigen has been convincingly demonstrated in mesangial deposits in a patient with atypical membranoproliferative glomerulonephritis associated with chronic hepatitis B infection and AIDS (19).

Yoshikawa et al. (121) have recently described findings that may help to differentiate hepatitis B associated membranous glomerulonephritis from the idiopathic form and that also suggest that different pathogenetic mechanisms may be involved. In patients with hepatitis, mesangial or subendothelial deposits were found by electron microscopy, and hypocomplementemia was also frequently observed. These are findings of type I membranoproliferative glomerulonephritis, more typical features of which are seen in some patients with hepatitis B infection.

Association between Membranous Glomerulonephritis and Malignant Tumors

An association between membranous glomerulonephritis and malignant tumors has been reported, most often with carcinoma of the intestine or lung (1,46). It is not certain, however, that the association exceeds what might occur by chance. Although there are reports in which tumor-associated antigens or antibodies against such antigens have been described in glomerular deposits, the documentation is unconvincing. Evidence that resolution of the glomerular disease may occur following removal of the tumor is also equivocal (1). From a practical point of view, it may be unnecessary to perform a workup for malignancy in a patient with membranous glomerulonephritis (1).

De Novo Membranous Glomerulonephritis

De novo membranous glomerulonephritis develops in renal allografts more often than can be accounted for by chance (27,38,105) (see Chapter 7). It is necessary to know the nature of the patient's original disease to determine whether the condition in the allograft is *de novo*, since recurrence has also been observed, although only rarely (22,27,64). Membranous glomerulonephritis in allografts is of considerable interest with respect to pathogenesis, but it is not a major problem in renal transplantation.

Membranous Glomerulonephritis

Membranous glomerulonephritis is classified as *idiopathic* when evidence of the associated conditions or causes listed above is lacking. For the past several years, it has been widely believed that the deposits in membranous glomerulonephritis form locally because of the resemblance of the lesions to the experimental model Heymann nephritis, in which *in situ* formation has been established (see Chapter 2), and because of the lack of evidence of circulating immune complexes in most patients. However, attempts to demonstrate antibrush border antibodies or brush border related antigens in glomerular deposits, as in Heymann nephritis, have been reported in only a few cases (28,79) and were not found in several large studies (18,108,113). Recently, evidence of a different sort has been obtained that links the human disease and Heymann nephritis; antibodies eluted from glomeruli of a specimen of idiopathic membranous glomerulonephritis have been shown to react with deposits in some other specimens with the disease but not with other forms of immune complex nephritis. They have also been shown to react with renal glycoproteins isolated in the same manner as used for the preparation of nephritogenic antigens of Heymann nephritis (80). There is at present, however, no practical way for detecting such antibodies in the serum for diagnostic purposes.

IgA NEPHROPATHIES

A group of diseases, known as IgA nephropathies, (or IgA associated nephropathies), have conspicuous IgA containing glomerular deposits, primarily in mesangial regions (Fig. 2). The conditions may be restricted to the kidney (IgA nephropathy or Berger's disease) or associated with systemic diseases, notably Henoch-Schönlein purpura, as well as hepatic and gastrointestinal disorders (42). Patients with IgA nephropathies associated with gastrointestinal or hepatic disorders often have no clinical evidence of renal disease, which may reflect the lack of glomerular deposition of IgG, IgM and C3 (31).

Certain conditions in which IgA may be conspicuous in glomeruli are excluded from the category of IgA nephropathy because they are classifiable as some other form of glomer-

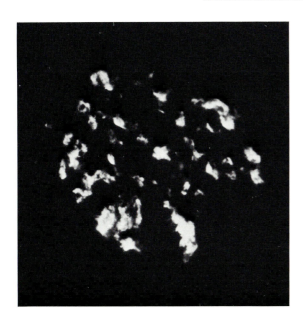

FIG. 2. IgA nephropathy. Large irregular deposits of IgA are seen in mesangial regions.

ulonephritis; a notable example is lupus nephritis, in which IgG is almost always predominant. And at least one case of anti-GBM nephritis has been reported in which the predominant anti-GBM antibodies were of the IgA class (10). In addition, some cases with prominent IgA deposits have features characteristic of type I membranoproliferative glomerulonephritis and it is not always clear how they should be classified (45).

Idiopathic IgA Nephropathy (Berger's Disease)

In cases of Berger's disease, IgA appears to be the predominant immunoglobulin class, as judged by the intensity of immunofluorescence staining, although in some instances, the intensity of staining for IgG and IgA appear to be nearly equal. Of the other classes, IgM is also often found, and C3 is present in the deposits in most cases, but Clq is generally absent (its presence suggests lupus nephritis).

It is obvious that the finding of a predominance of IgA in glomerular deposits does not define a disease entity and it appears likely that the condition classified as idiopathic IgA nephropathy is itself heterogeneous. Certainly the patients have a wide range of clinical and pathological manifestations. Originally described as a relatively benign condition, IgA nephropathy generally manifested itself by recurrent hematuria, but with stable renal function. It is now known, however, that about 20 to 30% of patients eventually develop progressive renal failure. Moreover, some patients have the nephrotic syndrome, and this appears to be associated with a poor prognosis (54). IgA nephropathy encompasses patients with or without macroscopic hematuria, and there are conflicting reports as to whether those with macroscopic hematuria have a poorer or better prognosis than those without (6,8). To what extent the variable clinical manifestations reflect basic disease differences is unknown. A study from Japan (53a) provides some evidence for different underlying host factors: patients with severe and progressive disease were found to have an association with HLA DR4, whereas this was not seen in patients with mild disease. Progress in the subclassification of idiopathic IgA nephropathy awaits the discovery of distinctive hallmarks, such as specific antigens or primary immunopathogenetic mechanisms.

At present, the subdivision of idiopathic IgA nephropathy can only be done at the descriptive level. A wide range of histologic abnormalities are found in cases classified as IgA nephropathy. Various histologic classifications have been proposed, no one of which is agreed upon by all (47,59,63). It is, however, generally accepted that the patients with the most severe histologic abnormalities have the poorest prognosis. Patients with glomeruli that appear normal or with only minimal mesangial abnormalities have generally had a benign course, especially if young (although further follow-up may reveal that some eventually develop renal failure) (47). Findings that have been associated with progression are severe glomerular tuft hypercellularity (especially if diffuse), crescent formation, glomerular sclerosis, glomerular subendothelial deposits (best detected by electron microscopy), and tubulointerstitial and arteriolar lesions (hyalinosis, sometimes with IgA deposits) (30, 35,45,77). Since there is no effective treatment for IgA nephropathy, this type of information is only of prognostic value.

Source and Nature of IgA in Glomerular Deposits in IgA Nephropathy

The IgA in glomerular deposits of IgA nephropathy is probably largely of mucosal origin (31). For one thing, J (joining) chains have been detected in the deposits in some cases. (Specimens without IgM, which also have J chains, must be studied). J chains are found in polymers (especially dimers) of IgA, as in IgA of mucosal origin. In addition, binding of free secretory components to glomerular deposits *in vitro* has been demonstrated, although secretory component itself is not found in deposits (89). Furthermore, the frequent association of episodes of hematuria with pharyngitis implicates mucosal infection.

Evidence concerning the origin of IgA in glomeruli has also been sought by investigating the two IgA subclasses in the deposits. Since IgA2 is produced mainly in mucosal sites, its presence would favor mucosal origin. In an early report in which rabbit antibodies against human IgA subclasses were used, it was concluded that IgA2 was the major subclass (2). In several later studies, however, based largely on monoclonal antibodies, IgA1 has generally been found to be the main subclass (20,89), although IgA2 has also been demonstrated in a few cases (65).

Because of the greater specificity of monoclonal antibodies, the results obtained with these antibodies are given greater weight than those employing polyclonal antibodies. A recent study by Melvin et al. (73), however, points to a potential pitfall, which results from the fact that monoclonal antibodies recognize epitopes (antigenic determinants) and not macromolecules. If the epitope is hidden or altered, the antigen will not be detected. Melvin et al. (73) have shown that an IgA epitope recognized by a particular monoclonal antibody is masked in certain deposits, presumably because the determinant is in the hinge region of the immunoglobulin, which is likely to be altered in immune complexes. It has not been shown, however, that the monoclonal antibodies that have been used to detect IgA2 in IgA nephropathy are directed against epitopes that are masked in immune complexes, and it appears that IgA1 is in fact the predominant subclass.

It appears likely that IgA deposits in glomeruli result from trapping of circulating immune complexes or IgA polymers, since the mesangial pattern resembles that seen after intravenous injections of preformed complexes or aggregated proteins in animals (67). Furthermore, elevated levels of circulating IgA containing complexes or polymeric IgA have been reported in some patients with IgA nephropathy, although similar findings have sometimes been noted in patients without evidence of glomerular disease (21,91,119). Food antigens, in particular bovine serum albumin, have been demonstrated in circulating complexes in a few patients with IgA nephropathy (119), and bovine protein antigens and possibly soy bean proteins have been described in mesangial deposits in some specimens (90). Further studies are needed to define the role of food or other exogenous antigens in the pathogenesis of IgA nephropathy. Serum antibodies that react with collagen IV alpha chains and also with types I and II collagen (14) have been detected in some patients with IgA nephropathy; their pathogenetic significance, if any, is unknown.

Henoch-Schönlein Purpura

The distinction between idiopathic IgA nephropathy and that of Henoch-Schönlein purpura cannot be made on the basis of renal biopsy findings. The diagnosis of Henoch-Schönlein purpura rather than idiopathic IgA nephropathy is made when the patient has nonthrombocytopenic purpura, often with arthralgia and abdominal pain. It has been suggested that Henoch-Schönlein purpura and IgA nephropathy are part of a spectrum of the same disease, but in the absence of knowledge of causative agents or basic pathogenetic mechanisms, this hypothesis must be considered unproved (24,78). A number of authors have attempted to define features with prognostic value in the nephropathy of Henoch-Schönlein purpura (58,72,100,120). In general, as in idiopathic IgA nephropathy, the more severe the histologic changes, the worse the prognosis. Extensive crescent formation is associated with a particularly poor prognosis.

IDIOPATHIC CRESCENTIC GLOMERULONEPHRITIS

One of the most important groups of renal disease the pathologist has to diagnose are those usually classified as crescentic glomerulonephritis. Immunofluorescence is of major importance in subclassifying this group. Extensive crescent formation occurs in a variety of glomerular diseases, including several idiopathic glomerular diseases and some forms associated with infectious or systemic diseases. The term crescentic glomerulonephritis is generally applied to the idiopathic forms. Some object to the designation since other glomerular abnormalities are often found, especially necrosis of the tufts or severe tubulo-interstitial changes; in some cases classified as crescentic glomerulonephritis, these features appear to be more prominent than the crescents. Furthermore, there is no general agreement as to how many crescents have to be present: some require that more than 60% to 70% of glomeruli be involved, whereas others require no more than 25% (42,43,103,106). Moreover, crescents vary in size. It is obvious, therefore, that even from a morphologic point of view, crescentic glomerulonephritis is heterogeneous.

If crescents are sufficiently large and numerous, the clinical picture is that of rapidly progressive renal failure, often with oliguria or anuria. A synonym for crescentic glomerulonephritis is rapidly progressive glomerulonephritis. This term is acceptable, but only if there is pathologic confirmation, since there are other causes of rapidly progressive renal failure, such as acute interstitial nephritis or vascular disease.

Histologic features do not provide reliable guidelines for subdivision of idiopathic crescentic glomerulonephritis, although crescents appear to be more extensive and necrosis less

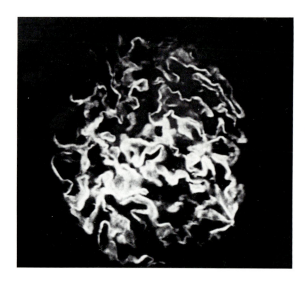

FIG. 3. Anti-GBM nephritis. There is linear staining for IgG along the GBM. The areas that do not appear to be stained are out of the plane of focus.

prominent in anti-GBM nephritis than in the other forms. Subclassification depends primarily on immunofluorescence findings. On this basis, three forms are generally recognized, as described below.

Idiopathic Crescentic Glomerulonephritis Type I (Anti-GBM Nephritis)

Anti-GBM nephritis is commonly classified as idiopathic crescentic glomerulonephritis, type I, but can also simply be referred to as anti-GBM nephritis. Anti-GBM nephritis is part of a spectrum of conditions with anti-basement membrane antibodies that affect the kidneys and lungs. When associated with lung hemorrhage, the condition is referred to as Goodpasture's syndrome; however, unrelated diseases—notably Wegener's granulomatosis, systemic lupus erythematosus, and periarteritis nodosa—can also produce the syndrome of rapidly progressive renal failure and lung hemorrhage.

Problems in the Diagnosis of Anti-GBM Nephritis

The diagnosis of anti-GBM glomerulonephritis requires the demonstration of anti-GBM antibodies. The characteristic linear accumulation of immunoglobulin (almost always IgG) along the GBM provides evidence for *in vivo* bound anti-GBM antibodies (Fig. 3). However, nonimmunologically bound IgG can produce a similar picture, as is frequently seen in autopsy tissue or in biopsy specimens from diabetics. In many such cases, bright linear GBM staining for albumin is also seen. Studies of eluates from diabetic kidneys have shown that the recovered immunoglobulins have no reactivity with the GBM (40). Accordingly, when linear GBM staining for IgG is found, tests should be performed to detect anti-GBM antibodies in the circulation or, when sufficient tissue is available, in eluates of renal tissue. Confirmation is particularly important if the staining is not intense and if the clinical and histological features are not those usually associated with anti-GBM nephritis: namely, rapidly progressive renal failure with or without lung hemorrhage and severe crescentic glomerulonephritis, often with linear tubular basement membrane (TBM) de-

posits of IgG and tubulointerstitial nephritis (3). Rarely, however, patients with well-documented anti-GBM antibodies have mild glomerular disease without crescents (7).

In early studies circulating anti-GBM antibodies were generally detected by indirect immunofluorescence, using normal kidney as the substrate, but recently described radio-immunoassay or ELISA procedures appear to be more sensitive and specific (39,112,117). Over 90% of patients with proved anti-GBM disease have circulating antibodies, as measured by radioimmunoassays employing collagenase-solubilized GBM preparations (117). Unfortunately, these assays are not widely available, nor are they uniform from one laboratory to another. Methods employing other techniques, such as hemagglutination, or other types of antigen preparations, such as guanidine hydrochloride extracts, have yielded positive results in conditions other than anti-GBM nephritis, including IgA nephropathy and lupus nephritis (14,115).

Measurement of anti-GBM antibody titers using collagenase-solubilized antigen preparations may be of value in monitoring the disease. Some findings suggest that plasma exchange, combined with immunosuppressive therapy, reduces the level of circulating anti-GBM antibodies and ameliorates the renal damage in nonoliguric patients (84), especially those with relatively mild histologic abnormalities (52). In view of this and because the disease can progress very rapidly, it is important to establish the diagnosis as quickly as possible.

Nature of Goodpasture Antigens

It has generally been believed that the relevant antigens ("Goodpasture antigens") in anti-GBM nephritis are present in noncollagenous basement membrane components (because they survive collagenase treatment). Wieslander et al. (114) have recently obtained evidence that is contrary to this belief. They have found that the antigens reside in collagenase-resistant sequences (M2 peptides) in the NCl globular domain at the carboxy-terminal end of type IV collagen. Anti-GBM antibodies in most patients are apparently heterogeneous, since they show variable reactivity with renal tubular basement membranes, Bowman's capsule, lung, and choroid plexus by indirect immunofluorescence. Some of this variability may be due to masking of the relevant antigens in certain tissues (116,122). However, studies using immunoblotting techniques have shown that some Goodpasture sera identify components of the globular domain with several molecular weights (53). On the other hand, the anti-GBM antibodies in some patients appear to react effectively with only a limited number of determinants; thus, a monoclonal anti-GBM antibody apparently competes appreciably with certain human antibodies (88). The studies concerned with the specificity of anti-GBM antibodies have dealt with small numbers of patients, and the full range of reactivity of antibodies remains to be determined (55).

Pathogenetic Role of Anti-GBM Antibodies

Although it is almost universally accepted that anti-GBM antibodies are the primary immunopathogenetic agents in anti-GBM nephritis (61) (often referred to as anti-GBM antibody mediated nephritis), the evidence for this view is not unassailable (98), and it seems likely that the interaction of sensitized T cells with basement membrane antigens initiates or contributes to glomerular and tubulointerstitial injury.

Causative Factors in Anti-GBM Nephritis

What initiates the formation of the anti-GBM autoantibodies is unknown. The evidence that exposure to hydrocarbons or viral infection may be responsible is inconclusive (7, 117). Genetic factors may be important in susceptibility as shown by an association of anti-GBM disease with HLA-DR2 in patients studied in Great Britain (84). Of interest is the additional finding that the possession of B7, which is in linkage disequilibrium with DR2, appears to be accompanied by a very poor prognosis (84). In any case, the auto-immune response in most patients is transient, so that if a patient can survive the initial period without irreparable renal damage, recovery is possible.

Some special forms of anti-GBM nephritis have been described. A few cases have been reported in which anti-GBM antibodies and crescentic glomerulonephritis have been seen in association with membranous glomerulonephritis (57,85). In addition, anti-GBM nephritis may recur in allografts, especially if transplantation is performed while circulating anti-GBM antibodies are still present (117). Anti-GBM nephritis has also been observed to develop *de novo* in renal allografts in some patients with familial nephritis (Alport's syndrome), apparently because the recipients had not established tolerance against certain GBM antigens that are absent from their own kidneys (71,76). (See Chapter 7.) Serum antibodies in such Alport patients recognize a Goodpasture antigen, but the reactivity may be more restricted than that of serum antibodies in some patients with Goodpasture's syndrome (53). Thus, antibodies from a patient with Alport's syndrome recognized only a 26,000 molecular weight monomer derived from globular domain of type IV collagen, whereas three Goodpasture's sera reacted with two additional components (53).

Idiopathic Crescentic Glomerulonephritis with Immunoglobulin Deposits Type II

In some patients with idiopathic crescentic glomerulonephritis, granular deposits of immunoglobulins (IgG and/or IgM) are found, either in mesangial regions, along glomerular capillary walls, or in both locations (9,17). Deposits of C3 may or may not be found. The extent of the deposits is variable in cases classified as type II idiopathic crescentic glomerulonephritis and is often quite scanty. By electron microscopy, scattered electron dense deposits are found in the mesangium and in the subendothelial space in some cases (17,42). This form of idiopathic crescentic glomerulonephritis is generally thought to be mediated by immune complexes. Aside from the deposits other evidence that has been cited as favoring a pathogenetic role of immune complexes is the presence of circulating complexes and hypocomplementemia in some cases (42). If the glomerular deposits do actually represent immune complexes, it is difficult to understand how they can account for the severe necrotizing and crescentic lesions that accompany them, since more abundant deposits are often seen in other glomerular diseases lacking these features. It is possible that cell mediated mechanisms are required for the glomerular injury, although there is no evidence for this. The antigens that may be present in the deposits are unknown.

Idiopathic Crescentic Glomerulonephritis without Immunoglobulin Deposits (Type III)

In some cases of idiopathic crescentic glomerulonephritis, no immunoglobulin-containing deposits are found in glomeruli. The frequency of this type is uncertain (42). Stilmant et al. (106) have found this group to be more common than either anti-GBM

nephritis or the presumed immune complex form. In contrast, Cohen et al. (17) report finding immunoglobulin-containing deposits in all cases. Undoubtedly, differences in techniques and in interpretation of immunofluorescence findings are important; small focal, segmental deposits may be considered as insignificant by some (with the result that the cases are classified as type III) or as indicative of immune complexes by others. Stilmant et al. (106) found no evidence of circulating immune complexes in any of their patients with idiopathic crescentic glomerulonephritis without immune deposits. The primary pathogenetic mechanisms in this group are obviously unknown; it is possible that cell mediated mechanisms are involved, but direct evidence is lacking.

DIFFERENTIAL DIAGNOSIS OF IDIOPATHIC CRESCENTIC GLOMERULONEPHRITIS (TYPES II AND III)

The immunofluorescence and histological findings in idiopathic crescentic glomerulonephritis with scanty or absent immunoglobulin accumulation (type III and some cases of type II) and in the glomerulonephritis of Wegener's granulomatosis or periarteritis nodosa are generally indistinguishable. Although it has been widely held that both of the latter conditions are mediated by immune complexes, the evidence for this view is scanty, and conspicuous granular deposits of immunoglobulins are rarely found in glomeruli. Indeed, when they are found, the diagnosis of these conditions should be questioned. Only in rare instances are typical granulomatous lesions or necrotizing arteritis found in renal biopsy specimens. Thus, the diagnosis of Wegener's granulomatosis or periarteritis nodosa usually depends on demonstration of characteristic lesions in extrarenal tissue. In many patients in which these diagnoses are suspected on clinical grounds because of pulmonary lesions, fever, elevated erythrocyte sedimentation rate, or other signs of "multisystem disease," pathologic confirmation is not obtained (111). Perhaps a search for anti-leukocytic cytoplasmic antibodies will help to diagnose and monitor disease activity in Wegener's granulomatosis (109), but whether it will help differentiate Wegener's granulomatosis from idiopathic crescentic glomerulonephritis, or periarticular nodosa is not clear. The distinction between these three conditions is not entirely academic, because they may differ in their response to therapy (34,43,111). Since the diseases can progress rapidly, early diagnosis is important.

DIFFERENTIAL DIAGNOSIS OF ACUTE GLOMERULONEPHRITIS AND MEMBRANOPROLIFERATIVE GLOMERULONEPHRITIS, TYPES I AND II (DENSE DEPOSIT DISEASE)

The distinction between acute (poststreptococcal) glomerulonephritis and membranoproliferative glomerulonephritis (types I and II) is important and often difficult, both on clinical and histologic grounds. All three conditions may present with clinical features of acute glomerulonephritis (the acute nephritic syndrome), often with hypocomplementemia. Histologically, these diseases are generally characterized by diffuse hypercellularity of glomerular tufts. Although distinctive abnormalities are found in peripheral capillary walls and mesangial regions in the majority of cases of types I and II membranoproliferative glomerulonephritis, these features are not always discernible in histologic preparations, especially in patients biopsied shortly after apparent onset. Immunohistochemical studies for mononuclear cell markers might be of help in making the differential diagnosis, since in acute glomerulonephritis there is an accumulation of monocytes, and to a lesser extent of lymphocytes (83), whereas this does not occur in membranoproliferative glomerulo-nephritis (37). The practical value of this approach has not been assessed, however.

Immunofluorescence findings often permit a definitive diagnosis in this group. In acute glomerulonephritis, the findings are somewhat variable and include mesangial deposits of IgG and C3, as well as the more characteristic large, granular, deposits of Ig and C3 (or of C3 alone) along the glomerular capillary walls (110) (Fig. 4). The peripheral deposits are usually scattered, but may be contiguous ("garland pattern") (102). In type I membra-noproliferative glomerulonephritis, C3 is found as irregular, often broad deposits outlining peripheral capillary walls and as irregular mesangial deposits (62) (Fig. 5); IgM and IgG are found in about two-thirds of cases and IgA in a smaller percentage (which, as noted earlier, may cause confusion with IgA nephropathy). In type II membranoproliferative glomerulonephritis (dense deposit disease), the predominant finding is accumulation of C3 in the form of large globules in mesangial regions and often in a broad ribbon-like or double linear pattern along parts of the glomerular capillary walls, Bowman's capsule, and tubular basement membrane (26) (Fig. 6). Immunoglobulins, especially IgG, are usually lacking.

The combined immunofluorescence and histological findings are, however, not always conclusive. In such cases electron microscopy will often help establish the diagnosis (15). In acute glomerulonephritis, characteristic epimembranous dense deposits, "humps," are usually found. In type I membranoproliferative glomerulonephritis, broad, subendothelial deposits of electron dense material are seen, and in type II membranoproliferative glomer-ulonephritis, large segments of the basement membrane are occupied by extremely electron dense material, which is regarded as the most definitive pathologic finding in dense deposit disease. In occasional cases, however, even electron-microscopic findings are not defini-tive, largely for the following reasons: (a) humps may be seen in type I and II membrano-proliferative glomerulonephritis and even more so in what some classify as type III (13, 107); (b) subendothelial and even intramembranous deposits may be found in acute glomer-ulonephritis (13,110); and (c) intramembranous deposits are not always diagnostic of dense

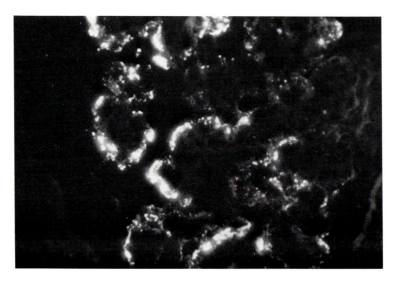

FIG. 4. Acute poststreptococcal glomerulonephritis. Irregular granular staining for IgG is shown along the glomerular capillary wall.

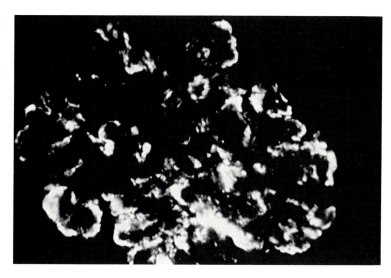

FIG. 5. Membranoproliferative glomerulonephritis, type I. Broad, irregular deposits of C3 are present along glomerular capillary walls.

deposit disease, especially when small and irregular. In cases where the combined histologic, initial clinical, immunofluorescence, and electron-microscopic findings do not lead to a definite diagnosis, the course of the disease may provide a partial answer: disappearance of renal abnormalities and return of complement levels to normal favor the diagnosis of poststreptococcal glomerulonephritis. No doubt some cases diagnosed on renal biopsy as acute glomerulonephritis before the widespread use of immunofluorescence or electron microscopy were in fact examples of membranoproliferative glomerulonephritis, and this type of error resulted in exaggerated pessimism about the prognosis of poststreptococcal glomerulonephritis.

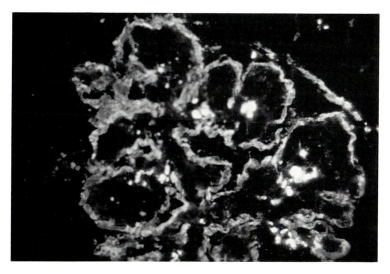

FIG. 6. Membranoproliferative glomerulonephritis, type II. C3 is present along the GBM and Bowman's capsule, in some places in bilaminar form, as well as in mesangial regions as intensely stained globules.

IDIOPATHIC MIXED CRYOGLOBULINEMIA

The histologic features of idiopathic mixed cryoglobulinemia can also be confused with those of acute glomerulonephritis and even with types I or II membranoproliferative glomerulonephritis; however, because of the associated clinical and laboratory findings in mixed cryoglobulinemia—in particular purpura, arthralgia, neuritis—the differential diagnosis is usually not a problem. Although the diagnosis requires evidence of circulating mixed cryoglobulins, this may also be present in poststreptococcal glomerulonephritis and type I membranoproliferative glomerulonephritis (42,43). The finding in biopsy specimens of eosinophilic intracapillary masses, which characteristically stain for IgG, IgM, IgG and C3, is suggestive of mixed cryoglobulinemia. In most cases, granular deposits containing IgG, IgM, and C3 are found also along the GBM. It is possible to demonstrate rheumatoid factor (anti-IgG) activity in the deposits, by demonstration of reactivity of fluorescein-labeled, aggregated IgG with glomerular deposits, but this approach is not often used for diagnostic purposes. By electron microscopy, deposits with characteristic cylindrical structures are seen in some cases (36). Numerous mononuclear phagocytes have been demonstrated in the glomeruli in mixed cryoglobulinemia, which should be of value in the differentiation from membranoproliferative glomerulonephritides, but not from acute poststreptococcal glomerulonephritis (37).

LUPUS NEPHRITIS

The characteristic immunofluorescence findings in most forms of lupus nephritis are rarely required for the diagnosis, since the histological and serological evidence of systemic lupus erythematosus usually suffice to establish the diagnosis. Rarely, however, membranous glomerulonephritis may be the first manifestation of systemic lupus erythematosus (95,96).

In most cases of lupus nephritis, conspicuous immune deposits are found that almost always contain IgG, Clq, C3, and usually IgM, and often IgA as well. Even IgE is sometimes seen (42,43). Peritubular deposits are commonly present (see below). Immunofluorescence is of considerable value in the subclassification of lupus nephritis as seen in Table 1 (5,69). In general, the severity of the glomerular histologic abnormalities appears to correlate with the extent and degree of immune deposits, and in particular with subendothelial deposits. However, severe active lupus glomerulonephritis has been observed with only mild, focal mesangial deposits, which suggests that mechanisms other than immune complex accumulation are sometimes involved in pathogenesis (93).

SYSTEMIC LIGHT CHAIN DISEASE (LIGHT CHAIN NEPHROPATHY)

The condition known as systemic light chain disease nephropathy has been widely recognized only recently (41,94,97). Some use the term *light chain deposition disease*, to distinguish the condition from Bence Jones nephropathy, in which light chains also play a role (33). Light chain nephropathy has been reported in association with multiple myeloma, with lymphoproliferative disorders, and in patients without overt evidence of neoplasia.

The two most common types of renal lesions in patients with multiple myeloma are amyloidosis and the so-called myeloma kidney (with tubular cell damage, usually with characteristic casts and giant cell formation). The lesions referred to as light chain nephrop-

l. The lesions frequently cause scar formation. The histo-
ns reveals a subepidermal blister with an inflammatory cell
ytes and neutrophils. The histological differential diagnosis
mative gingivitis, and aphthous stomatitis. The immuno-
in resolving the differential diagnostic dilemma. The therapy usually includes an immunosuppressive regimen.

Direct immunofluorescence of perilesional mucosa shows linear deposition of IgG or
C3, and in 80% of cases IgA, IgM, and IgE may be seen (5,89). Some cases classified as
cicatricial pemphigoid have the only IgA in a linear pattern in mucous membranes. These
cases probably should be separated and called linear IgA bullous disease, but the issue has
yet to be resolved (34). Immunoelectron microscopy has localized the immunoreactants to
the lamina lucida, but the antigen has not been isolated (59). Indirect immunofluorescence
reveals circulating IgG anti-basement membrane zone antibodies in only 10% to 25% of
cases (5,81).

Herpes Gestationis

Herpes gestationis is a self-limited bullous skin disease characterized by intensely pruritic, grouped vesicobullous lesions in pregnant women (usually in their third trimester or
during postpartum) and newborn infants. The histological examination of lesional skin
reveals a subepidermal bulla with eosinophils. Early lesions may show a superficial and
deep perivascular and interstitial mixed cell infiltrate with papillary dermal edema. Histological differential diagnosis includes allergic contact dermatitis, insect bites, and pruritic
urticarial papules and plaques of pregnancy. Immunopathological studies are important in
evaluation of these lesions.

Direct immunofluorescence of perilesional skin shows linear deposition, C3 in 100% of
cases, and IgG in 30% to 50% of cases (46). IgM and IgA are only rarely identified.
Immunoelectron microscopy has demonstrated that the immunoreactants are present in the
lamina lucida and diffusely on the dermal face of the basal cell plasma membranes (88).
This ultrastructural localization is subtly different from that of bullous and cicatricial
pemphigoid in that the distribution is more uniform rather than associated with hemidesmosomes. These findings, as well as the clinical features, support the view that herpes
gestationis is a distinct entity. The antigen has not been isolated.

Routine indirect immunofluorescence demonstrates circulating IgG anti-basement membrane zone antibodies in up to 25% of patients (46). Complement fixation tests, which
employ indirect immunofluorescence with an added complement source step and test for
complement fixation, are more sensitive and can demonstrate circulating antibodies in 85%
of patients (46).

The expression of herpes gestationis appears to be modulated by hormonal factors. In
some patients, after their pregnancy-related eruption has resolved, clinical exacerbations
have been noted during the ovulatory period and the premenstrual period of the menstrual
cycle. These times are associated with increased estrogen and decreased progesterone,
respectively. In addition, in one study, herpes gestationis patients receiving oral contraceptives containing estrogens and progesterones have had exacerbations, while patients receiving progesterone only have had no exacerbations (35). This study would support the argument that estrogens promote the disease, while progesterone is inhibitory.

Epidermal Bullous Aquisita

Epidermolysis bullous aquisita (EBA) is a bullous skin disease, characterized by tense bullae and erosions, scarring, milia, and nail dystrophy. Histological examination shows subepidermal blisters with variable inflammatory cell infiltrates. The histological differential diagnosis includes bullous pemphigoid, porphyria cutanea tarda, and allergic contact dermatitis. The immunopathological studies are helpful in the differential diagnosis. The therapy usually includes immunosuppressive therapy.

Direct immunofluorescence of perilesional skin reveals linear deposition of IgG and/or C3 in the basement membrane zone in 100% of cases (87). IgA, IgM may be seen. False positive studies are very rare. Immunoelectron microscopy localizes the immunoreactants to the sublamina densa area (87). Indirect immunofluorescence demonstrates circulating IgG anti-basement membrane zone antibodies in 50% of cases (87).

The routine histological and immunopathological evaluation of patients with EBA cannot definitively distinguish this entity from bullous pemphigoid. Previously, the only definitive study was immunoelectron microscopy (87), which is expensive, time-consuming, and not readily available. The development of the sodium chloride-split skin method of indirect immunofluorescence has addressed this problem (24). Normal human skin is incubated in 1.0 M NaCl until a split occurs through the lamina lucida. This NaCl-split, normal human skin is used as the substrate for indirect immunofluorescence. Bullous pemphigoid antibodies react with the epidermal side (Fig. 6) or both the epidermal and dermal sides of the split. Epidermolysis bullous acquisita sera, which localizes to the sublamina densa area, stains only the dermal side of the split skin (Fig. 7). This simple test has made differentiation of EBA and bullous pemphigoid readily available. Retrospective and prospective

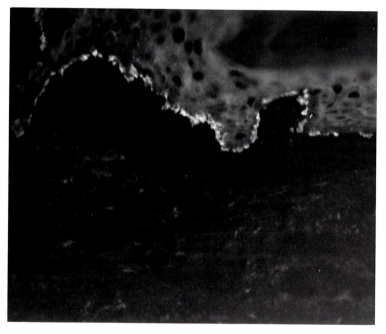

FIG. 6. Localization of bullous pemphigoid antibodies to the epidermal side of NaCl-split normal skin [indirect immunofluorescence (IgG), × 100].

branes and skin may be affected. The lesions frequently cause scar formation. The histological examination of the lesions reveals a subepidermal blister with an inflammatory cell infiltrate, composed of lymphocytes and neutrophils. The histological differential diagnosis includes lichen planus, desquamative gingivitis, and aphthous stomatitis. The immunopathological studies are helpful in resolving the differential diagnostic dilemma. The therapy usually includes an immunosuppressive regimen.

Direct immunofluorescence of perilesional mucosa shows linear deposition of IgG or C3, and in 80% of cases IgA, IgM, and IgE may be seen (5,89). Some cases classified as cicatricial pemphigoid have the only IgA in a linear pattern in mucous membranes. These cases probably should be separated and called linear IgA bullous disease, but the issue has yet to be resolved (34). Immunoelectron microscopy has localized the immunoreactants to the lamina lucida, but the antigen has not been isolated (59). Indirect immunofluorescence reveals circulating IgG anti-basement membrane zone antibodies in only 10% to 25% of cases (5,81).

Herpes Gestationis

Herpes gestationis is a self-limited bullous skin disease characterized by intensely pruritic, grouped vesicobullous lesions in pregnant women (usually in their third trimester or during postpartum) and newborn infants. The histological examination of lesional skin reveals a subepidermal bulla with eosinophils. Early lesions may show a superficial and deep perivascular and interstitial mixed cell infiltrate with papillary dermal edema. Histological differential diagnosis includes allergic contact dermatitis, insect bites, and pruritic urticarial papules and plaques of pregnancy. Immunopathological studies are important in evaluation of these lesions.

Direct immunofluorescence of perilesional skin shows linear deposition, C3 in 100% of cases, and IgG in 30% to 50% of cases (46). IgM and IgA are only rarely identified. Immunoelectron microscopy has demonstrated that the immunoreactants are present in the lamina lucida and diffusely on the dermal face of the basal cell plasma membranes (88). This ultrastructural localization is subtly different from that of bullous and cicatricial pemphigoid in that the distribution is more uniform rather than associated with hemidesmosomes. These findings, as well as the clinical features, support the view that herpes gestationis is a distinct entity. The antigen has not been isolated.

Routine indirect immunofluorescence demonstrates circulating IgG anti-basement membrane zone antibodies in up to 25% of patients (46). Complement fixation tests, which employ indirect immunofluorescence with an added complement source step and test for complement fixation, are more sensitive and can demonstrate circulating antibodies in 85% of patients (46).

The expression of herpes gestationis appears to be modulated by hormonal factors. In some patients, after their pregnancy-related eruption has resolved, clinical exacerbations have been noted during the ovulatory period and the premenstrual period of the menstrual cycle. These times are associated with increased estrogen and decreased progesterone, respectively. In addition, in one study, herpes gestationis patients receiving oral contraceptives containing estrogens and progesterones have had exacerbations, while patients receiving progesterone only have had no exacerbations (35). This study would support the argument that estrogens promote the disease, while progesterone is inhibitory.

Epidermal Bullous Aquisita

Epidermolysis bullous aquisita (EBA) is a bullous skin disease, characterized by tense bullae and erosions, scarring, milia, and nail dystrophy. Histological examination shows subepidermal blisters with variable inflammatory cell infiltrates. The histological differential diagnosis includes bullous pemphigoid, porphyria cutanea tarda, and allergic contact dermatitis. The immunopathological studies are helpful in the differential diagnosis. The therapy usually includes immunosuppressive therapy.

Direct immunofluorescence of perilesional skin reveals linear deposition of IgG and/or C3 in the basement membrane zone in 100% of cases (87). IgA, IgM may be seen. False positive studies are very rare. Immunoelectron microscopy localizes the immunoreactants to the sublamina densa area (87). Indirect immunofluorescence demonstrates circulating IgG anti-basement membrane zone antibodies in 50% of cases (87).

The routine histological and immunopathological evaluation of patients with EBA cannot definitively distinguish this entity from bullous pemphigoid. Previously, the only definitive study was immunoelectron microscopy (87), which is expensive, time-consuming, and not readily available. The development of the sodium chloride-split skin method of indirect immunofluorescence has addressed this problem (24). Normal human skin is incubated in 1.0 M NaCl until a split occurs through the lamina lucida. This NaCl-split, normal human skin is used as the substrate for indirect immunofluorescence. Bullous pemphigoid antibodies react with the epidermal side (Fig. 6) or both the epidermal and dermal sides of the split. Epidermolysis bullous acquisita sera, which localizes to the sublamina densa area, stains only the dermal side of the split skin (Fig. 7). This simple test has made differentiation of EBA and bullous pemphigoid readily available. Retrospective and prospective

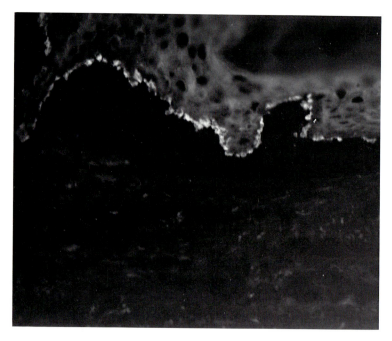

FIG. 6. Localization of bullous pemphigoid antibodies to the epidermal side of NaCl-split normal skin [indirect immunofluorescence (IgG), × 100].

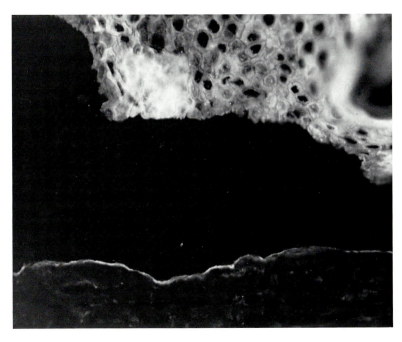

FIG. 7. Localization of epidermolysis bullosa acquisita antibodies to the dermal side of NaCl-split normal skin [indirect immunofluorescence (IgG), × 100].

studies of sera of patients with antibodies localized to the basement membrane zone are widening the definition of EBA to include cases that were previously thought to be bullous pemphigoid (84). The clinical and therapeutic implications have yet to be fully evaluated.

Linear IgA Bullous Dermatosis

Linear IgA bullous dermatosis is a bullous skin disease with a clinical presentation that is similar to bullous pemphigoid (i.e., large, tense bullae) or dermatitis herpetiformis (i.e., grouped papulovesicular lesions). The histological features include a subepidermal bullae with neutrophils at the dermal-epidermal junction. The differential diagnosis includes dermatitis herpetiformis and bullous lupus erythematosus. Immunopathological studies are helpful in the differential diagnosis. The therapy usually includes sulfapyridine or the sulfones. These patients are not responsive to a gluten-free diet.

Direct immunofluorescence of perilesional skin shows linear IgA in the basement membrane zone in 100% of cases and linear C3 in 20% to 25% of cases (15,51); IgG and IgM are occasionally found. Immunoelectron microscopy demonstrates immunoreactants in three patterns. The immunoreactants can be located in the lamina lucida, below the lamina densa, or both in the lamina lucida and below the lamina densa (53,85). False positive and false negative studies are rare.

Indirect immunofluorescence identifies circulating IgA anti-basement membrane zone antibodies in 10% to 25% of cases (15,51). False positive indirect immunofluorescence studies are rare.

Deposits in Dermal Papillae

Dermatitis Herpetiformis

Dermatitis herpetiformis is a systemic disease characterized by pruritic papulovesicular lesions on the extensor surfaces bilaterally and a gluten-sensitive enteropathy. Histological findings include a subepidermal blister and neutrophils in the tips of the dermal papillae. The histological differential diagnosis includes bullous lupus erythematosus and linear IgA bullous dermatosis. Immunofluorescence studies are helpful in confirming the diagnosis. Therapy may include a gluten-free diet, sulfones, and sulfapyridine.

Direct immunofluorescence of perilesional or nonlesional skin reveals granular deposits of IgA in the dermal papillae (Fig. 8) in 100% of cases (23,47). These deposits may be focal; therefore, multiple levels should be examined (normally do nine). In 70% of cases C3 is found, and IgG, IgM, IgD, and IgE may also be seen. Immunoelectron microscopy demonstrates that the IgA deposits are associated with the microfibrillary bundles of elastic fibers in the papillary dermis (86). False positive and false negative studies are rare.

Indirect immunofluorescence for circulating IgG or IgA antibodies selective for the dermis are negative. Circulating IgA anti-endomysial antibodies have been identified in 70% of cases of dermatitis herpetiformis and in 100% of cases with a gluten-sensitive enteropathy (1). Ciculating IgG and IgA anti-gluten (50) and anti-reticulin (49) antibodies have been identified in 70% to 90% and 50% to 67% of cases, respectively. Circulating immune complexes have been identified in 30% to 40% of cases (31).

The cause of dermatitis herpetiformis is gluten hypersensitivity (52). The mechanism by which gluten is able to provoke the lesions of dermatitis herpetiformis has not been resolved. There appears to be a genetic predisposition to the disease. The ingestion of gluten leads to alterations in the intestine and the production of antibodies specific for gluten. The deposition of immune complexes in the skin and the recruitment of inflammatory cells produce the skin lesions (89).

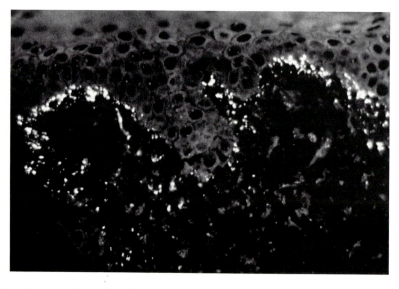

FIG. 8. Granular deposition of IgA in dermal papillae in dermatitis herpetiformis [direct immunofluorescence (IgA), × 100].

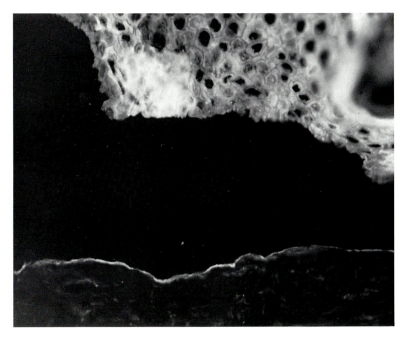

FIG. 7. Localization of epidermolysis bullosa acquisita antibodies to the dermal side of NaCl-split normal skin [indirect immunofluorescence (IgG), × 100].

studies of sera of patients with antibodies localized to the basement membrane zone are widening the definition of EBA to include cases that were previously thought to be bullous pemphigoid (84). The clinical and therapeutic implications have yet to be fully evaluated.

Linear IgA Bullous Dermatosis

Linear IgA bullous dermatosis is a bullous skin disease with a clinical presentation that is similar to bullous pemphigoid (i.e., large, tense bullae) or dermatitis herpetiformis (i.e., grouped papulovesicular lesions). The histological features include a subepidermal bullae with neutrophils at the dermal-epidermal junction. The differential diagnosis includes dermatitis herpetiformis and bullous lupus erythematosus. Immunopathological studies are helpful in the differential diagnosis. The therapy usually includes sulfapyridine or the sulfones. These patients are not responsive to a gluten-free diet.

Direct immunofluorescence of perilesional skin shows linear IgA in the basement membrane zone in 100% of cases and linear C3 in 20% to 25% of cases (15,51); IgG and IgM are occasionally found. Immunoelectron microscopy demonstrates immunoreactants in three patterns. The immunoreactants can be located in the lamina lucida, below the lamina densa, or both in the lamina lucida and below the lamina densa (53,85). False positive and false negative studies are rare.

Indirect immunofluorescence identifies circulating IgA anti-basement membrane zone antibodies in 10% to 25% of cases (15,51). False positive indirect immunofluorescence studies are rare.

Deposits in Dermal Papillae

Dermatitis Herpetiformis

Dermatitis herpetiformis is a systemic disease characterized by pruritic papulovesicular lesions on the extensor surfaces bilaterally and a gluten-sensitive enteropathy. Histological findings include a subepidermal blister and neutrophils in the tips of the dermal papillae. The histological differential diagnosis includes bullous lupus erythematosus and linear IgA bullous dermatosis. Immunofluorescence studies are helpful in confirming the diagnosis. Therapy may include a gluten-free diet, sulfones, and sulfapyridine.

Direct immunofluorescence of perilesional or nonlesional skin reveals granular deposits of IgA in the dermal papillae (Fig. 8) in 100% of cases (23,47). These deposits may be focal; therefore, multiple levels should be examined (normally do nine). In 70% of cases C3 is found, and IgG, IgM, IgD, and IgE may also be seen. Immunoelectron microscopy demonstrates that the IgA deposits are associated with the microfibrillary bundles of elastic fibers in the papillary dermis (86). False positive and false negative studies are rare.

Indirect immunofluorescence for circulating IgG or IgA antibodies selective for the dermis are negative. Circulating IgA anti-endomysial antibodies have been identified in 70% of cases of dermatitis herpetiformis and in 100% of cases with a gluten-sensitive enteropathy (1). Ciculating IgG and IgA anti-gluten (50) and anti-reticulin (49) antibodies have been identified in 70% to 90% and 50% to 67% of cases, respectively. Circulating immune complexes have been identified in 30% to 40% of cases (31).

The cause of dermatitis herpetiformis is gluten hypersensitivity (52). The mechanism by which gluten is able to provoke the lesions of dermatitis herpetiformis has not been resolved. There appears to be a genetic predisposition to the disease. The ingestion of gluten leads to alterations in the intestine and the production of antibodies specific for gluten. The deposition of immune complexes in the skin and the recruitment of inflammatory cells produce the skin lesions (89).

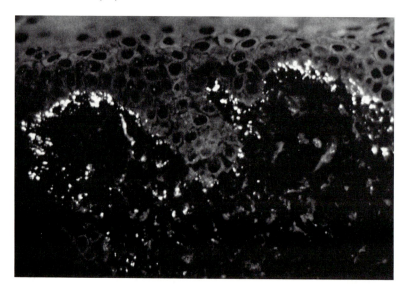

FIG. 8. Granular deposition of IgA in dermal papillae in dermatitis herpetiformis [direct immunofluorescence (IgA), × 100].

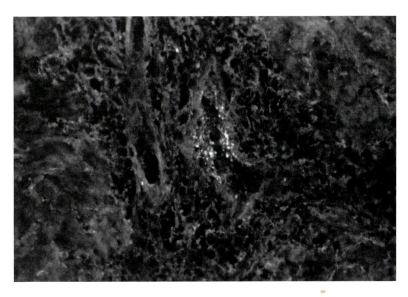

FIG. 9. Granular deposition of C3 in vessels walls in Henoch-Schönlein purpura [direct immunofluorescence (C3), × 100].

Vascular Deposits

Henoch-Schönlein Purpura

Henoch-Schönlein purpura is a systemic disease, characterized by palpable purpuric skin lesions, arthralgia, gastrointestinal and renal bleeding. The histopathology of the skin lesions is that of leukocytoclastic vasculitis, usually involving the superficial and deep blood vessels. The histological differential diagnosis includes leukocytoclastic vasculitis, whether idiopathic or in association with another etiologic entity.

Direct immunofluorescence of perilesional skin shows exclusively or predominantly granular IgA in the vessel walls (4). In addition, C3 may be present (Fig. 9). It is important to look at perilesional or normal skin rather than the lesion itself. The lesional skin shows a mixture of immunoreactants secondary to vascular injury (T.J. Flotte, *unpublished observation*).

Other Forms of Vasculitis

The role of immunofluorescence studies in the evaluation of vasculitis is controversial. There is deposition of IgM and C3 in the vessel walls of most vasculitides early in the course of inflammation. Some believe that these findings are not specific for vasculitis and may be seen in many conditions in which there is vascular injury. Therefore, the immunofluorescent findings do not enter into our differential diagnosis of vasculitis. The one exception to this philosophy is Henoch-Schönlein purpura. The question is not whether this represents a vasculitis, because that distinction is made by H&E sections, but whether the vasculitis is the cutaneous manifestation of Henoch-Schönlein purpura. This diagnosis is made by direct immunofluorescence examination of perilesional skin for IgA deposits.

Henoch-Schönlein purpura is important because of the possible renal complications. There are studies showing deposition of IgA in the skin of patients with renal involvement. Unfortunately, there are not any good prospective studies of the predictive value of skin deposits of IgA for the development with renal disease. Early studies that suggested IgA deposits in cutaneous vessels of normal skin in Berger's disease have not been confirmed (see Chapter 3). Vascular deposition of immunoglobulin has been noted in lesional and clinically normal skin (30% to 95% of biopsies in systemic lupus erythematosus, and 0% to 38% in discoid lupus erythematosus patients) (32).

Inherited Diseases

Epidermolysis Bullosa

Epidermolysis bullosa represents a group of genetic diseases characterized by spontaneous or trauma-induced blister formation which is noninflammatory. The diseases range from mild blisters of the hands and feet to widespread bullae. There are at least 16 different variants. A discussion of these diseases is beyond the scope of this book. One of the important pieces of information that is needed in evaluating such patients is the location of the blister. They are generally grouped into intraepidermal, junctional, and dermal locations. Traditionally, a biopsy is taken for electron microscopical evaluation. Recent understanding of the organization of the basement membrane zone has led to the ability to use antibodies to normal constituents of the basement membrane zone to determine the location of the split by light microscopy. Table 2 illustrates the findings of these various reagents (22,44).

Another approach to epidermolysis bullosa has been to try to identify alterations in the structural components of the skin. Three monoclonal antibodies, KF-1, AF-1, and AF-2, have been described. The antibody, KF-1, reacts with a non-collagenous component of the lamina densa. It is absent in the recessively inherited form of dystrophic epidermolysis bullosa and markedly reduced in the dominantly inherited form of dystrophic epidermolysis bullosa. Antibodies, AF-1 and AF-2, react with anchoring fibrils (21) and do not stain the normal or blistered skin of patients with the recessive form of dystrophic epidermolysis bullosa. The relevant antigens are present in the skin of patients with the dominant form of dystrophic epidermolysis bullosa as well as normal controls (29).

Alport's Syndrome

Several families with Alport's syndrome have been shown to lack an epitope on a basement membrane component, probably type IV collagen. The epitope can be detected by acid urea denaturation, using anti-GBM serum (see Chapter 3).

TABLE 2. *Localization of basement membrane zone antigens in the bullae of epidermolysis bullosa*

Location	Bullous Pemphigoid Antigen	Laminin	Type IV Collagen
Intraepidermal	Floor	Floor	Floor
Junctional	Roof	Floor	Floor
Dermal	Roof	Roof	Roof

Granular Deposits along the Basement Membrane Zone

Lupus Band Test

The lupus band test was first described in 1963 by Burnham et al. (11). In this study, a band of immunoglobulins was localized at the dermal-epidermal junction in skin lesions of patients with both discoid and systemic lupus erythematosus. However, they did not find immunoglobulins in nonlesional skin in a patient with discoid lupus, nor in one patient with systemic lupus erythematosus (11). In 1964, Cormane demonstrated that certain patients with systemic lupus erythematosus had a band of immunoglobulins at the dermal-epidermal junction in visibly normal skin (16). Subsequently, a number of investigators have examined not only the type of band, but also the incidence of a positive band in lesional as well as nonlesional, sun-exposed and sun-protected skin. These studies attempted to determine the sensitivity and specificity of the positive band with regard to the diagnosis of lupus, as well as disease activity and prognosis.

The lupus band test is a direct immunofluorescence test that can be reliably performed on cryostat sections of either fresh frozen tissue or tissue that has been transported in a solution of ammonium sulfate, N-ethylmaleimide, and magnesium sulfate (54,60). The tissue sections are then stained with fluorescein-conjugated antisera monospecific to IgG, IgM, IgA, and C3 and viewed through an immunofluorescence microscope (8).

In either lesional or nonlesional skin, all of the classes of immunoglobulins as well as the early and late complement components—properdin, properdin factor B, and fibrin—have been noted (32,65). A lupus band test is only considered to be positive, however, when there is a bright band of immunoglobulin and/or C3 at the dermal-epidermal junction (Fig. 10). According to some authors, it is necessary for either IgM or IgG to be present, either alone or with other immunoglobulins and complement. Others consider the test to be positive when the band is composed of immunoglobulin or C3 in any combination (32,39).

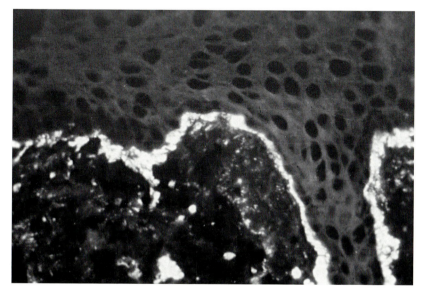

FIG. 10. Granular and homogeneous deposition of IgM at the dermo-epidermal junction in Lupus Erythematosus [direct immunofluorescence (IgM), × 100].

TABLE 3. *Incidence of positive lupus band tests**

Disease	Lesion	Normal Skin	
	%	Sun Exposed	Sun Protected
Lupus Erythematosus			
Discoid	70–90	<5	<5
Systemic	70–90	50–80	50
Subacute cutaneous	60	46	26
Mixed connective tissue disease	78	50	33
Other connective tissue diseases	<5	<5	<5

*Personal communication, J.-C. Bystryn.

The pattern of the band is either homogenous or granular, and it consists of closely spaced fibrils, threads, or stipples (32). It is felt by some authors that the band morphology is dependent on the skin examined (42).

By electron microscopy and immunoelectron microscopy immunoglobulins and complement have been seen as electron dense granular deposits, subjacent to the epidermal basement membrane zone. Small amounts have also been noted in the lamina lucida and basal lamina, as well as in blood vessel walls and along collagen bundles (32).

The lupus band test is most often positive, and thus maximally sensitive, in sun-exposed lesional skin in either discoid or systemic lupus erythematosus and in perilesional skin in bullous systemic lupus erythematosus (61). It is also positive, to a lesser extent, in subacute cutaneous lupus erythematosus and mixed connective tissue disease (32,75). The lupus band test is less sensitive, but more specific in noninvolved sun-exposed or sun-protected skin (32,75) (Table 3). Furthermore, the results vary with the duration of a lesion, treatment, and within the same site (38,39) (Table 4).

False positive reactions occur in less than 1% of the cases and have been reported in rosacea with telangiectasia, porphyria cutanea tarda, vasculitis, polymorphous light erup-

TABLE 4. *Lupus band test reactions at the dermal epidermal junction in lesional skin biopsy specimens of patients with discoid lupus erythematosus**

Cases Examined	% Positive
All forms with typical lesions	84
Sun-exposed lesions	87
Unexposed lesions	35
Duration of lesions	
1 month or less	30
1 to 2 months	80
2 to 6 months	80
6 to 36 months	87
over 6 months	86
Untreated cases	95
Treated with corticosteroids at time of biopsy	35
Edematous lesions	47

*Modified with permission from Jablonska, S., Chorzelski, T.P., and Beutner, E.H. (1979): Indication for skin and serum immunofluorescence in dermatology. In: *Immunopathology of the Skin, 2nd Edition*, edited by E.H. Beutner, T.P. Chorzelski, and S.F. Bean, p. 17, John Wiley and Sons, New York.

tion, drug eruptions, senile keratosis, squamous cell carcinoma, cutaneous infarctions, rheumatoid arthritis, and lichen planus (38,56).

An additional observation made on direct immunofluorescence is speckled nuclear and nucleolar staining. The speckled epidermal nuclear staining recognizes RNase-resistant (Sm) extractable nuclear antigen (ENA) (18,27,73). In 15 patients with mixed connective tissue disease and a high titer, speckled ANA, as well as RNase-sensitive (RNP) ENA that ranged from 1 : 32,000 to > 1 : 500,000 there was speckled epidermal nuclear staining in 100% of the cases whereas the lupus band test on noninvolved volar forearm skin was only positive in 33% of the cases (26). It is presumed that the intracellular staining occurs as a result of cellular disruption during tissue processing. Vascular deposits are common as noted earlier (32).

The incidence of a positive lupus band test is greater in lesional than in nonlesional skin and is also seen more frequently in sun-exposed versus non-sun-exposed. In general, lesional skin tends to have a greater amount of immunoglobulin and complement than nonlesional skin (9,10). In view of these findings it is felt that both local and systemic factors play a role in the development of a positive lupus band.

There are two mechanisms that have been invoked to explain the deposition of immunoglobulin along the basement membrane. First, immunoglobulin and complement are deposited at the basement membrane zone as a preformed circulating immune complex disease composed of various nuclear and perhaps cytoplasmic components (type III injury). The immune complexes, made up of these antigens and their corresponding antibodies, are deposited at the dermal-epidermal junction as a result of their passing across the microvasculature, analogous to what is postulated in the kidney (see Chapters 2 and 3). It is not obvious, however, why such complexes should accumulate in the basement membrane of the epidermis (rather than in the vessels). Indeed, epidermal deposits are not a feature of chronic serum sickness (see Chapter 2). Furthermore, the difference in the incidence of a positive lupus band test in different areas of the body argues against this possibility (65).

Secondly, a positive lupus band test is probably the result of local immune complex formation (type II B injury). Epidermal proliferation and injury, whether induced by sunlight or other factors, leads to the release of DNA and nuclear products, which subsequently diffuse across the basement membrane zone and encounter anti-nuclear antibodies from the systemic circulation. An experiment that has given some credibility to this hypothesis is the finding that normal mice injected with antibodies against denatured DNA develop a positive lupus band test only if subsequently exposed to ultraviolet light (58). Furthermore, higher frequency of a positive lupus band test occurs in areas of the skin with epidermal proliferation (increased DNA synthesis). This hypothesis does not explain the correlation between a positive lupus band test and renal disease (65). Perhaps both are influenced by the magnitude or specificity of the autoantibodies, or the skin may be an important source of nuclear antigens in the circulation.

Although most investigators agree that the lupus band test is useful in the diagnosis of lupus erythematosus, some differ as to its usefulness as a prognostic indicator. In some series IgG, either alone or in combination with other immunoreactants, is seen much more frequently than IgM. In other series the reverse is true (42,79,80). This is important because some investigators have noted that in noninvolved sun-protected skin, a lupus band with IgG, either alone or in combination with other immunoreactants, is associated with more severe disease, while IgM alone or a negative test in noninvolved sun-protected skin correlated with milder disease (2,62,74). Tuffanelli states that patients with large amounts of complement have more active disease, and that there is no relationship between clinical status and the presence of IgG or IgM (80). Authors do agree that the finding of a positive lupus band in noninvolved, sun-protected skin is associated with a worse prognosis, as is an elevated anti-*n*DNA, low complement levels, lymphopenia, and an elevated sedimentation rate (19,30).

Both the presence and the absence of a correlation between the lupus band test and renal disease have been noted (18,25,72,82). Some of the differences may be due to the small number of patients in the studies, inadequate follow-up, and the lack of histopathology. Gilliam and Dantzig and their colleagues noted that a lupus band, principally composed of IgG and IgM, was associated with severe renal disease in 81% to 83% of the cases and mild renal disease in 18% to 23% of the cases. Furthermore, although the incidence of renal disease is less if the lupus band test is negative in noninvolved, sun-protected skin, at least one group has found an incidence as high as 39% (25).

In addition to the controversy over the presence and type of immunoreactants in a lupus band test in noninvolved, sun-protected skin and its correlation to renal disease, some (25), but not all authors (66) found that a positive lupus band test in a noninvolved, sun-protected area is associated with more severe forms of renal disease (diffuse proliferative and membranous glomerulonephritis), whereas a negative lupus band test is associated with more mild renal disease (focal proliferative glomerulonephritis or normal histopathology).

With the advent of serologic tests for *n*DNA, Sm, RNP, Ro and La, as well as the ANA, complement, sedimentation rate, and lymphocyte count, it appears that the lupus band test is still useful in the diagnosis of lupus, but is, in the opinion of many, less useful in the prognostication of this disease. Instead, because none of these tests are completely specific, confirmation of the diagnosis and some insight into the prognosis are best achieved when a panel of laboratory tests is performed, including the lupus band test. For example, in one study where the lupus band test was evaluated with *n*DNA and Sm, it was found that at least one of these tests could be abnormal in patients with a connective tissue disease other than systemic lupus erythematosus, but that in 80% of patients with systemic lupus erythematosus, at least two of the tests were positive (55).

REFERENCES

1. Accetta, P., Kumar, V., Beutner, E. H., Chorzelski, T. P., and Helm. F. (1986): Anti-endomysial antibodies. A serologic marker of dermatitis herpetiformis. *Arch. Dermatol.*, 122:459–462.
2. Ahmed, A. R., and Provost, T. T. (1979): Incidence of a positive lupus band test using sun-exposed and un-exposed skin. *Arch. Dermatol.*, 115:228–229.
3. Anhalt, G. J., Labib, R. S., Voorhees, J. J., Beals, T. F., and Diaz, L. A. (1982): Induction of pemphigus in neonatal mice by passive transfer of IgG from patients with the disease. *N. Engl. J. Med.*, 306:1189–1196.
4. Baart de la Faille-Kuyper, E. H., Kater, L., Kooiker, C. J., and Dorhout Mees, E. J. (1973): IgA deposits in cutaneous blood vessel walls and mesangium in Henoch-Schönlein syndrome. *Lancet*, 1:892-893.
5. Bean, S. F. (1974): Cicatricial pemphigoid: Immunofluorescent studies. *Arch. Dermatol.*, 110:552–555.
6. Beutner, E. H., and Jordon, R. E. (1964): Demonstration of skin antibodies in sera of pemphigus vulgaris patients by indirect immunofluorescent staining. *Proc. Soc. Exp. Biol. Med.*, 117:505–510.
7. Beutner, E. H., Jordon, R. E., and Chorzelski, T. P. (1968): The immunopathology of pemphigus and bullous pemphigoid. *J. Invest. Dermatol.*, 51:63–80.
8. Beutner, E. H., Nisengard, R. J., and Kumar, V. (1979): Defined immunofluorescence: Basic concepts and their application to clinical immunodermatology. In: *Immunopathology of the Skin*, 2nd Edition, edited by E. H. Beutner, T. P. Chorzelski, and S. F. Bean, pp. 31–35. John Wiley and Sons, New York.
9. Burnham, T. K., and Fine, G. (1973): The immunofluorescent "band" test for lupus erythematosus III. Employing clinically normal skin. *Arch. Dermatol.*, 102:24–32.
10. Burnham, T. K., Fine, G., and Neblett, T. R. (1970): Immunofluorescent "band" test for lupus erythematosus II. Employing skin lesions. *Arch. Dermatol.*, 102:42–50.

11. Burnham, T. K., Neblett, T. R., and Fine, G. (1963): The application of fluorescent antibody technique to the investigation of lupus erythematosus and various dermatoses. *J. Invest. Dermatol.*, 41:541–456.
12. Bystryn, J. -C., Abel, E., and DeFeo, C. (1974): Pemphigus foliaceus: Subcorneal intercellular antibody of unique specificity. *Arch. Dermatol.*, 110:857–861.
13. Bystryn, J. -C., and Rodriguez, J. (1978): Absence of intercellular antigens in the deep layers of the epidermis in pemphigus foliaceus. *J. Clin. Invest.*, 61:339–348.
14. Chorzelski, T. P., Beutner, E. H., and Jarzabek, M. (1970): Passive transfer of pemphigus in experimental animals. *Int. Arch. Allergy*, 39:106.
15. Chorzelski, T. P., and Jablonska, S. (1979): IgA linear dermatosis of childhood (chronic bullous disease of childhood). *Br. J. Dermatol.*, 101:535–542.
16. Corman, R. H. (1964): "Bound" globulin in the skin of patients with chronic discoid lupus erythematosus and systemic lupus erythematosus. *Lancet*, 1:534–535.
17. Dahl, M. V. (1983): Usefulness of direct immunofluorescence in patients with lupus erythematosus. *Arch. Dermatol.*, 119:1010–1017.
18. Danzig, P. I., Mauro, J., Rayhanzadeh, S., and Rudofsky, U. (1975): The significance of a positive cutaneous immunofluorescence test in systemic lupus erythematosus. *Br. J. Dermatol.*, 92:531–537.
19. Davis, B. M., and Gillam, J. (1984): Prognostic significance of subepidermal immune deposits on uninvolved skin of patients with SLE: A 10-year longitudinal study. *J. Invest. Dermatol.*, 83:242–247.
20. Farb, R. M., Dykes, R., and Lazarus, G. S. (1978): Anti-epidermal-cell-surface pemphigus antibody detaches viable epidermal cells from culture plates by activation of proteinase. *Proc. Natl. Acad. Sci. USA*, 75:459–463.
21. Fine, J. -D., Breathnach, S. M., and Katz, S. I. (1984): KF-1 monoclonal antibody defines a specific basement membrane antigenic defect in dystrophic forms of epidermolysis bullosa. *J. Invest. Dermatol.*, 82:35–38.
22. Fine, J. -D., and Gay, S. (1986): LDA-1 monoclonal antibody. *Arch. Dermatol.*, 122:48–51.
23. Fry, L, and Seah, P. P. (1974): Dermatitis herpetiformis: An evaluation of diagnostic criteria. *Br. J. Dermatol.*, 90:137–146.
24. Gammon, W. R., Briggaman, R. A., Inman, M. S., Queen, L. L., and Wheeler, C. E. (1984): Differentiating anti-lamina lucida and anti-sublamina densa anti-BMZ antibodies by indirect immunofluorescence on 1.0 M sodium chloride-separated skin. *J. Invest. Dermatol.*, 82:139–144.
25. Gilliam, J. N., Cheatum, D. E., Hurd, E. R., Stastory, P., and Ziff, M. (1974): Immunoglobulin in clinically uninvolved skin in systemic lupus erythematosus associated with renal disease. *J. Clin. Invest.*, 53:1434–1440.
26. Gilliam, J. N., and Prystowsky, S. D. (1977): Mixed connective tissue disease syndrome: Cutaneous manifestations of patients with epidermal nuclear staining and high titre serum antibody to ribonuclease-sensitive extractable nuclear antigen. *Arch. Dermatol.*, 113:583–587.
27. Gilliam, J. N., Smiley, J. D., and Ziff, M. (1974): Correlation between serum antibody to extractable nuclear antigen and immunoglobulin localization in epidermal nuclei. *Clin. Res.*, 22:611, (A).
28. Gilliam, J. N., Smiley, J. D., and Ziff, M. (1975): Association of mixed connective tissue disease (MCTD) with immunoglobulin localization in epidermal nuclei of biopsies from areas of normal skin. *Clin. Res.*, 23:229, (A).
29. Goldsmith, L. A., and Briggaman, R. A. (1983): Monoclonal antibodies to anchoring fibrils for the diagnosis of epidermolysis bullosa. *J. Invest. Dermatol.*, 81:464–466.
30. Halberg, P., Ullman, S., and Jorgensen, F. (1982): The lupus band test as a measure of disease activity in systemic lupus erythematosus. *Arch. Dermatol.*, 118:572–576.
31. Hall, R. P., Lawley, T. J., Heck, J. A., and Katz, S. I. (1980): IgA containing circulating immune complexes in dermatitis herpetiformis, Henoch-Schönlein purpura, systemic lupus erythematosus and other diseases. *Clin. Exp. Immunol.*, 40:431–437.
32. Harrist, T. J., and Mihm, M. C., Jr. (1980): The specificity and clinical usefulness of the lupus band test. *Arthritis Rheum.*, 23:479–490.
33. Hashimoto, K., Shafran, K. M., Webber, P. S., Lazarus, G. S., and Singer, K. H. (1983): Anti-cell surface pemphigus antibody stimulates plasminogen activator activity. *J. Exp. Med.*, 157:259–272.
34. Hietanen, J., Rantala, I., and Reunala, T. (1985): Benign mucous membrane pemphigoid with linear IgA deposits in oral mucosa. *Scand. J. Dent. Res.*, 93:46–51.
35. Holmes, R. C., and Black, M. M. (1983): Herpes gestationis. *Dermatol. Clin.*, 1:195.
36. Huff, J. C., Golitz, L. E., and Kunke, K. S. (1985): Intraepidermal neutrophilic IgA dermatosis. *N. Engl. J. Med.*, 313:1643–1645.
37. Jablonska, S., Chorzelski, T. P., Blaszczyk, M., and Maciejewski, W. (1977): Pathogenesis of pemphigus erythematosus. *Arch. Dermatol. Res.*, 258:135–140.
38. Jablonska, S., Chorzelski, T. P., and Beutner, E. H. (1979): Indication for skin and serum immunofluorescence in dermatology. In: *Immunopathology of the Skin*, 2nd Edition, edited by E. H. Beutner, T. P. Chorzelski, and S. F. Bean, p. 17. John Wiley and Sons, New York.

39. Jacobs, M. I., Schned, E. J., and Bystryn, J. -C. (1983): Variability of the lupus band test. *Arch. Dermatol.*, 119:883–889.

40. Jones, J. C., Yokoo, K. M., and Goldman, R. D. (1986): Further analysis of pemphigus autoantibodies and their use in studies on the heterogeneity, structure, and function of desmosomes. *J. Cell Biol.*, 102:1109–1117.

41. Jordon, R. E. (1976): Complement activation in pemphigus and bullous pemphigoid. *J. Invest. Dermatol.*, 67:366–371.

42. Jordon, R. E., Schroeter, A. L., and Winkelman, R. K. (1975): Dermal-epidermal deposition of complement components and properdin in systemic lupus erythematosus. *Br. J. Dermatol.*, 92:263–271.

43. Jordon, R. E., Triftshauser, C. T., and Schroeter, A. L. (1971): Direct immunofluorescent studies of pemphigus and bullous pemphigoid. *Arch. Dermatol.*, 103:486–491.

44. Katz, S. I. (1984): The epidermal basement membrane zone—structure, ontogeny, and role in disease. *J. Am. Acad. Dermatol.*, 11:1025–1037.

45. Katz, S. I., Halprin, K. M., and Inderbitzin, T. M. (1969): The use of human skin for the detection of antiepithelial autoantibodies. *J. Invest. Dermatol.*, 53:390–399.

46. Katz, S. I., Hertz, K. C., and Yaoita, H. (1976): Herpes gestationis: Unopathology and characterization of the HG factor. *J. Clin. Invest.*, 57:1434–1446.

47. Katz, S. I., and Strober, W. (1978): The pathogenesis of dermatitis herpetiformis. *J. Invest. Dermatol.*, 70:63–75.

48. Kawana, S., Geoghegan, W. D., and Jordon, R. E. (1985): Compliment fixation of pemphigus antibody. II. Complement enhanced detachment of epidermal cells. *Clin. Exp. Immunol.*, 61:517–525.

49. Lancaster-Smith, M., Kumar, P., Clark, M. L., Marks, R., and Johnson, G. D. (1975): Antireticulin antibodies in dermatitis herpetiformis and coeliac disease. *Br. J. Dermatol.*, 92:37–42.

50. Lane, A. T., Huff, J. C., Zone, J. J., and Weston, W. L. (1983): Class specific antigluten antibodies in dermatitis herpetiformis. *J. Invest. Dermatol.*, 80:402–405.

51. Leonard, J. N., Haffenden, G. P., Ring, N. P., McMinn, R. M. H., Sidgwick, A., Mowbray, J. F., Unsworth, D. J., Holborow, E. J., Blenkinsopp, W. K., Swain, A. F., and Fry, L. (1982): Linear IgA disease in adults. *Br. J. Dermatol.*, 107:301–316.

52. Leonard, J., Haffenden, G., Tucker, W., Unsworth, J., Swain, F., McMinn, R., Holborow, J., and Fry, L. (1983): Gluten challenge in dermatitis herpetiformis. *N. Engl. J. Med.*, 308:816–819.

53. Leonard, J. N., Ring, N., Haffenden, G. P., and Fry, L. (1982): Ultrastructural localization of IgA deposits in adult linear IgA disease. *J. R. Soc. Med.*, 75:237–241.

54. Michel, B., Milner, Y., and David, K. (1973): Preservation of tissue-fixed immunoglobulins in skin biopsies of patients with lupus erythematosus and bullous diseases—preliminary report. *J. Invest. Dermatol.*, 59:449–452.

55. Moses, S., and Barland, P. (1979): Laboratory criteria for a diagnosis of systemic lupus erythematosus. *J.A.M.A.*, 242:1039–1043.

56. Muijs van de Moer, W. W., and Cats, A. (1967): Immunofluorescence of the skin in patients with rheumatoid arthritis. *Dermatologica*, 134:351–355.

57. Naito, K., Morioka, S., Ikeda, S., and Ogawa, H. (1984): Experimental bullous pemphigoid in guinea pigs: The role of pemphigoid antibodies, complement, migrating cells. *J. Invest. Dermatol.*, 82:227–230.

58. Natali, P. B., and Tan, E. M. (1973): Experimental skin lesions in mice resembling systemic lupus erythematosus. *Arthritis Rheum.*, 16:579–589.

59. Nieboer, C., Boorsma, D. M., and Woerdeman, M. J. (1982): Immunoelectron microscopic findings in cicatricial pemphigoid: Their significance in relation to epidermolysis bullosa acquisita. *Br. J. Dermatol.*, 106:419–422.

60. Nisengar, R. J., Blaszczyk, M., Chorzelski, T., and Beutner, E. (1978): Immunofluorescence of biopsy specimens: Comparison of methods of transportation. *Arch. Dermatol.*, 114:1329–1332.

61. Olansky, A. J., Briggaman, R. A., Gammon, W. R., Kelly, T. F., and Sams, W. M., Jr. (1982): Bullous systemic lupus erythematosus. *J. Am. Acad. Dermatol.*, 7:511–520.

62. Pennebaker, J. B., Gilliam, J. N., and Ziff, M. (1977): Immunoglobulin classes of DNA binding activity in serum and skin in systemic lupus erythematosus. *J. Clin. Invest.*, 60:1331–1338.

63. Person, J. R., Rogers, R. S., and Perry, H. O. (1976): Localized pemphigoid. *Br. J. Dermatol.*, 95:531–534.

64. Peterson, L. L., and Wuepper, K. D. (1984): Isolation and purification of the pemphigus vulgaris antigen from human epidermis. *J. Clin. Invest.*, 73:1113–1120.

65. Provost, T. T. (1979): Lupus Band Test. In: *Immunopathology of the Skin*, 2nd Edition, edited by E. H. Beutner, T. P. Chorzelski, and S. F. Bean, p. 401. John Wiley and Sons, New York.

66. Provost, T. T. (1979): Lupus Band Test. In: *Immunopathology of the Skin*, 2nd Edition, edited by E. H. Beutner, T. P. Chorzelski, and S. F. Bean, p. 404. John Wiley and Sons, New York.

67. Provost, T. T., and Tomasi, T. B. (1974): Immunopathology of bullous pemphigoid. *Clin. Exp. Immunol.*, 18:193–200.

68. Prystowsky, S. D., Gilliam, J. N., and Tuffanelli, D. L. (1978): Epidermal nucleolar IgG deposition in clinically normal skin. *Arch. Dermatol.*, 114:536–538.

69. Sams, W. M., and Jordon, R. E. (1971): Correlation of pemphigoid and pemphigus antibody titers with activity of disease. *Br. J. Dermatol.*, 84:7–13.
70. Schaumburg-Lever, G., Rule, A., Schmidt-Ullrich, B., and Lever, W. F. (1975): Ultrastructural localization of *in vivo* bound immunoglobulins in bullous pemphigoid. *J. Invest. Dermatol.*, 64:47–49.
71. Schiltz, J. R., and Michel, B. (1976): Production of epidermal acantholysis in normal human skin in vitro by the IgG fraction from pemphigus serum. *J. Invest. Dermatol.*, 67:254–260.
72. Schrager, M. A., and Rothfield, N. F. (1976): Clinical significance of serum properdin levels and properdin deposition in the dermal-epidermal junction in systemic lupus erythematosus. *J. Clin. Invest.*, 57:212–221.
73. Shu, S., and Beutner, E. (1976): Studies on apparent reactivity of ANA with viable cells. *Fed. Proc.*, 35:512, (A).
74. Sontheimer, R. D., and Gilliam, J. N. (1979): A reappraisal of the relationship between subepidermal immunoglobulin deposits and DNA antibodies in systemic lupus erythematosus: A study using Crithida luciliae immunofluorescence anti-DNA assay. *J. Invest. Dermatol.*, 72:29–32.
75. Sontheimer, R. D., Thomas, J. R., and Gilliam, J. N. (1979): Subacute cutaneous lupus erythematosus: A cutaneous marker for a distinct lupus erythematosus subset. *Arch. Dermatol.*, 115:1409–1415.
76. Stanley, J. R., Hawley-Nelson, P., Yuspa, S. H., Shevach, E. M., and Katz, S. I. (1981): Characterization of bullous pemphigoid antigen—a unique basement membrane protein of stratified squamous epithelia. *Cell*, 24:897–904.
77. Stanley, J. R., Koulu, L., Klaus-Kovtun, V., and Steinberg, M. S. (1986): A monoclonal antibody to the desmosomal glycoprotein desmoglein 1 binds the same polypeptide as human autoantibodies in pemphigus foliaceus. *J. Immunol.*, 136:1227–1230.
78. Stanley, J. R., Koulu, L., and Thivolet, C. (1984): Distinction between epidermal antigens binding pemphigus vulgaris and pemphigus foliaceus autoantibodies. *J. Clin. Invest.*, 74:313–320.
79. Ten Have-Opbroek, A. A. W (1966): Demonstration of immunoglobulins and complement in the skin of patients with lupus erythematosus. *Acta Dermatol. Venereol.*, 46:68–71.
80. Tuffanelli, D. L. (1978): Clinical cutaneous immunopathology. *J. Clin. Exp. Dermatol.*, 16:19–39.
81. Tuffanelli, D. L. (1971): Cutaneous immunopathology: Recent observations. *J. Invest. Dermatol.*, 65:143–153.
82. Wertheimer, D., and Barland, P. (1976): Clinical significance of immune deposits in the skin in SLE. *Arthritis Rheum*, 19:1249–1255.
83. Westgate, G. E., Weaver, A. C., and Couchman, J. R. (1985): Bullous pemphigoid antigen localization suggests an intracellular association with hemidesmosomes. *J. Invest. Dermatol.*, 84:218–224.
84. Woodley, D. T., Briggaman, R. A., O'Keefe, E. J., Inman, A. O., Queen, L. L., and Gammon, W. R. (1984): Identification of the skin basement-membrane autoantigen in epidermolysis bullosa acquisita. *N. Engl. J. Med.*, 310:1007–1013.
85. Yamasaki, Y., Hashimoto, T., and Nishikawa, T. (1982): Dermatitis herpetiformis with linear IgA deposition: Ultrastructural localization of *in vivo* bound IgA. *Acta Dermatovener*, 62:401–405.
86. Yaoita, H. (1978): Identification of IgA binding structures in skin of patients with dermatitis herpetiformis. *J. Invest. Dermatol.*, 71:213–216.
87. Yaoita, H., Briggaman, R. H., Lawley, T. J., Provost, T. T., and Katz, S. I. (1981): Epidermolysis bullosa acquisita: Ultrastructural and immunological studies. *J. Invest. Dermatol.*, 76:288–292.
88. Yaoita, H., Gullino, M., and Katz, S. I. (1976): Herpes gestationis. Ultrastructure and ultrastructural localization of *in vivo*-bound complement. *J. Invest. Dermatol.*, 66:383–388.
89. Zone, J. J., and Petersen, M. J. (1986): Dermatitis herpetiformis. In: *Pathogenesis of Skin Disease*, edited by B. H. Thiers and R. L. Dobson, pp. 159–183. Churchill Livingstone, New York.

Diagnostic Immunopathology,
edited by R.B. Colvin,
A.K. Bhan, and R.T. McCluskey.
Raven Press, New York © 1988.

5 / *Autoantibodies*

C. Lynne Burek and Noel R. Rose

The Johns Hopkins University School of Hygiene and Public Health, Department of Immunology and Infectious Diseases, Baltimore, Maryland 21205

Humans frequently develop autoantibodies, although the pathologic significance of these antibodies in many cases is uncertain. Consequently, the demonstration of autoantibodies is not necessarily synonymous with autoimmune disease. In the normal human population, autoantibody formation appears to be related to age and sex, the highest prevalence being in older females and the lowest in younger males.

The term *autoimmune disease* is properly reserved for those conditions in which the autoimmune process contributes significantly to the pathogenesis of the disease. Criteria for the designation of a human autoimmune disease were proposed by Witebsky et al. in 1957 (114). They include the demonstration of relevant antibodies or of cell-mediated immunity operating under physiologic conditions. The responsible antigen should be defined, isolated, and used to induce an immunologic response in experimental animals. Pathologic changes similar to those seen in human disease should appear in the corresponding tissue of the immunized animal.

There is considerable controversy over the role of autoantibodies in the particular diseases in which they are found. Antibodies clearly have been shown to be responsible for disease in only a few systems. These instances include autoantibodies that are directed to the erythrocyte surface (autoimmune hemolytic anemia), to thyroid stimulating hormone (TSH) receptors (Graves' disease), to acetylcholine receptors of the neuromuscular junctions (myasthenia gravis), to the glomerular basement membrane (see Chapter 3) and to the epidermis (see Chapter 4). Even in these cases, the stimuli are largely unknown and continue to be investigated.

Autoantibodies can also arise after an initial infection or other tissue injury, as in postinfarction syndrome or postinfectious encephalomyelitis. In these situations, demonstration of autoantibodies may be valuable in recognizing and distinguishing an autoimmune state from the initial injury. The empirical association between an autoantibody and a particular disease may provide a clinically useful diagnostic tool, even in the absence of a cause-and-effect relationship. An example is the demonstration of cardiolipin antibody as a serological test for syphilis. This is still a valuable first step in identifying disease due to *Treponema pallidum* infection. In another example, the presence of cold hemagglutinins is useful for the diagnosis of *Mycoplasma pneumoniae*.

Human diseases associated with autoantibody production range from strictly organ-specific conditions to more generalized disorders. There is a tendency for more than one autoimmune disorder to occur in the same individual. The overlaps are generally within the same category of disease, as seen in patients with multiple endocrine disorders (such as thyroiditis and adrenalitis) or multiple "connective tissue" diseases (such as Sjögren's keratoconjunctivitis sicca and lupus). In addition, there is a significantly higher incidence of autoantibodies to unrelated organ-specific antigens in patients with an autoimmune disease. For example, one-quarter of patients with thyroiditis have antibodies to gastric parietal cells, while almost half of patients with pernicious anemia have antibodies to a thyroid antigen. Antibodies to thyroid antigens occur in 25% of patients with Addison's disease (adrenal insufficiency) and in 20% of patients with diabetes mellitus, suggesting that a shared autoimmune factor is involved in those diseases. The aggregation of auto-immune responses to immunologically distinct organ-specific antigens cannot be explained except as a genetic predisposition to the development of autoimmune responses.

This chapter will highlight the most frequently detected autoantibodies, review their methods of measurement, and discuss their interpretation. The field is changing with the use of more sensitive detection methods, coupled with the increasing availability of puri-fied antigens.

METHODS

The method for demonstrating autoantibodies is dictated by the position and properties of the antigen and the level of sensitivity desired. Historically, agglutination and precipita-tion were the first methods employed for demonstrating autoantibodies in human sera. Agglutination tests use stable suspensions of beads or cells, especially erythrocytes, either uncoated or coated with appropriate soluble antigens. The direct Coombs antiglobulin test for immunoglobulin on the surface of red blood cells is the cornerstone of the diagnosis of autoimmune hemolytic anemia. Indirect hemagglutination is frequently used for detection of thyroid autoantibodies. Soluble antigens can also be used in latex fixation tests. Latex agglutination is still the most widely used test for the measurement of rheumatoid factor. Although less sensitive than agglutination, precipitation in fluid or gels is still useful for the demonstration of antibodies to soluble antigens. Immunodiffusion is often employed for detection of certain nuclear antibodies.

The most commonly used test for detection of antibodies directed against tissue antigens is indirect immunofluorescence (IIF) (see Chapter 16). A screening test based on IIF is useful for the discovery of unanticipated antibodies that may prove to be a significant correlate of disease. Therefore, IIF is valuable in testing for autoantibodies for which the antigen has not yet been characterized. The only necessity is a tissue substrate, containing the particular antigen in its immunochemically reactive state. Having broad applications, IIF can be utilized under conditions where more than one type of antibody may be present, such as with antinuclear antibodies (ANA). If tests using only purified nuclear antigens are employed, reactions with minor nuclear antigens may be missed. Indirect immunoperoxi-dase is similar to IIF in concept, but uses an enzyme, such as horseradish peroxidase, rather than a fluorescent marker (see Chapter 17).

Radioimmunoassay (RIA) has long been used to detect autoantibodies at very low levels. These assays are limited by a requirement for defined antigens and the use of radioiso-topes. There is a trend to replace radiolabeled compounds with enzyme-labeled substances. Therefore, many of the former RIAs have been converted to enzyme immunoassays (EIA), such as the enzyme-linked immunosorbent assay (ELISA). When antigens have been identified and partially purified, such as some of the nuclear antigens, they are readily incorporated into EIA technology.

Another test system that has recently been introduced for clinical diagnosis is the Western immunoblot. It does not require that the antigen be pure, but is relatively slow and expensive.

For many of the immunoassays, commercial packages or "kits" are available. They may be purchased as complete systems or as component parts. While many of the products are excellent, there is frequently considerable variation in performance between kits of different manufacturers, even when testing for the same antibody. Some of these differences may be due to variations in substrate. Problems can still occur with kits because of poor product quality control or operator errors.

CLASSIFICATION OF AUTOANTIBODIES

Autoantibodies can be classified into two broad categories. One group is characterized by reactivity to generally distributed nuclear or cytoplasmic constituents, not demonstrating any tissue or organ specificity. Examples of these include antinuclear antibody (ANA), rheumatoid factor (RF) and antimitochondrial antibody. These are called non-organ-specific autoantibodies. The other group of autoantibodies demonstrates tissue restriction. Among these are the autoantibodies to endocrine organs, muscle, gastric parietal cells, and certain cell surface receptors. These are considered as organ-specific autoantibodies.

NON-ORGAN-SPECIFIC AUTOANTIBODIES

Screening Assay for Antibodies to Nuclear Antigens

The development of autoantibodies to nuclear antigens is an important feature of many systemic rheumatic or connective tissue diseases and may also reflect a heightened immunological reactivity in other autoimmune disorders. Therefore, detection of circulating autoantibody to components of cell nuclei is an important first step for investigation and diagnosis of the disorders. Although several tests are available for the determination of autoantibodies to individual nuclear antigens, IIF is the most widely used screening assay. In conjunction with several special substrates, IIF provides information on antibody specificity without the necessity for more elaborate tests. The reading of IIF is subjective, however, and semiquantitative at best.

There are now at least 21 reported specificities of ANA, as presented in Table 1. With the advent of improved techniques for isolation of macromolecules, certain of the antigens have been isolated and characterized by biochemical and immunologic procedures. The isolated antigens have then been incorporated into RIAs or EIAs to aid in the diagnosis of specific systemic disorders. Many of the reactions are of minor clinical value and are as yet only research tools. The assignment of antigen must be considered putative. For example, some anti-DNA antibodies cross-react with cardiolipin and lymphocyte surfaces.

The autoantibodies to nuclear constituents are not organ or species restricted, so that frozen sections of any nucleated animal tissue may theoretically be used as substrate. The most important variables involved in producing a standardized technique are (a) type of substrate, including source, storage, and preparation; (b) duration of staining and washing;

TABLE 1. *Antigenic reactivity of ANA*[a]*

Antibody	Disease in which antibodies seen	Characteristic of antigenic determinants	Pattern observed by direct immunofluorescent test	Other tests used to detect specific antibody
Antibody to DNA				
1. Reacts only with double-stranded DNA	Characteristic of SLE; few cases reported	Double-strandedness of DNA essential	Rim, homogeneous, or both	RIA, ID, CIE, HA, CF, EIA, and special IF
2. Reacts with both double- and single-stranded DNA[b]	High levels in SLE; lower levels in other rheumatic diseases	Related to deoxyribose, purines, and pyrimidines, but not dependent on double helix	Same as no. 1	Same as no. 1
3. Reacts only with single-stranded DNA	Rheumatic, nonrheumatic diseases	Related to purines and pyrimidines, with ribose and deoxyribose equally reactive	Not detected on routine screen; special treatment necessary	RIA, ID, CIE, HA, EIA, and CF
Deoxynucleoprotein, soluble form	LE cell antibody in SLE, drug-induced LE	DNA-histone complex; dissociated components are nonreactive	Rim, homogeneous, or both	RIA, ID, EIA, latex, HA, bentonite, and LE cell
Histone (H1, H2A, H2B, H3, H4)	SLE, drug-induced SLE, RA	Different classes of histones may have different determinants	Homogeneous, rim, or both	CF, special IF test, RIA, EIA
Histone (H3)	Undifferentiated connective-tissue disease	H3	Variable large speckles[c]	RIA, EIA
Smith[b] (Sm)	Highly diagnostic of SLE	Small nuclear RNP (U2-U4 RNP)	Speckled	ID, CIE, HA, EIA, and CF
Nuclear RNP[b] (Mo)	High levels in mixed connective-tissue disease and SLE; lower levels in other rheumatic diseases	RNA-protein complex (U1 RNP)	Speckled	ID, CIE, HA, EIA, and CF
Cytoplasmic RNP (Mu)	SLE	Ribosomal fraction	Nucleolar, cytoplasm	ID
Scl-70	Highly diagnostic of scleroderma	DNA Topoisomerase I	Atypical speckled	ID
Centromere[b] (kinetochore)	CREST variant scleroderma, less frequently in Raynaud's phenomenon and other rheumatic diseases	Protein	Discrete speckled[d]	None
SS-A (Ro)[b]	High prevalence in Sjögren's syndrome sicca complex, subacute cutaneous lupus and	Protein (?RNA complex)	Negative	ID, EIA, CIE using spleen, human thymus, or WiI$_2$ extracts

Antigen	Disease association	Nature of antigen	Immunofluorescence pattern	Test
SS-B (La, Ha)[b]	High prevalence in Sjögren's syndrome sicca complex; neonatal lupus syndrome, and SLE; lower prevalence in other rheumatic diseases	Protein (?RNA complex)	Speckled	ID, EIA, CIE
Ma	SLE	Chemical nature unknown	?	ID
RANA	Present in RA and Sjögren's syndrome with RA	Epstein-Barr virus-related protein	Negative	ID, using Wil$_2$ or Raji cell extracts
SL	SLE/Sjögren's syndrome overlap	?	? Speckled	ID
PM-1 (PM/Scl)	Myositis/scleroderma overlap	Chemical nature unknown	Variable, speckled	ID
Jo-1	Polymyositis	Histidyl tRNA synthetase	?[d] Cytoplasmic	
Mi-1	Dermatomyositis	?	?	
Ku	Polymyositis	?	?	
PCNA (Ga, LE-4)	SLE	33-kDa protein (?cyclin)	Variable-sized speckles in some cells[d]	ID
NSpl, NSpII	Various rheumatic diseases, Sjögren's syndrome	Protein	Speckled[d]	None
Nucleolar	High prevalence in progressive systemic sclerosis; SLE	4–6S RNA, other nucleolar RNA, and RNP	Nucleolar	
Nuclear matrix	SLE, undifferentiated connective-tissue disease	HnRNA + matrix protein	Large speckles[d]	None

[a]CF, complement fixation; CIE, counterimmunoelectrophoresis in agar gel; EIA, enzyme-linked immunoassay; HA, passive hemagglutination; HnRNA, heterogeneous nuclear RNA; ID, agar gel double immunodiffusion; IF, immunofluorescence; kDa, kilodalton; LE, lupus erythematosus; PM, polymyositis; RA, rheumatoid arthritis; RANA, rheumatoid arthritis nuclear antigen; RIA, radioimmunoassay; Scl, scleroderma.

[b]Prototype sera available from Centers for Disease Control, Atlanta, Georgia.

[c]On acetone-fixed mouse kidney substrate.

[d]On HEp-2 and other cell culture substrates.

*Reprinted with slight modification from M.J. Fritzler (35).

and (c) specificity and sensitivity of the conjugate. An essential part of each test is the incorporation of known positive and negative reactive sera as controls.

The most readily available substrate tissue for IIF antinuclear antibody tests is liver from young mice or rats. The animal is exsanguinated and the liver immediately removed, divided into cubes about 5 mm thick and quickly frozen, using dry ice or liquid nitrogen. These tissue blocks can be used for long periods of time (either unmounted or mounted), if they are stored at −70°C and sealed well to prevent drying. Tissue blocks are cut 4 microns thick with a cryostat, placed on a clean slide, and air dried fixation. Other fixation procedures may denature and lower the reactivity of certain antigens. Some of the antigens (e.g., Sm or RNP, see below) are soluble in buffer. Fixation for 10 minutes in acetone at room temperature (35) improves the preservation of these antigens. Because of their large nucleus, HEp-2 cells are a frequent substrate for the IIF assay. This substrate is discussed further in the section on special substrates.

Rabbit or goat antibodies, prepared by immunization with human globulin or with individual classes of immunoglobulins (e.g., heavy chains) conjugated to fluorescein isothiocyanate (FITC), are used to locate the site of the reaction between the tissue substrate and antibody from the patient's serum. The conjugated antibodies should be characterized for sensitivity and specificity (see Chapter 16).

Plasma is unsuitable for use in IIF, because the fibrinogen causes considerable nonspecific fluorescence of tissue substrate; therefore, only serum should be tested. Since concentrated serum will also cause nonspecific staining and result in unclear results, an initial serum dilution of 1 : 10 or greater is recommended, depending upon the sensitivity of the assay. Screening of patient sera is conducted routinely at 2 or more dilutions. Positive sera may be retested using serial dilutions until an endpoint is reached. Until standard sera are generally available, each laboratory will have to establish its own set of standards with regard to quantitation. On a limited basis, sera for standardization can be obtained through the Centers for Disease Control, Atlanta, Georgia or through the College of American Pathologists, Skokie, Illinois.

Each assay run should include controls for autofluorescence of tissue and conjugate specificity, as well as known positive and negative sera for each recognized pattern (described below). FITC conjugate combined with an optional counterstain of rhodamine B-BSA (Rh B-BSA) will provide good contrast to the FITC conjugate. Twenty μl reconstituted Rh B-BSA is added per ml of the appropriate dilution of FITC-conjugated antiserum. Another counterstain frequently used is Evans blue.

Commonly Identified Patterns

Different patterns of nuclear staining (or combinations thereof) may be encountered. The most frequent patterns are homogeneous, speckled, peripheral, and nucleolar; the pattern depends on the constituent(s) of the nucleus to which the antibody is directed.

Homogeneous Pattern

In the homogeneous pattern (Fig. 1A), the entire nucleus is stained uniformly, except that in some cases a small round dark spot appears, representing the nucleolus. Antibodies producing the homogeneous pattern are directed primarily against nuclear histone but sometimes to a histone-DNA complex.

Speckled Pattern

Speckled staining (Fig. 1B) may have a variable appearance ranging from small bright dots to fluorescent threads and variably sized clumps in irregular arrangement. The antibodies associated with speckled staining are those directed against various nuclear proteins and are impossible to distinguish using this assay. Assays for autoantibodies to particular nuclear antigens are described below.

Peripheral Pattern

In the peripheral pattern (Fig. 1C), the staining appears as a bright fluorescent rim surrounding the dark, unstained center of the nucleus. Antibodies producing this pattern are frequently directed against native (ds) DNA.

Nucleolar Pattern

The nucleolar pattern (Fig. 1D) appears as one or more bright, round structures, variable in size, within the unstained nuclei. The antigen contains RNA and possibly associated protein.

In some cases the patterns may be mixed. Dilution of the sample may reveal another pattern that is weaker. (For example, homogeneous fluorescence may mask a speckled pattern.) Sometimes they can be seen together. Assays using special substrates or isolated nuclear antigens may provide additional information.

The titer is considered to be the reciprocal of the highest dilution, still giving a result that is definitely positive when compared to the normal (negative) serum control.

Special Substrates

Crithidia luciliae, a hemoflagellate protozoan, contains a modified giant kinetoplast with a large concentration of well-characterized, double-stranded DNA in a circular configuration (61). The kinetoplast DNA is not associated with RNA or other nuclear proteins (26,61), thereby providing a simple and convenient substrate for detecting anti-DNA antibodies by IIF without the need for chemical purification of the DNA (1). The organism is nonpathogenic for man and may be maintained in culture (8) or be obtained from several commercial sources already on slides. A positive test appears as a brightly staining kinetoplast, which is somewhat smaller than the nucleus and is usually located at the periphery of the organism. Frequently, the nucleus will also be stained, if the serum contains antibodies to other nuclear antigens. An excellent detailed report for using *Crithidia luciliae* was presented by Ballou and Kushner (8).

Culture preparations of HEp-2 cells are an alternative substrate to mouse/rat liver for detection of ANA. There are several commercial sources for these specimens. The nuclei of HEp-2 cells are large and may contain certain antigens in greater concentration than mouse/rat liver. The small ribonucleic protein SS-A (Ro) antigen, which is cytoplasmic in rodent tissue is intranuclear in HEp-2 cells (46). Antigens of rapidly dividing cells are also found in HEp-2 cells. The antibodies that bind to proliferating cell nuclear antigen (PCNA) are found in 5% of SLE patients (78). Antibodies to the centromeric antigen are reported in

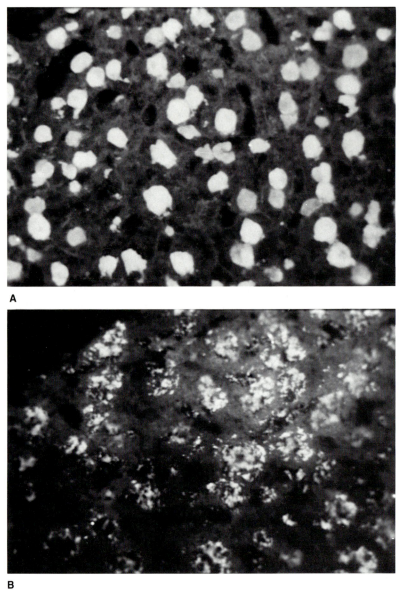

FIG. 1. Indirect immunofluorescence test for antinuclear antibody. Frozen sections of rat liver are used as tissue substrate. **A.** Homogeneous pattern. **B.** Speckled pattern. (*Figure continues*.)

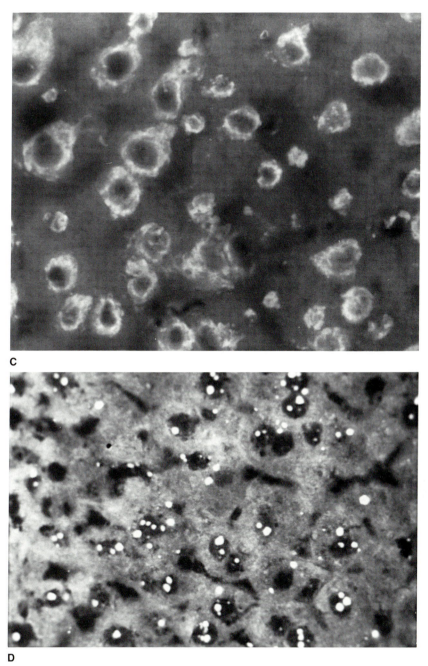

FIG. 1 (*continued*). **C.** Peripheral pattern. **D.** Nucleolar pattern.

90% of patients with the CREST syndrome (calcinosis, Raynaud's phenomenon, esophageal dysfunction, sclerodactyly, and telangiectasia) (54).

Acid-extracted tissue substrate can be used in IIF for the detection of antibodies to histones. These antibodies are found frequently in cases of drug-induced SLE (36). Briefly, acetone-fixed mouse kidney cells are treated with 0.1N HCl for 30 minutes at room temperature, which extracts or denatures most of the nuclear antigens (102). The sections are washed with 0.01 M PBS pH 7.3, and then reconstituted with 25 μg/ml of histone H-2 fraction, (Worthington Biochemical Corporation, Freehold, New Jersey), followed by another PBS wash. The tissue sections can be used as substrate for IIF. Criteria for positive histone antibodies suggested by Epstein and Barland (32) are (a) a greater than twofold fall in the ANA titer following acid extraction of the kidney substrate, and (b) a greater than twofold return of the activity after histone reconstitution. The work of Portanova et al. (85) indicates that the IIF histone reconstitution assay only measures antibodies directed against the histone H2A-H2B fraction, most frequently found in patients with procainamide-induced SLE (32). Therefore, the interpretation of the histone-reconstitution assay must be made cautiously, in case there are antibodies directed to other histone fractions.

Interpretation

Although sensitive, IIF testing for ANA is not diagnostically specific. Two general considerations should be made when interpreting the results of a positive ANA test: the pattern of the reaction and the titer of the antibody. The best correlation between ANA and a disease is in systemic lupus erythematosus (SLE). Over 90% of patients with SLE have positive ANA tests, with a predominance of homogeneous and peripheral patterns (10,21). Speckled patterns are seen as well, but to a lesser degree, and are often associated with a variant of SLE, known as mixed connective tissue disease (21,51,60). Many cases of seronegative SLE have subsequently been found to have antibodies to one of the more obscure nuclear antigens, necessitating the use of special substrates (72). Certain reports state that a correlation exists between the presence of anti-dsDNA antibodies (peripheral pattern) and lupus nephritis in patients with active disease (22,104). The prognosis for these subjects is poorer than that for other SLE patients. Those patients with drug-induced SLE tend to develop antibodies to DNA histones. The clinical course of SLE is sometimes reflected by a changing titer of ANA. Those patients treated effectively or those in remission often have diminished levels of ANA.

Sera from patients with rheumatoid arthritis (RA), scleroderma, or Sjögren's disease also show a high prevalence of ANA, although less frequently and with lower titer than in SLE. Titer and pattern are not as well correlated with severity of disease as in SLE. Many laboratories report a higher incidence of speckled or nucleolar patterns in scleroderma patients. The sera of RA patients show speckled and homogeneous patterns, with a lower incidence of peripheral patterns.

Other connective tissue disorders or conditions associated with autoimmune phenomena exhibit a low incidence of ANA, generally of a low titer. These diseases include chronic thyroiditis, chronic active hepatitis, discoid lupus erythematosus, pernicious anemia, idiopathic leukopenia, chronic interstitial pneumonia, myasthenia gravis, and Felty's syndrome (21,51,60).

A low titered ANA is also associated with various nonimmune disorders. Even sera from a normal population of blood group donors show a low incidence of ANA. The interpretation of the test in the diagnosis of disease must therefore be based on other clinical findings and not solely on the results of this test.

The IIF technique for ANA is important as a screening test in the identification and localization of antibodies directed against nuclear antigens. Even as a screening technique, however, IIF has serious limitations. The tissue substrate is composed of many antigens. There is no separation of the nuclear components, and the reaction can often be unclear, especially if antibodies are directed to more than one nuclear constituent.

Positive serum can be titered in a semiquantitative fashion, but the evaluation of the final reaction is often subjective. The intensity of fluorescence judged by different individuals can vary considerably. Each laboratory must establish criteria for endpoint titers, and these may not correspond with criteria from other laboratories. Many different substrates are used, which vary in nuclear components. These substrates include cultured fibroblasts, cultured tumor cells, or imprints of tumor cells, spleen cells, and liver cells (21,40).

It is understandable that correlations between pattern and disease (other than those with SLE) are difficult to establish using IIF patterns as criteria. For example, speckled patterns may be produced by antibodies reacting to several different non-histone nuclear antigens (97,101). Procedures using isolated products from cell nuclei have been initiated and have a twofold purpose: to identify antibody specificity and to improve quantitation.

Tests for ANA Using Specific Nuclear Antigens

DNA

The IIF test using *Crithidia luciliae* has been mentioned previously. While this test is highly specific, it lacks sensitivity in comparison to ligand-based assays.

The DNA-binding assay quantitatively measures serum for antibodies to DNA. This assay has been adapted from the ammonium sulfate globulin precipitation technique of Farr (33) and is highly specific and sensitive (83,115). The principle of the assay is that free antigen has a different solubility than that of antigen bound to antibody after precipitation by addition of saturated ammonium sulfate to a final concentration of 37% saturation. The use of radiolabeled DNA allows rapid and accurate quantitation of the final precipitate.

Solid-phase ELISA methods, which generally show good agreement with the method described above, are an alternative to techniques using radioactive compounds. The most important feature of an ELISA for anti-DNA antibodies is a DNA preparation that is essentially free of single-stranded regions. Antibodies to single-stranded DNA (ss-DNA) are found in a wide variety of autoimmune conditions in addition to SLE, whereas antibodies to native or double-stranded DNA (dsDNA) are found almost exclusively in SLE patients (87). Thus, the presence of ss-DNA reduces specificity. A detailed protocol for an anti-DNA antibody ELISA is presented by Rubin (93). Briefly, dsDNA is adsorbed to polystyrene microtiter plates precoated with methylated bovine serum albumin (m-BSA). The m-BSA is necessary to improve the binding of dsDNA, which normally does not adsorb well to plastics. Single-stranded sites are removed by S1 nuclease incubation of the microtiter wells just prior to the assay, and unoccupied sites on the plastic are blocked with 0.1% gelatin in PBS. Serum dilutions are incubated in the wells, excess proteins are washed away, and the wells are incubated with an anti-immunoglobulin reagent conjugated to an enzyme. The enzymes most frequently used are either horseradish peroxidase (HRP) or alkaline phosphatase (AP). After an appropriate incubation period, excess antiglobulin is removed by washing, and enzyme substrate is added. The color change of the substrate is read using an ELISA reader (i.e., a spectrophotometer), using the wave length appropriate to the enzyme-substrate reactivity. Controls are very important in this assay. It is necessary to include positive sera reference standards in every assay to control for intra-assay variation. Normal sera should also be evaluated to establish the baseline or background binding of the assay, and it is also important to include sera from patients with ss-DNA antibodies, as controls for specificity.

Another method for the detection of specific nuclear antigens is tanned cell hemagglutination (19). Briefly, sheep red blood cells are modified by treatment with a weak solution of tannic acid, washed, and then exposed to the specific antigen. The coated cells should only be used on the day of preparation. This technique has been adapted from the method used for years for the detection of autoantibodies to thyroid-specific antigens. For use as an antigen, DNA is prepared from a commercial source (no. D-1501 deoxyribonucleic acid from calf thymus, type 1, Sigma Chemical Co., St. Louis, MO). Treatment with S1-nuclease (93) ensures specificity for dsDNA. This technique lends itself well to laboratories without expensive readers, but as with any similar test, care is required in the preparation of the coated cells, and appropriate controls must be included. The sera should be tested in parallel against tanned-but-uncoated cells to exclude reactivity to the treated red cells themselves.

SLE patients generally have dsDNA antibodies (77), especially when the disorder is complicated with lupus nephritis, and the serum titers correlate with disease activity (88,96). The pathogenic action of DNA antibodies is attributed to immune complex formation (see Chapters 2 and 3). A method has recently been proposed to measure DNA-anti-DNA complexes directly in the serum. The procedure measures an increase in detectable anti-DNA antibodies in serum (by DNA binding) after DNase digestion of the serum sample (22).

Histones

Five histones have been identified in calf thymus by polyacrylamide gel electrophoresis: H1, H2A, H2B, H3, and H4 (15). Sera from patients with various rheumatic or autoimmune disorders may contain antibodies to one or more of these antigens. The histone-reconstitution IIF assay, described previously, is limited because autoantibodies to histone H3 and H4 are not measured (94). More recently, an ELISA screening technique has been established that will measure autoantibodies to total histones (93). With the use of isolated histones as antigens, the ELISA can be adapted to measure individual antihistone antibodies. These specific histone antibodies may have diagnostic value, as in the case of patients with procainamide-induced SLE. The use of uncontaminated antigen preparations in the ELISA is critical (93); a good preparation of total histones is available from (Calbiochem-Behring and United States Biochemical Corp., Cleveland, OH). All histone preparation should be considered to be contaminated with DNA and digested with DNase in the presence of phenymethylsulfonyl fluoride to inhibit endogenous proteases (93). The assay itself is similar to that described for the DNA ELISA. Details of the procedure are presented by Rubin (93).

Nonhistone Proteins

Serum autoantibodies to nonhistone nuclear antigens produce a "speckled" appearance in IIF. Sometimes the speckles are large and variable, and sometimes small and uniform.

Burnham described some 17 different speckled patterns (21). There are many different nonhistone antigens to which autoantibodies are directed; some have been identified and characterized biochemically. In some cases the identification is relevant to clinical diagnosis or prognosis.

Smith (Sm) and nuclear ribonucleic protein (nRNP) are two nonhistone antigens extracted from soluble fractions of cell nuclei, and both are part of what was originally designated as "extractable nuclear antigen" or ENA (50). The antigen known as the Sm antigen was described first and was found in precipitation reactions in a high percentage of SLE sera (104). Both antigens are resistant to DNase. The Sm antigen is resistant to RNase and partially sensitive to trypsin digestion. The nRNP activity is destroyed by both RNase and trypsin (81). Heat (at 56°C for 60 min) destroys nRNP but not Sm reactivity. The Sm and nRNP antigens consist of RNA and protein constituents (68). The RNA molecules belong to the small nuclear RNA present in the nucleus. Antibodies to Sm antigen bind to the U1, U2, U4, U5 and U6-RNA moieties, whereas antibodies to nRNP bind only to the U1-RNA (95).

Autoantibodies to Sm antigen are found in approximately 30% of patients with SLE. This antibody has been considered a highly specific marker of SLE because it has not been identified in either normals or patients with a variety of other systemic rheumatic diseases. Antibodies to nRNP are found in patients with various systemic rheumatic disorders; however, if a high titer of anti-nRNP is found with no other ANA specificities, the mixed connective tissue disease syndrome is suspected (97).

Antibodies to the Sm antigen can be detected by complement fixation or more commonly by immunodiffusion or tanned cell hemagglutination. Autoantibodies to Sm and nRNP have also been detected by counterimmunoelectrophoresis (CIE). Although this technique was described several years ago, it has not been used widely (17,58). A recent evaluation for anti-Sm and anti-nRNP assays reports that CIE is less specific than either immunodiffusion or hemagglutination but is more suited for quantitation (79). Recently, an ELISA for Sm antigen has been reported (73,84), but the purified antigens required for this assay are not yet widely available.

The tanned cell hemagglutination procedure is a technique that can be adapted easily for identifying autoantibodies to ENAs. Briefly, human group O red cells are coated with a preparation of ENA prepared from calf thymus (97). Autoantibodies to both Sm and nRNP will hemagglutinate this preparation. To determine specificity, the red cells are treated with RNase, which digests the nRNP part of the antigen coating the red cell. The hemagglutination is performed again, and the results are compared to the original test. If there is no change in titer, only antibodies to Sm are present. If there is a reduction in titer, antibodies to both Sm and nRNP are present.

The immunodiffusion test for antibodies to Sm and nRNP has been well described by Wilson and Nitsche (112). The immunodiffusion can be set up for these antigens and other nonhistone nuclear antigens at the same time. With a more sensitive method such as the ELISA, Sm antibody was detected in about 50% to 60% of SLE patients, compared to 25% to 30% by immunodiffusion, and it was also found in 25% of patients with progressive systemic sclerosis (PSS) and in 23% of patients with rheumatoid arthritis (73). Since both nonprecipitating and nonhemagglutinating antibodies can be detected, ELISA has an advantage (84).

An innovative technique employs Western blotting as a method to detect antibodies to nonhistone nuclear antigens (111). The method compares well to CIE and immunodiffusion if both anti-IgG and anti-IgM specific reagents are used. It also detects nonprecipitating antibodies. The limitations are the scarcity of purified antigens and appropriate equipment. Also, running gels and performing the electrotransfers requires expertise.

Ro (SS-A) and La (SS-B)

Autoantibodies to Ro (SS-A) and La (SS-B) in systemic rheumatic diseases are most prevalent in SLE and Sjögren's syndrome. Frequently, these antibodies are closely associated with one another. Anti-Ro (SS-A) has been reported in 60% to 70% of patients with Sjögren's syndrome and in 30% to 40% of patients with SLE (71) when detected by immunodiffusion. Anti-La (SS-B) is reported in approximately 60% of Sjögren's patients and in only 15% of those with SLE. Anti-Ro (SS-A) antibodies distinguish a group of small ribonuclear particles, consisting of a single RNA molecule complexed with protein. This complex resides primarily in the cytoplasm of rodent tissue cells (66). Anti-La (SS-B) antibodies are directed to a specific group of small nuclear ribonucleoproteins (65).

While antibodies to La (SS-B) and Ro (SS-A) can be measured by IIF (using mouse or rat liver substrate), their speckled appearance is indistinguishable from that due to antibodies to Sm or nRNP. Immunodiffusion is the most common test for these antibodies, performed in the same manner as for antibodies to Sm or nRNP. The interpretation depends on lines of identity (or nonidentity) with reference sera of known specificity (112).

A newly developed test for detection of autoantibodies to small nuclear and cytoplasmic ribonucleoproteins (67) and well described by Hardin (43) utilizes an electrophoretic identification of immunoprecipitated RNA molecules. Briefly, Hela cells are incubated with $^{32}PO_4$, and the radiolabeled nucleoproteins are solubilized and exposed to Sepharose-protein A beads, coated with IgG from the test serum. The IgG-coated beads bind to specific RNP, which is then recovered by phenol extraction. The isolated RNPs are separated by polyacrylamide gel electrophoresis and visualized by autoradiography. Their identity establishes the antibody specificity in the patient's serum. The concept of this assay is directly analogous to the concept of affinity absorption. There is no need to obtain isolated or purified antigen, as there is in ELISA techniques. The test has been used to detect a number of autoantibodies, such as Sm, nRNP and Ro (SS-A), La (SS-B), and others. It is a powerful tool for identifying almost the entire range of autoantibodies to ribonucleoproteins. It is more sensitive and more discriminatory than either immunodiffusion or HA, although the results are only semiquantitative. Because of the complex nature of the test, however, few laboratories currently have the resources to perform this assay.

Recent purification of Ro (SS-A) and La (SS-B) by affinity chromatography has lead to the development of an ELISA for these antibodies (45,116). Using this technique, Harley et al. (44) found that of 86 patients with Sjögren's syndrome, more than 96% had anti-Ro (SS-A) and 87% had anti-La (SS-B), much higher percentages than reported previously. The investigators were able to quantitate these antibodies and correlate high levels of antibodies with a subset of patients with purpura, leukopenia, lymphopenia, and increased polyclonal gammaglobulins.

Scl-70

The autoantibodies to the antigen Scl-70 (originally called Scl-1) (103) appear to be markers of progressive systemic sclerosis (PSS). The antigen was characterized as a basic nuclear protein with a molecular weight of 70,000 daltons (30). Anti-Scl-70 is commonly detected by a precipitin reaction in agar gel, as described previously for anti-Sm or anti-nRNP autoantibodies. Recently, Shero et al. (98) presented evidence from Western blotting, suggesting that the Scl-70 antigen is a DNA topoisomerase I which is involved with DNA replication and transcription. The immunoblotting technique is several times more sensitive in detecting anti-Scl-70 than is immunodiffusion.

Miscellaneous Nonhistone Nuclear Antigens

Autoantibodies are found to a number of other nuclear antigens, but with much less frequency (see Table 1). The methods to detect most of these autoantibodies are either IIF (using special substrates), or immunodiffusion. They include autoantibodies to other nuclear antigens including centromeres (54), rheumatoid-associated nuclear antigen (RANA) present in EBV transformed cells, MA, Jo-1, and PM-1 (112).

Cytoplasmic Antigens

Autoantibodies to mitochondria are found frequently in patients with primary biliary cirrhosis and less frequently in patients with systemic lupus erythematosus (12). They are most often detected by IIF on rat kidney tissue substrate, since the tubules of the kidney are rich in mitochondria. The appearance of the IIF is presented in Fig. 2. Autoantibodies to other generally distributed cytoplasmic components are found in chronic active hepatitis (cytoskeleton) (see below).

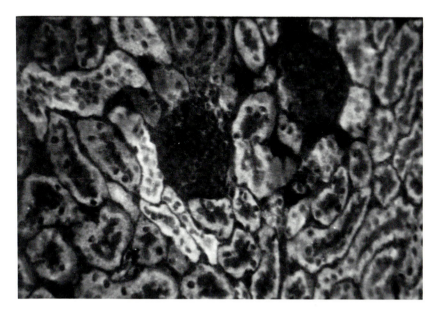

FIG. 2. Indirect immunofluorescence test for autoantibodies to mitochondria. Frozen sections of rat kidney are used as substrate. The fluorescent staining appears in the cytoplasm of the tubules. Glomeruli are negative.

Rheumatoid Factor

Rheumatoid factors (RF) are antibodies that react with antigenic determinants on the Fc portion of immunoglobulin. The phenomenon was first noted by Waaler (109), who found that serum from patients with rheumatoid arthritis would agglutinate sheep red blood cells (SRBC), sensitized by rabbit anti-SRBC. This observation became the basis of the Waaler-Rose test (92), described in detail elsewhere (19). Methods using latex beads (99) are the basis of the most widely used tests today and are described in detail by Linker and Williams (70). These tests utilize Cohn fraction II from human serum as the source of IgG antigen.

New techniques for demonstrating RF include nephelometry and ELISA. Laser nephelometry and rate nephelometry utilize the changes in light-scattering properties of aggregated IgG when exposed to sera containing RF (34,110). These tests are equally sensitive and specific, are more reproducible than agglutination techniques, and can be automated. The ELISA techniques for RF have an additional advantage: not only are they quantitative, but also they can be adapted to identify specific isotypes of RF. Although RF is commonly IgM, RF of almost any isotype can be found. The ELISA will also pick up RF that is nonagglutinating. The ELISA is a double-antibody method in which IgG is bound to microtiter wells. The wells are exposed to test serum containing the possible RF, washed, and then incubated with a purified antibody directed to a specific human isotype and conjugated to an enzyme. The level of RF in the serum is directly proportional to the color after hydrolysis of enzyme substrate. A detailed protocol is presented by Linker and Williams (70).

Rheumatoid factor is most frequently used for differentiating rheumatoid arthritis from other chronic arthritic conditions. A certain number of patients with SLE, Sjögren's syndrome, chronic active hepatitis, other connective tissue diseases, and some chronic infections may have these factors. With the latex fixation test, RFs are found in 1% to 4% of the general population, and the prevalence can be as high as 20% in individuals over 65 years of age (70). Therefore, any clinical correlation should be approached with caution, and results should be assessed in the light of other symptoms and physical signs suggestive of rheumatoid arthritis.

ORGAN-SPECIFIC ANTIBODIES: INTRACELLULAR AND SECRETED ANTIGENS

Organ-specific autoantibodies develop in several disease processes. The prototypes are the autoantibodies to thyroid antigens in patients with chronic thyroiditis or other thyroid diseases. They provide a valuable exclusionary test, because over 95% of thyroiditis patients have autoantibodies directed against either the epithelial cell microsomes, thyroglobulin, or both. A negative test can virtually exclude a diagnosis of thyroiditis. A positive test, however, does not eliminate the diagnosis of such conditions as adenocarcinoma or hyperthyroidism, since 20% of these patients have antibodies to thyroid antigen, although titers are generally lower than in those patients with thyroiditis. Other organs to which autoantibodies correlate with disease include the adrenal glands, pancreas, ovary, stomach, kidney (see Chapter 3) and skin (see Chapter 4). They are much less prevalent than thyroid autoantibodies but, if present, help with differential diagnoses.

Muscle (smooth or striated) is a tissue to which autoantibodies develop. These autoantibodies may be considered as a transition between the non-organ-specific antibodies, such as ANA, and the organ-specific autoantibodies that are produced in response to disease within a specific organ, such as the thyroid. These antibodies are directed to tissue-specific antigens, which are widely distributed, so the autoantibody may signify a disease process that nominally has no connection with a specific organ. For example, patients with chronic active hepatitis (CAH) frequently develop antibodies that bind to smooth muscle. Actin is the putative antigen, but the relationship between a chronic liver disorder and autoantibodies to actin is unclear. Nevertheless, these autoantibodies are useful for confirmation of diagnosis of the autoimmune form of chronic active hepatitis, distinguishing it from the virus-mediated disease.

Autoantibodies to cell-surface receptors are a relatively recent discovery. The two examples in which measurement of these autoantibodies has the greatest impact are in Graves' disease and in myasthenia gravis. In these instances the autoantibodies themselves contribute directly to disease. These antibodies are discussed in a later section.

The most widely used test to detect organ-specific autoantibodies is IIF. The procedure is similar to that described for antinuclear antibodies, except that the tissue substrate is selected for the particular antigen. Immunofluorescence is advantageous because the reaction site can be visualized and the locale of the cellular antigen can be determined. In addition, a single tissue can sometimes be used for several autoantibody reactions. For example, thyroid tissue will react with antinuclear antibody, antithyroid microsomal antibody, and antithyroglobulin antibody. Some laboratories perform screening tests on a "composite tissue block" made up of several different tissues.

In a few cases, the autoantigen associated with a particular autoimmune disorder has been isolated, and more quantitative tests, such as hemagglutination, ELISA, or RIA, have been developed using the isolated antigen fraction.

Thyroid-Specific Antigens

Sera from patients with autoimmune thyroid disease, such as chronic lymphocytic thyroiditis (Hashimoto's thyroiditis), spontaneous myxedema of the adult, and Graves' disease, frequently contain autoantibodies to various thyroid antigens. While there is controversy over the role of antibodies in the initiation of disease, and in their participation in immunological reactions that perpetuate the inflammation and cellular infiltration of the thyroid (20), autoantibodies to thyroid antigens at the least may be viewed as markers of autoimmune thyroid disease.

The antigens to which most autoantibodies are developed are thyroglobulin and the thyroid microsomal fraction. Thyroglobulin, a glycoprotein of approximately 650 Kd, is the primary component of the thyroid colloid contained within the thyroid follicle and is the storage form of the thyroid hormones. The microsomal antigen is contained within the "microsomal fraction" of the cytoplasm of the thyroid epithelial cell, and until recently, very little was known about its nature.

Thyroglobulin

Several methods have been used to detect autoantibodies to thyroglobulin. Precipitation in fluid or gelified medium is a simple but insensitive method. A microscopic slide agglutination test employing latex particles as a carrier for thyroglobulin is more sensitive but lacks specificity. Although used commonly to detect thyroglobulin autoantibodies, the sensitivity of IIF is low. A high degree of sensitivity without loss of specificity is achieved by tanned cell hemagglutination and more recently by the chromic chloride hemagglutination test using modified human group O erythrocytes coated with thyroglobulin. An ELISA with considerable sensitivity has also been developed.

Indirect immunofluorescence

To detect autoantibodies against thyroglobulin using IIF, tissue sections must be fixed with absolute methanol for 10 minutes at 56°C, since the soluble thyroglobulin would otherwise leak out of the follicle while being washed in buffered saline. Positive sera elicit any of the following patterns (7): (a) "three dimensional" floccular pattern (usually seen in patients with precipitin-positive sera), (b) crazed pattern with dull staining of colloid spaces and bright fluorescence at the edges and cracks (tanned cell hemagglutination positive sera), and (c) a uniformly bright-staining colloid pattern (negative by precipitin, tanned cell hemagglutination, and complement fixative tests). The last pattern is attributed to a second colloid antigen (CA2) not detected by other tests.

Hemagglutination

The trivalent metallic cation chromium (Cr^{3+}) will bind protein nonspecifically to red cells. Because of this property, chromic chloride ($CrCl_3$) solutions have been employed in the coating of antigens on group O erythrocytes that are subsequently used for indirect or passive hemagglutination. The method for preparation of the cells has been described elsewhere (37). One advantage is that the preparation of erythrocytes is considerably faster than that used in the tanned cell method. The nonspecific agglutination of the control non-antigen-coated cell found with tanned-only cells is considerably diminished using chromic chloride-treated red cells. Another advantage is the stability of the cells following antigen coating. We have successfully used cells coated with thyroglobulin up to 2 weeks following their preparation, whereas tanned cells can be only used on the day of preparation.

Preparations of tanned cells coated with thyroglobulin are commercially available (Ames, Kankakee, IL). The cells are lyophilized and have a limited shelf life after rehydration. The performance of the test is adequate compared to other tanned cell tests, and it has the advantage of being readily available. We have compared the commercial tanned cell assay to our $CrCl_3$ hemagglutination and have found that the $CrCl_3$ test is approximately tenfold more sensitive. Using a commercially available tanned cell kit, we were unable to detect thyroglobulin antibodies in the sera of many of the patients with chronic lymphocytic thyroiditis that showed low titers by the $CrCl_3$ assay.

Hemagglutinating antibodies to thyroglobulin have been found in most patients with Hashimoto's thyroiditis (75% to 80%). At least one-fourth of them have titers of 1,000 or more. Autoantibodies to thyroglobulin are found regularly in patients with other forms of thyroiditis, but with a lower incidence and a lower titer (113). About 60% of patients with Graves' disease and 30% of thyroid cancer patients have hemagglutinating autoantibodies, but less than 10% have titers of 1,000 or more (5,113). The frequency of thyroglobulin antibodies in normal subjects is greater in women than in men, and the incidence increases with age. As many as 35% of women and 15% of men 50 to 70 years old have detectable antibody, although usually in low titer (27).

ELISA

For measuring autoantibodies to thyroglobulin, ELISA also has been employed (108). The method is especially useful for large scale studies. The sensitivity of the ELISA is slightly less than that of our $CrCl_3$ assay, but it can detect a few subjects who have thyroid autoantibodies which are not hemagglutinating antibodies. An advantage of the ELISA is that specific isotypes of the thyroglobulin antibody can be determined (82,91). Although this should be regarded as a research tool at the moment, additional investigation of isotypes may provide insight into the subsets of the disease.

Microsomal Antigen

The microsomal antigen was discovered by Holborow (49) and found to be an integral part of the smooth endoplasmic reticulum (89). Later, Mariotti et al. (75) showed an intimate association between microsomal antigen and the lipid bilayer of the membrane. Microsomal antigen is available on the membrane in thyroid cell cultures, where it is located on the apical surface of acinar cells (55), but it can also appear on the basal side under certain experimental conditions (42). The microsomal antigen was also found on the surface of cultured rat thyroid cells (24), although its expression was dependent on the presence of thyroid stimulating hormone (TSH) in the medium. Thyroid peroxidase (TPO) has been identified as an antigen that reacts with human antimicrosomal antibodies (26,86). Antibody to the microsomal antigen binds complement and may participate in complement-mediated cytotoxicity (56) as well as in antibody dependent cell-mediated cytotoxicity (ADCC) (14). Recent studies have provided some information on the biochemical and immunochemical character of the antigen. There are difficulties in purifying the antigen, since after isolation and solubilization of the microsomes, contaminating substances (especially thyroglobulin) have been found (9,38,41,75). Despite this problem, two independent groups of investigators used immunoprecipitation (9,41) and Western immunoblotting (41) techniques to identify a protein with a molecular weight of about 105 Kd that binds to antimicrosomal antibody from patients with autoimmune disease. Intrachain disulfide bonds may be present, since Banga et al. (9) found a difference in the mobility of the antigen in polyacrylamide gel electrophoresis when comparing reducing versus nonreducing conditions. At least two epitopes bind antibodies from patient sera. One of the antigenic sites is a sequential epitope, while the other may be a conformational epitope dependent upon the integrity of the intrachain disulfide bonds.

Historically, the test of choice for many years for the detection of microsomal antigens was the complement fixation test using an optimal dilution of thyrotoxic thyroid extract (49). The immunofluorescence method that supplanted this test was found to be more sensitive, and IIF remains one of the most commonly used tests for microsomal autoantibody. The substrate consists of frozen human or monkey thyroid tissue which is air dried and unfixed. A positive test of patient sera on unfixed slides appears as bright fluorescence of the follicular epithelial cells (Fig. 3).

Clinical Correlations

Patients with chronic forms of thyroiditis may have antibodies either to thyroglobulin or to microsomal antibodies or to both, so a complete analysis of the patient's status should

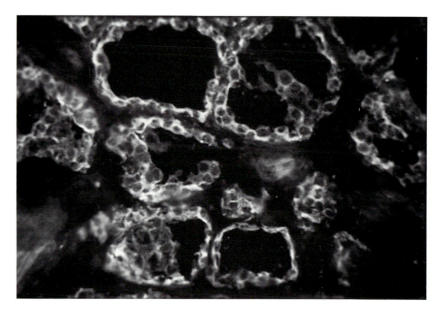

FIG. 3. Indirect immunofluorescence for autoantibodies directed to thyroid microsomes. The substrate consists of air-dried, unfixed, frozen sections of primate tissue. The fluorescent staining is confined to the cytoplasm of the thyroid follicle epithelial cell. Nuclei are negative.

include testing for both antibodies. Autoantibody to microsomal antigen is more closely associated with active clinical disease than is antithyroglobulin (28).

In our own studies, we found that virtually all juveniles with chronic lymphocytic thyroiditis, and many with Graves' disease, had antibody to thyroglobulin (18). Their clinically normal siblings often had antithyroglobulin, and a few also had microsomal antibodies. Interestingly, several of the siblings with both antibodies later developed biochemical evidence of thyroid disease (18).

Although antimicrosomal antibody has been strongly correlated with clinically apparent disease, its role *in vivo* is still unknown. Hypothetically, there may be two stages to autoimmune thyroid disease. An initial event leading to the development of antithyroglobulin may be followed by the development of antimicrosomal antibody. Previous work (6) showed that when monkeys were immunized with purified monkey thyroglobulin and adjuvant, the monkeys first developed antithyroglobulin followed by antimicrosomal antibody. The production of the two antibodies could be separate events, each increasing the severity of thyroid damage, with the autoimmune response to microsomal antigen a consequence of the inflammation caused by autoimmunity to thyroglobulin.

Gastric Parietal Cell

Autoantibodies to gastric parietal cells are frequently found in patients with pernicious anemia (90%) or atrophic gastritis (60%) (12). The presence of these antibodies is helpful in confirming the clinical diagnosis, but the absence of antibodies is not informative. These antibodies are also found in patients with chronic thyroiditis, Sjögren's disease, or gastric ulcer, but at a reduced prevalence (15% to 33%) (12). The method of choice for detection of parietal cell autoantibodies is IIF (Fig. 4). The cells of the gastric mucosa, however, are

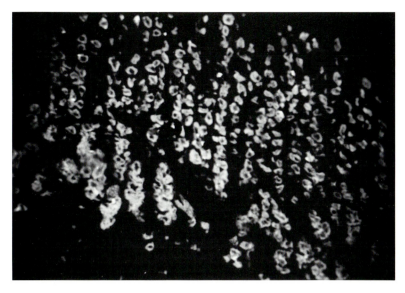

FIG. 4. Indirect immunofluorescence for gastric parietal cell autoantibodies. Frozen sections of the mucosa of mouse/rat stomach is used as tissue substrate. Columns of positive cells are stained with the fluorescent marker.

rich in mitochondria, and antimitochondrial antibodies will also react with these cells. Therefore, simultaneous testing of patient serum with kidney tissue will control for possible antimitochondrial activity. If the kidney tubules are negative and the gastric mucosa is positive, there is a specific parietal cell reaction.

Adrenal Autoantibodies

The idiopathic form of primary adrenocortical insufficiency (Addison's disease) is frequently associated with autoimmune phenomena. Autoantibodies to the adrenal cortex can be demonstrated by indirect immunofluorescence on primate adrenal tissue substrate (Fig. 5) in approximately 50% of these patients (38% to 64% in various studies). Patients with forms of Addison's disease due to exogenous etiology (e.g., tuberculosis) infrequently develop these antibodies. Based on prospective studies, the presence of adrenal autoantibodies in "normal" individuals may serve as a predictive sign of incipient adrenal failure (11). The autoantibodies may react with individual zones or with all three zones of the cortex. Idiopathic Addison's disease is frequently associated with other autoimmune conditions and their respective autoantibodies. In certain patients the autoantibodies cross-react with steroid-secreting cells of the theca interna of the ovary or with the Leydig cells of the testes. In Addison patients and in patients with primary ovarian failure, clinical evidence of ovarian failure is correlated with the presence of these autoantibodies.

Pancreatic Islets

Autoantibodies to pancreatic islet cells have been recognized as a feature of certain forms of diabetes mellitus, and this association has revolutionized the classification of diabetes. Autoantibodies to islet cells are almost entirely restricted to type I diabetes,

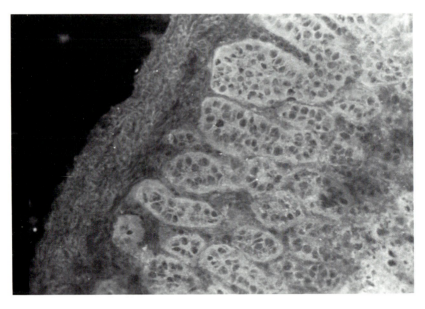

FIG. 5. Indirect immunofluorescence for anti-adrenal antibodies on frozen sections of monkey adrenal. The cells of the glomerulosa, the fasciculata, and the reticularis (not shown) are all positive. Nuclei and the capsule of the adrenal are negative.

which is insulin dependent and usually of juvenile onset (16,52,63). These antibodies are detected by indirect immunofluorescence on human (blood group O) or other primate pancreas tissue. Although the disease is the result of failure of the insulin-secreting β cells of the pancreas, antibodies usually react to the entire islet (Fig. 6). The autoantibodies are found most frequently at the time of diagnosis. The prevalence drops dramatically within a year after diagnosis, except in a small proportion of patients with multi-endocrine auto-immune syndromes. The reason for such a sharp decline is unclear. Antibodies persist only in those few positives who are highly predisposed to organ-specific autoimmunity. The antibodies are primarily IgG and are capable of binding complement. Testing for these autoantibodies helps to classify disease, and may help to identify first degree relatives who are at higher risk for development of disease (100). The presence of islet cell antibodies can help to identify those patients with type II (non-insulin dependent) diabetes who may later develop insulin dependence (39).

Muscle

Patients with chronic active hepatitis (CAH) frequently develop autoantibodies that react with smooth muscle antigens. They can best be detected by indirect immunofluorescence on smooth muscle tissue substrate (Fig 7). A high titer of these antibodies (> 80) may help to distinguish CAH from other types of liver disorders. However, the absence of antibody is not helpful, because the frequency of the antibodies in CAH is 40% to 70% (12). Smooth muscle antibodies are not specific for CAH, as many individuals with acute viral infections or even normal individuals may have smooth muscle antibodies, although the titer rarely exceeds 80. While the main antigenic component is actin, antibodies to other cytoskeletal components may also be produced (59). The assays for antibodies to

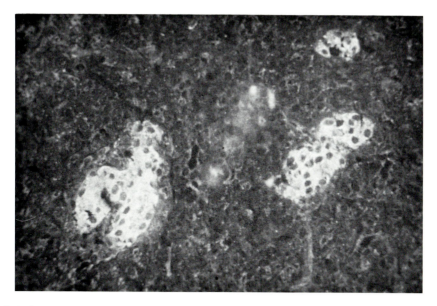

FIG. 6. Indirect immunofluorescence for antibodies to pancreas islets on frozen sections of monkey tissue. Islets picking up the fluorescent stain stand out among the negative exocrine pancreas.

individual components of the cytoskeleton have not been well defined and are mostly dependent upon IIF, using different cell lines that may contain various cytoskeleton components (107) or cells treated with metabolic poisons. Until purified components of the cytoskeletal system are widely available for use in solid state assays, the detection of these antibodies will remain in the province of research.

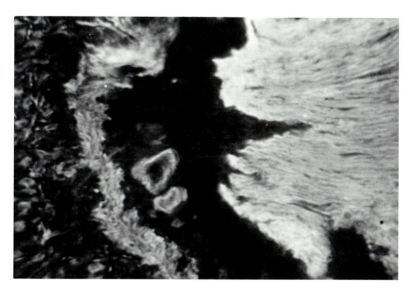

FIG. 7. Indirect immunofluorescence test for smooth muscle antibodies using frozen section of rat stomach. The muscle fibers of the muscularis mucosa and the muscularis are positive. An edge of the mucosa can be seen and is negative.

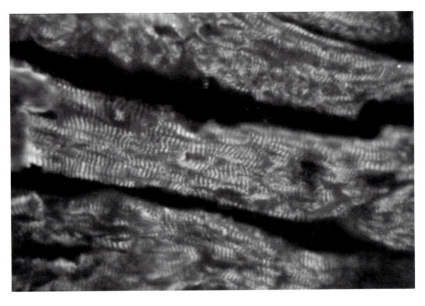

FIG. 8. Indirect immunofluorescence for striated muscle autoantibodies. Frozen sections of rat cardiac tissue (also skeletal muscle as control) are used to detect autoantibodies to heart antigens. Antifibrillary antibodies are positive.

Antibodies to striated muscle in many patients with myasthenia gravis have been shown to be unrelated to diagnosis or to the mechanism of the disease. The acetylcholine receptor appears to be the predominant autoantigen in this condition.

There is a recent interest in autoantibodies that react to striated cardiac muscle in patients with cardiomyopathy. The presence of striated anti-cardiac muscle antibodies in these patients may help to distinguish autoimmune cardiomyopathies from other etiologic forms of myocarditis (74). This in turn may influence therapy. These antibodies, as shown in Fig. 8, are detected by IIF. The most severe cases in our laboratory have been associated with high titers of IgG antibodies specific for striated cardiac muscle but not for skeletal muscle (90). Many normal individuals may have low titers of anti-striated muscle antibodies, primarily IgM that reacts with both types of striated muscle.

ORGAN SPECIFIC AUTOANTIBODIES: CELL SURFACE RECEPTORS

Autoantibody production to surface receptors is now recognized as the basis of several endocrine and neurological conditions. The most widely understood disorders associated with receptor autoantibodies are myasthenia gravis and Graves' disease. The salient features of these and the other conditions associated with receptor antibodies, such as extreme insulin resistance and a variant of bronchial asthma, are presented in Table 2.

The autoantibodies to surface receptors may produce clinical symptoms by altering one of two basic functions. The first occurs when the surface target receptor is bound, and there is either blocking of the normally reactive substance (e.g., insulin resistance) or accelerated degradation of the receptor (e.g., myasthenia gravis), both of which lead to decreased function. In the second case, autoantibodies bind to receptors and mimic the

TABLE 2. *General features of anti-receptor autoimmune diseases**

	Myasthenia gravis	Graves' disease	Insulin resistance with acanthosis nigricans	Ataxia telangiectasia	Bronchial asthma
Antigen	Acetylcholine receptor	Thyrotropin (TSH) receptor	Insulin receptor	Insulin receptor	β-Adrenergic receptor
Antibody	IgG	IgG	IgG	IgM	IgG
Prevalence of autoantibodies	90–100%	50–95%	100%	100%	5%
Clinical effects	Muscle weakness	Hyperthyroidism or hypothyroidism	Hyperglycemic diabetes mellitus or hypoglycemia	Hyperglycemic diabetes mellitus	Bronchospasm
Immunopathogenesis	Increased degradation of receptor	TSH mimetic or blocker	Insulin blocker or mimetic	Insulin blocker	β-blocker
Polyautoimmune associations	Yes	Yes	Yes	Probably	Probably
Major HLA associations	B-8, DR-3	B-8, DR-3	?	?	?
Sex predominance	Female	Female	Female	?	None

*Reprinted with slight modification M. Blecher (13).

action of the agonist (e.g., Graves' disease) resulting in uncontrolled increased function. Cytotoxicity is another possible consequence, with lysis of the target cell.

Acetylcholine Receptor

Myasthenia gravis is a disease characterized by weakness and fatigability of the voluntary muscles. Autoantibodies to acetylcholine receptors are found in myasthenia gravis, where they interact with the receptors on the postsynaptic membrane of the neuromuscular junction at or near the binding site of acetylcholine. There is a reduction in the number of receptors, reportedly owing to the antibody cross-linking the receptors followed by their accelerated internalization and degradation. In addition, there may be blocking of some receptors and a destruction of others due to the action of antibody and complement.

The basis of most assays for autoantibodies to acetylcholine receptors depends upon a toxin, alpha bungarotoxin from *Bungarus multicinctus*, which binds to the acetylcholine receptor at a site distinct from that used by acetylcholine. A source of acetylcholine receptors, such as the electric organ of *Torpedo californica*, is also required for the assay. Initially, RIA (12,23,69,80,105) and later the ELISA techniques (47,57) were employed for the measurement of these autoantibodies.

RIA can be used either as a measurement of the inhibition by patient antibody of toxin binding to isolated receptors or more commonly as a double antibody assay employing a radio-labeled neurotoxin-receptor complex. This second assay (immunoprecipitation) is described in detail by Bigazzi et al. (12). Briefly, ^{125}I-labeled toxin-receptor complex is incubated with a dilution of patient serum. Antibodies bind to the receptor at a site or sites other than the neurotoxin-binding site, as previously mentioned. A sufficient excess of anti-human IgG is added to precipitate all human IgG, which is then separated by centrifugation and washed. The radioactivity is measured by a gamma counter. The counts are directly related to the quantity of autoantibody.

Positive reactions have been reported in up to 95% of sera from myasthenia gravis patients (62). Variations in prevalence are due to differences in methods and reagents, such as the source of acetylcholine receptor. Initially, the receptors were from the electric organ of *Torpedo californica*, but greater success has now been achieved using human skeletal muscle from amputees with conditions that lead to muscle denervation (e.g., diabetes) (12). There are also variations in antibody. The immune response is heterogeneous with respect to the fine specificity of the individual antibody populations, but in some cases there may be antibodies to the site of toxin binding. This may occur in up to 30% of patients (64), although rarely (< 1%) is this the only antibody found. Currently, there is no correlation between the severity of disease and the pattern of antibody specificity. Similarly, the correlation between the severity of clinical symptoms and concentration of antibody is low, but it appears to be higher if changes of titer within individual patients are taken into account (12). The traditional immunoprecipitation assay, as described above, has been used in combination with a second assay to provide additional information about the "functional" status of the antibodies. Drachman et al. (31) measured the ability of the autoantibodies to accelerate the degradation of the acetylcholine receptors in skeletal muscle tissue culture. Together, information from the two assays was combined to produce an "index of immunoglobulin activities" which correlated with the clinical severity of disease in most of the patients tested.

TSH Receptor

Autoantibodies to the TSH receptor on the surface of thyroid epithelial cells are believed to be the direct cause of the hyperthyroid state in Graves' disease. The autoantibodies bind near or at the site of TSH and mimic its action, but without its negative feedback control, result in uncontrolled stimulation. These autoantibodies appear to be heterogeneous and are primarily described by the assay used for their evaluation, as summarized in Table 3. The prevalence of these antibodies in the sera of patients with Graves' disease ranges from 55% to 95%, depending on the test used for their detection.

Initially called long-acting thyroid stimulator (LATS), the antibody was identified as a stimulatory serum factor present in a few patients with Graves' disease, when measured by bioassay in mice (2,76); however, not all antibodies bound to mouse thyroid—the basis of the LATS bioassay. Another subset of these receptor antibodies, called long-acting thyroid stimulator-protector (LATS-P), was found to bind only human thyroids and not mouse thyroids. Named for its "function," LATS-P prevented or "protected" neutralization of LATS when human thyroid tissue was added to sera prior to the LATS bioassay (4). Later, a more general term, *thyroid-stimulating antibodies (TSAb)* (sometimes called thyroid stimulating immunoglobulins (TSI)) has been applied to the autoantibodies, which stimulate human thyroid tissue *in vitro*, resulting in an increase in cyclic AMP (3). If antibodies are evaluated by their ability to block the binding of TSH to the receptor rather than their stimulatory activity (i.e., an increase in cyclic-AMP), the term *thyrotropin binding-inhibiting immunoglobulin (TBII or TBI)* is more properly applied. The TSAb and TBII may represent different specificities of autoantibodies to the thyroid epithelial cell surface on or

TABLE 3. *Assays for anti-thyrotropin receptor autoantibodies**

Method	Recommended term for antibody	Parameter measured	Thyroid tissue source
Bioassays			
McKenzie	LATS	Iodine uptake	Mouse
Cyclic AMP	TSAb	Increase in cAMP in cultured FRTL-5 cells	Rat
		Increase in cAMP in primary thyroid cell cultures	Human
		Adenylate cyclase activation in plasma membranes	Human
Thyroid cell growth	None	Stimulation of growth of cultured FRTL-5 thyroid cells	Rat
Binding assays			
LATS-P	LATS-P	Prevention of binding of LATS by thyroid tissue	Human
Radioreceptor assay	TBI	Inhibition of binding of ^{125}I-TSH to particulate or solubilized plasma membranes	

LATS, long-acting thyroid stimulator; TSAb, thyroid-stimulating antibodies; LATS-P, long-acting thyroid stimulator protector; TBI, thyrotropin-binding inhibitor; TSH, thyrotropin (thyroid-stimulating hormone).
*Reprinted with slight modification from M. Blecher (13).

near the TSH receptor. The heterogeneity of the autoantibodies and the diversity of the assays for their demonstration has created some confusion.

Assays for TSAb are primarily of two types, as listed in Table 3. They are either bioassays or binding assays. Most of the bioassays have limited usefulness because they are cumbersome and require special materials, such as viable human thyroid tissue. Bioassays measure a functional component of the effect of the antibodies as their endpoint, such as adenylate cyclase activation or cyclic AMP increase (117). The binding assays depend upon competition between labeled TSH and patient immunoglobulin for binding to thyroid preparations.

An assay using a cloned line of rat thyroid cells (FRTL-5) is very promising, as these cells can be maintained in tissue culture. The assay is based on the stimulation of adenylate cyclase in the cell membranes of FRTL-5 by patient sera. The amount of cAMP is measured and compared to the effect of normal sera, and a "TSI index" is calculated. At least two groups of investigators have found good correlation between elevated index and Graves' disease (53,106). Kits for cAMP measurement are available commercially.

Diagnosis of hyperthyroidism is dependent upon the demonstration of elevated thyroid hormones and may not always be due to autoimmune disease. The TSAb assay may be useful in cases where results of conventional tests are equivocal, or clinical signs and symptoms are minimal (e.g., exopthalmos in the absence of other features). The TSI assay is usually negative in patients with thyrotoxicosis in association with thyroid nodules, with cancer, or in patients with subacute thyroiditis (53). Therefore, a positive test allows diagnosis of Graves' disease with a high level of confidence. Successful treatment of Graves' disease with propylthiouracil may result in gradually lowered antibody levels (53). Therefore, the test could be used to monitor treatment of the disease. The test for TSI may also be useful in diagnosis of neonatal thyrotoxicosis in which the parental antibodies cross the placenta and cause thyrotoxicosis of the infant. There is at least one reported case of a hypothyroid mother whose newborn child suffered severely from this disorder (48). Upon testing the mother, a high level of TSAb was found, a completely unexpected finding based on her medical history.

CONCLUSION

Detection of autoantibodies as an aid in diagnosis or prognosis is well established, although certain systems are more highly characterized than others. The relationship between the autoantibodies and the pathogenesis of many diseases is less clear. The mechanism by which these autoantibodies are developed is the subject of continuing research. In many cases, there is a strong genetic influence on the antibody response. The situation may be analogous to atopy; that is, a predisposition to several forms of immunologic disease. From studies in animal models, however, it can be shown that even nonpredisposed strains will develop an autoimmune response if given sufficient stimulation. Many external or environmental influences (infectious agents, drugs, pollutants, volatile chemicals) may also drive an individual toward an autoimmune response. A long-range goal of research in this field is to evaluate these responses, correlate them with disease, and if possible, determine the mechanism by which they occur to improve diagnostic and therapeutic strategies.

ACKNOWLEDGMENTS

This work was supported by grants R23-AR35383, R01-AG04362, R01-HL33878, and R01-AM31632, from the National Institutes of Health.

REFERENCES

1. Aarden, L. A., deGroot, E. R., and Feltkamp, T. E. W. (1975): Immunology of DNA. III. *Crithidia luciliae*, a simple substrate for the determination of anti-dsDNA with the immunofluorescence technique. *Ann. N.Y. Acad. Sci.*, 254:505–515.
2. Adams, D. C. (1958): The presence of an abnormal thyroid stimulating hormone in the serum of some thyrotoxic patients. *J. Clin. Endocrinol. Metab.*, 18:699–712.
3. Adams, D. D., Dermkis, S., and Doniach, D. (1975): Nomenclature of thyroid stimulating autoantibodies. *Lancet i*:1201–1205.
4. Adams, D. D., Kennedy, T. H. (1971): Evidence to suggest that LATS protector stimulates the human thyroid gland. *J. Clin. Endocrinol. Metab.*, 33:47–51.
5. Anderson, J. W., McConahey, W. M., Alarcon-Segovia, D., Emslander, R. F., and Wakim, K. G. (1967): Diagnostic value of thyroid antibodies. *J. Clin. Endocr.*, 27:937–944.
6. Andrada, J. A., Rose, N. R., and Kite, J. H., Jr. (1968): Experimental thyroiditis in the Rhesus monkey. IV. The role of thyroglobulin and cellular antigens. *Clin. Exp. Immunol.*, 3:133–151.
7. Balfour, B. M., Doniach, D., Roitt, I. M., and Couchman, K. G. (1961): Fluorescent antibody studies in human thyroiditis: Auto-antibodies to an antigen of the thyroid distinct from thyroglobulin. *Br. J. Exp. Pathol.*, 42:307–316.
8. Ballou, S. P., and Kushner, I. (1986): *Crithidia luciliae* immunofluorescence test for antibodies to DNA. In: *Manual of Clinical Laboratory Immunology*, 3rd Edition, edited by N. R. Rose, H. Friedman, and J. Fahey, pp. 740–743. American Society for Microbiology, Washington, D.C.
9. Banga, J. P., Pryce, G., Hammond, L., and Roitt, I. M. (1985): Structural features of the autoantigens involved in thyroid autoimmune disease: The thyroid microsomal/microvillar antigen. *Mol. Immunol.*, 22:629–642.
10. Bartholomew, B. A. (1974): Antinuclear antibody tests as a clinically selected procedure. *Am. J. Clin. Pathol.*, 61:495–499.
11. Betterle, C., Zanette, F., Zanchetta, R., Pedini, B., Trevisan, A., Mantero, R., and Rigon, F. (1983): Complement-fixing adrenal autoantibodies as a marker for predicting onset of idiopathic Addison's disease. *Lancet*, 1:1238–1241.
12. Bigazzi, P. E., Burek, C. L., and Rose, N. R. (1986): Antibodies to tissue-specific endocrine, gastrointestinal, and neurological antigens. In: *Manual of Clinical Laboratory Immunology*, 3rd Edition, edited by N. R. Rose, H. Friedman, and J. Fahey, pp. 762–770. American Society for Microbiology, Washington, D.C.
13. Blecher, M. (1984): Receptors, antibodies, and disease. *Clin. Chem.*, 30:1137–1156.
14. Bogner, U., Schleusener, H., and Wall, J. R. (1984): Antibody-dependent cell mediated cytotoxicity against human thyroid cells in Hashimoto's thyroiditis but not Graves' disease. *J. Clin. Endocrinol. Metab.*, 59:734–738.
15. Boehm, F. L., Strickland, W. N., Strickland, M., Theraits, B. H., Van Der Westhuizen, D. R., and Von Holt, C. (1973): Purification of the five main calf thymus histone fractions by gel exclusion chromatography. *FEBS Lett.*, 34:217–221.
16. Bottazo, G. F., Florin-Christensen, A., and Doniach, D. (1974): Islet-cell antibodies in diabetes mellitus with autoimmune polyendocrine deficiencies. *Lancet ii*:1279–1283.
17. Bresnihan, B., Bunn, C., Snaith, M. L., and Hughes, G. R. V. (1977): Antiribonucleoprotein antibodies in connective tissue diseases: Estimation by counterimmunoelectrophoresis. *Br. Med. J.*, 1:610–611.
18. Burek, C. L., Hoffman, W. H., and Rose, N. R. (1982): The presence of thyroid autoantibodies in children and adolescents with autoimmune thyroid disease and in their siblings and parents. *Clin. Immunol. Immunopathol.*, 25:395–404.
19. Burek, C. L., and Rose, N. R. (1980): Detection of Autoantibodies. In: *Gradwohl's Clinical Laboratory Methods and Diagnosis*, 8th Edition, edited by A. C. Sonnenwirth and L. Jarett, pp. 1257–1278. C. V. Mosby Co., St. Louis.
20. Burek, C. L., and Rose, N. R. (1986): Cell-mediated immunity in autoimmune thyroid disease. *Hum. Pathol.*, 17:246–254.
21. Burnham, T. K., and Bank, P. W. (1974): Antinuclear antibodies I. Patterns of nuclear immunofluorescence. *J. Invest. Dermatol.*, 62:526–534.
22. Carr, R. I., Harbeck, R. J., Hoffman, A. A., Pirofsky, B., and Bardana, E. J. (1975): Clinical studies on the

significance of DNA: Anti-DNA complexes in the systemic circulation and cerebrospinal fluid (CSF) of patients with systemic lupus erythematosus. *J. Rheumatol.*, 2:184–193.

23. Carter, B., Harrison, R., Lunt, G. G., Morris, H., Savage-Marengo, T., and Stephenson, F. A. (1981): An assessment of RIA procedures for determination of ACh receptor antibodies in sera of patients with MG. *Ann. Clin. Biochem.*, 18:146–152.

24. Chiovato, L., Vitti, P., Lombardi, A., Kohn, L. D., and Pinchera, A. (1985): Expression of the microsomal antigen on the surface of continuously cultured rat thyroid cells is modulated by thyrotropin. *J. Clin. Endocrinol. Metab.*, 61:12–16.

25. Crowe, W., and Kushner, I. (1977): An immunofluorescent method using *Crithidia luciliae* to detect antibodies to double-stranded DNA. *Arthritis Rheum.*, 20:811–814.

26. Czarnocka, B., Ruf, J., Ferrand, M., Carayon, P., and Lissitzky, S. (1985): Purification of the human thyroid peroxidase and its identification as the microsomal antigen involved in autoimmune thyroid disease. *FEBS Lett.*, 190:147–152.

27. Doniach, D., and Roitt, I. M. (1973): Autoimmune thyroid disease. In: *Textbook on Immunopathology*, Vol. 2, 2nd Edition, edited by P.A. Miescher, and H.J. Muller-Eberhard, pp. 715–735. Grune & Stratton, New York.

28. Doniach, D., and Roitt, I. M. (1975): Thyroid auto-allergic disease. In: *Clinical Aspects of Immunology*, 3rd Edition, edited by P.G.H. Gell, R.R.A. Coombs, and P.J. Lachmann, pp. 1355–1368. Blackwell Scientific Publications, Oxford.

29. Doniach, D., and Walker, J. G. (1974): Mitochondrial antibodies. *Gut*, 15:664–668.

30. Douvas, A. S., Achten, M., and Tan, E. M. (1979): Identification of a nuclear protein (Scl-70) as a unique target of human antinuclear antibodies in scleroderma. *J. Biol. Chem.*, 254:10514–10522.

31. Drachman, D. B., Adams, R. N., Josifek, L. F., and Self, S. G. (1982): Functional activities of autoantibodies to ACh receptors and the clinical severity of MG. *N. Engl. J. Med.*, 307:769–775.

32. Epstein, A., and Barland, P. (1985): The diagnostic value of antihistone antibodies in drug-induced lupus erythematosus. *Arthritis Rheum.*, 28:158–162.

33. Farr, R. S. (1958): A quantitative immunochemical measure of the primary interaction between I*BSA and antibody. *J. Infect. Dis.*, 103:239–262.

34. Finley, P. R., Hicks, M. J., Williams, R. J., Hinlicky, J., and Lichtl, D. A. (1979): Rate nephelometric measurement of rheumatoid factor in serum. *Clin. Chem.*, 25:1909–1914.

35. Fritzler, M. J. (1986): Immunofluorescent antinuclear antibody tests. In: *Manual of Clinical Laboratory Immunology*, 3rd Edition, edited by N.R. Rose, H. Friedman, and J. Fahey, pp. 733–739. American Society for Microbiology, Washington, D.C.

36. Fritzler, M. J., and Tan, E. M. (1978): Antibodies to histone in drug-induced and idiopathic lupus erythematosus. *J. Clin. Invest.*, 62:560–567.

37. Gold, E. R., and Fudenberg, H. H. (1967): Chromic chloride: A coupling reagent for passive hemagglutination reactions. *J. Immunol.*, 99:859–866.

38. Goodburn, R., Williams, D. L., and Marks, V. (1982): The preparation of thyroid microsomal antigen for use in the indirect micro-ELISA method for the detection of anti-thyroid microsomal autoantibody. *Clin. Chim. Acta*, 119:291–297.

39. Groop, L. C., Bottazzo, G. F., and Doniach, D. (1986): Islet cell antibodies identify latent type I diabetes in patients aged 35–75 years at diagnosis. *Diabetes*, 35:237–241.

40. Hahon, N., Eckert, H. L., and Stewart, L. (1975): Evaluation of cellular substrates for antinuclear antibody determinations. *J. Clin. Microbiol.*, 2:42–45.

41. Hamada, N., Grimm, C., Mori, H., and DeGroot, L. J. (1985): Identification of a thyroid microsomal antigen by western blot and immunoprecipitation. *J. Clin. Endocrinol. Metab.*, 61:120–128.

42. Hanafusa, T., Pujol-Borrell, R., Chiovato, L., Doniach, D., and Bottazzo, G. F. (1984): *In vitro* and *in vivo* reversal of thyroid epithelial polarity: Its relevance for autoimmune thyroid disease. *Clin. Exp. Immunol.*, 57:639–646.

43. Hardin, J. A. (1986): Autoantibodies to small nuclear ribonucleoproteins and small cytoplasmic ribonucleoproteins. In: *Manual of Clinical Laboratory Immunology*, 3rd Edition, edited by N.R. Rose, H. Friedman, and J. Fahey, pp. 755–758. American Society for Microbiology, Washington, D.C.

44. Harley, J. B., Alexander, E. L., Bias, W. B., Fox, O. F., Provost, T. T., Reichlin, M., Yamagata, H., and Arnett, F. C. (1986): Anti-Ro (SS-A) and anti-La (SS-B) in patients with Sjögren's syndrome. *Arthritis Rheum.*, 29:196–206.

45. Harley, J. B., Yamagata, H., and Reichlin, M. (1984): Anti-La/SSB antibody is present in some normal sera and is coincident with anti-Ro/SSA precipitins in systemic lupus erythematosus. *J. Rheumatol.*, 11:309–314.

46. Harmon, C. E., Deng, J-S., Peebles, C. L., and Tan, E. M. (1984): The importance of tissue substrate in the SS-A/Ro antigen/antibody system. *Arthritis Rheum.*, 27:166–173.

47. Hinman, C. L., Burek, C. L., Hudson, R. A., Goodlow, G., and Rauch, H. C. (1983): An ELISA for measuring antibody against acetylcholine receptor. *J. Neurosci. Methods*, 9:141–155.

48. Hoffman, W. H., Sahasrananan, P., Ferandos, S. S., Burek, C. L., and Rose, N. R. (1982): Transient thyrotoxicosis in an infant delivered to a long-acting thyroid stimulator (LATS)- and LATS protector-negative, thyroid-stimulating antibody-positive woman with Hashimoto's thyroiditis. *J. Clin. Endocrinol. Metab.*, 54:354–356.

49. Holborow, E. J., Brown, P. C., Roitt, I. M., and Doniach, D. (1959): Cytoplasmic localization of "complement-fixing" auto-antigen in human thyroid epithelium. *Brit. J. Exp. Pathol.*, 40:583–588.

50. Holman, H. R. (1965): Partial purification and characterization of an extractable nuclear antigen which reacts with SLE sera. *Ann. N.Y. Acad. Sci.*, 124:800–806.

51. Husain, M., Neff, J., Daily, E. Townsend, J., and Lucas, F. (1974): Antinuclear antibodies: Clinical significance of titers and fluorescence patterns. *Am. J. Clin. Pathol.*, 61:59–65.

52. Irvine, W. J., McCallum, C. J., Gray, R. S., Campbell, C. J., Duncan, L. J. P., Farquhar, J. W., Vaughan, H., and Morris, P. J. (1977): Pancreatic islet cell antibodies in diabetes mellitus correlated with the duration and type of diabetes, coexistent autoimmune disease, and HLA-type. *Diabetes*, 26:138–147.

53. Jiang, N-S., Fairbanks, V. F., and Hay, I. D. (1986): Assay for thyroid stimulating immunoglobulin. *Mayo Clin. Proc.*, 61:753–755.

54. Kallenberg, C. G. M., Pastoor, G. W., Wanda, A. A., and The, T. H. (1982): Antinuclear antibodies in patients with Raynaud's phenomenon. Clinical significance of anticentromere antibodies. *Ann. Rheum. Dis.*, 41:382–387.

55. Khoury, E. L., Bottazzo, G. F., and Roitt, I. M. (1984): The thyroid "microsomal" antibody revisited. *J. Exp. Med.*, 159:577–591.

56. Khoury, E. L., Hammond, L., Bottazzo, G. F., and Doniach, D. (1981): Presence of the organ-specific 'microsomal' autoantigen on the surface of human thyroid cells in culture: Its involvement in complement-mediated cytotoxicity. *Clin. Exp. Immunol.*, 45:316–328.

57. Kobayashi, H., Sugita, H., Terada, E., Ghoda, A., Okudaira, H., Ogita, T., and Miyamoto, T. (1984): A solid-phase enzyme immunoassay for anti-acetylcholine receptor antibody in myasthenia gravis patients. *J. Immunol. Methods.*, 73:267–272.

58. Kurata, N., and Tan, E. M. (1976): Identification of antibodies to nuclear acidic antigens by counterimmunoelectrophoresis. *Arthritis Rheum.*, 19:574–580.

59. Kurki, P., and Virtanen, I. (1984): The detection of human antibodies against cytoskeletal components. *J. Immunol. Methods.*, 67:209–223.

60. Lange, A. (1972): Antinuclear antibodies in some internal diseases, especially autoimmune diseases. *Arch. Immunol. Ther. Exp.*, 20:209–226.

61. Laurent, M., Van Assel, S., and Steinert, M. (1971): Kinetoplast DNA. A unique macromolecular structure of considerable size and mechanical resistance. *Biochem. Biophys. Res. Commun.*, 43:278–284.

62. Lefvert, A. K., Bergstrom, K., Matell, G., Osterman, P. O., and Pirskanen, R. (1978): Determination of acetylcholine receptor antibody in myasthenia gravis: Clinical usefulness and pathogenetic implications. *J. Neurol. Neurosurg. Psychiatry*, 41:394–403.

63. Lendrum, R., Walker, G., and Gamble, O. R. (1975): Islet cell autoantibodies in juvenile diabetes mellitus of recent onset. *Lancet*, i:880–882.

64. Lennon, V. A. (1982): MG. Diagnosis by assay of serum antibodies. *Mayo Clin. Proc.*, 57:723–729.

65. Lerner, M. R., Boyle, J. A., Hardin, J. A., and Steitz, J. A. (1981): Two novel classes of small ribonucleoproteins detected by antibodies associated with lupus erythematosus. *Science*, 211:400–402.

66. Lerner, E. A., Lerner, M. R., Hardin, J. A., Janeway, C. A., and Steitz, J. A. (1982): Deciphering the mysteries of RNA-containing lupus antigens. *Arthritis Rheum.*, 25:761–766.

67. Lerner, E. A., Lerner, M. R., Janeway, C. A., Jr., and Steitz, J. A. (1981): Monoclonal antibodies to nucleic acid-containing cellular constituents: Probes for molecular biology and autoimmune disease. *Proc. Natl. Acad. Sci. USA*, 78:2737–2741.

68. Lerner, M. R., and Steitz, J. A. (1979): Antibodies to small nuclear RNAs complexed with proteins are produced by patients with systemic lupus erythematosus. *Proc. Natl. Acad. Sci. USA*, 76:5495–5499.

69. Lindstrom, J. M. (1977): An assay for antibodies to human ACh receptor in serum from patients with MG. *Clin. Immunol. Immunopathol.*, 7:36–43.

70. Linker, J. B., III., and Williams, R. C., Jr. (1986): In: *Manual of Clinical Laboratory Immunology*, 3rd Edition, edited by N.R. Rose, H. Friedman, and J. Fahey, pp. 759–761. American Society for Microbiology, Washington, D.C.

71. Maddison, P., Mogavero, H., Provost, T. T., and Reichlin, M. (1979): The clinical significance of autoantibodies to a soluble cytoplasmic antigen in systemic lupus erythematosus and other connective tissue diseases. *J. Rheumatol.*, 6:189–195.

72. Maddison, P. J., Provost, T. T., and Reichlin, M. (1981): Serological findings in patients with 'ANA negative' systemic lupus erythematosus. *Medicine*, 60:87–94.

73. Maddison, P. J., Skinner, R. P., Vlachoyiannopoulous, P., Brennand, D. M., and Hough, D. (1985): Antibodies to nRNP, Sm, Ro(SS-A) and La(SS-B) detected by ELISA: Their specificity and inter-relations in connective tissue disease sera. *Clin. Exp. Immunol.*, 62:337–345.

74. Maisch, B., Trostel-Soeder, R., Stechemesser, E., Berg, P. A., and Kochsiek, K. (1982): Diagnostic relevance of humoral and cell-mediated immune reactions in patients with acute viral myocarditis. *Clin. Exp. Immunol.*, 48:533–545.
75. Mariotti, S., Pinchera, A., Marcocci, C., Vitti, P., Urbano, C., Chiovato, L., Tosi, M., and Baschieri, L. (1979): Solubilization of human thyroid microsomal antigen. *J. Clin. Endocrinol. Metab.*, 48:207–212.
76. McKenzie, J. M., and Zakarija, M. (1977): LATS in Graves' disease. *Recent Prog. Horm. Res.*, 33:29–53.
77. Miniter, M. F., Stollar, B. D., and Agnello, V. (1979): Reassessment of the clinical significance of native DNA antibodies in systemic lupus erythematosus. *Arthritis Rheum.*, 22:959–968.
78. Miyachi, K., Fritler, M., and Tan, E. M. (1981): Autoantibody to nuclear antigen in proliferating cells. *J. Immunol.*, 121:2228–2234.
79. Molden, D. P., Suzuki, H., and Nakamura, R. M. (1985): Assays for Sm and RNP antibodies: Pitfalls and technical considerations. *Diagn. Immunol.*, 3:24–28.
80. Monnier, V. M., and Fulpius, B. W. (1977): A radioimmunoassay for the quantitative evaluation of anti-human acetylcholine receptor antibodies in myasthenia gravis. *Clin. Exp. Immunol.*, 29:16–22.
81. Northway, J. D., and Tan, E. M. (1972): Differentiations of antinuclear antibodies giving speckled staining patterns in immunofluorescence. *Clin. Immunol. Immunopathol.*, 1:140–154.
82. Parkes, A. B., McLachlan, S. M., Bird, P., and Rees-Smith, B. (1984): The distribution of microsomal and thyroglobulin antibody activity among the IgG subclasses. *Clin. Exp. Immunol.*, 57:239–243.
83. Pincus, T., Schur, P. H., Rose, J. A., Decker, J. L., and Talal, N. (1969): Measurement of serum DNA-binding activity in systemic lupus erythematosus. *N. Engl. J. Med.*, 281:701–705.
84. Pollard, K. M., and Tan, E. M. (1985): Purification of the Sm nuclear autoantigen. Detection and clinical significance of IgM antibody. *Clin. Exp. Immunol.*, 60:586–596.
85. Portanova, J. P., Rubin, R. L., Joslin, F. G., Agnello, V. D., and Tan, E. M. (1982): Reactivity of anti-histone antibodies induced by procainamide and hydralazine. *Clin. Immunol. Immunopathol.*, 26:67–79.
86. Portmann, L., Hamada, N., Heinrich, G., and DeGroot, L. J. (1985): Anti-thyroid peroxidase antibody in patients with autoimmune thyroid disease: Possible identity with anti-microsomal antibody. *J. Clin. Endocrinol. Metab.*, 61:1001–1003.
87. Reichlin, M. (1981): Current perspectives in serological reaction in SLE patients. *Clin. Exp. Immunol.*, 44:1–10.
88. Reichlin, M., and Mattioli, M. (1972): Correlation of a precipitin reaction to an RNA protein antigen and low prevalence of nephritis in patients with systemic lupus erythematosus. *N. Engl. J. Med.*, 286:908–911.
89. Roitt, I. M., Ling, N. R., Doniach, D., and Couchman, K. G. (1964): The cytoplasmic auto-antigen of the human thyroid I. Immunological and biochemical characteristics. *Immunology*, 7:375–393.
90. Rose, N. R., Beisel, K. W., Herskowitz, A., Neu, N., Wolfgram, L. J., Alvarez, F., Traystman, M. D., and Craig, S. W. (1987): Cardiac myosin and autoimmune myocarditis. In: *Autoimmunity and autoimmune disease. Ciba Foundation Symposium 129*, edited by D. Evered, pp. 3–24; Wiley, Chichester.
91. Rose, N. R., Outschoorn, I. M., Burek, C. L., and Kuppers, R. (1987): IgG subclass distribution of anti-Tg antibodies among thyroid disease patients and their relatives and in high and low responder mouse strains. In: *Thyroid Autoimmunity—Thirtieth Anniversary: Memories and Perspectives*, Plenum Publishing Co., New York.
92. Rose, H. M., Ragan, C., Pearce, E., Lipman, M. O. (1948): Differential agglutination of normal and sensitized sheep erythrocytes by sera of patients with rheumatoid arthritis. *Proc. Soc. Exp. Biol. Med.*, 68:1–6.
93. Rubin, R. L. (1986): Enzyme-linked immunosorbent assay for anti-DNA and antihistone antibodies. In: *Manual of Clinical Laboratory Immunology*, 3rd Edition, edited by N. R. Rose, H. Friedman, and J. Fahey, pp. 744–749. American Society for Microbiology, Washington, D.C.
94. Rubin, R. L., Joslin, F. G., and Tan, E. M. (1982): A solid phase radioimmunoassay for anti-histone antibodies in human sera: Comparison with an immunofluorescence assay. *Scand. J. Immunol.*, 15:63–70.
95. Sekeris, C. E., and Guialis, A. (1981): In: *The Cell Nucleus*, edited by H. Busch. Academic Press, New York.
96. Sharp, G. C., Irvin, W. S., LaRoque, R. L., Velez, C., Daly, V., Kaiser, A. D., and Holman, H. R. (1971): Association of antibodies to different nuclear antigens with clinical patterns of rheumatic disease and responsiveness to therapy. *J. Clin. Invest.*, 50:350–359.
97. Sharp, G. C., Irvin, W. S., Tan, E. M., Bould, R. G., and Holman, H. R. (1972): Mixed connective tissue disease: An apparently distinct rheumatic disease syndrome associated with specific antibody to an extractable nuclear antigen. *Am. J. Med.*, 52:148–159.
98. Shero, J. H., Bordwell, B., Rothfield, N. F., and Earnshaw, W. C. (1986): High titers of antibodies to topoisomerase I (Scl-70) in sera from scleroderma patients. *Science*, 231:737–740.
99. Singer, J. M., and Plotz, C. M. (1956): The latex fixation test. I. Application to the serologic diagnosis of rheumatoid arthritis. *Am. J. Med.*, 21:888–892.
100. Srikanta, S., Ganda, O. P., Rabizadeh, A., Soeldner, J. S., and Eisenbarth, G. J. (1985): First-degree relatives of patients with type I diabetes mellitus. *N. Engl. J. Med.*, 313:461–464.
101. Tan, E. M., and Kunkel, H. G. (1966): Characteristics of a soluble nuclear antigen precipitating with sera of patients with systemic lupus erythematosus. *J. Immunol.*, 96:464–471.

102. Tan, E. M., Robinson, J., and Robitaille, P. (1976): Studies on antibodies to histones by immunofluorescence. *Scand. J. Immunol.*, 5:811–817.

103. Tan, E. M., and Rodman, G. P. (1976): Profile of antinuclear antibodies in progressive systemic sclerosis (PSS), abstracted. *Arthritis Rheum.*, 18:430.

104. Tan, E. M., Shur, P. H., Carr, R. I., and Kunkel, H. G. (1966): Deoxyribonucleic acid (DNA) and antibodies to DNA in the serum of patients with systemic lupus erythematosus. *J. Clin. Invest.*, 45:1732–1740.

105. Tindall, R. S. A., Kent, M., and Wells, L. (1981): A rapid immunoadsorbent RIA for anti-ACh receptor antibody. *J. Immunol. Methods.*, 45:1–14.

106. Vitti, P., Rotella, C. M., Valente, W. A., Cohen, J., Aloj, S. M., Laccetti, P., Ambesi-Impiombato, F. S., Grollman, E. F., Pinchera, A., Toccafondi, R., and Kohn, L. D. (1983): Characterization of the optimal stimulatory effects of Graves' monoclonal and serum immoglobulin G on adenosine 3',5'-monophosphate production in FRTL-5 thyroid cells: A potential clinical assay. *J. Clin. Endocrinol. Metab.*, 57:782–791.

107. Virtanen, I., Lehto, V. P., Lehtonen, E., Vartio, T., Stenman, S., Kurki, P., Wagner, O., Small, J. V., Dahl, D., and Badley, R. A. (1981): Expression of intermediate filaments in cultured cells. *J. Cell Sci.*, 50:45–63.

108. Voller, A., Bidwell, D. E., and Burek, C. L. (1980): An enzyme-linked immunosorbent assay (ELISA) for antibodies to thyroglobulin. *Proc. Soc. Exp. Biol. Med.*, 163:402–405.

109. Waaler, E. (1940): On the occurrence of a factor in human serum activating the specific agglutination of sheep blood corpuscles. *Acta Pathol. Microbiol. Scand.*, 17:172–188.

110. Weinblatt, M. D., and Schur, P. C. (1980): Rheumatoid factor detection by nephelometry. *Arthritis Rheum.*, 23:777–779.

111. Williams, D. G., Stocks, M. R., Charles, P. J., and Maini, R. N. (1986): Antibodies to La, Jo-1, nRNP and Sm detected by multi-track immunoblotting using a novel filter holder: A comparative study with counter-immunoelectrophoresis and immunodiffusion using sera from patients with systemic lupus erythematosus and Sjögren's syndrome. *J. Immunol. Methods*, 91:65–73.

112. Wilson, M. R., Nitsche, J. F. (1986): Immunodiffusion assays for antibodies to nonhistone nuclear antigens. In: *Manual of Clinical Laboratory Immunology*, 3rd Edition, edited by N.R. Rose, H. Friedman, and J. Fahey, pp. 750–754. American Society for Microbiology, Washington, D.C.

113. Witebsky, E., and Rose, N. R. (1963): Autoimmunity and its relationship to thyroid diseases. *N.Y. State J. Med.*, 63:56–59.

114. Witebsky, E., Rose, N. R., Terplan, K., Paine, J. R., and Egan, R. W. (1957): Chronic thyroiditis and autoimmunization. *JAMA*, 164:1439–1447.

115. Wold, R. T., Young, F. E., Tan, E. M., and Farr, R. S. (1968): Deoxyribonucleic acid antibody: A method to detect its primary interaction with deoxyribonucleic acid. *Science*, 161:806–807.

116. Yamagata, H., Harley, J. B., and Reichlin, M. (1984): Molecular properties of the Ro/SSA antigen and ELISA for quantitation of antibody. *J. Clin. Invest.*, 74:625–633.

117. Zakarija, M., and McKenzie, J. M. (1981): Assays for thyroid-stimulating antibody and their clinical application. In: *Physiopathology of endocrine diseases: Mechanisms of hormone action*, edited by R.J. Soto, A. De Nicola, and J. Balqier, pp. 147–152. Liss, New York.

Diagnostic Immunopathology,
edited by R.B. Colvin,
A.K. Bhan, and R.T. McCluskey.
Raven Press, New York © 1988.

6 / *Inherited and Acquired Immunodeficiency Disorders*

David T. Purtilo, James Linder, and Thomas A. Seemayer*

*Departments of Pathology and Microbiology, Pediatrics, and the Eppley Institute
for Research in Cancer and Allied Diseases, University of Nebraska Medical Center,
Omaha, Nebraska 68105; and *Department of Pathology, Montreal Children's Hospital,
and McGill University, Montreal Children's Hospital Research Institute,
Montreal, Quebec, H3H 1P3 Canada*

Recognition by Colonel Ogden Bruton in 1952 that recurrent and persistent pyogenic infections in a young man were due to lack of antibodies marked a major milestone in immunology. This initial step toward dissecting the immune system provided a foundation for defining the roles of cellular and humoral components in the resistance to infection. The molecular bases of inherited (primary immunodeficiency disorders and the role of lymphotropic viruses such as human immunodeficiency virus (HIV) in the induction of the acquired immune deficiency syndrome (AIDS) are now being elucidated. In this chapter, the clinical and histopathological features of selected immunodeficiency disorders are summarized and illustrated. Mechanisms of virus-induced immunodeficiency and opportunistic infectious diseases and malignant neoplasms will be considered in the context of defective immune surveillance.

Observations leading to the recognition of dual components of the immune system were initially based on studies of autopsy or surgical biopsy specimens of lymphoid tissues from children with inherited immune defects (1,2,62) (Fig. 1). The ablation of the thymus in mice or the bursa of Fabricius in chickens (19) indicated that these organs were essential for T or B cell development, respectively, in peripheral lymphoid tissues. These studies permitted recognition of the clinical significance of depletion of the T cell or thymus-dependent and/or B cell populations in lymphoid tissues in immune deficient patients (10). The association between autoimmunity, immunodeficiency, and lymphoma within an individual or among family members is well known (17,27).

An expert committee of the World Health Organization (WHO) has classified the primary immunodeficiency disorders (Table 1) (51,52). Specific diseases have been selected to illustrate pathognomonic or highly suggestive immunopathologic features of certain distinct entities. Undoubtedly, many immune deficiency disorders arise as the result of multiple genetic, physiologic (sex, age), and environmental (nutrition, infection, toxin) influences (44). Even though the etiological basis of the immunodeficiency is unknown for many patients, certain conclusions can be drawn by correlating the clinical and laboratory findings of a patient. The types of opportunistic infections immunocompromised individuals develop provide clues to the functional roles of T cells, antibodies and phagocytic

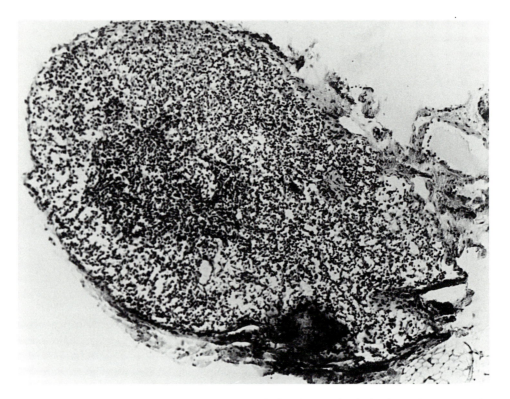

FIG. 1. Lymph node from a patient with agammaglobulinemia showing lack of germinal centers. No plasma cells are evident. X40. Published with permission of M. Lanning and Scandanavian Journal of Infectious Diseases.

leukocytes of the immune system (Table 2). This information can guide the diagnosis of immune deficiency.

At least a dozen X-linked traits are immunologically manifested. Among these are Bruton's agammaglobulinemia, severe combined immunodeficiency, Wiskott-Aldrich syndrome, chronic granulomatous disease, immunodeficiency with increased IgM, XLP, and others listed in McKusick's catalogues (37). The present challenge is to identify the genes in the X chromosome responsible for these immune deficiencies (32b), most of which probably also contribute to the more active immune response in women to most infectious agents (47).

DEVELOPMENT OF THE IMMUNE SYSTEM

Pre-B cells can be detected in the human fetal liver and later in the bone marrow. In the adult, the bone marrow is presumed to be the bursa-equivalent. The B cells enter the circulation and migrate to secondary lymphoid tissues (lymphoid follicles in the lymph nodes, spleen, Peyer's patches) (see Chapter 10). The chorioamniotic membranes normally exclude exogenous antigens that might drive immunoglobulin production in utero. Fetal B cells are able to produce IgM in response to intrauterine infections. Passive protective immunity is conferred by transport of maternal IgG by the trophoblast (other classes are not

TABLE 1. *Classification of primary immunodeficiency diseases*

Predominant antibody defects
  X-linked agammaglobulinemia
  X-linked hypogammaglobulinemia with growth hormone deficiency
  Autosomal recessive agammaglobulinemia
  Immunoglobulin deficient with increased IgM (and IgG)
  IgA deficiency
  Selective deficiency of other immunoglobulin isotypes
  Kappa chain deficiency
  Antibody deficiency with normal gamma globulin levels or hypergammaglobulinemia
  Immunodeficiency with thymoma
  Transient hypogammaglobulinemia of infancy
  Common variable immunodeficiency with predominant B-cell defect
    Nearly normal B cell number with $\mu+$, $\delta+$, with $\mu+$ $\delta+$, $\mu+$ $\gamma+$, $\gamma+$, or $\alpha+$ cells
    Very low B cell number
    $\mu+$ $\gamma+$ or γ "nonsecretory" B cells with plasma cells
    Normal or increased B cell number with $\mu+$ $\delta+$ $\gamma+$, $\alpha+$ $\mu+$ $\delta+$, $\alpha+$, and $\alpha+$ β cells
  Common variable immunodeficiency with predominant immunoregulatory T cell disorder
    Deficiency of helper T cells
    Presence of activated suppressor T cells
  Common variable immunodeficiency with autoantibodies to B or T cells
Predominant defects of cell-mediated immunity
  Combined immunodeficiency with predominant T cell defect
  Purine-nucleoside phosphorylase deficiency
  Severe combined immunodeficiency with adenosine deaminase deficiency
  Severe combined immunodeficiency
    Reticular dysgenesis
    Low T and B cell numbers
    Low T cell and normal B cell numbers (Swiss)
    "Bare-lymphocyte syndrome"
  Immunodeficiency with unusual response to Epstein-Barr virus[a]
Immunodeficiency associated with other defects
  Transcobalamin 2 deficiency
  Wiskott-Aldrich syndrome
  Ataxia-telangiectasia
  Third- and fourth-pouch/arch (DiGeorge's syndrome)

World Health Organization Classification.
[a]X-linked lymphoproliferative syndrome.

actively transported). Production of IgM and IgG commences in response to environmental antigens. Adult levels of immunoglobulin are reached sequentially: IgM at approximately 1 year, IgG at 5 to 7 years, and IgA at puberty (10 to 14 years) (51). The nadir serum IgG level is about 350 mg/dl, reached 3 to 6 months after birth. Responsiveness to polysaccharide antigens (as in vaccines) occurs later in infancy than that to protein antigens (51).

The lymphoid progenitor cells of the thymus-dependent system arise within the blood islands of the yolk sac at approximately 3 weeks of gestation. At about 6 weeks, the 3rd and 4th pharyngeal arches bud outwards and migrate caudally to form the thymus, and 2 weeks later the first wave of stem cells arrives (51). The thymus weighs about 70 g at birth, peaks at about 10 years, and then as adipose tissue replaces lymphoid tissue, the size decreases eventually to about 3 g in the elderly (51). The thymic microenvironment, especially the dendritic and epithelial cells, plays an essential but still enigmatic role, selecting immunocompetent cells that are self-tolerant. The epithelial thymus produces hormones which likely modulate the maturation of pre-T cells with T suppressor/cytotoxic or T helper/inducer capabilities (23,24) (see Chapter 10). Antigen-presenting cells (mac-

TABLE 2. *Opportunistic pathogens in immunodeficient patients*

Defective component of immune defense	Pathogens
B cell humoral responses	Pneumococcus sp. *Hemophilus influenzae* Streptococcus sp. Meningococcus sp. *Pseudomonas aeruginosa* Hepatitis B virus *Pneumocystic carinii* *Giardia lamblia* Echovirus
T cell responses	Rubeola Varicella Epstein-Barr virus Cytomegalovirus *Mycobacterium tuberculosis* Herpes simplex virus JC virus with progressive multifocal leukoencephalopathy *Mycobacterium avium intracellularis* *Candida albicans* *Histoplasma capsulatum* Cryptospordium *Pneumocystis carinii* *Strongyloides stercoralis* *Entoamoeba histolytica* *Toxoplasma gondii* *Cryptoccocus neoformans*
Phagocytic leukocytes	*Staphylococcus aureus* Klebsiella sp. *Candida albicans* Aspergillus sp. *Nocardia asteroides*

rophages) interact with the T helper/inducer cells, and together they evoke immature B cells and generate immunoglobulin secretion. These carefully orchestrated interactions are described in Chapters 1 and 10.

The lymphocyte count rises from about 5,500/µl at birth to 7,500 at 8 to 10 months. The levels then decline to the normal adult levels of 2,500/µl by about age 20 (39b). Levels below 1,500/µl in a child less than 4 years old or below 1,100/µl in an adult are abnormal (> 2 standard deviations from normal) and suggest an underlying immunodeficiency (39b).

The use of monoclonal antibodies against surface molecules of T and B cells has confirmed that the T cells in lymph nodes reside chiefly in the paracortex (Chapter 1); failure to develop cellularity in this area is characteristic of thymic deficiency. The B cells are found chiefly in the germinal centers and the medullary cords of lymph nodes; these are absent in patients with congenital agammaglobulinemia (Fig. 1). The administration of antithymocyte globulin to mice and humans depletes the thymus dependent areas immediately adjacent to the penicillar arteries in the spleen and the paracortex of lymph nodes.

PRIMARY IMMUNE DEFICIENCY DISEASES

B Cell Immunodeficiency Disorders

X-linked Agammaglobulinemia (Bruton's)

Individuals with this disorder, who are almost always males, develop infection early in childhood, characteristically after maternal antibody dissipates at 3 to 6 months after birth. Pyogenic bacterial infections result in otitis, sinusitis, pneumonitis, meningitis, or conjunctivitis. Malabsorption associated with *Giardia lamblia* may also ensue. Affected maternal male relatives can be found in about 20% (51,62).

The laboratory diagnosis requires a serum IgG of less than 200 mg/dl and markedly reduced or absent other immunoglobulin classes. Mature B cells with surface Ig are absent from the blood, although pre-B cells with small amounts of cytoplasmic IgM may be present. A lack of response to immunization with tetanus or other antigens and decreased ABO antibodies are observed. Biopsy of lymphoid tissues reveals absence of B cells and plasma cells (Fig. 1). In contrast, T cell numbers and responses are normal (mitogenic response to phytohemagglutinin, delayed-type hypersensitivity). The lack of B cells and the lack of a progressive rise in serum IgM and IgA distinguish agammaglobulinemia from transient hypogammaglobulinemia of infancy (52).

Although some heterogeneity is noted among patients with X-linked agammaglobulinemia (33), the disease is probably a single entity (51). The defect resides in the B cell. The postulated mechanism is a failure to translocate the V_H region genes resulting in a lack of maturation of pre-B cells to B cells capable of producing immunoglobulin (51). A restriction fragment-length polymorphism has localized the gene to the region Xq21.3-Xq22 on the long arm of the X chromosome (32b).

Intramuscular or intravenous immunoglobulin therapy is the cornerstone to treatment. Antibiotics or fresh frozen plasma may be added to the therapy when persistent or recurrent infections are found. Anaphylactoid reactions can occur to aggregates of IgG if present in the intravenous preparations. Although these individuals usually enjoy a long lifespan, pyogenic infections can lead to long-term sequelae, such as bronchiectasis or postmeningitis syndromes.

Selective IgA Deficiency

Selective IgA deficiency is a common disorder occurring in approximately 1 in 700 individuals. Although the majority of the patients are healthy, an increased frequency of reccurrent sinopulmonary infections, allergies, gastrointestinal tract disease, and autoimmune disease has been reported (51,52). Exposure to certain drugs, such as phenytoin or penicillamine, can induce a transient IgA deficiency that mimics this disorder, apparently due to induction of T cells that suppress IgA production.

The diagnosis is made by serum IgA levels < 5 mg/dl and normal levels of other Ig classes (some may have IgG subclass deficiencies, see below). Circulating B cells express surface IgA but fail to mature into IgA plasma cells *in vivo* or *in vitro*. A substantial fraction of these patients have antibodies to IgA, even without prior administration of blood products. Some may develop a severe anaphylactic response to transfused blood (or IgA containing fractions) and should be given washed red cells if transfusion is needed.

Normally, a differential distribution of IgA1 and IgA2 populations of lymphocytes is found in various tissues. Approximately 90% of plasma cells in bone marrow are of the IgA1 subclass, whereas equal numbers of the two subclasses are in the intestine. Most patients with IgM deficiency lack both subclasses. The minority that lack only IgG1 have abundant IgA2-producing plasma cells in the gut but a low serum IgA level (51,52). A patient that lacked secretory piece (needed for IgA secretion by epithelium) had normal serum IgA but decreased secretory IgA.

Other Class and Subclass Deficiencies

A primary, selective decrease in IgM has been associated with meningococcemia and other infections (52). Deficiency of IgM can also result from gluten enteropathy (52). One or more IgG subclass deficiencies, often with IgA deficiency has been noted. The patients lack IgG2, IgG4 or IgE (52). The subclass deficiency would be missed on routine analysis of total IgG levels, since overall IgG levels can be normal (52). Some normal persons have absent IgE (52).

Common Variable Immunodeficiency

Males and females develop variable immunoglobulin deficiency with equal frequency at any age. Three types of diseases have been identified: intrinsic B cell defects, immunoregulatory T cell disturbances, and autoantibodies to T or B cells (52). These patients have low or normal numbers of B cells and low CD4/CD8 T cell ratios, suggesting that suppressor T cells may prevent production of immunoglobulin (51). The increased CD8 cells, however, may be a response to the opportunistic infections these individuals experience, rather than the cause of the hypogammaglobulinemia.

T Cell Immunodeficiency Disorders

With the exception of DiGeorge's syndrome, most of the T cell immunodeficiency disorders also significantly involve the humoral limb because T cells regulate B cell function. Furthermore, many disorders which manifest primarily as a cellular immunodeficiency are actually a combined genetic defect that involves B and T cells.

Third- and Fourth- Pouch/Arch Syndrome (DiGeorge's Syndrome)

In 1965, DiGeorge (11) described neonatal hypocalcemic tetany resulting from hypoparathyroidism, associated with coarctation of the aorta, a small mandible, and immunodeficiency with absence of the thymus. These patients are especially susceptible to viral infection. The cause of the syndrome is thought to be an exogenous insult to the embryo at the end of the 6th week of gestation which prevents the third and fourth pharyngeal pouches/arches from giving rise to the parathyroids, thymus, portions of the neck, aortic arch, and great vessels. Experimental ablation of a portion of the cephalic portion of the neural crest in a stage 9 or 10 chick embryo markedly reduces the size of the thymus gland and may result in thymic aplasia; parathyroid, thyroid, and heart defects may also arise. This finding supports the view that diGeorge's syndrome may result from a failure of neural crest derivatives to migrate and interact properly with the pharyngeal pouch ento-derm (3).

Diagnosis relies on the characteristic clinical picture supported by hypocalcemia and absence of a thymic shadow on a lateral chest film. Marked diminution of numbers of circulating mature T cells with nearly normal levels of serum immunoglobulins and B cell populations are found. Most often the syndrome is incomplete, resulting in a hypoplastic or "a form fruste" thymus. The T cell-dependent regions of the lymph nodes and spleen are depleted of cells. Successful treatment has been achieved with fetal thymus transplantation, but even untreated patients show slow acquisition of CD4 cells and T cell function with time (52).

Mixed Immunodeficiencies

Severe Combined Immune Deficiency Syndrome

Typically, infants with severe combined immune deficiency syndrome (SCID) become ill within the first few months of life, even while maternal antibodies remain. These in-dividuals fail to grow and may have a morbilliform rash during the first few days of life. The rash may be a manifestation of graft versus host (GVH) disease due to transfer of maternal T cells (52). Early and frequent onset of infections with viruses, fungi, bacteria, and protozoan microorganisms occur. When vaccinated with live viruses, adverse reactions are common. *Pneumocystis carinii* infection may develop.

The laboratory features of severe combined immunodeficiency include serum IgG lev-els of < 150 mg/ld (unless younger than 6 months) with absent IgM, IgA, IgG, and IgE isotypes. No antibody responses to injected antigens are found. Severe lymphopenia (< 1000/μl) is usual, with reduced or absent circulating T and B cells and decreased phytohemagglutinin and mixed leukocyte responses. Patients may have circulating T cells with various phenotypes (52).

Etiology

A syndrome caused by a variety of distinct underlying defects, SCID leads to profound impairment of T and B cell function (Table 3). About half of the autosomal inherited cases are due to deficient production of adenosine deaminase, vital in the purine salvage path-way, which leads to lymphocytotoxic accumulation of adenosine. Engraftment of maternal lymphocytes in the fetus can also lead to SCID because of thymic destruction from a GVH reaction (56). The bare lymphocyte syndrome is the result of lack of expression of HLA-Class I antigens (52).

TABLE 3. *Major types of severe combined immune deficiency syndromes*

Type	Inheritance
Swiss type	X-linked, autosomal recessive
Adenosine deaminase deficiency	Autosomal recessive
Nucleoside phosphorylase deficiency	Autosomal recessive
Bare lymphocyte syndrome	Autosomal recessive
Reticular dysgenesis	Unknown inheritance
Sporadic	Maternal-fetal T lymphocyte engraftment

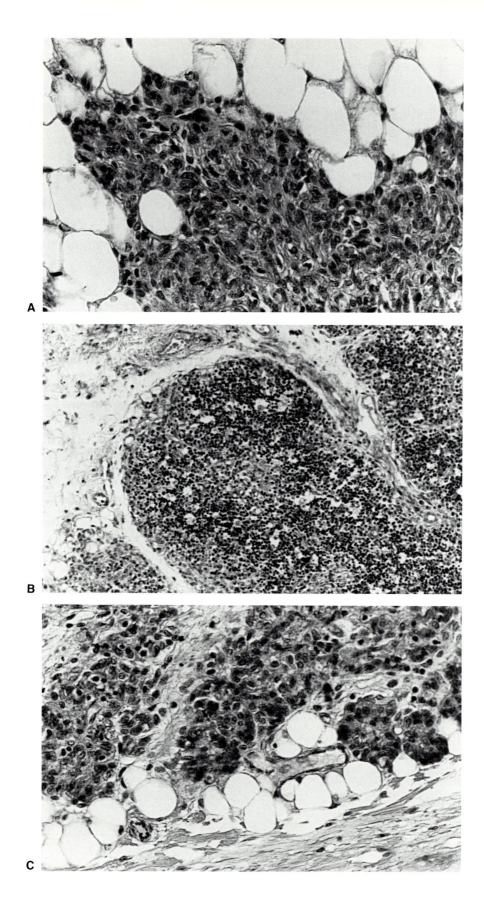

Thymic lesions in SCID

Recent descriptions of the thymus glands from patients with SCID permits discrimination of the lesions from acquired thymic changes. Although 2.5 g has been suggested as a cutoff point to distinguish thymuses congenitally (genetically) defective from acquired involution, weight alone is not a reliable discriminant. More important are the histopathologic findings described recently by Nezelof (41) of untreated or unsuccessively treated SCID. The adjectives, dysplastic or hypoplastic, are used to connote an arrest in the embryological development of the thymus, whereas degenerative and atrophic thymic changes are observed in involuted glands.

Nezelof has proposed (41) four categories of thymic histology in SCID. *Simple Dysplasia*, the most common form, resembles lesions in the nude mouse. Thymic lobules are small, separated by abundant adipose or fibroadipose tissue, and composed of polyhedral cells with scanty, poorly defined, eosinophilic cytoplasm and an ovoid nucleus (Fig. 2A). Corticomedullary demarcation and Hassall's corpuscles are not identified, and lymphoid cells are sparse. *Dysplasia with stromal corticomedullary differentiation* is characterized by larger lobules than the foregoing. Corticomedullary differentiation is evident despite the lack of lymphocytes and Hassall's corpuscles (Fig. 2B). *Dysplasia with a pseudoglandular appearance* is a rare, primitive pattern, wherein epithelial cells are arranged in clusters reminiscent of groups of acini in a glandular pattern (Fig. 2C). No Hassall's corpuscles or lymphoid cells can be observed. A pattern *similar to atrophy* is occasionally seen. The lobules are similar in size and shape to the simple dysplastic SCID thymus, but sometimes larger. Hassall's corpuscles are present in reduced numbers and lymphocytes tend to be concentrated to the medulla giving an "inverted" thymic pattern.

Nezelof (41) has suggested that thymic morphology varies with the age of death of the patient. The patterns seen, arranged from youngest to oldest are: (a) dysplasia with pseudoglandular pattern, (b) dysplasia with corticomedullary demarcation, (c) simple dysplasia, and (d) atrophic pattern. Nezelof has suggested that these thymic changes progress with the duration of the disease. As expected, the lymph nodes in patients with SCID are small or absent. Only sparse periarteriolar lymphoid tissue is seen in spleen.

Monoclonal antibodies reactive with the epithelial component of the thymus have disclosed an arrest in the development of the endocrine-associated epithelium of patients with SCID (34). During ontogeny, partitioning of the epithelium into cortical and medullary zones occurs at about 14 weeks of gestation; Hassall's corpuscles appear during the next 2 weeks as derivatives of medullary epithelium. Monoclonal antibodies reactive with epithelium in the medullary show complete absence of reactivity in the thymus of SCID patients. This supports the notion of an arrested development of thymic epithelium before the development of Hassall's corpuscles at 14 to 16 weeks (23).

Treatment

Successful treatment of SCID by histocompatible bone marrow transplantation was accomplished in 1968 by Gatti and Good (19). This therapy has prevented opportunistic

---

FIG. 2. A. Thymus. Severe combined immune deficiency. Simple dysplasia. No corticomedullary demarcation is seen. The lobule is constituted by immature epithelial cells. Hematoxylin and eosin X400. **B.** Thymus. Severe combined immune deficiency. Dysplasia similar to severe atrophy but stromal corticomedullary demarcation is noted. Hematoxylin and eosin X400. **C.** Thymus. Severe combined immune deficiency. Thymic dysplasia with pseudoglandular appearance. Acinar pattern of epithelial components of thymic lobule. Hematoxylin and eosin X400.

infection and malignant lymphoma (29,40). These patients may also require intramuscular gammaglobulin and antibiotics if reconstitution is not complete (16). Limited benefit has resulted from transplantation of fetal liver, thymus, or cultured thymic epithelium (4,40,52). Replacement with marrow argues for a stem cell defect rather than a thymic defect. Reconstitution with bone marrow from HLA incompatible donors, depleted of T cells with lectins or monoclonal antibodies, has also been successful (52). These patients are exquisitely sensitive to GVH disease (52) and have frequently developed Epstein-Barr virus (EBV) positive lymphomas (35,39a).

Wiskott-Aldrich Syndrome

Males with this rare ($4/10^6$ male births) X-linked recessive disorder present with severe eczema and may have hemorrhage due to microthrombocytopenia and defective platelet function. Also, they manifest complex immunodeficiencies due to defective T-B cell and T-T cell interactions (19,38).

Recurrent infections with pyogenic microorganisms are common as an eczema and autoimmune disturbance. A 128-fold increased risk of extranodal lymphoma compared to nonimmunodeficient patients has been noted. By the 4th decade, nearly 100% of the patients develop malignant lymphoma (14). The serum contains decreased levels of IgM but elevated (IgA, IgE) or normal (IgG) levels of the other immunoglobulin. Curiously, these patients do not make an antibody response to polysaccharide antigens, including ABO antigens; thus, their serum lacks isohemagglutinins (52). By age 6 years, T lymphopenia develops. A 115 kd protein is absent from T cells and glycoprotein Ib from platelets (52).

Antibiotic treatment is required to prevent infection by encapsulated pyogenic bacteria. Immunoglobulin therapy may be problematic because of thrombocytopenia. Steroids and splenectomy are cautioned against because of increased susceptibility to sepsis. Bone marrow transplantation can restore the T cell and B cell function, with cure of the eczema, but the thrombocytopenia persists (52).

Ataxia-telangiectasia

This autosomal recessive, multisystem disease is characterized by cerebellar ataxia, telangiectasia of the sclera and nasal skin, recurrent sinopulmonary infections, and variable immunodeficiency. The patients may also manifest gonadal dysgenesis and mental retardation (36,60).

Diagnosis is based on finding variable immune deficiency in conjunction with the hematologic and clinical findings. In approximately 40% of the cases, IgA is absent, and IgG subclass deficiency is frequently seen. Variable antibody responses are found following immunization. Curiously, elevated serum alpha fetoprotein often occurs, possibly as a manifestation of a mesenchymal defect.

Lymphomas occur with increased frequency, predominantly non-Hodgkins lymphomas. However, T and B lymphocytic leukemia, Hodgkin's disease, and carcinomas of the gastrointestinal tract and other organs also arise at increased frequency in these patients. Prospective studies of patients with ataxia-telangiectasia have revealed an increased percentage of lymphocytes containing translocations involving band 14q12, the region of the α chain of the T cell antigen receptor (59b) towards the centromere of the long arm of chromosome 14 (28). Ataxia-telangiectasia, as well as Bloom's syndrome and Fanconi's anemia, are among the clastogenic syndromes that are characterized by chromosomal fragility (44). Some leukemias and lymphomas arising in these patients are probably related to the chromosomal translocations occurring in lymphoid cells. The B-cell lymphomas, however, are more likely associated with defective immune surveillance to EBV (53).

X-linked Lymphoproliferative Syndrome (Duncan's Syndrome)

The X-linked lymphoproliferative syndrome (XLP) is characterized by immune deficiency to Epstein-Barr virus (EBV). Life-threatening or fatal infectious mononucleosis (about 63% of cases), acquired hypogammaglobulinemia (25%), or malignant B-cell lymphomas (23%) invariably arise following primary infection with the virus (46).

Diagnosis

The affected males in our XLP Registry have ranged from 5 months to 40 years of age. The mortality is 85% by the third decade and apparently, 100% by 40 years. The occurrence of the above three phenotypes in maternally related males less than 40 years of age is presumptive evidence that XLP is responsible. Investigation of lymphoid tissues using molecular probes reveals the EBV genome. Serum of patients with acute infectious mononucleosis contain EBV specific antibodies, usually of low titer. Atypical lymphocytosis with polyclonal activation of B cells leads to hypergammaglobulinemia. The lymphocytosis predominantly involves $CD8^+$ T cells and natural killer (NK) cell phenotypes. Long-term survivors usually lack antibodies to EB nuclear-associated antigen (EBNA). Generally, the patients manifest no increased susceptibility to infection prior to encountering EBV. However, affected males challenged with a prototype antigen, bacteriophage φX174, fail to switch from IgM to IgG on secondary challenge (42). Shown in Figure 3 are the hypothesized chronological events occurring in patients with this genetic defect. A few females

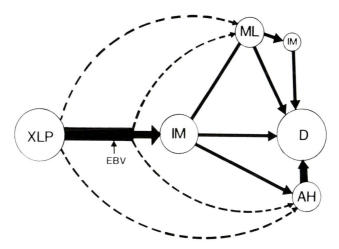

FIG. 3. Hypothesized events in the pathogenesis of X-linked lymphoproliferative syndrome (XLP). The size of the circles and arrows indicate the relative number of patients who have the phenotypes. IM = infectious mononucleosis; AH = acquired hypogammaglobulinemia; ML = malignant lymphoma; D = death; and EBV = Epstein-Barr virus. From Purtilo, D.T. (1987): Immunoglobulin therapy in the x-linked lymphoproliferative syndrome. *Vox Sanguinis*, 52:4, with permission of S. Karger AG, Basel.

have been described with a similar EBV syndrome; the relationship to the putative X-linked form is not clear (52).

Histopathology

Following EBV infection, the lymphoid tissue shows a biphasic response: first an explosive lymphoproliferation and then hypoplasia. The thymus gland shows destruction of Hassall's corpuscles. Multinucleated giant cells may be present in the medulla. During the lymphoproliferative phase, the thymus is invaded by EBV-infected B cells (Fig. 4), which are surrounded by CD8[+] T cells and NK cells. In the liver, a similar B cell infiltrate with CD8[+] T cells and NK cells in the periportal regions is likely responsible for fulminant hepatitis. The virus-associated hemophagocytic syndrome may occur. Approximately 90% of the deaths are due to hemorrhage or infection.

The B cell lymphomas can follow a protracted course of infectious mononucleosis or emerge without antecedent IM. The lymphomas are all extranodal, have a good prognosis, and often have concomitant acquired hypogammaglobulinemia and low CD4/CD8 blood T cell ratios (21).

Treatment

Prevention of the life-threatening EBV diseases in XLP is based on detecting the defect before the EBV infection in siblings, using φX174 challenge (42). The affected seronegative males should be placed on prophylactic immunoglobulin therapy because 100% of patients

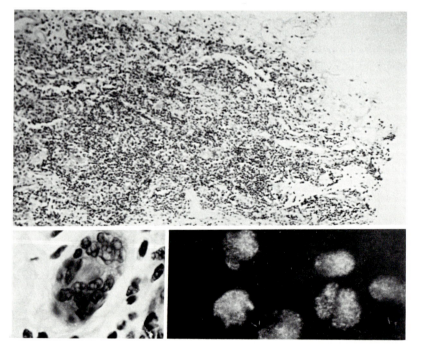

FIG. 4. Thymus from a patient with the fatal IM phenotype of XLP showing lymphoproliferation with loss of corticomedullary demarcation. Inset demonstrates a multinucleated giant cell and another inset EB nuclear antigen staining of B cells infiltrating the gland.

have died by 40 years of age. Bone marrow transplantation from HLA-matched donors has restored immunity to EBV and the number of T cells and immunoglobulin levels returned to nearly normal in two males within 6 weeks; however, both subsequently died with sepsis after the grafts had been established (15).

Chediak-Higashi Syndrome

This autosomal recessive condition involves multiple systems and is manifested by partial albinism, giant lysosomes of leukocytes, increased susceptibility to bacterial infections, and lymphoproliferation. The patients characteristically have defective NK cell activity and elevated antibodies to EBV (38). An accelerated lymphoproliferative phase frequently leads to death of the patients before 10 years of age.

At autopsy, the thymus is devoid of epithelium and depleted of lymphoid cells (32a). A lymphoid infiltrate with plasma cell differentiation involves periportal regions of liver and these cells disseminate throughout the body. Although EBV genome (K. McClain, *personal communication*) has been detected in one case, the clonality of the proliferation is unclear. No treatment other than supportive antibiotic therapy has been available for these patients.

ACQUIRED OR SECONDARY IMMUNODEFICIENCY DISEASES

Acquired immune deficiency disorders occur much more commonly than do primary immune deficiency disorders. Many agents and conditions can conspire to induce immune deficiency (Table 4). Protein-calorie malnutrition, infectious diseases, especially viruses, (20) and catabolic states, such as cancer, severe burns, or chronic renal or hepatic failure, are a few of the common disorders characterized by acquired immunodeficiency.

Protein-calorie Malnutrition

During the past century, a marked decline in prevalence of infectious disease has occurred, owing largely to improvements in nutrition and sanitation in developed countries. In contrast, protein-calorie malnutrition (PCM) prevails in several hundred million preschool-aged children in the third world. Kwashiorkor, a form of PCM, in the Ga language of Ghana, literally means "one-two." The malnutrition results when a child is displaced from its mother's breast by a newborn sibling. Another form of PCM, marasmus, means "withering." Kwashiorkor results from a deficiency primarily of protein, while total

TABLE 4. *Acquired or secondary immunodeficiency diseases*

Infections, especially parasitic, viral intracellular, bacterial, fungal, and spirochetal
Immunosuppressive or cytotoxic therapy including corticosteroids, cytotoxic agents, and irradiation
Trauma including surgery and burns
Pregnancy
Catabolic states including protein-losing enteropathy, lymphangiectasia, chronic renal, or hepatic
　disorders
Autoimmune disorders
Protein-calorie malnutrition

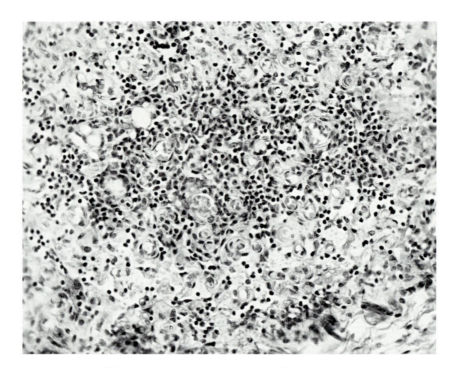

FIG. 5. Thymus from a child with severe protein-calorie malnutrition displaying marked depletion of lymphoid cells with a loss of corticomedullary demarcation, coalescence of Hassall's epithelial bodies and edema in the intralobular connective tissues. Hematoxylin and eosin X350.

caloric intake is adequate, whereas marasmus is a deprivation of both protein and calories. Both disorders show atrophy of the immune system concomitantly with other organs.

Nutritional thymectomy occurs in patients with extensive PCM (49,58a). Histopathologic patterns range from normal histology to acute or chronic involution of the thymus. Usually, thymic lobules are small due to reduced numbers of lymphocytes and a loss of the corticomedullary demarcation. The atrophic thymus shows lobules with indented edges, a lack of corticomedullary differentiation, few lymphocytes, and mostly fibroblast-like cells (Fig. 5) (12,49). The Hassall's corpuscles may be cystic and occasionally calcified. As a consequence of lymphoid cell depletion, the Hassall's corpuscles tend to coalesce into the central medullary portion. The connective tissue surrounding the lobules often is fibrotic and/or edematous. The findings in PCM are comparable to stress-induced atrophy. The thymus-dependent periarteriolar lymphoid sheath in the spleen can be substantially depleted, as are paracortical regions of lymph nodes. The nodal sinuses are generally expanded by edema or filled with histiocytes. Laboratory evaluation shows global (T cell and B cell) deficiency in severe PCM (Table 5). Therefore, it is not surprising to find an array of microbes and nematodes that exact substantial morbidity and mortality (57).

Within 2 to 3 weeks following nutritional replenishment, the number of T lymphcytes in the peripheral blood returns to normal. In contrast, serum albumin does not approach normal levels until approximately 6 weeks (8). Whether permanent damage to the immune system remains in individuals with extensive PCM and nutritional thymectomy who survive is unknown (61).

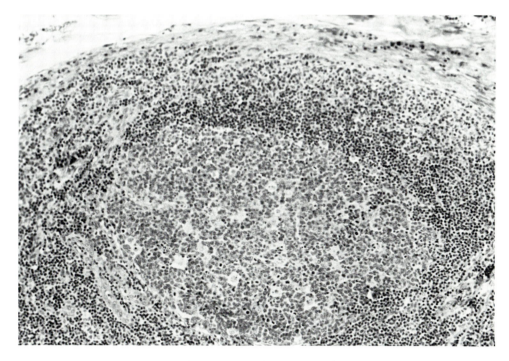

FIG. 6. Lymph node biopsy from AIDS patients may show explosive follicular hyperplasia with both regularly and irregularly shaped follicles. Numerous tangible body macrophages are present. Hematoxylin and eosin X250. Published with permission of W.B. Saunders Co.

TABLE 5. *Immune defects secondary to malnutrition*

Humoral immunity
    Serum complement decreased (hence, deficient killing of gram-negative bacteria)
    Serum transferrin decreased (thus, loss of this bacteriostatic defense)
    Immunoglobulins increased during infection; secretory IgA, however, decreased
    Antibody-forming capacity reduced (cannot mount antibodies against bacteria)

Cellular immunity
    Atrophic thymus and lymphoid organs. Increased vulnerability to intracellular microbes results in death
        from certain bacterial (i.e., tuberculosis), viral (i.e., measles), and nematode (i.e., Strongyloides)
        infections
    Interferon

Phagocytes
    Neutrophils fail to migrate, phagocytose, digest, and kill bacteria
    Macrophages fail to kill bacteria

From Seshi, B. and Purtilo, D.T. (1984): Humoral immune responses in parasitized, malnourished children. In: *Nutrition, Disease Resistance, and Immune Function,* edited by R.R. Watson, pp. 71–86. Marcel Dekker, New York. Published with permission of Marcel Dekker.

Stress-induced Involution of Thymus

Acute illness can lead to involution of the thymus within hours to days. A study of 200 cases revealed four progressive stages (25). Stage I, involving the initial lesion, appears within 12 to 24 hours and consists of lymphophagocytosis. Advanced lymphophagocytosis develops between 24 to 28 hours (stage II). Stage III appears by 47 to 72 hours and consists of cortical lymphocytic depletion. Beyond 3 days the thymus displays lobular shrinkage, and the medulla contains more lymphocytes than the cortex (so-called "inversion") and has an increased amount of interlobular connective tissue (stage IV). Thymic epithelium usually remains intact; calcification of some Hassall's corpuscles may be found. Similar thymic histology is seen after radiation, corticosteroid or cytotoxic chemotherapy.

Virus-induced Immune Suppression

Four mechanisms have been described by which viruses cause immune suppression (20): (a) induction of suppressor macrophages that temporarily effect anergy as in hepatitis B, cytomegalovirus (CMV), and EBV infections (22,48); (b) selective destruction, inactivation, or arrested maturation of helper or effector T cells has been identified in experimental animals infected by specific viruses and in humans with HIV (see below); (c) soluble suppressor factors (such as prostaglandins) elaborated by lymphocytes or macrophages are produced during viral infections; and (d) inactivation of macrophages can occur during acute influenza infection.

Acquired Immune Deficiency Syndrome (AIDS)

Caused by the human immunodeficiency virus (HIV), AIDS emerged in the late 1970s and was formerly known as HTLV-III or lymphadenopathy-associated virus (LAV). It has a tropism for T helper/inducer cells and other cells bearing the CD4 molecule (18) and is characterized by severe immunologic deficiency, opportunistic infectious diseases, Kaposi's sarcoma, and non-Hodgkin's lymphoma (9,50). The epidemiology, clinical and laboratory findings, histopathology, etiological bases, prevention, and treatment of AIDS will be briefly reviewed. Owing to the rapid pace of new information, our review is incomplete.

Definition

Requests for Pentamidine from physicians in New York City and San Francisco for treatment of *Pneumocystis carinii* pneumonia led to recognition of a new immune deficiency syndrome in 1981 (6,7). Epidemiologists from the Centers for Disease Control (CDC) found homosexual men were predominantly affected. The CDC has developed evolving diagnostic criteria, which until June 1981, did not include results of serologic tests.

The clinical definition of AIDS requires that a patient have a reliably diagnosed disorder that is indicative of an underlying cellular immunodeficiency and that no other known cause of cellular immune deficiency or reduced resistance associated with particular diseases be present (50). Pediatric AIDS is similarly defined with the exclusion of congenital infections (i.e., toxoplasmosis or Herpes simplex virus infection in the first month after birth or CMV infection in the first 6 months after birth). Primary immunodeficiency diseases and secondary immunodeficiency associated with immunosuppressive therapy, lymphoreticular malignancy, or starvation must be excluded.

The CDC has further refined the case definition of AIDS to include patients with any of the following diseases, if the patient has a positive serologic or virologic test for HIV:

- disseminated histoplasmosis (not confined to lungs or lymph nodes)
- isosporosis, causing chronic diarrhea (over 1 month)
- bronchial or pulmonary candidiasis
- non-Hodgkin's lymphoma of high-grade type (diffuse, undifferentiated) of B cell or unknown immunologic phenotype
- histologically confirmed Kaposi's sarcoma in patients who are 60 years of age or younger when diagnosed.

To increase the specificity of the case definition, cases are excluded if they have a negative result on testing for serum antibody to HIV, have no other type of HIV test with a positive result, and do not have a low number of CD4$^+$ lymphocytes or a low ratio of CD4/CD8 lymphocytes. In the absence of results of HIV tests, patients satisfying all other clinical criteria in the definition will continue to be included.

Definition of AIDS-related complex

It was recognized that the same population at risk for AIDS—homosexual men, intravenous drug abusers, and recipients of HIV-contaminated blood products such as hemophiliacs—was being affected by a syndrome consisting of generalized lymphadenopathy, fatigue, fever, night sweats, and weight loss (50). This has been defined as the AIDS-related complex (ARC), which is a combination of clinical signs/symptoms and laboratory abnormalities (50), as presented in Table 6. As time passes and experience is gained in integrating results of HIV serology, we can anticipate that the definitions of AIDS and ARC will continue to be refined (Table 7) (55).

TABLE 6. *Definition of AIDS-related complex*

Clinical
    Fever: ≥100°F, intermittent or continuous, for at least 3 months, in the absence of other identifiable causes
    Weight loss: ≥10% or ≥15 lbs
    Lymphadenopathy: persistent for at least 3 months, involving two extrainguinal node-bearing areas
    Diarrhea: intermittent or continuous, ≥3 months, in the absence of other identifiable causes
    Fatigue, to the point of decreased physical or mental function
    Night sweats: intermittent or continuous, ≥3 months, in the absence of other identifiable causes

Laboratory
    Decreased numbers of helper T cells (≥2 standard deviations below mean)
    Decreased T-helper/T-suppressor ratio (≥2 standard deviations below mean)
    At least one of the following: leukopenia, thrombocytopenia, absolute lymphopenia or anemia
    Elevated concentrations of serum immunoglobulins
    Depressed lymphocyte blastogenesis (pokeweed and PHA)
    Anergy in standard skin tests (using Multi-test or equivalent)

At least two of the above *clinical* signs/symptoms lasting 3 or more months plus two or more of the above *laboratory* abnormalities, occurring in a patient having no underlying infectious cause for the symptoms and who is in a cohort at increased risk for developing AIDS. From Purtilo, D.T. et al. (1986): Acquired immune deficiency syndrome (AIDS). *Clin. Lab. Med.,* 6:3. Published with permission of W.B. Saunders Co.

TABLE 7. *Summary of classification system for HIV[a] infections*

Group I	Acute infection (transient symptoms with seroconversion)
Group II	Asymptomatic infection
Group III	Persistent generalized lymphadenopathy
Group IV	Other manifestations
	Chronic constitutional disease
	Neurologic disease
	Specified secondary infections
	Specified secondary cancers
	Other conditions

[a]HIV, human immunodeficiency virus.
From Selik, R.M. et al. (1986): CDC's definition of AIDS. *N. Engl. J. Med.* 315:761. Published with permission of New England Journal of Medicine.

Epidemiology of AIDS

When recognized as a syndrome, the number of cases doubled every 6 months and were generally confined to various high risk groups (9). More recently, the doubling time has increased to about 1 year. This suggests some slowing in the spread of AIDS, yet the pool of individuals that have been exposed to the virus is enormous. Cases have occurred in Europe, Africa, Asia, and South America. The syndrome has become the leading cause of death in young men in Manhattan, and retrospective studies have revealed that 40% HIV seropositive homosexual men in Manhattan developed AIDS during a three-year period of study (13). Estimates are that from 3 to 10 million Africans and about 1.5 million Americans are seropositive for HIV. An estimated 275,000 cases of AIDS will likely occur by 1991 in the United States (13).

Clinical and laboratory findings

The presenting symptoms of AIDS and ARC include: unexplained fever associated with opportunistic infection; cutaneous or visceral Kaposi's sarcoma; cough and dyspnea from the opportunistic pulmonary infections; diarrhea associated with parasites and bacteria; lymphadenopathy from viral, mycobacterial infections, and lymphoma; hematological disorders due to cytopenias; and headaches and neurological changes associated with malignant lymphoma and viral, fungal and parasitic infection of the brain.

Hematopathology of AIDS

Since the CD4$^+$ cell is the major target of HIV, it is not surprising that lymphoreticular organs are markedly damaged in AIDS. Recognizing lesions prevalent in AIDS is potentially useful for diagnosing AIDS, as well as understanding its pathogenesis.

Lymph nodes. Lymph node biopsy specimens from patients with ARC and AIDS may show three major histologic patterns: "explosive" follicular hyperplasia, follicular involution, and a combination of explosive follicular hyperplasia and follicular involution. The characteristic HIV particles can be seen by electron microscopy.

Explosive follicular hyperplasia is characterized by distortion of nodal architecture by lymphoid follicles which are increased in both size and number. The germinal centers have irregular shapes and serrated margins. Elongated or dumbbell configurations are common. Numerous tangible body macrophages are present within the germinal centers, imparting a starry sky pattern at low magnification (Fig. 6). In the parafollicular areas of the lymph nodes immunoblasts and blood vessels proliferate. Sinus histiocytosis with macrophages containing engulfed nuclear debris and polymorphonuclear leukocytes is seen. This pattern occurs in approximately 70% of lymph node biopsy specimens.

Follicular involution occurs in approximately 25% of biopsies. In striking contrast to the explosive follicular hyperplasia, the follicles are small, hypocellular, and frequently hyalinized (Fig. 7). Vascular proliferation is more prominent in this pattern. The interfollicular cells are polymorphous with numerous immunoblasts, plasmacytoid lymphocytes, and small lymphocytes. The remaining 5% of patients have a mixed histology of follicular hyperplasia and follicular hyperplasia can evolve to a pattern of follicular involution.

Immunophenotyping of lymph nodes from patients with AIDs or ARC discloses decreased numbers of CD4$^+$ T cells, paralleling the inverted CD4/CD8 ratio of peripheral blood lymphocytes. Immunofluorescence or immunoperoxidase stains of lymph nodes with B cell-antisera reveals a mixed population of cells which possesses all classes of heavy and light chain immunoglobulins. These morphologic changes likely reflect underlying defective immunoregulation secondary to infection by HIV. The severity of the immune defect parallels the histologic pattern: follicular involution is associated with a profound depression of the CD4/CD8 ratio. These patients are at great risk for severe infection, Kaposi's sarcoma or malignant lymphoma.

Approximately 15% of patients with AIDS develop non-Hodgkin's lymphomas, which are usually of high histologic grade, such as undifferentiated or immunoblastic lymphoma. Burkitt's lymphomas (BL) or BL-like lesions having t(8;14) karyotypes and EBV-DNA within the tumors frequently occur (Fig. 8). The underlying immune defect in AIDS

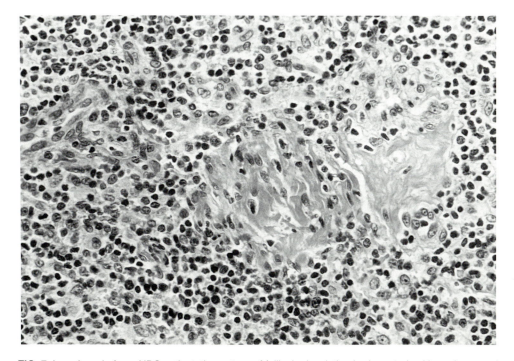

FIG. 7. Lymph node from AIDS patient; the pattern of follicular involution is characterized by a decreased number of follicles, a paucity of cells in T-cell zones, and frequently hyalinization of follicular centers. Hematoxylin and eosin X400. Published with permission of W.B. Saunders Co.

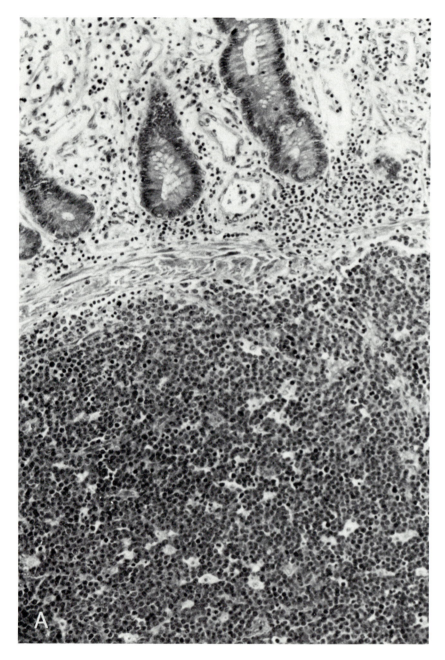

FIG. 8. A. Small bowel biopsy of 24-year-old man with AIDS reveals submucosa expanded by a monotonous proliferation of lymphoid cells. X250. (*Figure continues*)

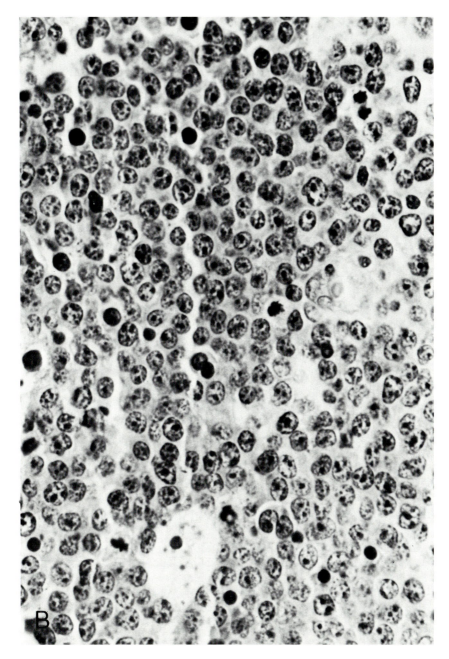

FIG. 8 (*continued*). **B.** Monotonous lymphoid cells have smooth contours and prominent chromocenters intermixed with tangible body macrophages. These features are typical of Burkitt's lymphoma. X750. Published with permission of W.B. Saunders Co.

permits uncontrolled proliferation of EBV-infected B cells. In some AIDS patients angio-immunoblastic lymphadenopathy with dysproteinemia precedes the development of malignant lymphoma. Molecular and cytogenetic alteration in B cell may occur due to mechanisms analogous to that proposed by Kelin in Africans developing Burkitt's lymphoma (30).

Lymph nodes from AIDS patients may harbor small foci of metastatic Kaposi's sarcoma (KS). Extensive serial sectioning of lymph nodes may be necessary to identify subcapsular aggregations of spindle-shaped tumor cells.

The life-threatening infections typical of AIDS, such as disseminated *Mycobacterium avium intracellulare*, may evoke granulomatous inflammation or aggregates of epithelioid histiocytes filled with organisms in lymph nodes. Likewise, systemic fungal or toxoplasmal infections may be detected in the lymph node biopsy. Lymphadenopathy of suspected infectious origin may be evaluated by fine-needle aspiration to obtain material for microbial culture or stained smears. Needle aspiration may also identify malignant lymphoma or metastic KS, although the focality of this latter lesion limits the sensitivity of this technique.

Bone Marrow. The bone marrow of the AIDS patient is frequently abnormal. Granulocytic hyperplasia or plasmacytosis may occur secondary to infection. Lymphohistocytic aggregates secondary to mycobacterial infection may mimic malignant lymphoma. *M. avian intracellulare* may be within macrophages, without developing well-formed granulomas, so that acid-fast stains of all marrow aspirates or biopsies ought to be examined.

Spleen. The spleen may exhibit lymphoid hyperplasia or lymphoid depletion, analogous to that occurring in the lymph nodes. Because morphologic examination of the spleen does not occur until autopsy, most patients have advanced lymphoid depletion. An onionskin appearance of collagen around arterioles, reminiscent of systemic lupus erythematosus, is common (Fig. 9). Many of the follicles are hyalinized, reflecting a depleted stage of the immune system. The red pulp is typically congested and contains plasmacytoid cells. If infection is present, numerous polymorphonuclear leukocytes may be seen. Erythrophagocytosis and extramedullary hemotpoiesis are often identified.

Thymus. The thymus can be so markedly damaged in AIDS that it may be impossible to identify at autopsy. When the gland is present, marked lymphoid depletion is seen. Hassall's corpuscles may or may not be evident and, if present, they may be calcified. The gland assumes a rudimentary morphology, similar to that seen in graft versus host disease, severe combined immune deficiency and several immune deficiency conditions (Fig. 10). Patients with AIDS have deficient circulating thymic hormones. These findings suggest that thymic damage may play a role in the evolution of AIDS. Biopsy of the thymus in children with AIDS has shown similar histology to the adult patients (26).

Pathogenesis

A retrovirus closely related to lentiviruses, HIV is highly mutable. Thus, a patient may be infected with different strains of HIV (59). The virus produces severe crippling of the immune system by infecting T cells through binding to the CD4 molecule, which acts as a receptor for the virus. It is apparent that not only T cells bearing the CD4 molecule, but other cells including macrophages, B cells, endothelial cells and cells in the brain may also be infected. In some cases, this has related to surface CD4 expression (macrophages). The consequent immune defects that can occur in the infected individual are thought to be due to the direct viral infection producing lysis of $CD4^+$ cells. The net effect is a quantitative

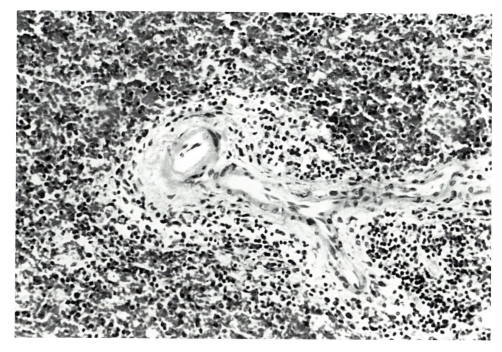

FIG. 9. Depletion of periarteriolar lymphocytes of the spleen is common in AIDS. Blood vessels may show hyalinization of their walls. The splenic parenchyma is congested with red blood cells. X250. Published with permission of W.B. Saunders Co.

TABLE 8. *Immune dysfunction in AIDS*

Cutaneous anergy
Lymphopenia predominantly due to a selective defect in the helper/inducer subset (OKT4, Leu-3) or T-lymphocytes
Decreased *in vivo* T cell function
    Susceptibility to opportunistic neoplasms
    Susceptibility to opportunistic infections
    Decreased delayed-type hypersensitivity
Altered *in vitro* T cell function
    Decreased blast transformation
    Decreased alloreactivity
    Decreased specific and natural killer cytotoxicity
    Increased numbers of cells marking with HNK1 antibody
    Decreased ability to provide help to B lymphocytes
    Decreased thymosin alphal levels
    Increased acid-labile interferon levels
B cell dysregulation
    Due to polyclonal B cell activation by HIV, and/or EBV, CMV
    Inability to mount a *de novo* serologic response to a new antigen
    Refractoriness to B cell activation by pokeweed mitogen and to EBV
    Decreased population of cells with EBV receptors
    Circulating immune complexes

Modified from Purtilo, D.T. et al. (1986): Acquired immune deficiency syndrome (AIDS). *Clin. Lab. Med.,* 6:3. Published with permission of W.B. Saunders Co.

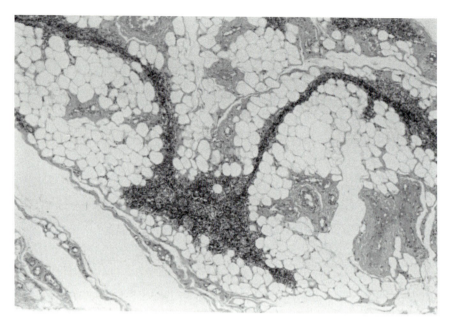

FIG. 10. Thymus gland of patient with acquired immune deficiency syndrome. Marked depletion of lymphocytes in cortex and precocious involution of Hassall's bodies are seen. Hematoxylin and eosin X40.

decrease in helper/inducer T cells, decreased immunologic responses to soluble antigens, and decreased induction of virus-specific cytotoxic cells. Paradoxically, polyclonal activation of B cells occurs with elevation (often marked) of serum IgG and IgM. Recently, Schnittman and colleagues (54) have presented convincing evidence that HIV itself acts as a polyclonal activator *in vitro*. However, the ubiquitous EBV could also contribute to the hyperimmunoglobulinemia, as it and other infectious agents are polyclonal B cell activators.

Immunologic findings

Individuals with ARC or AIDS have cellular immune deficiency dominated by decreased total T cells and CD4$^+$ T cells. The most characteristic of the cellular abnormalities is a depletion of the absolute number of circulating T cells of the CD4$^+$ phenotype. Concurrently, there is a lowered CD4/CD8 ratio. A gradation from extensive loss (ratio < 0.2) to slight depletion (0.8–1.0) is seen. The CD4/CD8 ratios in ascending order are: opportunistic infections < Kaposi's sarcoma < AIDS-related immune complex. Indeed, the observation of diminished CD4 cell populations led to the hypothesis that the etiology of AIDS was a virus that destroyed these cells. Monocyte adherence, B cell numbers, and delayed hypersensitivity responses are also depressed. Immunoglobulin concentrations are elevated in a polyclonal fashion. Often serum interferon levels, especially acid-labile alpha-interferon, are elevated. Immune complexes and various other immunological perturbations (summarized in Table 8) are found in a majority of patients.

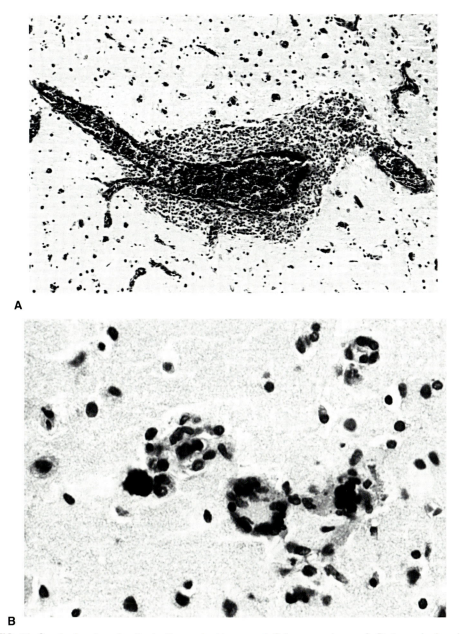

FIG. 11. Cerebral cortex of patient with acquired immune deficiency syndrome. **A.** Perivascular lymphoid infiltrate. Hematoxylin and eosin X75. **B.** Multinucleated giant cells. Hematoxylin and eosin X450.

Infective lesions of the central nervous system.

A variety of neurological disorders are associated with AIDS (5). Nearly one-third of patients with AIDS have premortem neurological abnormalities and over 75% of autopsy subjects have histologic evidence of neurological involvement. In addition to opportunistic infections by *Toxoplasma gondii*, fungi, and other agents, JC virus and herpes simplex may infect the CNS. Progressive dementia and cerebral atrophy are common. Concomitant infection by HIV has been incriminated as being responsible for the syndrome. Viral particles resembling HIV occur in giant multinucleated histiocytes or astrocytes in brains of encephalopathic patients (5) (Fig. 11). Human immunodeficiency virus has been identified in macrophages by virus isolation, *in situ* hybridization, immunocytochemistry and transmission electron microscopy (31). The diagnostic feature is the presence of multinucleated cells.

Multinucleated giant cells have been described, in addition to the brain, in lymph nodes and lungs *in vivo* in patients with AIDS and ARC. Multinucleated T cells form *in vitro* in response to HIV, mediated by the CD4 molecule. Possibly, the monocyte/macrophage serves as a major virus reservoir. Infection of other cells such as glia, neurons and endothelial cells could also play a role in the pathogenesis of AIDS dementia.

Mortality with AIDS

The morbidity and mortality of patients with AIDS is substantial: almost all patients have died within two years after diagnosis. Unless a cure for AIDS becomes available, all patients with AIDS will likely die. Many experimental drugs are being tested; Azidothymidine (AZT) has shown initial promise.

AIDS-associated opportunistic malignancies

Table 9 summarizes the major forms of opportunistic malignancies occurring in individuals with AIDS. Kaposi's sarcoma (KS) may be etiologically associated with the ubiquitous CMV (45). Kaposi's sarcoma occurs in elderly individuals of Mediterranean and Jewish descent and males in tropical Africa. However, the Kaposi's sarcoma of most

TABLE 9. *Virus-associated malignant neoplasms in immune deficient patients[a]*

Group	Malignancies	Postulated viruses and cofactors
Inherited	B cell lymphoma	EBV
	Leukemia	Chromosome breakage
	Hepatocellular carcinoma	HBV, anabolic steroids
Acquired renal transplant	Squamous cell carcinoma	HPV, ultraviolet light
	B cell lymphoma	EBV
	Kaposi's sarcoma	CMV
	Cervical carcinoma	HPV
Male homosexuals	B cell lymphoma	EBV, chromosome breakage
	Oral squamous cell carcinoma	HPV, HSV
	Cloagenic carcinoma	HSV, HPV
	Hepatocellular carcinoma	HBV
Africans	Hepatocellular carcinoma	HBV, aflatoxin
	Kaposi's sarcoma	CMV
	Burkitt's lymphoma	EBV
	Squamous cell carcinoma	HPV

[a]HBV, hepatitis B virus; HPV, human papilloma virus; EBV, Epstein-Barr virus.

Africans is not associated with obvious immune deficiency or HIV. It is noteworthy that immunosuppressed renal transplant recipients have an increased risk of Kaposi's sarcoma (43) (Chapter 7). Kaposi's sarcoma in AIDS patients and transplant recipients may be induced by CMV. This virus was implicated as a cause of Kaposi's sarcoma as early as 1972.

As noted earlier, non-Hodgkin's lymphomas are the second most frequent malignancy in patients with AIDS. Epstein-Barr virus (EBV) has been isolated in these tumors and we have detected EBV gnome from lymph nodes from male homosexuals with ARC. Patients with ARC and AIDS may show an unusual lesion on the lateral surface of the tongue, termed hairy leukoplakia. This consists of shaggy gray-white patches of hyperkeratotic squamous epithelium. Koiliocytosis (a pale halo around the squamous cell nuclei) suggests the presence of papilloma virus. Surprisingly EBV genome is present in the lesions (50).

Less commonly occurring cancers in AIDS patients are squamous cell carcinomas involving the mouth and anus. Sexually active homosexual males may have condylomatous lesions associated with human papilloma virus. Squamous cell carcinomas are prevalent in immunosuppressed transplant patients (Chapter 7). Defective immune surveillance in patients with AIDS likely permits ubiquitous viruses such as EBV and papilloma virus to induce malignancies in target cells transformed by these or other ubiquitous viruses. Inherited or acquired immune deficiency may be a key factor in permitting escape of a proliferating cell from host immune surveillance (45).

ACKNOWLEDGMENTS

This work was supported in part by PHS CA30196, awarded by the National Cancer Institute, DHHS, NCI Laboratory Research Center Support Grant CA36727, the State of Nebraska Department of Health, LB506, and the Lymphoproliferative Research Fund.

REFERENCES

1. Barre-Sinoussi, F., Chermann, J. C., and Rey, F. et al. (1983): Isolation of a T-lymphotropic virus from a patient at risk for acquired immune deficiency syndrome (AIDS). *Science*, 220:868–871.
2. Bergsma, D., Good, R. A., Finstad, J., and Paul, N. A. (1985): Immunodeficiency in Man and Animals. Birth Defects Original Article Series, Vol. 11, No. 1, Sinauer Associates, Inc., Sunderland, MA.
3. Bockman, D. E., and Kerby, M. L. (1984): Dependence of thymus development on derivatives of the neural crest. *Science*, 220:498–500.
4. Borzy, M. S., Hung, R., Horowitz, S. D., Gilbert, E., Kaufman, D., DeMendonca, W., Oxelius, V. A., Dictor, M., and Pacham, L. (1979): Fatal lymphoma after transplantation of cultured thymus in children with combined immunodeficiency disease. *N. Engl. J. Med.*, 301:565–568.
5. Carne, C. A., Smith, A., Elkington, S. G., Preston, F. E., Tedder, R. S., Sutherland, S., Daly, H. M., and Craske, J. (1985): Acute encephalopathy coincident with seroconversion for anti-HTLV-III. *Lancet*, 2:1206–1208.
6. Centers for Disease Control (1981): Pneumocystis pneumonia—Los Angeles. *Morbid. Mortal. Rev.*, 30:250–253.
7. Centers for Disease Control (1981): Kaposi's sarcoma and Pneumocystis pneumonia among homosexual men—New York City and California. *Morbid. Mortal. Rev.*, 30:305–308.
8. Chandra, R. K. (1983): In: *Malnutrition in Primary and Immunodeficiency Disorders*, edited by R.K. Chandra, pp. 187–203. Churchill-Livingstone, London.
9. Curran, J. W., Morgan, W. M., Hardy, A. M., Jaffee, H. W., Darrow, W. W., and Dowdle, W. R. (1985): The epidemiology of AIDS. Current status and future prospects. *Science*, 229:1352–1357.
10. DeSousa, M. (1980): Lymphocyte maldistribution and immunodeficiency. *Hosp. Pract.*, 15:71–87.
11. DiGeorge, A. M. (1965): Discussion. In: *A New Concept of the Cellular Basis of Immunity*, edited by M.D. Cooper, R.D.A. Peterson, R.A. Good, *J. Pediatr.*, 67:907–908.

12. Durov, N. Thymic atrophy and immune deficiency in malnutrition. In: *Malnutrition in Primary and Immunodeficiency Disorders*, edited by R.K. Chandra, pp. 127–150. Churchill-Livingstone, London.
13. Ebbesen, P. (1986): The global epidemic of AIDS. *AIDS Res.* 2 [Suppl. 1]:23–28.
14. Filipovich, A. H., Frizzera, G., Gferer, J., Zerbe, A. and Jordan-Heinitz, K. (1988): Cancer in Wiskott-Aldrich syndrome: Report of the Immunodeficiency—Cancer Registry. Submitted for publication.
15. Filipovich, A. H., Blazar, B. R., Ramsay, N. K. C., Kersey, J. H., Zelkowitz, L., Harada, S., and Purtilo, D. T. (1986): Allogeneic bone marrow transplantation for X-linked lymphoproliferative syndrome. *Transplantation*, 42:222–224.
16. Friedrich, W., Goldman, S. F., Ebell, W., Blutters-Sawatzki, R., Gaedick, G., Ragahavachar, A., Peter, H. H., Belohradsky, B., Kreth, W., Kubanek, B. (1985): Severe combined immunodeficiency: Treatment by bone marrow transplantation in 15 infants using HLA haploid identified donors. *Eur. J. Pediatr.*, 144:125–130.
17. Fudenberg, H. H. (1966): Immunologic deficiency, autoimmune disease, and lymphoma: Observations, implications and speculations. *Arthritis Rheum.*, 9:464–472.
18. Gallo, R. C., Salahuddin, S. Z., and Popvic, M., Shearer, G. M., Kaplan, M., Haynes, B. F., Palker, T. S., Redfield, R., Oleske, J., Safai, B., White, G., Foster, P., Malkham, P. D. (1984): Frequent detection and isolation of cytopathic retroviruses (HTLV-III) from patients with AIDS and at risk for AIDS. *Science*, 224:500–503.
19. Gatti, R. A., and Good, R. A. (1970): The immunological deficiency diseases. *Med. Clin. North America*, 54:281–307.
20. Gilmore, N., Wainberg, M. A., editors (1985): *Viral Mechanisms of Immune Suppression*. Alan R. Liss, Inc., New York.
21. Harrington, D., Weisenburger, D. D., and Purtilo, D. T. (1988): Malignant lymphomas in the X-linked lymphoproliferative syndrome. *Cancer* (in press).
22. Haynes, B. F., Schooley, R. T., Grouse, J. E., Payling-Wright, C. R., Dolin, R., and Fauci, A. S. (1979): Characterization of thymus-derived lymphocyte subsets in acute Epstein-Barr virus-induced infectious mononucleosis. *J. Immunol.*, 122:699–702.
23. Haynes, B. F., Warren, R. W., Buckley, R. H., McClure, J. E., Goldstein, A. L., Henderson, F. W., Hensley, L. L., and Eisenbarth, G. S. (1983): Demonstration of abnormalities in expression of thymic epithelial surface antigens in severe cellular immunodeficiency diseases. *J. Immunol.*, 130:1182–1188.
24. Haynes, B. F. (1986): The role of the thymic microenvironment in promotion of early stages of human T cell maturation. *Clin. Res.*, 34:422–431.
25. Huber, J., and Van Baarlen, J. (1986): Thymus-histology as a parameter of duration of illness or stress. International Academy of Pathology, Vienna.
26. Joshi, V. V., Oleske, J. M., Saad, S., Gadol, C., Connor, E., Bobila, R., and Minnefor, A. B. (1986): Thymus biopsy in children with acquired immunodeficiency syndrome. *Arch. Pathol. Lab. Med.*, 110:837–842.
27. Kadin, M. E., Berard, C. W., Naba, K., and Yakasa, H. (1983): Lymphoproliferative diseases in Japan and Western countries. *Hum. Pathol.*, 14:745–772.
28. Kaiser, C., McCaw, B., Hetch, F., Harnden, D. G., and Tepletts, R. L. (1975): Somatic rearrangement of chromosome 14 in human lymphocytes. *Proc. Natl. Acad. Sci. USA*, 72:2071–2075.
29. Kleihauer, E. (1985): Severe combined immunodeficiency: treatment by bone marrow transplantation in infants using HLA haplo-identical donors. *Europ. J. Pediatr.*, 144:125–130.
30. Klein, G., and Klein, E. (1986): Conditioned tumorigenicity of activated oncogenes. *Cancer Res.*, 46:3211–3224.
31. Koenig, S., Gendelman, H. E., Orenstein, J. M., Dal Canto, M. C., Pezeshkpour, C. H., Ungbluth, M., Janotta, F., Aksamit, A., Martin, M. A., and Fauci, A. S. (1986): Detection of AIDS virus in macrophages in brain tissue from AIDS patients with encephalopathy. *Science*, 233:1089–1091.
32a.Krueger, G., Bedoya, V., and Grimley, P. M. (1971): Lymphoreticular tissue lesions in Steinbrinck-Chediak-Higashi syndrome. *Virchow's Arch.*, 353:273–288.
32b.Kwan, S. P., Kunkel, L., Bruns, G., Wedgwood, R. J., Latt, S., Rosen, F. S. (1986): Mapping of the X-linked agammaglobulinemia locus by use of restriction fragment-length polymorphism. *J. Clin. Invest.*, 77:649–652.
33. Landreth, K. S., Englehard, D., Anasetti, C., Kapoor, N., Kincade, P. W., and Good, R. A. (1985): Pre-B cells in agammaglobulinemia: Evidence for disease heterogeneity among affected boys. *J. Clin. Immunol.*, 5:84–89.
34. Lobach, D. F., Scearce, R. M., and Haynes, B. F. (1985): The human thymic microenvironment, phenotypic characterization of Hassall's bodies with the use of monoclonal antibodies. *J. Immunol.*, 134:250–257.
35. McClain, K. L., Shapiro, R. S., Ramsay, N., and Filipovich, A. H. (1985): Virologic studies in four patients with post-transplant lymphomas following T-depleted mismatched bone marrow transplantation (BMT). *Proc. Am. Soc. Hematol.* (in press).
36. McFarland, D. E., Stroper, W., and Waldmann, T. A. (1972): Ataxia-telangiectasia. *Medicine*, 51:281–314.
37. McKusick, V. A., editor (1983): *Mendelian inheritance in man. Catalogs of autosomal dominant, autosomal recessive, and X-linked phenotypes*, 6th Edition. The Johns Hopkins University Press, Baltimore.
38. Merino, F, Henle, W., and Ramirez-Duque, P. (1986): Chronic active Epstein-Barr virus infection in patients with Chediak-Higashi syndrome. *J. Clin. Immunol.*, 6:299–305.

39a. Meuwissen, H. J., and Purtilo, D. T. (1984): Epstein-Barr virus and marrow transplantation recipients. In: *Immune Deficiency and Cancer: Epstein-Barr Virus and Lymphoproliferative Malignancies*, edited by D. T. Purtilo, pp. 457–470. Plenum Press, New York.

39b. Miale, J. D. (1982): *Laboratory Medicine—Hematology*, 6th Edition, pp. 658–688. C.V. Mosby Co., St. Louis.

40. Neudorf, S. L., Filipovich, A. H., and Kersey, J. H. (1984): Immunoreconstitution by bone marrow transplantation decreases lymphoproliferative malignancies in Wiskott-Aldrich and severe combined immune deficiency syndrome. In: *Immune Deficiency and Cancer: Epstein-Barr Virus and Lymphoproliferative Malignancies*, edited by D.T. Purtilo, pp. 471–480. Plenum Press, New York.

41. Nezelof, C. (1986): Pathology of the thymus in immunodeficiency states. In: *The Human Thymus: Histophysiology and Pathology*, edited by H.K. Muller-Hermelink, C.L. Berry, and E. Grundmann, pp. 151–177. Springer-Verlag, Berlin.

42. Ochs, H. D., Sullivan, J. L., Wedgwood, R. J., Seeley, J. K., Sakamoto, K., and Purtilo, D. T. (1983): X-Linked Lymphoproliferative Syndrome: Abnormal antibody responses to bacteriophage φX174. In: *Primary Immunodeficiency Disease*, edited by R. Wedgwood and F. Rosen, pp. 321–323. Alan R. Liss, New York.

43. Penn, I. (1984): Allograft transplant cancer registry. In: *Immune Deficiency and Cancer: Epstein-Barr Virus and Lymphoproliferative Malignancies*, edited by D. T. Purtilo, pp. 281–308. Plenum Press, New York.

44. Purtilo, D. T., Pacquin, L. A., and Gindhart, T. (1978): Genetics of neoplasia: Impact of ecogenetics on oncogenesis. *Am. J. Path.*, 91:609–688.

45. Purtilo, D. T. (1984): Defective immune surveillance in viral oncogenesis. *Lab. Invest.*, 51:373–385.

46. Purtilo, D. T., Yang, J. P. S., Cassel, C. K., Harper, P., Stephenson, S. R., Landing, B. H., and Vawter, G. F. (1975): X-linked recessive progressive combined variable immunodeficiency (Duncan's disease). *Lancet*, i:935–950.

47. Purtilo, D. T., and Sullivan, J. L. (1979): Immunological bases for superior survival of females. *Am. J. Dis. Child.*, 133:1251–1253.

48. Purtilo, D. T. (1986): Lymphotropic viruses, Epstein-Barr virus (EBV) and human T lymphotropic virus-I (HTLV-I)/adult T cell leukemia virus (ATLV) and HTLV-III/human immune deficiency virus (HIV) as etiological agents of malignant lymphoma and immune deficiency. *AIDS Res.* (in press).

49. Purtilo, D. T., and Connor, D. H. (1975): Fatal infections in protein-calorie malnourished children with thymolymphatic atrophy. *Arch. Dis. Child.*, 50:149–152.

50. Purtilo, D. T., Linder, J., and Volsky, D. J. (1986): Acquired immune deficiency syndrome. *Clin. Lab. Med.*, 6:3–26.

51. Rosen, F. S., Cooper, M. D., and Wedgwood, R. J. P. (1984): The primary immunodeficiencies. Part I. *N. Engl. J. Med.*, 311:235–242.

52. Rosen, F. S., Cooper, M. D., and Wedgwood, R. J. P. (1984): The primary immunodeficiencies. Part II. *N. Engl. J. Med.*, 311:235–242.

53. Saemundsen, A. K., Berkel, A. I., Henle, W., Henle, G., Anvret, M., Sanal, O., Ersoy, F., Caglar, M., and Klein, G. (1981): Epstein-Barr-virus-carrying lymphoma in a patient with ataxia telangiectasia. *Br. Med. J.*, 82:425–427.

54. Schnittman, S. M., Lane, H. C., Higgins, S. E., Folks, T., and Fauci, A. S. (1986): Direct polyclonal activation of human B lymphocytes by the acquired immune deficiency syndrome virus. *Science*, 233:1084–1086.

55. Selik, R. M., Jaffe, H. W., Solomon, S. L., and Curran, J. W. (1986): CDC's definition of AIDS. *N. Engl. J. Med.*, 315:761.

56. Seemayer, T. A., Laroche, C., and Russo, P., Malebranche, R., Arnoux, E., Guerin, J.-M., Pierre, G., Dupuy, J.-M., Gartner, J. G., Lapp, W. S., Spira, T. S., and Elie, R. (1985): Precocious thymic involution manifest by epithelial injury in the acquired immune deficiency syndrome. *Human Pathol.*, 15:469–474.

57. Seshi, B., and Purtilo, D. T. (1983): Humoral immune responses in parasitized malnourished children. In: *Nutrition, Disease Resistance and Immune Function*, edited by R.R. Watson, pp. 71–86. Marcel Dekker, New York.

58a. Smythe, P. M., Brereton-Stiles, G. G., Grace, M., Mafoyane, A., Schonland, M., Coovaidia, H. M., Loening, W. E., Parent, M. A., and Vos, G. H. (1971): Thymolymphatic deficiency and depression of cell-mediated immunity in protein-calorie malnutrition. *Lancet*, ii:939–943.

58b. Toyonaga, B., and Mak, T. W. (1987): Genes of the T-cell antigen receptor in normal and malignant cells. *Ann. Rev. Immunol.*, 5:585–620.

59. Volsky, D. J., Sakai, K., Stevenson, M., and Dewhurst, S. (1986): Retroviral etiology of the acquired immune deficiency syndrome (AIDS). *AIDS Res.* 2 [Suppl. 1]:35–48.

60. Waldman, T. A., Misiti, J., Nelson, D. L., and Kraemer, K. H. (1983): Telangiectasia: A multisystem hereditary disease with immunodeficiency, impaired organ maturation, X-ray hypersensitivity and a high incidence of neoplasia. *Ann. Int. Med.*, 99:367–379.

61. Watson, R. R., and Stinnett, J. D. (1983): Nutrition and the Immune Response. CRC Press, Boca Raton, Florida.

62. Wedgwood, R. J., Rosen, F. S., and Paul, N. W., editors (1983): *Primary Immunodeficiency Diseases*, Vol. 19, No. 3, Alan R. Liss, New York.

Diagnostic Immunopathology,
edited by R.B. Colvin,
A.K. Bhan, and R.T. McCluskey.
Raven Press, New York © 1988.

7 / *Renal Allografts*

Robert B. Colvin

*Immunopathology Unit, Department of Pathology, Massachusetts General Hospital and Harvard
Medical School, Boston, Massachusetts 02114*

Clinical and laboratory studies establish the diagnosis of renal allograft dysfunction. Of these, the renal biopsy remains the most definitive, yet it has become more difficult to interpret since the advent of cyclosporine with its attendant nephrotoxicity. This chapter reviews the pathogenesis of the various forms of injury, the practical aspects of renal biopsy interpretation, and alternative immunopathologic tests.

MECHANISMS OF ALLOGRAFT REJECTION

Antigens

Primary immunologic rejection of organ allografts results from the recognition by T lymphocytes of individual-specific antigens ("alloantigens") on donor cells that differ from the recipient (222). The principal targets are the highly polymorphic, major histocompatibility antigens—products of the major histocompatibility complex (MHC)—present in probably all vertebrates (222). The human MHC (termed HLA for human leukocyte antigen) spans 3,000 kilobases on the short arm of chromosome 6 and contains multiple genes (Fig. 1) (138). The dominance the HLA locus is indicated by the observation that grafts from an HLA-identical sibling survive longer than those from an HLA-nonidentical sibling (222). The exquisite sensitivity of the immune system to these antigens has been elegantly demonstrated using K^{bm} mutant mice. Skin grafts from donors that differ from the recipient in only 1 to 3 amino acids in a single MHC molecule are promptly rejected (214,222). Two chemically and functionally different classes (I and II) of histocompatibility molecules are encoded in the MHC (8). Disparity of either is sufficient to cause graft rejection, as shown in the bm mutant mice (214).

The class I antigens consist of a polymorphic transmembrane 45 kilodalton (kd) α glycoprotein chain associated with β2-microglobulin, a monomorphic 12 kd serum protein. Multiple alleles at each of the 3 class I α loci (A,B,C) have been defined with alloantibodies; the B locus is the most polymorphic with at least 40 alleles (128). Further allelic diversity can be defined using T cell recognition and genetic probes (8). Class I antigens are usually said to be on all nucleated cells, but their concentration on the cell surface varies widely, even to the point of undetectability by standard immunohistochemical techniques (e.g., placental and Langerhans cells) (128). In the normal human kidney, the

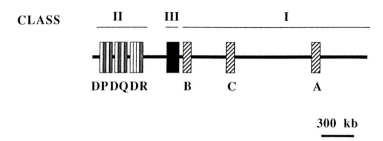

FIG. 1. Scaled diagram of the HLA gene complex (138). The class II α genes are solid; class II β genes open, and class I α genes stippled. Potential class II genes DZ(α) and DO(β) are between DP and DQ but their products have not been identified. Genes in the class III region are C2, factor B, C4, tumor necrosis factor (α/β), and steroid 21-hydroxylase (8). Nonpolymorphic class I related loci are present to the right (3′) of **A** (138).

vascular endothelium (arteries, veins, capillaries) stains most intensely for class I antigens; the tubular epithelium is moderately positive (59,85,266,279).

The class II antigens consist of 2 noncovalently associated transmembrane proteins of 25 to 28 and 29 to 34 kd, with most of the polymorphism on the smaller β chain. Three gene families (DP, DQ, DR), each with 1 to 2 α and 2 to 3 β genes have been identified. Four heterodimers are known to be expressed on cell surfaces (DPαβ, DQ αβ, DR αβ1 and DR αβ2). The distribution of class II antigens is more restricted than those of class I and varies by species and class II family. In humans, class II antigens are normally found on B cells, dendritic cells, capillary endothelium, monocytes, Langerhans cells, and activated T cells (60,128). In the kidney, DR but not DQ is demonstrable on capillary endothelium, including glomeruli; both are on dendritic cells (Fig. 2). Proximal tubules normally have less intense staining for HLA-DR and no DQ or DP (71,85,266,279). Normal arterial endothelium has little or no class II antigens. Class II antigens are not detectable on murine endothelium in tissue (238).

The only established function of the class I and II molecules is to "present" exogenous antigen to T cells. Specific class II molecules bind certain antigens more avidly and thereby present these antigens more effectively (19,267). The class II genes, termed "immune response" (Ir) genes, were discovered by virtue of their critical role in determining whether an animal would respond to specific exogenous antigens (19). The rich assortment of binding specificities caused by MHC polymorphism provides a selective advantage for the species by increasing the likelihood that some individuals will be able to develop protective immunity to any particular new pathogen (128). The T cells are normally selected ("educated") in the thymus for recognition of self MHC molecules, so that their response is "restricted" to antigen presented by self MHC antigens (227). The T cells recognize an altered conformation of self MHC molecules plus the associated antigen (267). Antigen unassociated with MHC molecules is generally invisible to T cells.

According to this conception, graft rejection occurs because the T cells recognize the foreign MHC antigens as if they were self MHC molecules altered by association with some "X" antigen (the altered self hypothesis) (67,160). This mimicry of normal antigen presentation would explain the high frequency of alloreactive cells (0.1% to 0.2%) (128) and thereby the reason that the MHC is the "major" determinant of allograft survival

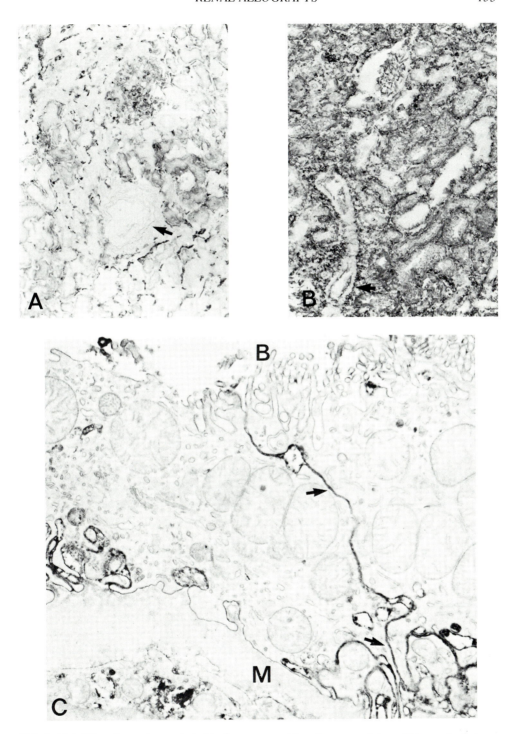

FIG. 2. HLA-DR antigens demonstrated by immunoperoxidase in a normal donor kidney prior to transplantation (**A**) and during an acute cellular rejection (**B**). The normal peritubular and glomerular capillaries are HLA-DR+, as are interstitial dendritic cells. The arterial endothelium (*arrows*) stains in rejection but not in the normal kidney. The proximal tubules (T) have increased HLA-DR in rejection, and the interstitial mononuclear cells are positive. **C.** By electron microscopy the staining is detected on the baso-lateral surfaces of the proximal tubular cells (*arrows*). The brush border (**B**) is focally positive. M, tubular basement membrane. Courtesy of E.E. Schneeberger. × 4,500.

(160,176). T cells can also react with alloantigens processed and presented by autologous cells (such as dendritic cells or infiltrating macrophages), as with other protein antigens (231). This response could potentially cause rejection by the action of lymphokines, but not by direct cytotoxicity.

Many so-called weak or "minor" histocompatibility antigens exist, defined simply by an ability to elicit graft rejection and a genetic locus outside the MHC. These antigens cause graft rejection between MHC-identical congenic mice and HLA-identical siblings (222). Their chemical nature and distribution are largely unknown. Some are tissue-specific differentiation antigens, such as an endothelial-monocyte alloantigen in man (44). In mice, minor antigens include a male-specific antigen encoded on the Y chromosome (237) and a variant $\beta2$-microglobulin (211). Minor histocompatibility antigens are recognized by T cells in conjunction with self MHC antigens.

The expression of MHC molecules on the cell surface is dynamic and under the control of inflammatory mediators, such as the interferons (IFN) and tumor necrosis factor (TNF) (49,203). Made by macrophages and fibroblasts in response to viral infection and other stimuli, IFNα/β induces class I antigens on a variety of cells; endothelial and glomerular cells are highly responsive (149,203). In contrast, IFNγ, a lymphokine produced by antigen activated T-cells, induces both class I and class II MHC antigens (238). The proximal tubular epithelium is the most responsive in murine kidneys (238). Increased surface density of MHC molecules enhances the susceptibility to T cell mediated lysis and the ability to present antigen (159). One would predict that induction of graft MHC molecules would promote rejection, but this has not been proved.

Effectors

T Cells

The primary effectors (antigen-specific) of allograft rejection in a previously nonsensitized recipient are T cells (222). This has been shown by cell transfer experiments in which T cells, but not antibodies, are able to promote rejection in animals (155,222,282). In man, the incontrovertible evidence is that monoclonal antibodies (OKT3) to a T cell antigen receptor component (CD3) dramatically reverse graft rejection (55,192).

The antigen recognition structure (Ti) on T cells consist of a heterodimer of 45 to 50 kd, with a variable and constant regions on each chain, homologous to immunoglobulin V domains (151). The Ti associates with CD3 (T3) and certain other molecules to form the active antigen receptor complex (151). Most T cells (both cytotoxic and helper) use an α/β chain; a minor population ($< 5\%$), of unknown function, use a different dimer (γ/δ) (32) The Vβ may have affinity for specific MHC antigens (28). Thus, the T cell repertoire may be biased in favor of the MHC molecules due to intrinsic properties of the antigen receptor variable regions (28).

Upon recognition of antigen on a cell surface, the T cells can make at least two different responses: direct cytotoxic killing of the presenting cell or secretion of peptide mediators (lymphokines), which affect the behavior of nearby cells. Delayed-type hypersensitivity to exogenous protein antigens is mediated by the latter mechanism (see Chapter 1). The competing theories of graft rejection were based on these two responses, once thought to involve mutually exclusive cell types (helper and cytotoxic) (155,250). Since the realization that many T cell clones have both properties (cytotoxicity and lymphokine production), the theories must be revised so that the division applies to cellular mechanisms, not to cell type. Indeed, the cells that have both functions may be the most potent in graft rejection (215).

One indelible property of a T cell is the class of MHC antigen recognized, which is strongly correlated with the presence of CD4 or CD8 on the cell surface (Chapter 1). $CD4^+$ cells respond preferentially to class II molecules and $CD8^+$ cells respond to class I molecules (146,258). Expression of CD4 and CD8 correlates more stringently with MHC class recognition than function (help, cytotoxicity) (146,258). The CD4 and CD8 molecules are members of the immunoglobulin supergene family that also includes the MHC antigens and the T cell antigen receptor (listed in Table 2, Chapter 18). Antibodies to CD4 or CD8 are able to block function *in vitro*, although higher affinity Ti may be resistant (146). The CD4 and CD8 molecules probably bind to nonpolymorphic parts of the class II and I MHC antigens, respectively, to enhance cellular adhesion (146). Direct evidence for this has been obtained for CD4 and DR (74,146). Only occasional exceptions to the CD4 class II and CD8-class I rule have been reported, and those with individual T cell clones or hybridomas. The exceptions may be more apparent than real, since some can be explained by $CD8^+$ clones that recognize class II molecules presented by class I molecules (146,231).

The T cells of either the $CD4^+$ or $CD8^+$ subset are sufficient to transfer rejection of murine skin grafts, provided the graft and recipient differ in class II or class I antigens, respectively (214,248). In most circumstances, however, both $CD4^+$ and $CD8^+$ cells participate and probably collaborate to mediate graft rejection. In mice disparate at the whole MHC or in nonhuman primates, either anti-CD4 or anti-CD8 antibodies can inhibit rejection (48,56,115). In monkeys, the CD4 antibodies are efficacious only when given before rejection is initiated, while the anti-CD8 antibodies can quench an ongoing rejection (56,115). The $CD4^+$ cells are essential for the generation of primed $CD8^+$ cells and subsequent graft rejection in some circumstances (48,215). These data argue that the $CD4^+$ cells ordinarily function in the early phase of rejection to promote $CD8^+$ expansion and differentiation, while the later injury is $CD8^+$ cell dependent.

By recombinant DNA techniques, several lymphokines have materialized from misty "factors" as sequenced molecules. Two are known to be highly relevant to graft rejection. Interleukin 2 (IL-2) stimulates T cell division after interaction with a specific IL-2 receptor (78). An antibody that inhibits T cell activation by binding to the interleukin 2 receptor can prevent rejection of human renal allografts (246). IFNγ is the major T cell macrophage activating factor (182), as well as a potent modulator of HLA antigen expression. Important, but still at the "factor" stage of understanding, are the macrophage procoagulant stimulatory factor (98) and the soluble factors that cause vasoconstriction and increased vascular permeability. Both $CD4^+$ and $CD8^+$ cells are able to produce most, if not all, lymphokines, although there are clonal and subset differences. For example, two types of CD4 clones have been described in the mouse: one produces IL-2 and IFNγ and is able to transfer delayed-type hypersensitivity reactions (T_H1) and the other produces IL-4 (T_H2) (46).

Antibodies

Antibodies to class I and class II antigens are demonstrable in recipients of allografts, although their role is uncertain (222,282). While there is no evidence that alloantibody is important in first set rejection, antibody may contribute to more chronic graft injury, including the vascular damage in arteries and glomeruli (see below).

Passively transferred humoral antibodies to MHC antigens generally fail to induce rejection of allografts in rodents (lymphoid tissue is a notable exception), and under some circumstances enhance graft survival (43,282). Rodent xenografts can be readily rejected by passive antibodies, owing to deposition of antibodies on the vascular endothelium (36, 116), analogous to hyperacute rejection in man (see below). The difference in susceptibility between murine xenografts and allografts is probably because of the density of the target antigens on the endothelium.

Secondary Mediators

Various nonspecific mediators can be activated by T cells or antibodies and thus contribute to graft damage. These include the clotting, complement and kinin systems, and other inflammatory cells, such as macrophages, granulocytes, and natural killer cells (see Chapters 1 and 2).

Macrophages

Universally present in rejecting grafts, macrophages may be particularly important by virtue of their interaction with T cells. Macrophages cause cell and matrix damage by release of proteases and reactive oxygen species (2). Cytocidal activity is induced in macrophages by IFNγ and endotoxin (2,182). Furthermore, macrophages secrete a panoply of mediators that promote inflammation (prostaglandins, leukotrienes, procoagulants) and stimulate fibroblast collagen production and division (2,230). Several of these monokines can contribute to the chronic phase of injury, particularly interleukin 1 (IL-1) and the growth factors related to or identical with platelet-derived growth factor (PDGF) and transforming growth factor β.

Natural Killer (NK) Cells

Natural killer cells may contribute to the immunologically nonspecific graft injury, by virtue of their ability to kill target cells, but this is unproved (185). In human blood most of the NK activity is by cells that display the CD16 marker (Leu 11) and lack CD3; some have low density CD8 and/or HNK-1 (Leu 7) (136). Convincing identification of NK cells in tissues awaits the discovery of a unique differentiation marker.

Long-term Adaptation to Graft

For largely unknown reasons, severe rejection episodes become less frequent with time. In kidneys, most losses from rejection occur during the first 3 months. The critical immunoregulatory adaptations of the immune system that permit acceptance of an allograft are not fully understood and will be discussed here only briefly. Donor specific T suppressor cells (122) and anti-idiotype antibodies (174) that block the T cell antigen receptor have been demonstrated and are among the leading theoretical possibilities. Adaptation within the graft may also promote long survival. Rodent skin xenografts can be accepted by the host indefinitely and become resistant to passive antibody. This has been attributed to substantial replacement of the microvasculature by host vessels (116). However, vessels remain sensitive to donor-specific antibody in *organ* xenografts (36). In human liver allografts DR positive donor Kupffer cells disappear during early rejection episodes and are replaced by recipient cells (77). It has been reported that class I and II antigens become decreased on endothelial cells, as judged in aspirates from long-term stable renal grafts (95). Endothelial HLA expression and replacement in accepted grafts deserves further evaluation with allospecific monoclonal antibody.

DIAGNOSTIC INTERPRETATION OF BIOPSIES

Hamburger pointed out over 20 years ago that graft rejection cannot be attributed merely to different intensities of a single type of immune response (82). The major variables are the effectors (T cells and antibody), the tissue target, and the therapy. As therapy has changed over the last two decades, so has the pathology. Certain types of rejection, such as hyperacute and accelerated rejection, have become less common, while new lesions, such as cyclosporine toxicity, have appeared. A working classification of the lesions that arise from immunologic and nonimmunologic mechanisms in renal allografts is given in Table 1. This classification is based on published reports and a personal experience of over 500 graft biopsies.

TABLE 1. *Diagnostic classification of renal allograft biopsies*

I. Immunologic rejection
  A. Antibody Mediated
    1. Hyperacute allograft rejection
    2. Necrotizing arteritis (accelerated rejection)
  B. T Cell Mediated
    1. Acute cellular allograft rejection
      a. Tubulointerstitial
      b. Vascular
      c. Glomerular (acute allograft glomerulopathy)
  C. Mixed or Unknown Pathogenesis
    1. Chronic allograft rejection
      a. Tubulointerstitial
      b. Vascular
      c. Glomerular
    2. De novo glomerulonephritis

II. Nonimmunologic injury
  A. Acute ischemic injury (ATN)
  B. Perfusion injury
  C. Cyclosporine A nephrotoxicity
    1. Acute Cyclosporine A toxicity
      a. Tubular
      b. Arterial
      c. Hemolytic-uremic syndrome
    2. Chronic Cyclosporine A toxicity
  D. Major vessel occlusion/stenosis
  E. Obstruction
  F. Infection
III. Recurrent primary disease
  A. Immunological
  B. Metabolic

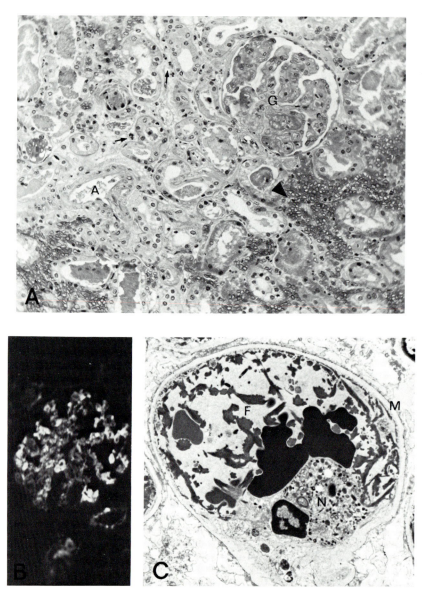

FIG. 3. Hyperacute rejection in a patient with circulating antibody to HLA-DR reactive to the donor (3). **A**. At 24 hours after transplantation, light microscopy shows hemorrhage (*arrowhead*), interstitial edema and neutrophils (*arrows*) and occlusion of glomerular capillaries by fibrin and swollen endothelial cells (G). Arteries (**A**) are spared. These lesions correspond to the distribution of HLA-DR in the normal kidney (Fig. 2). × 200. **B**. IgM is demonstrated in a glomerulus and focally in a small vessel by immunofluorescence. **C**. Electron microscopy shows a glomerular capillary filled with fibrin (F) and a neutrophil (N). The basement membrane (M) is denuded of endothelium. × 3,600.

Antibody Mediated Rejection

Hyperacute Rejection

If the recipient has circulating antibodies to certain alloantigens expressed on the graft endothelium, "hyperacute" rejection can occur within minutes after perfusion with recipient blood. During the operation, the kidney rapidly becomes cyanotic and flaccid and urine output ceases (or never begins). This lesion rarely develops after the first 2 days (189). Postoperative signs are anuria, high fever, thrombocytopenia, and increased circulating fibrin split products.

By light microscopy the early lesions show neutrophil and platelet margination along damaged endothelium of small arteries, arterioles, glomeruli and peritubular capillaries (Fig. 3). The endothelium is stripped off the underlying basal lamina, and the interstitium becomes edematous and hemorrhagic. Intravascular coagulation occurs and cortical necrosis ensues over 12 to 24 hours without evidence of mononuclear cell participation. The medulla is relatively spared. Immunofluroescence typically shows immunoglobulin (especially IgM) and complement components in the vascular and glomerular lesions (39, 157,178,249,280) (Fig. 3). Antibody sometimes cannot be detected in the tissues, perhaps because the endothelial cells have disintegrated and the membrane-bound antibody has been washed away or degraded.

Hyperacute rejection is caused by the binding of antibodies on the surface of endothelial cells, fixation of complement, platelet activation, lysis of the endothelium, and activation of the clotting system with thrombosis (116,282). T cell mediated hyperacute rejection has not been reported in man, but has been described in presensitized pigs with no detectable humoral antibody; the early lesion consists of lymphocytes attached to the arterial endothelium (125).

The first identified targets of hyperacute rejection were the ABO blood group antigens (249,280). In the kidney, the ABO antigens are on the endothelium and distal convoluted tubules (and on the collecting ducts with secretors) (14). Almost universally, ABO antibodies are present in individuals lacking the A or B antigen. Blood group A_2 is an exception, since "natural" antibodies to this determinant do not occur, and these kidneys behave as type O (35). Rarely A_1 or B kidneys have survived in incompatible hosts, presumably because pre-existing antibodies were below the minimal threshold.

Removal of circulating ABO antibody by extracorporeal immunoabsorption (13) or plasmapheresis (4) has permitted successful transplantation of ABO incompatible kidneys from HLA-identical siblings (13), provided splenectomies are performed. Survival of greater then 1 year has been achieved, even though high titers of IgG and IgM antibodies return in the circulation (4). It would be quite interesting to determine the reason for the remarkable lack of immune-mediated damage in this setting.

Targets of hyperacute rejection can include HLA class I (126,178,249,280) and some class II (3) antigens. Anti-HLA antibodies have been eluted from a few hyperacutely rejected kidneys (170). The HLA antibodies arise from immunization by whole blood transfusion, previous transplantation, or pregnancy. The rapid graft destruction in humans by anti-MHC antibodies contrasts to that in rodents and may be explained by the fact that normal murine endothelium has little, if any, class I or class II antigens (238).

Cold-reactive IgM antibodies have been implicated in immediate injury in kidneys that are not rewarmed before blood flow is re-established (147,256). The lesions have relatively few neutrophils, resembling *ex vivo* perfusion injury (see below). Cold agglutinins, espe-

cially those reactive at 22°C, can also cause immediate graft dysfunction due to intravascular aggregation and thrombosis, as described in 5 cases (228).

Hyperacute rejection is fortunately preventable and rare, encountered in < 0.2% of
transplants in our experience. Prevention requires a crossmatch between donor lymphocytes and recipient serum taken close to the time of transplantation, with a sensitive technique (282). To detect antibodies to class II antigens, B cells or T cell blasts are needed. If
the titer of HLA antibodies diminishes to undetectable levels, transplantation has been
safely undertaken, even though antibodies were previously present (41,72).

Necrotizing Arteritis

Necrotizing arteritis was commonly recognized in the early studies of allografts (236).
This form of allograft rejection, also termed "accelerated" or "vascular" rejection, has a
uniformly poor prognosis (12,101,110,158). The arterial media shows myocyte necrosis,
fragmentation of elastica and accumulation of brightly eosinophilic material called "fibrinoid" (Fig. 4). A scant neutrophilic infiltrate and thrombosis may also be present. The
lesions may occur with little associated mononuclear infiltrate in the interstitium or vessels.
Immunofluorescence shows the "fibrinoid" deposits contain immunoglobulin (usually IgG
and IgM), C3 and fibrin (39,166) (Fig. 4). This lesion is not dissimilar to microscopic
polyarteritis. Presensitized recipients show rapid development of this lesion, which appears
to be mediated primarily by humoral antibody. The vascular lesions can occur at any time
(although usually in the first 6 weeks) and occur even in HLA-identical grafts. This pattern
of rejection was found in 7% of biopsies (14/204) in the pre-cyclosporine era (158), but is
now less common, at least in our experience. The current diagnostic problem is that cyclosporine toxicity also causes arterial lesions (see below).

T Cell Mediated Rejection

Acute Cellular Rejection

This is the common form of rejection that develops classically 1 to 3 weeks after transplantation, but may erupt at any time, even after many years (152). The onset is heralded
by fever, graft tenderness and swelling, and a rising creatinine. The urine contains lymphocytes, fibrin split products, and tubular cell components (265). The clinical features can be
muted by cyclosporine, particularly the allograft swelling. The kidney appears pale and
enlarged, indicative of ischemia and edema. In severe cases, focal infarction or rupture can
occur (157). The sites of acute cellular rejection are the interstitium/tubules, the arterial
endothelium, and the glomeruli. These may be involved separately or in combination.

Tubulo-interstitial rejection

Light and electron microscopy. The characteristic microscopic feature is a pleomorphic
interstitial infiltrate of mononuclear cells (Fig. 5), accompanied by interstitial edema and a
variable amount of hemorrhage. The earliest lesion in our experience is a perivascular infiltrate around the arcuate vessels at the corticomedullary junction, and a rather inconspicuous intertubular infiltrate without edema. Perhaps not coincidentally, these are the normal
locations of dendritic cells (279). The mononuclear cells commonly invade tubules and are

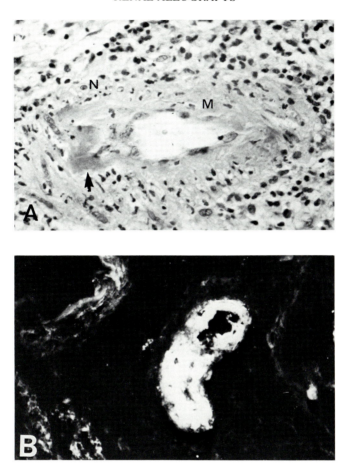

FIG. 4. Necrotizing allograft arteritis (accelerated rejection) in an allograft at 6 weeks. **A.** Fibrinoid necrosis (F) of a small artery with loss of smooth muscle (M) and nuclear debris (N). **B.** Immunofluorescence of another case (165) shows IgG in the arterial wall. Reprinted with permission from ref. 165.

found insinuated between tubular epithelial cells (Figs. 5–7). This "tubulitis" occurs in other forms of acute interstitial nephritis, such as drug-induced allergic interstitial nephritis (54).

The infiltrating mononuclear cells have increased cytoplasmic basophilia and mitotic figures may be present, indications of increased synthetic and proliferative activity (Fig. 7). Numerous lymphoblasts, with prominent nucleoli and abundant free cytoplasmic polyribosomes are seen by electron microscopy. The mononuclear cells are frequently found in close contact with each other, tubular epithelium or endothelium (Figs. 7,8). By ultrastructural criteria, the other cells are small lymphocytes, with dense nuclear chromatin and little cytoplasm, and macrophages/monocytes, with numerous phagolysosomes. A minority of the cells have extensive rough endoplasmic reticulum, resembling plasma cell precursors (180,278). Basophils comprise a minor component of the infiltrate which invade tubules, and can be the predominant granulocyte (up to 5% of the infiltrate) (51) (Fig. 5). Eosinophils are rarely more than 2% to 3% of the infiltrate (276). It is our impression that these cells are more commonly present in patients on cyclosporine, but this has not been sys-

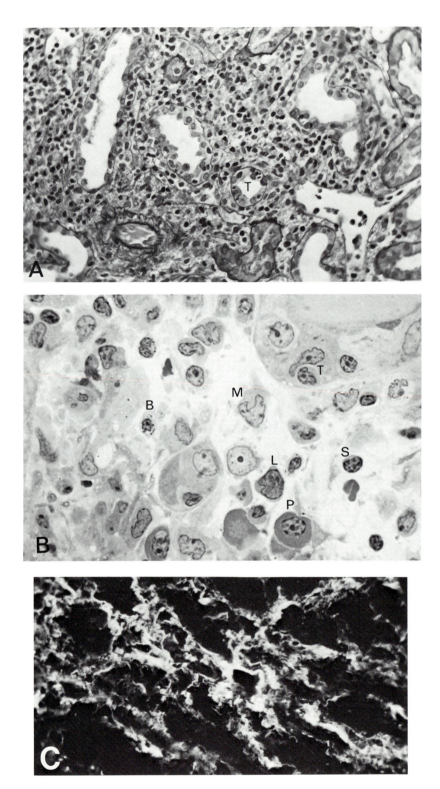

FIG. 5. Acute cellular allograft rejection. **A**. Light microscopy shows an intense mononuclear cell interstitial infiltrate with focal invasion of tubules (T) and edema. PAS stain, × 313. **B**. One micron epon embedded section reveals the morphology of the infiltrate quite clearly (165). Small lymphocytes (S), lymphoblasts (L), macrophages (M) and basophilic leukocytes B are seen in the interstitium. Lymphocytes invade the tubules (T). Giemsa stain, reprinted with permission. **C**. Immunofluorescence shows abundant interstitial fibrin.

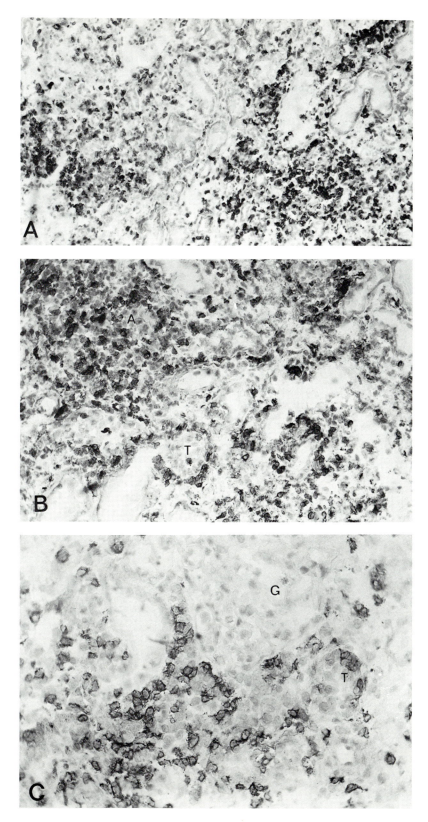

FIG. 6. Acute cellular allograft rejection stained for T cell markers with immunoperoxidase. **A**, CD3 (leu 4); **B**, CD4 (leu 3a); and **C**, CD8 (OKT8). The interstitial infiltrate consists principally of CD3+ cells. CD4+ and CD8+ cells invade tubules (T). CD4+ tend to form aggregates (A), while CD8+ cells infiltrate diffusely. A glomerulus (G) shows no T cells. **A**. × 125, **B**. × 200, **C**. × 313.

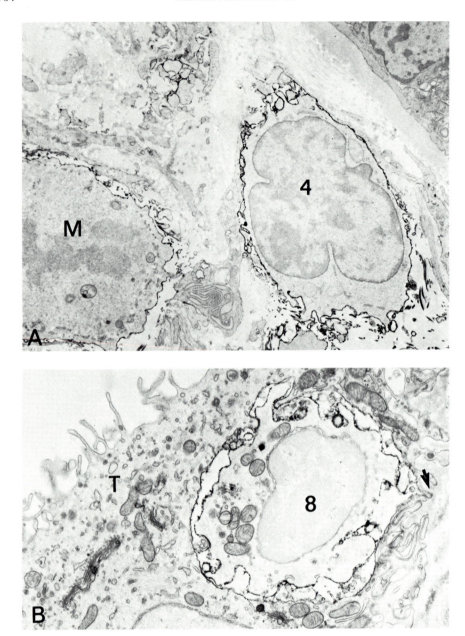

FIG. 7. Acute cellular allograft rejection stained for T cell markers with immunoperoxidase, using immu-noelectronmicroscopy. **A**. Stains for CD4 show a positive lymphocyte (4) and a positive cell in mitosis (M) in the interstitium. × 5,780. **B**. Stains for CD8 reveal a positive lymphocyte (8) invading across the tubular basement membrane (*arrow*) into a tubule (T). × 10,260. Courtesy of E.E. Schneeberger.

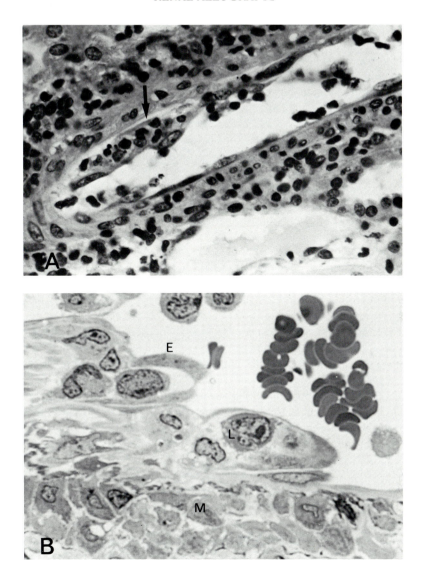

FIG. 8. Acute cellular allograft arteritis. **A**. Light microscopy shows invasion under the arterial endothelium by lymphocytes (*arrow*). Other lymphocytes appear attached to the surface. **B**. One micron section shows the subendothelial cells include lymphoblasts (L) (165). Endothelium (E), media (M). × 1,240. Reprinted with permission from ref. 165.

tematically studied. Neutrophils can be focally prominent and rarely form intratubular casts that mimic acute pyelonephritis (unpublished observations).

Arterial endothelium commonly has attached mononuclear cells and injury (Fig. 8). By electron microscopy endothelial loss and deposition of fibrin may be observed in the peritubular capillaries, sometimes with extravasation of neutrophil granules (39,189). In most cases, the glomeruli are spared; a few scattered mononuclear cells and segmental endothelial damage are sometimes present. By electron microscopy, the glomeruli are usually unremarkable, but may show segmental accumulation of low density amorphous material under the endothelium, sometimes with fibrillar deposits and occasional effacement of podocyte foot processes (189).

Immunofluorescence microscopy. Fibrin is typically present in the interstitium (38,39,166) (Fig. 5). The fibrin-rich interstitial edema probably causes the allograft swelling, analogous to the fibrin gel that causes induration in delayed hypersensitivity reactions (53). The fibrin deposition derives from increased vascular permeability and activation of the clotting system, perhaps by T cell induction of macrophage procoagulants (98).

Little, if any, immunoglobulin deposition is found and eluates from acutely rejected kidneys usually yield no detectable HLA antibodies (170). Soulillou found only 15% of eluates from 34 grafts rejected in the first 3 months had anti-T cell cytotoxic antibodies, mostly IgG3; anti-B cell (presumably class II reactive) antibodies were found in 21% (245). Eluates also occasionally contain antibodies to GBM, TBM, and DNA (245). C3 commonly accumulates along the TBM in segmental linear deposits, as an exaggeration of the normal pattern. The local activation of the complement system is probably caused by release of components from injured tubular cells, but this has not been established.

Mononuclear cell phenotype. Immunoperoxidase studies have revealed that about 30% to 50% of infiltrating cells are T cells, as judged by the CD3 marker (26,142,168,200, 225,266) (Figs. 6,7). Both $CD8^+$ and CD4 T cell subsets are always present, although in varying proportions. Both $CD8^+$ and $CD4^+$ cells invade tubules to a similar degree, suggesting both class I and II antigens are targets (266). $CD8^+$ cells usually predominate and typically infiltrate diffusely in the renal cortex (225,266); $CD4^+$ cells can be more numerous in perivascular aggregates and early biopsies (81,142,225,266). Analogous observations have been made in unmodified human skin graft rejection, in which the $CD4^+$ cells remain as perivascular aggregates and the $CD8^+$ cells infiltrate into the epithelium (24) (see Chapter 1). In cardiac allografts, a rise in the CD4/CD8 ratio in the infiltrate sometimes precedes myocyte necrosis by a week (108). The CD4/CD8 ratio in the graft does not correlate well with the ratio in the blood (26,269,275). Some of the $CD4^+$ cells are macrophages, which also express CD4 (see Chapter 2). The $CD4^+$ T cells can be calculated from the difference between $CD3^+$ and $CD8^+$ cells (71,266).

No major differences have been noted in the composition of the infiltrating cells in patients on cyclosporine, compared with those on azathioprine. Some note fewer $CD3^+$ cells (168) and more $CD4^+$ cells (275) during rejection on cyclosporine, but most find no difference (26,66,168,266). The infiltrate in cyclosporine toxicity may have more $CD4^+$ cells than in rejection (130,202), but more studies are needed to determine whether this is diagnostically useful.

Macrophages rival T cells in abundance and may be the predominate leukocyte (71). Macrophages display markers of activation, including tissue-factor, procoagulant-related antigen A1-3 (84,86), FMC33 (86), and a fibronectin receptor (266). Macrophages expressing the tissue, procoagulant-related antigen were commonly associated with interstitial fibrin deposits (84). Few studies have used a macrophage specific marker (86,142, 266). Since it is also on granulocytes, NK cells, and some suppressor cells, CD11 (OKM1, Leu 15) is an unreliable indicator of macrophages.

Small numbers of other cell types are present. About 5% have the Leu 7 (HNK-1) marker (21,71,84,266). The $Leu 7^+$ cells are more common (17%) in early biopsies (days 3 to 4) (84). Invasion of tubules by $Leu 7^+$ cells can be demonstrated in paraffin sections and has been proposed as a feature that distinguishes cellular rejection from ATN or stable grafts (21). Whether these are NK cells is unknown because Leu 7 is also on subpopulations of CD8$^+$ and CD4$^+$ T cells, including CD8$^+$ cytotoxic effectors (198). Studies of IL-2 dependent cells derived from biopsies of acutely rejecting grafts have revealed little NK activity (209), although some T cells clones also kill NK targets (251). Despite cells with the appearance of plasma cells by electron microscopy, B cells are exceedingly uncommon in the acute phase of graft rejection (26,142,266).

The T cells express activation markers in a characteristic sequence *in vitro*, with the IL-2 receptor (CD25) followed by the transferrin receptor and CD38 (T10), the class II antigens and the late antigens (133,137). In later phases of activation DR/DQ may be present with little IL-2 receptor (209). Activation of the infiltrating cells at all stages has been demonstrated by the presence of IL-2 receptors (84), tranferrin receptor (275), and HLA class II antigens (26,266,275), and CD38 (Fig. 2). The IL-2 receptor has been reported on 15% of the leukocytes in rejection (84), and the transferrin receptor on 2% to 8% (275). HLA-DQ (Leu 10) was on 11% to 27% of the cells (275). Since it is absent from peritubular capillary endothelium (266), HLA-DQ is a better marker of T cell activation than DR; however, both are on macrophages and B cells. Dual markers will improve the information obtained from the activation markers, since none is subset or even cell type specific.

MHC Antigens. Increased tubular DR antigen expression correlates strongly with the presence of a T cell infiltrate and presumably is a local response to IFNγ produced by these cells (26,71). Increased tubular DR is characteristic of acute cellular rejection (16,26,71, 81,275), as distinguished from ATN (275) or cyclosporine toxicity (16) (Fig. 2). Quantitative grading of tubular DR has permitted the diagnosis of 94% of rejection episodes, with no false positives among those with cyclosporine toxicity or stable function (27). However, even during rejection episodes, patients on cyclosporine have less tubular cell DR than those on azathioprine (26,71). During rejection, DR is increased in the endothelium of larger vessels, which normally has little or no class II antigen (71).

Acute cellular arteritis

Mononuclear cells infiltrating arterial and arteriolar endothelium are the pathognomic lesions of acute cellular rejection, as first noted by Dammin (61) (Fig. 8). In our opinion, the cellular arteritis is a usual and probably significant manifestation of cellular rejection. The biologic and diagnostic significance of this lesion has been emphasized in the past (165) and is widely accepted (37,189,234). The "endothelialitis" (234) can be detected in at least half of the biopsies of acute rejection (48% in one series) (234). Such lesions have been widely observed in diverse allograft organs and species, including murine kidney (219), human heart (239), and liver (241). If present, the endarteritis permits a certain diagnosis of active rejection (37,234).

The inflammatory cells associated with the endothelium include lymphocytes, lymphoblasts, and monocytes, but seldom granulocytes. Both CD8$^+$ and CD4$^+$ cells invade the intima in early grafts, but later, CD8$^+$ cells predominate (266), suggesting that class I antigens are the primary target. The endothelial cells are typically reactive with increased cytoplasmic volume and basophilia. They may be lifted off the subendothelial basement membrane (difficult to distinguish from artifact unless mononuclear cells undermine them), necrotic or absent. The media usually shows little change. Frank necrosis of the wall or thrombosis is unusual. Immunofluorescence studies sometimes show focal fibrin deposition, but little or no immunoglobulin.

The evidence is quite convincing that the acute cellular endarteritis is mediated by T cells rather than antibodies. The lesion contains T cells but not antibodies. The cellular arteritis occurs in the absence of humoral antibody and has not been produced by passive transfer of antibodies in animals (116,282). Finally, in man, rejection with vascular infiltrates can be reversed with OKT3 (55, and R. B. Colvin, *unpublished observations*).

Cellular arteritis should not be confused with necrotizing arteritis, characteristic of accelerated rejection and probably due to antibody (see above). Some have not separated these two lesions, regarding both types of "vascular rejection" as predominantly humoral (148, 206). Cellular arteritis has a much better rate of reversal than necrotizing arteritis (61% versus 29% one-year graft survival) (158), and practical grounds alone justify separation of the two lesions.

Acute allograft glomerulopathy

In 1981 Richardson and his colleagues drew attention to a distinctive, acute allograft glomerulopathy, characterized by hypercellularity, injury and enlargement of endothelial cells, and infiltration of glomeruli by mononuclear cells and by webs of periodic acid Shiff (PAS) positive material (213) (Fig. 9). Affected patients presented with azotemia, often with moderate proteinuria, a low blood CD4/CD8 ratio and frequently lost their graft (50). This glomerulopathy has been observed by others in 4% to 7% of biopsies taken for allograft dysfunction, typically 1 to 4 months after transplantation (10,102,153,213) and has been termed "pseudo-glomerulitis" (287).

The principal target of the damage is the glomerular endothelium, as judged by the severe injury and reactive changes of these cells. In addition, arterial endothelium was affected in 92% of our cases, as manifested by infiltration of arterial endothelium by mononuclear cells and intimal proliferation (50,153,266). The glomeruli contain numerous $CD3^+$ and $CD8^+$ T cells and monocytes (104,266) (Fig. 9). The lymphocytes have an activated phenotype, as judged by the presence of IL-2 receptor and HLA-DR. Others have noted the accumulation of monocytes in glomeruli especially in severe rejection (84,90, 190,287). The glomeruli have increased staining for HLA class I antigens (266). By immunofluorescence, fibrin and scant immunoglobulin and complement deposits are found in glomeruli.

The pathogenesis of acute allograft glomerulopathy has been the subject of controversy. The lesions have been strongly correlated with cytomegalovirus (CMV) infection in our patients (5,50,213,226), and to a lesser degree (or not at all) by others (5,10,102,153). Among patients with CMV viremia in three series the incidence ranges from 13% to 70% (5,50,213). The frequent occurrence of CMV infection in allograft recipients and the fact that only a minority of the CMV infected patients develop the lesion could obscure any association. Serial, frequent routine viral cultures, and stringent criteria for temporal association were used to detect the association in our original studies (213,226). Puzzling features that must be explained are the sequential occurrence in two allografts, each during CMV viremia (213), occurrence in HLA-identical kidneys (50,213,266), presentation as a distinct episode following conventional rejection (213), and relative resistance to OKT3 (*unpublished observation*).

Even if associated with the glomerulopathy, CMV must exert its putative effect indirectly and only in renal allografts. Acute glomerulopathy has not been observed in bone marrow transplant recipients with CMV infection (102, *unpublished observations*) or neonatal CMV infection (201). Furthermore, viral particles or antigens have not been found in the glomeruli (213,266). Only 1% of graft biopsies have CMV infected intraglomerular

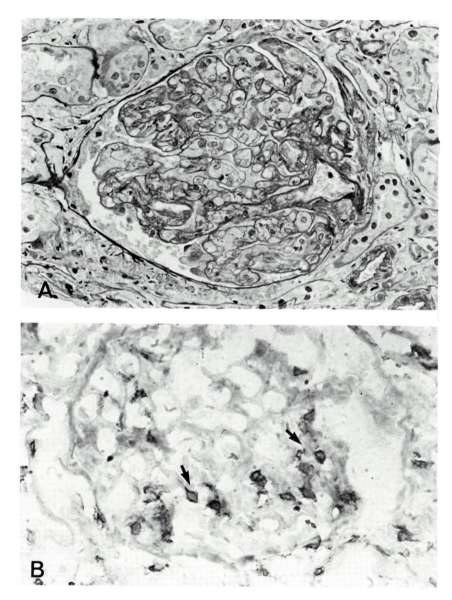

FIG 9. Acute allograft glomerulopathy. **A**. Glomerular capillaries are occluded by swollen endothelial cells, mononuclear cells and webs of PAS positive material. The interstitium has little infiltrate (266). PAS stain × 313. **B**. Immunoperoxidase stain with OKT8 reveals many intraglomerular CD8+ cells. × 500. Reprinted with permission from ref. 266.

cells, as judged by *in situ* DNA hybridization, even though 41% had infected tubular epithelium (131).

Acute allograft glomerulopathy is probably an unusual variant of cellular rejection. Some regard the lesion as a form of humoral rejection, and the mononuclear cells have not always been recognized (153); however, T cells, rather than antibodies, are detected in the glomeruli immunohistochemically (104,266). Since florid glomerulopathy may occur with little interstitial infiltrate, the glomerular lesions are not simply a manifestation of an unusually severe interstitial rejection. Rather, the rejection becomes focused on glomerular components. An element of acute allograft glomerulopathy may occur in other grafts, since occasional reactive endothelial cells and mononuclear cells are present.

We have hypothesized that IFN, especially IFNα/β produced in response to viral infection, focuses the rejection process on the glomerulus and arterial endothelium (266). Glomerular and arterial injury can be precipitated in allografts (but not autologous kidneys) by high dose recombinant IFNα, given for viral prophylaxis (132). Nephrotic range proteinuria occurred in 3 of 8 patients, and a biopsy of one showed "intracapillary proliferative glomerulonephritis". The cells of the glomerulus and the arterial endothelium are more responsive than those of the tubule to class I induction by IFN-α/β (149). In a host with inhibited T cell function, a viral infection might promote a relatively selective response of IFN-α/β, rather IFN-γ. The proposed pathogenesis is compatible with the increased HLA class I expression and the accumulation of CD8$^+$ cells observed. This theory would explain how CMV infection promotes glomerular injury indirectly and only in allografted kidneys. Furthermore, the theory would predict that stimuli of IFN release other than CMV, possibly other viruses or the rejection reaction itself, could cause the same lesion.

Prognosis

Certain pathologic features of acute rejection have prognostic significance either individually or in combination (68,110) (Table 2). In the pre-cyclosporine era, only 10% of kidneys with either medial arterial necrosis, acute glomerular lesions or interstitial hemorrhage remained functional at one year (101); others confirmed the importance of these lesions (12,110,158). Similarly, the presence of infarction or glomerular or arterial thrombi in the first 60 days was a reliable harbinger of graft loss within a year (123); these are occasionally found in well-functioning grafts, possibly dating from the time of transplantation (242).

Cellular endarteritis is significantly associated with later loss of function in kidneys (101), hearts (239), and livers (241). However, the loss rate was similar to tubulo-interstitial rejection without arteritis (61% versus 64% one-year kidney graft survival) (158). The two other types of vascular lesions, necrotizing arteritis and chronic intimal proliferation, are much more ominous (29% and 10% one-year graft survival, respectively) (158).

The intensity of the interstitial infiltrate has no correlation with the outcome of the graft (12,101,110,123); however, the relative proportion of CD8$^+$ cells is correlated with a poorer response to immunosuppressive therapy (26, 225, 266). By multivariate analysis, only the diffuse cortical CD8$^+$ infiltrate was associated with graft loss within 10 weeks, with a relative risk factor of 46 (excluding cases with vascular involvement) (225). The reason for this is unclear; the CD8$^+$ may be relatively resistant to the immunosuppressive drugs or may mediate more severe injury. In cardiac grafts, intractable rejection is characterized by CD8$^+$ and CD11$^+$ positive infiltrates (108). The numbers of CD3$^+$ or CD2$^+$ (T11) cells in the interstitial infiltrate correlate with the presence but not the prognosis of rejection (26,168,275). Eosinophil rich infiltrates ($> 2\%$) have also been associated with graft loss (276).

The intensity of tubular DR was greater in patients with irreversible rejection when biopsied during the rejection episode (71). In routine biopsies 90 days after transplantation, tubular cell DR was increased in non-cyclosporine treated patients (71% versus 9% on

TABLE 2. Renal allograft biopsy features that correlate with irreversible rejection

	Reference
Vessels	
Arterial/arteriolar thrombosis	123
Medial (fibrinoid) necrosis	12,101,110,158
Infarction	123
Interstitium	
Hemorrhage	12,101
CD8$^+$ cells	26,225,266,269
Eosinophils	276
Tubules	
Increased DR	71
Glomeruli	
Thrombosis	123
Necrosis	12,101
Acute glomerulopathy	50,213
Intraglomerular mononuclear cells	
CD3$^+$ T lymphocytes	26,266
CD8$^+$ lymphocytes	266
Monocytes	90,190

cyclosporine). All patients (14/14) with normal tubular cell DR at 90 days and functioning kidney at 2 years, while 33% (3/9) of those with increased DR subsequently lost grafts (71). The MHC increase may directly affect the susceptibility of the graft to rejection, or simply serve as a marker of the intensity of the reaction (71).

Acute glomerulopathy has a poor prognosis (213); in our combined series of 21 grafts 67% were lost (50,213,266). Graft loss correlates with the number of CD8$^+$ intraglomerular cells but not with the CD4$^+$ cells (266). Even in nonglomerulopathy cases, the presence of intraglomerular T cells (26) that are CD8$^+$ (266) and monocytes (90) correlate with subsequent graft loss. In contrast to tubulo-interstitial rejection, prognosis in the glomerulopathy is inversely related to the intensity of the interstitial infiltrate of CD8$^+$ cells.

Morphology of Normally Functioning Grafts

Biopsies of stable grafts taken in research protocols have demonstrated that a mononuclear interstitial infiltrate can be conspicuous, without obvious clinical evidence of rejection. This has been noted especially in biopsies within the first 4 weeks (37,168). By point count morphometry, the "normal" infiltrate occupied 11% to 12% of the cortex at 7 and 21 days and declined to 6% at 90 days. Patients treated with cyclosporine who had stable function had less infiltrate at day 21 (8%) than those on azathioprine (15%). Analogous "normal" infiltrates occur in endomyocardial biopsies used to monitor heart allografts (233) and in liver biopsies (196).

One may then ask what features distinguish clinical rejection on this background of a "normal" infiltrate. The infiltrate doubles in intensity in rejection to 18% to 21% of the cortex by point count (168) and to 2,269 cells/mm^2 by direct counting (37). However, the proportions of the CD8$^+$ cells, Leu 7$^+$ and CD3$^+$ cells are the same in rejecting and stable grafts (168). One group reported increased CD8$^+$ cells in rejection (83) and another, invasion of tubules by Leu 7$^+$ cells (21) (see above). One diagnostic feature not found in stable or ischemic grafts is acute cellular arteritis (37).

The common "subclinical" allograft infiltrate has practical and theoretical implications. Clearly, the presence of an interstitial infiltrate alone is not sufficient to diagnose rejection, although such cells may mediate subclinical graft injury. These "normal" allograft residents contribute to the infiltrate otherwise attributed to cyclosporine toxicity (234) (see below). The fascinating question raised by these studies is whether the infiltrate contains immuno-regulatory cells important in the adaptation of the host to the graft. In certain class I dispa-rate murine renal allografts, the intense infiltrate spontaneously disappears and is followed by indefinite graft survival (219). An answer may be found by functional analysis of lymphocytes cultured from stable grafts (163,209).

Chronic Allograft Rejection

Graft function may be lost gradually over a period of months to years, with or without episodes of acute rejection. The slowly rising creatinine is often accompanied by severe proteinuria or hypertension. Biopsies show chronic lesions of arteries, glomeruli, tubules, and interstitium, in varying degrees (197). Little is known of the pathogenesis of these chronic lesions, whether due to scarring and repair from acute rejection episodes or to fundamentally different mechanisms that proceed at a much slower pace. The primary injury probably arises from a combination of antibody and T cells reactive to histocom-patibility antigens, but infections and nonimmunologic injury may contribute.

Chronic Tubulo-interstitial Rejection

In many longstanding grafts, the cortical tubules show atrophy and loss, and the inter-stitium has patchy fibrosis with a sparse mononuclear infiltrate with small lymphocytes, plasma cells, and mast cells (51). There are no features which distinguish this from the chronic interstitial fibrosis of cyclosporine toxicity (see below) or for that matter benign nephrosclerosis. Superimposed current activity of rejection is indicated by edema, tubular invasion, or acute vascular lesions. Ischemia due to the chronic arterial lesions as well as recurrent episodes of cellular rejection at the level of the tubules and peritubular capillaries probably contribute to these lesions. Subcapsular biopsies in most grafts show fibrosis and are not representative samples.

Anti-TBM antibodies

Anti-TBM antibodies are detected in 1% to 6% of patients with renal allografts, usually as a manifestation of rejection (114,127,191,210,216,245). These antibodies may also arise in conjunction with recurrent anti-GBM (140) or TBM (117,127) disease or as a response to TBM alloantigens (281). The target is one of several TBM components, in-cluding the 48 to 54 kd collagenase-released fragment restricted to proximal TBM, as in idiopathic anti-TBM disease (47,54,283). Allograft patients may also have antibodies to other antigens of the distal or collecting TBM (216). Antibodies to TBM (and to peri-tubular capillaries) were produced *in vitro* by plasma cells derived from a rejected renal allograft in a patient with recurrent anti-TBM disease (117). Notably, these had deposited *in vivo* but were not detectable in the serum.

The anti-TBM antibodies usually have little clinical significance (216). Linear TBM deposits appeared in biopsies from 18 of 662 patients 3 to 13 months after transplantation.

Half (48%) of the biopsies with linear TBM deposits were from stable patients, and 32% had only "minimal" histological changes. Circulating IgG anti-TBM antibodies could be detected in 55% of the 18 in low titers (< 1 : 16). The deposits disappeared in a subsequent biopsy in 67%. Linear IgG did not correlate with previous rejection episodes or graft survival (although those with circulating antibodies were not separately analyzed).

Chronic Allograft Arteriopathy

The arteries show pronounced fibrous intimal thickening with myointimal cells, collagen fibrils, focal calcification, a sparse mononuclear infiltrate, and lipid-filled, foamy macrophages disposed characteristically against the external elastica, which is duplicated and disrupted. The intima also commonly contains fibrin and acid mucopolysaccharides, stainable with Alcian blue (189). In late lesions, the media is replaced by fibrous tissue, and the lumen is almost occluded. Recanalized thrombi are occasionally present. Some of the spindle-shaped cells that contribute to the intimal thickening are of host origin, but of unknown lineage (120). Immunofluorescence, often but not invariably, shows IgG, IgM, C3, and fibrin in the intima and media (38,113,145,166,197). Anti-HLA antibodies have been eluted from a minority of late rejected grafts; 13% of eluates from 24 chronically rejected grafts had anti-T cell, and 38% had anti-B cell cytotoxic antibodies (262).

The pathogenesis of this clinically important lesion is unknown, but is clearly part of the immunologic rejection, as first proposed by Porter (207). This arterial lesion is also seen in other allografted organs, notably the heart (120) liver (241). Recurrent deposition of mural fibrin-platelet thrombi on the subendothelium, exposed by endothelial loss with subsequent organization, is the likely pathogenesis, analogous to atherosclerosis. In allografts, however, the primary endothelial injury is probably due to T cells and/or antibody. The degree of intimal thickening correlates with alloantibodies to graft class I antigens (113), implying a pathogenetic role. However, it is not uncommon to find focally intense lymphocytic infiltrates in the intima and what appear to be intermediate stages of acute cellular arteritis with mixtures of lymphocytes, fibrin, and fibromuscular proliferation. Nonimmunological endothelial damage, especially that owing to cyclosporine toxicity, hypertension, and hyperlipidemia, probably synergize with the immunological intimal injury and may be equally important.

Chronic Allograft Glomerulopathy

Glomerular abnormalities were first recognized in long-term grafts and related to rejection by Porter (205). The most severe changes are associated with proteinuria, even nephrotic syndrome (89,205). The glomeruli have an increase in mesangial cells and matrix and thickening of the GBM, with various degrees of scarring and adhesions. Foot process effacement, focal mesangial cell interposition, and mesangiolysis may also be present (111). Loss of endothelial fenestrations is common in our experience (Fig. 10) and in published illustrations (111, 112, 206), but is rarely noted. Loss of this normal, differentiated structure of glomerular endothelial cells should decrease filtration. The GBM is duplicated and thickened by subendothelial rarefactions, microfibrils, and deposits (38,111,205, 288) and has been categorized by Olsen into 5 ultrastructural types (188). The electron-lucent subendothelial flocculent material (type 1) is common and is also seen in acute rejection. The granular electron dense deposits (type 2) are similar to immune complexes in

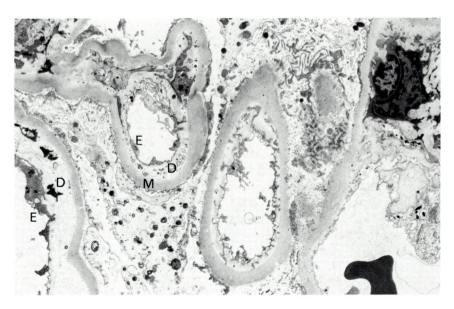

FIG. 10. Chronic allograft glomerulopathy. Electron microscopy shows marked widening of glomerular capillary walls with amorphorous deposits (D) containing a variety of cellular debris. This material accumulates between the glomerular basement membrane (M) and the endothelial cells (E), which show loss of fenestrations. × 2,880.

other diseases and are typically subendothelial or mesangial (188). The small (type 3) and large (type 4) vesicles were once thought to be viruses but are probably cell debris. The membranous ribbons (type 5) may be remnants of the slit diaphragms.

Immunofluorescence shows segmental or granular deposits of immunoglobulin (typically IgM and IgG, rarely IgA), C3, and sometimes fibrin in the capillary wall and in the mesangium (38,112,145,166,167,204). Extensive crescents, linear deposits of IgG, or subepithelial deposits are unusual and suggest recurrent or *de novo* glomerulonephritis (62,75,188,205).

Chronic glomerular lesions occur in patients without previous glomerular disease and thus are part of the response to the allograft, therapy, or infection. Histoincompatibility has an important influence. The lesions develop rarely in HLA identical sibling grafts (167, 217): none developed in 25 HLA-identical sibling grafts in one series (197). Immunofluorescence of the chronic lesions suggests an antibody-mediated component. In animals with chronic allogeneic disease, MHC antigens of the glomerular cells can be the target for *in situ* complex formation (76). The deposits sometimes contain cytotoxic antibodies to donor lymphocytes as shown in eluates from a singular case with similar deposits in the recipient kidney (17). In a few cases, repeat biopsies have shown this lesion to evolve after an episode of acute allograft glomerulopathy (153,213).

De Novo Glomerulonephritis

Patients without previous glomerular disease occasionally develop lesions in the allograft that resemble a primary glomerular disease, rather than the usual chronic allograft glomerulopathy just described. While some are undoubtedly coincidental, at least two are related to the allograft response: membranous glomerulonephritis and anti-GBM disease in Alport's syndrome.

Membranous glomerulonephritis (MGN)

Over 50 cases of *de novo* MGN in allografts have been reported (40,45). In a large survey, the frequency was 19/1,000 biopsies from 1,550 allografts (45). Six of the 13 cases of nephrotic syndrome among 1,282 transplant recipients were *de novo* MGN (106). The average time of appearance was 26 months after transplantation (range 2 to 58 months). No risk factors were identifiable (e.g., HLA matching or infections). A minority of patients (22%) with *de novo* MGN are HBs positive (270). The disease did not measurably shorten graft survival. We have seen 3 cases among about 600 transplant recipients, one discovered incidentally 10 years after transplantation. The ratio of *de novo* MGN to recurrent MGN is about 6 : 1 (106). Two cases had *de novo* MGN and recurrent amyloidosis (97).

Membranous glomerulonephritis can also arise in allografts from MHC identical rats (LEW.1D or LEW.1N to BN) (261). Immunoglobulin deposits in the allograft, not in the recipient kidney, indicate that the antigen is specific for the graft. The conclusion from these studies is that the target is a non-MHC glomerular alloantigen, presumably in the podocyte. If a similar pathogenesis applies to the human, the lesion is a form of rejection directed at minor histocompatibility antigens.

Anti-GBM nephritis

Anti-GBM nephritis has arisen in six grafts transplanted into patients with Alport's syndrome (119,164,173). In some well-documented cases of Alport's syndrome, an epitope on a noncollagenous domain of type IV collagen is absent, so that these patients can form alloantibodies to the normal GBM (119). The epitope is detectable in the GBM normally and in other basement membrane (BM) (TBM, epidermis, alveoli, and capillaries of the lung and placenta) after denaturation (119). In a large series, linear glomerular IgG deposits developed in 15% (5/34) of patients with Alport's syndrome and 1% (7/744) of others; however, none had overt glomerular injury or circulating antibodies (210); whether these have the same genetic defect is unknown.

Nonimmunological injury

Perfusion Injury

Immediate graft failure can result from perfusion injury (57,105,144,247). The kidney becomes cyanotic and soft immediately after re-perfusion, resembling hyperacute rejection. Biopsies taken 1 hour after reperfusion show loss of endothelial cells and plugs of platelet aggregates and fibrin in the microvasculature, especially in glomeruli (65,247). In contrast to hyperacute rejection, neutrophils are sparse in the early lesions. The loss rate is substantial: 43% of 21 grafts were lost, and only 14% had creatinines below 2 mg/dl at 1 month (247). The endothelial injury is thought to be due to abnormally high perfusion pressure or non-optimal perfusion solutions. Fortunately, this condition is now rare in most centers. Thrombosis of the main renal artery can also occur, as a consequence of trauma during perfusion (186).

Cyclosporine Toxicity

Cyclosporine has had a major beneficial effect on graft survival, yet acute and chronic nephrotoxicity remain significant clinical problems. Cyclosporine is a lipophilic cyclic endecapeptide isolated from a soil fungus, which has several N-methylated, nonpolar amino acids and a unique, unsaturated C-9 amino acid with an hydroxyl side group (30). The dramatic immunosuppressive effect can be explained in part by inhibition lymphokine production by T lymphocytes (IL-2, IFN-γ, macrophage procoagulant stimulating factor, and others) (103). Cyclosporine facilitates the generation of donor-specific suppressor cells by mechanisms that are still obscure (103,122).

Cyclosporine is converted by the liver cytochrome, P450 system to less toxic metabolites, and 95% is excreted in the bile. Inducers of the P450 system reduce nephrotoxicity (e.g., phenobarbitol) (221) and inhibitors, such as ketoconazole (277) and erythromycin (121), increase toxicity. Cyclosporine toxicity is enhanced experimentally by cyclo-oxygenase inhibitors (indomethacin), gentamicin, diuretics, ischemia, and graft irradiation (reviewed in 221). Toxicity correlates imperfectly with blood or serum levels, because the radioimmunoassay also reacts with cyclosporine metabolites and because individuals differ in sensitivity to the toxic effects.

Acute nephrotoxicity

Tubular injury. Acute toxicity usually presents as non-oliguric renal failure with sodium retention, hyperkalemia, and hyperchloremia. Hypertension is uncommon and fever is highly unusual (121). Physiologic studies in animals and humans have demonstrated that cyclosporine alters renal blood flow, metabolism of arachidonate derivatives, and renin-angiotensin regulation (121). Thus, cyclosporine shifts the balance of arachidonate pathways towards vasoconstriction and thrombosis (increased TxA2) and decreased vasodilation and anti-thrombosis (decreased PgI2 and prostacyclin) (184,286). In the early trials, higher doses (20mg/kg-day) caused oliguric renal failure in bone marrow recipients, who sometimes required dialysis (208).

In rats cyclosporine causes isometric vacuolization, giant mitochondria, and enlarged and irregular lysosomes in proximal tubules with dystrophic microcalcification, occasionally accompanied by a minimal focal mononuclear interstitial infiltrate (221). "Myelin figures" are not found, and tubular cell necrosis is uncommon (versus aminoglycoside toxicity). The tubular lesions, except for the microcalcification, are dose dependent and reversible within 10 days of stopping the cyclosporine.

The acute tubular lesions in humans are similar. The proximal tubules show the greatest morphologic changes: isometric vacuolization, giant mitochondria, enlarged multiple lysosomes, and microcalcification (171,172) (Fig. 11). The giant mitochondria stain with chromotrope aniline blue (121). Microcalcification and giant mitochondria occur in various conditions, including ischemic injury (257). Isometric vacuolization predominates in the straight portion of the proximal tubule (172), although we have seen it in the convoluted portion. The vacuoles contain aqueous fluid rather than lipid and are indistinguishable from those caused by osmotic diuretics. Necrotic cells are uncommon, but the dystrophic calcification presumably is a remnant of a necrotic epithelial cell.

The diagnosis of toxicity is difficult because none of these features is pathognomic for cyclosporine, and each occurs in other conditions, notably acute ischemic renal failure. Furthermore, cyclosporine toxicity may occur in the absence of morphologic changes

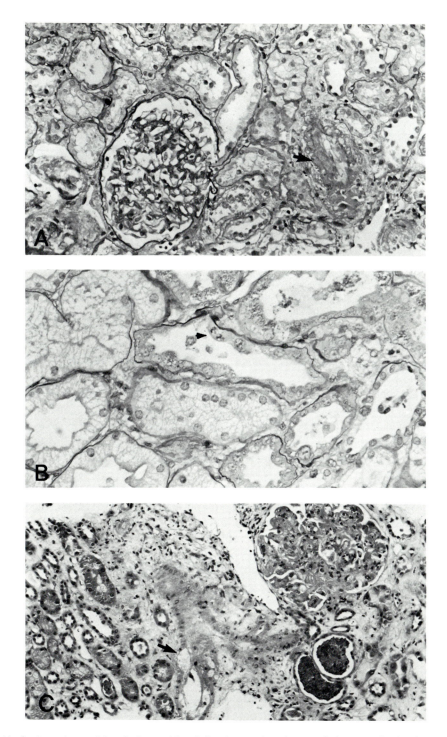

FIG. 11. Cyclosporine toxicity. **A**. Loss of brush borders and moderate tubular vacuolization is shown with focal arterial medial necrosis (*arrow*). The interstitial infiltrate is scant. The renal function recovered after cyclosoprine was decreased. × 200. **B**. Characteristic (but not diagnostic) isometric vacuolization of proximal tubular cells, which also show loss of brush border. A mitosis is present (*arrow*). PAS stain × 313. **C**. Hemolytic-uremic syndrome in an allograft recipient, which responded to decreased cyclosporine. The glomerular capillaries are occluded by swollen cells and fibrin. Arterial walls have ballooning necrosis of smooth muscle cells (*arrow*). × 125. **A** and **B** are from the same patient (255). Reprinted with permission from ref. 255.

(172). According to Mihatsch, however, the combination of vacuolization and giant mitochondria is more regularly observed in cyclosporine nephrotoxicity than any other known disease or drug nephropathy (172).

Difficulty arises in the distinction between rejection and cyclosporine toxicity and in the possibility that they may coexist. Interstitial infiltrates are minimal in autologous kidneys with nephrotoxicity (221), but are common in early allografts (37), and have no differential value unless minimal (66,234,260,271). Interstitial edema is typically slight in toxicity (172,234), but is an unreliable discriminator (66), as is the invasion of tubules by lymphocytes (234,271). Sibley noted that in cyclosporine toxicity, mononuclear cells tend to remain in the peritubular capillaries rather than infiltrate the interstitium, but this had limited differential value (234). In our experience and that of others (234,260), the only unequivocal evidence for rejection is acute cellular arteritis, which is not found in cyclosporine toxicity alone ($< 2\%$).

Immunoreactive cyclosporine in tubular cells correlates with cyclosporine toxicity (129, 273). A note of caution was raised by the finding that one anti-cyclosporine antiserum had no residual staining activity after absorption with normal tubular cells (221). In the most detailed study, toxicity correlated best with a "fine granular" tubular and diffuse interstitial cyclosporine antigen accumulation, as judged by immunoperoxidase staining of formalin-fixed, paraffin-embedded sections (129). Coarse granular tubular staining had no significance. The combination of intense cyclosporine deposition and little CD8 infiltrate identified cyclosporine toxicity correctly in 96% of the biopsies (129).

Arteriopathy. A spectrum of acute and chronic arteriopathy has been described by Mihatsch (172), ranging from acute, focal myocyte necrosis and mucoid intimal thickening to indolent, nodular hyaline deposits (Fig. 11). The vasculopathy may be less common in the current lower dose regimens, but is still seen. The vessels show deposits of IgM, C3 and fibrin, the last in early biopsies. Glomerular involvement is slight and focal, restricted to secondary ischemic changes and occasional fibrin-platelet thrombi. Later biopsies show progressive scarring of arterioles, intimal fibrosis, and segmental glomerular obsolescence. Arterial damage is not elicited by cyclosporine in normal animals, unless combined with other factors that cause vascular injury. Cyclosporine precipitates similar vascular lesions in the spontaneously hypertensive rat, with exudative fibrinoid necrosis and proliferative changes of the media of arterioles (221).

None of the vascular lesions is unique. However, we and others have found focal myocyte necrosis in the media of small arteries in the absence of intimal changes to be a reliable indicator of cyclosporine toxicity (66,255,260). These changes are probably related to the more dramatic endothelial/smooth muscle damage that results in the hemolytic-uremic syndrome.

Hemolytic-uremic syndrome. Hemolytic-uremic syndrome was first reported in bone marrow recipients (7,232) and subsequently in renal allografts (183,268). The patients develop acute renal failure, thrombocytopenia (platelet consumption in the kidney), red cell fragmentation, and hyperbilirubinemia. The presence of intravascular hemolysis is helpful in the differential diagnosis, since severe hemolysis is unusual in graft rejection. Hemolytic-uremic syndrome occurs under current regimens in 1% to 2% of our renal transplant recipients on cyclosporine, despite careful attention to blood cyclosporine levels.

The kidney has fibrinoid necrosis of arterioles and glomerular thrombi, with an interstitial infiltrate that varies from mild (243) to severe (121) (non-allografted kidneys have no infiltrate). Rejection alone may produce such lesions, since similar necrotizing arteritis was described in the pre-cyclosporine literature as accelerated rejection (39,243). The prognosis of the acute vasculopathy is poor; in one series of 16 renal allograft recipients, 75% lost their graft (121).

Two actions of cyclosporine which may promote the hemolytic-uremic syndrome are the inhibition of endothelial prostacyclin synthesis (184,286) and the enhancement of macrophage factor VII and thromboplastin synthesis in response to endotoxin (42). Other immune damage may be synergistic. Rabbits with acute serum sickness who are given cyclosporine develop acute renal failure with necrosis of afferent arterioles and thrombosis of glomerular capillaries (183), resembling the hemolytic-uremic syndrome (232).

By current techniques the pathologic changes of cyclosporine are indistinguishable from idiopathic hemolytic-uremic syndrome (Fig. 11). Indeed idiopathic hemolytic-uremic syndrome has been attributed to a familial deficiency in a plasma protein that induces prostacyclin synthesis (212). Recurrence of hemolytic-uremic syndrome in 2 patients on cyclosporine suggests that cyclosporine should not be used in this setting (96,141).

Chronic interstitial fibrosis. Loss of renal function in patients on long-term cyclosporine (> 1 year) was clearly demonstrated in cardiac allograft recipients (179). Biopsies show interstitial fibrosis and tubular atrophy, with a sparse infiltrate. Band-like zones of fibrosis ("striped") are said by some to be characteristic of cyclosporine (66,234), suggesting a vascular mechanism or damage to the medullary rays. The chronic scarring pattern is not distinctive enough to be distinguished from that commonly found in long-term renal allografts without cyclosporine therapy.

The pathogenesis of chronic nephrotoxicity is uncertain, because this lesion has not been produced in animals. Predisposing factors for the chronic lesions are renal ischemia and a history of acute nephrotoxicity (121). This is an element of individual sensitivity and the blood levels are not adequate predictors. About 10% of renal allograft recipients will not tolerate cyclosporine doses necessary to maintain adequate immunosuppression without chronic nephrotoxicity (121).

Other Pathology

The graft may be affected by other forms of injury, not unique to allografts, particularly ischemia (related to preservation or compromise of major vessels), obstruction (due to the ureteral anastomosis), drug reactions, and rarely acute pyelonephritis. The pathology of these is well described elsewhere (100,263,287).

RECURRENT RENAL DISEASE

Renal transplantation has provided insights into the basic mechanisms of renal disease. Many glomerular diseases have been shown to be caused by bloodborne factors, as demonstrated by their recurrence in the graft. In diseases unassociated with antibody deposition, the observation was quite unexpected (focal glomerular sclerosis and dense deposit disease). Failure to recur can be taken as evidence that the pathogenetic mechanisms are "burnt-out" (anti-GBM disease and SLE) or are intrinsic to the kidney (Alport's, adult polycystic disease, cystinosis, congenital nephrosis, and secondary focal sclerosis). The early pathologic events that precede clinical signs have been illuminated, as well as the reversibility of glomerular lesions present in the donor kidney.

The frequency and clinical significance of recurrence varies with the specific type of disease; most of the clinical cases involve glomerular disease (Table 3). Strong evidence

TABLE 3. *Recurrent glomerular disease[a]*

Recurrence	% recur	% lost	Number Patients	Reference
Usual				
Dense deposit disease	90[b]	15	75	40,64
Common				
Hemolytic-uremic syndrome	50	36	14	96
IgA nephropathy	48[b]	2	50	11,20,177
Henoch-Schönlein purpura	41[b]	>0	24	11,40
Focal glomerular sclerosis, 1°	39	13	124	80,143,254,285
Membranoproliferative GN (type I)	30	10	136	40
Idiopathic crescentic GN	28	14	21	40
Membranous glomerulonephritis	28	0	14	40,187
Amyloidosis	27	0	11	97
Occasional				
Anti-GBM disease	7	7	14	33,40
Wegener's granulomatosis	7	0	14	40,135
Systemic lupus erythematosus	(<2)	0	(>400)	40,169,134
Diabetes mellitus	(<1)	0	(>1,000)	154,161
No recurrence described				
Hereditary nephritis (Alport's)	0	0	34	210
Focal glomerular sclerosis, 2°	0	0	15	9,25,124
Congenital nephrotic syndrome	0	0	17	289

[a] Data selected and updated from Cameron (40). Individual case reports are omitted to minimize sampling error. Numbers in parentheses are estimates. GN, glomerulonephritis.
[b] As judged by biopsy.

for recurrence was found in 1% of 400 allografts in Olsen's experience (189). In contrast, the frequency of recurrence of glomerulonephritis (not completely characterized) was 61% in 18 isografts, without immunosuppression (75). Pathologic diagnosis of recurrence requires accurate classification of the original disease and the presence of lesions that can be distinguished from allograft glomerulopathy. This applies especially to those glomerular lesions that may appear in patients without primary glomerular disease, presumably as part of rejection (chronic allograft glomerulopathy resembling MPGN type I, membranous glomerulonephritis and focal glomerular sclerosis). The data in Table 3 are those of the larger series to minimize the overestimation inherent in individual case reports. Further citations and analysis are available in excellent reviews (34,40).

Focal Glomerular Sclerosis (FGS)

Primary FGS recurs frequently and is the most common cause of graft loss from recurrent disease (34,40). The combined frequency of recurrence in four large series was 39% (48/124 patients), with 13% graft loss from recurrence (80,143,254,285). The frequency of a second recurrence increases to 78% (107,254). The recurrence can be dramatic, with protein in the first drop of urine emerging from the ureter at surgery and over 40g excreted in the first 24 hr. The circulating factor has not been identified. The sequence of pathological changes in biopsies are widespread foot process loss and villous hypertrophy (1 to 2 weeks), podocyte detachment and proliferation (2 months), and segmental scars and foam cells (1 to 2 months) (272).

The risk factors for recurrent disease are rapid progression of the original disease (34,143, 199,254) and diffuse mesangial hypercellularity (150,254). For example, FGS recurred in 56% of 16 children who developed renal failure within 3 years, and 9% of the 11 who had a longer course (143). Plasmapheresis can diminish the proteinuria transiently, presumably by removing the circulating factor, but has little long-term benefit (284). Secondary FGS, arising as a late complication of other renal diseases, does not recur, indicating a different pathogenesis (probably hyperfiltration) (9,25,124).

IgA Nephropathy

As judged by immunofluorescence, IgA nephropathy recurs with a frequency of 48% (11,20,177). Only a minority of these patients have more than microscopic hematuria as the clinical consequence, and only rare kidneys are lost from recurrence (2%). Some apparent recurrences, particularly in HLA-identical sibling grafts, are probably asymptomatic IgA deposits in the donor (264). The IgA deposits in donor kidneys are reversible and disappear within a few months (8/8) (224,235).

Henoch-Schönlein Purpura

As in IgA nephropathy, subclinical recurrence can be detected by immunofluorescence, although the frequency varies widely (from 0/7 to 7/10) (40). Clinical glomerular disease is rare (4%) and usually associated with recurrence of the full syndrome (181). Graft loss from recurrence is rare but has been reported in 3 cases (40).

Membranous Glomerulonephritis (MGN)

Only a minority (<20%) of the cases of membranous glomerulonephritis in allografts arise in patients with previous MGN (see above) (109). Recurrent MGN can appear within 1 to 2 weeks after transplantation and 28% of cases develop it within 4 months (40,187). Later cases of "recurrent" MGN cannot be as reliably distinguished from *de novo* MGN. Of those that recurred within 4 months, 75% were in kidneys from HLA-matched, living, related donors (187). A known risk factor in primary MGN is HLA-DR3 (see Chapter 3), and HLA compatibility may be a risk factor in recurrence.

Anti-GBM Disease

Recurrence of anti-GBM disease is expected, if circulating antibodies are present in sufficient levels (not precisely defined). In the early experience, 41% (25/68) developed recurrent linear IgG deposition, but only 10% failed because of recurrence (206). Deposition of IgG on the GBM is thus insufficient to cause severe glomerular injury without other factors (presumably the inflammatory cell component inhibited by the immunosuppression). The anti-GBM autoantibody response is usually transient. Most recurrences can be prevented by postponing transplantation for 6 to 12 months, after the serum has become negative in a sensitive test for anti-GBM (radioimmunoassay or enzyme-linked immunosorbent assay) (33,40). Prior nephrectomy has no obvious beneficial effect (40).

Crescentic Glomerulonephritis

Wegener's granulomatosis is usually controlled by the conventional transplant immunosuppression, although cyclophosamide may be necessary for the occasional recurrence (1/9 in one series) (135). Primary (idiopathic) crescentic glomerulonephritis recurs with about the same frequency (29%) (40).

Dense Deposit Disease (DDD)

Dense deposit disease recurs in at least 90% of patients (40,64,224). Recurrence may not be inevitable; one recipient had a negative biopsy 8 years after transplantation (58). The glomerular dense deposits recur as early as 3 weeks after transplantation, preceding C3 accumulation (63), and are not necessarily symptomatic. Only 28% of the patients have clinical signs, and few have lost their kidneys from DDD (recent reports are less sanguine) (64). Abnormalities of the complement system do not predict outcome (40), but graft loss may be more common if the original disease had crescents (40,64).

Membranoproliferative Glomerulonephritis, Type I (MPGN)

Recurrence is particularly difficult to judge in this category, since chronic allograft glomerulopathy has a similar appearance. Hence, the rate of 30% is probably too high. As in DDD, crescents in the original disease are associated with graft loss, and complement levels are immaterial (40).

Hemolytic Uremic Syndrome

In the largest series, hemolytic-uremic syndrome recurred in 50% of 14 patients (96), from 1 day to 1 year after transplantation, with loss of the graft in 5. Since the lesions may also be seen as part of allograft rejection, definitive diagnosis requires the full syndrome (microangiopathic anemia and thrombocytopenia) (96). Cyclosporine can cause the same syndrome *de novo* (see above) and should be avoided in such patients, since a recurrence may be precipitated (96,141).

Systemic Lupus Erythematosus

Remarkably few cases of lupus nephritis have recurred, in over 400 lupus transplant recipients (40). None recurred in a series of 18, despite 4 with positive serology (169). As of 1987, only 5 cases of recurrence were found in the world literature (134). All 5 patients who had recurrence had a positive ANA at transplant, and 4/4 had a positive LE test; 2/4 had hypocomplementemia (134). The time to recur (1.5 to 9 years) correlates with the duration of dialysis, so that for every 4 months of pretransplant dialysis, the time to recur was increased by 1 year. While lupus activity appears to be "burnt-out" in many patients, the lack of recurrence in the presence of positive ANA has raised the possibility, at least to one astute observer, that "our present picture of the pathogenesis of lupus nephritis is wrong" (40).

Diabetic Nephropathy

Patients with diabetes develop arteriolar hyaline sclerosis more rapidly than nondiabetics, with 83% (10/12) showing this lesion by 2 to 5 years (versus none of 23 nondiabetics) (161). One suspects that cyclosporine may synergize with diabetic hyaline vascular disease. Thickening of the GBM by more than 50% of normal is common at 2 to 3 years (3/6) (29), but nodular diabetic glomerulosclerosis has been reported in only two cases so far (154,161). The long latency (5 to 9 years) means that more cases will be seen in the future. The thickening of the GBM should be preventable by pancreatic transplant, as suggested by the first two patients studied (29). Reversal of diabetic glomerulosclerosis in a donor kidney was documented by loss of proteinuria and mesangial hypercellularity at 7 months; cadaver kidneys with mild diabetic lesions might still be usable (1).

Other Diseases

Recurrence of systemic light chain disease, progressive systemic sclerosis, anti-TBM disease (216), and steroid sensitive nephrotic syndrome (162) have been described, but in less than 5 cases (40). Amyloidosis often recurs, but rarely contributes to graft loss (97). In 1975, a multicenter registry reported that primary oxalosis had a high rate of graft loss (92%) (13/14) and that patients with Fabry's disease often succumbed to their systemic disease (cardiac). Recurrence did not significantly affect the survival of transplanted kidneys in cystinosis or gout (6).

NEOPLASIA

The risk of cancer is increased in allograft recipients, regardless of the immunosuppressive drugs used (88,194), and is also increased in patients with genetic immunodeficiency (see Chapter 6). Overall, an average of 4% of transplant recipients have developed malignancies (194). The effect is remarkably selective for certain tumors (squamous carcinoma of the skin, lip and cervix, Kaposi's sarcoma, and B cell lymphoproliferative disease) (Table 4). The lesions include a dramatic polyclonal B cell proliferation often associated with a mononucleosis-like clinical picture (88). The risks of the more common adenocarcinomas (breast, lung, prostate, colon) are but little affected.

The incidence of tumors is influenced more by the intensity than the specific type of the immunosuppression. Of 5,500 patients, 0.4% on cyclosporine alone or with low-dose steroids developed lymphoma, while the frequency rose to 8% in those given cyclosporine with high-dose steroids, azathioprine and/or ATG (23). Lymphomas are relatively more frequent with cyclosporine therapy (41% versus 12% of tumors), and the latent period is shorter (11 versus 42 months) (195). Kaposi's sarcoma is also more frequent with cyclo-

TABLE 4. *Cancers with highest relative risk in allograft recipients*[a]

Type	Relative risk	Mean onset (yr)	Incidence (N/1,000/yr)	% of tumors
Kaposi's sarcoma	400–500	1	3	3.5
Lymphoma	40	2	10–20	13.8
Squamous carcinoma skin	20–36	1.5–4	10–140	26.9
Squamous carcinoma cervix	14	3	8	5.9

[a] Compiled from Hanto and Simons (88) and Penn (194)

sporine (8% versus 3%). Several of the specific tumors that occur with increased frequency are known to be associated with viral infection (EBV, human papilloma, CMV), which may be the essential common feature.

OTHER IMMUNOPATHOLOGIC DIAGNOSTIC TECHNIQUES

Fine Needle Aspiration

Diagnostic aspiration biopsy of renal allografts has been investigated extensively in Helsinki by Häyry and von Willebrand (93,95), since the original description by Pasternack (193). The key advantage is that the aspirates may be done frequently (even daily) with little or no risk, permitting assessment of the rate of change of the inflammation and response to therapy. The major disadvantages are that vessels cannot be evaluated and the spatial relationships of cells are lost. The technique is inadequate for assessing chronic changes, glomerular disease, or vascular injury.

The presence of mononuclear blasts and macrophages distinguish rejection from acute tubular necrosis (ATN) and cyclosporine toxicity (93,95). The inflammatory cells correlate with the infiltrate in needle biopsy, although macrophages are undersampled (18). In ATN, tubular cell swelling and vacuolization is present. In cyclosporine toxicity, the tubular and endothelial cells are markedly swollen, often containing amorphous cytoplasmic material and sometimes erythrocytes.

The interpretation of the cytologic smears is quite arcane and Häyry and von Willebrand recommend a week of training in a center with experts (95). The results are corrected mathematically for the inevitable blood contamination and for the different diagnostic weight given each of the 8 morphologic categories of mononuclear leukocytes (95). The adquacy of the sample is judged by the number of tubular epithelial cells obtained (18).

The technique is now done in many centers worldwide and continues to be refined. The addition of monoclonal antibodies permit more precise identification of cell types and their activation. The early results are mixed but encouraging. For example, DR expression on tubular cells distinguishes rejection from cyclosporine toxicity and nonrejection (27,94). Stable grafts have less than normal DR on tubular and endothelial cells (94). The CD4/CD8 ratio goes down in the aspirate 3 days before rejection and stays low if rejection is not reversed (259). This approach will probably find a niche in clinical management as further experience is gained.

Blood Tests

Many immunological blood tests have been evaluated in an attempt to develop an accurate, noninvasive specific test for rejection, infection and related conditions. While many assays correlate with rejection, none has yet proved superior to serum creatinine in evaluation of an individual patient. These assays include T cell proliferation and cytotoxicity (239), spontaneous blastogenesis (118), serum β2-microglobulin (15,69), cytotoxic antibodies (253), T cell subsets (220), and serum IL-2 receptor (52). The last two will be discussed here; the critical review by Smith is recommended for the other tests (240).

Flow Cytometry of Blood Leukocytes

The numbers of CD3$^+$, CD4$^+$ and CD8$^+$ T cells in the circulating blood have been analyzed extensively by flow cytometry in many transplantation centers worldwide, since the initial studies that showed correlations with frequency of rejection in ATG and azathioprine treated patients (55). In several studies, low CD4/CD8 ratios were associated with decreased risk of rejection, viral infection (due to CD8$^+$ lymphocytosis), and a poorer prognosis of rejection (220). Cyclosporine treated patients generally have less dramatic changes (229). In the largest series of cyclosporine therapy, patients with an average CD4/CD8 ratio of < 1.0 for the first 30 days had half as many rejection episodes (30/57) and graft losses (10/19) than those with ratios > 1.0 (122). Furthermore, the patients who had low ratios in the first month had better function at one year (serum Cr 1.8 versus 2.3). Donor-specific suppressor cells, which inhibit the proliferative response to donor but not third-party cells, were twice as common in those with ratios < 1.0 (60% versus 29%).

Unfortunately, the numbers and percentages of the CD4$^+$ and CD8$^+$ subsets do not reliably predict when or whether an individual patient will reject, and thus have limited use in patient management. Some have described a rise or fall in the CD4/CD8 ratio before rejection, but this has been inconsistent (220,229,252,259). Some argue that daily measurements must be taken to have diagnostic value, which seems impractical (92,175,259). At present the diagnostic use of these markers is largely limited to monitoring the adequacy of T lymphopenia during antibody therapy (ATGAM, OKT3), since patients with extremely low numbers of T cells (< 150/mm^2) seldom reject (55,79).

Blood lymphocyte studies will always be an imperfect mirror, at best, of the events in the graft. Only 1% of the lymphoid cells are in the circulation at any given time and these may not be representative of the relevant cells in the tissues and lymphoid organs. The CD4 and CD8 markers do not reveal the functional heterogeneity within each of these subsets. Furthermore, these markers give no indication of immunologic activity or antigen specificity. Until antigen and function specific markers are available, all that can be expected of the blood studies is an indication of immunologic activity, whether rejection, infection, or quiescence. This is not the ultimate goal, but may have considerable clinical value.

Current research efforts are digging more deeply, with measurement of activation markers and functionally homogenous "subsubsets", using 2 and 3 color fluorescence (see Chapter 16). Activation markers on T cells (DR and transferrin receptors) have been detectable in viral infections and graft rejection, usually as CD8$^+$DR$^+$ cells, by most (79,92,99, 269, R.B. Colvin, *unpublished observation*), but not all (99) investigators. Three to four days prior to rejection, CD2$^+$DR$^+$ decreased, then rose (92), providing evidence that frequent monitoring may be more sensitive. The initial studies of the "subsubsets" suggests that changes in the blood associated with rejection include a decrease in CD8$^+$CD11$^+$ (T suppressor) cells (79,91), an increase in CD8$^+$CD11$^-$ (T cytotoxic) cells (91), and a decrease in CD4$^+$Leu8$^-$ (T helper) cells (91). While long-term stable recipients have increased CD4$^+$Leu7$^+$ cells (139), CD8$^+$Leu7$^+$ cells rise in rejection and infection (31). Much work is needed to determine which combinations are most instructive and whether a more sophisticated approach will yield clinically useful monitoring methods.

Serum IL-2 Receptor

T cells release their IL-2 receptor β chain (CD25) in a soluble form during activation *in vitro* and *in vivo* (78,218). The molecule is about 10 kd smaller than the 55 kd cell surface molecule, but still binds IL-2 (218). Studies have begun to evaluate the diagnostic value of measurements of serum IL-2 receptor in transplantation, using a sandwich ELISA assay (52). Dialysis patients have elevated levels, which normally fall after transplantation and rise significantly in the serum/plasma in patients with acute rejection. In this respect, the IL-2 receptor behaves like creatinine and β2-microglobulin (69). A substantial rise, often to much higher levels than in rejecton, occurs in patients with viral infection, especially CMV, even without a rise in creatinine. The IL-2 receptor behaves quite differently from creatinine and β2-microglobulin, which rises in cyclosporine toxicity. As predicted, when the creatinine rises in cyclosporine toxicity, less elevation of IL-2 receptor occurs in cyclosporine toxicity, presumably due to suppression of IL-2 receptor synthesis. Occasionally, the rise in IL-2 receptor precedes the rise in Cr.

The greatest predictive value will probably result from combining the IL-2 receptor level with serum creatinine and using the incremental change in serial values (R.B. Colvin et al., *unpublished observation*). In cardiac allograft recipients, normal IL-2 receptor levels correlate with the absence of rejection as judged by the endomyocardial biopsy and might obviate the need for the latter invasive procedure (244). Further studies will determine the clinical usefulness of this assay.

Functional Studies of Biopsy Derived Cells

The culture of graft biopsies and aspirates is a research tool, capable of providing new pathogenetic insights. Early studies of fresh isolated cells from rejected allografts indicated that cytotoxic T cells were concentrated in the graft (262). The function and specificity of the infiltrating cells in acute cellular rejection can be further evaluated after expansion of the cells *in vitro*. Culture of fragments from biopsies in IL-2 stimulates growth of those T cells that express the IL-2 receptor (209), thus selecting for those cells that were activated *in vivo*. The cells cultured from biopsies with acute cellular rejection include both CD4$^+$ and CD8$^+$ cells, as well as a minor population of CD4$^+$CD8$^+$ cells. The CD4$^+$ cells generally lack Leu 8 (helper cell phenotype) and the CD8$^+$ cells lack CD11 (cytotoxic phenotype) (209). Both populations respond by proliferation to donor antigens and produce lymphokines, while cytotoxic activity is largely restricted to the CD8$^+$ cells (209). The T cells derived from human liver grafts show similar properties, with the most cytotoxic activity to class I antigens (73). The CD4$^+$CD8$^+$ cells produce ILZ and differentiate into CD4$^+$CD8$^-$ cells (209).

On a clonal level, all combinations of proliferative and cytotoxic responses to donor antigen are found among the CD4$^+$ and CD8$^+$ cells (251). A surprisingly large percentage of the clones harvested from nephrectomies of rejected renal grafts (10%) were donor specific, when recovered by limiting dilution immediately onto donor EBV cells (176). Southern blot analysis of the Ti β gene rearrangement in the mixed population of cells derived from rejecting allografts, indicates that dominant T cell clones are sometimes present (70,223). Such clonal dominance does not occur in mixed lymphocyte reactions, even after long-term culture *in vitro* (223). If confirmed as an accurate reflection of activated cells in the tissue, these data indicate a strong selection of the repertoire *in situ*, since a substantial fraction of T cells (0.1% to 0.2% of a mixed population, perhaps 10,000 different clones) proliferate in response to a particular MHC haplotype *in vitro* (128). the functional significance and relevance of the dominant clones remains to be established.

SUMMARY AND CONCLUSIONS

At present light microscopy of the renal biopsy remains the "gold standard" for diagnosis of rejection (242). In two studies of efficacy, the allograft biopsy changed the clinical diagnosis in 38% (275) and avoided the risk of increased immunosuppression in 40% to 44% of cases (156,275). Immunofluorescence adds diagnostic information in hyperacute rejection and recurrent disease. Electron microscopy is indicated for establishing the diagnosis of recurrent glomerular disease.

Immunoperoxidase marker studies can determine the cell types present, their location, and their functional status, but are unnecessary at present for diagnosis. Quantitation is tedious and techniques for multiple simultaneous markers, necessary to classify the activated cells and the "subsubsets" of T cells, have not yet been perfected (see Chapter 17). However, a panel of monoclonal antibodies to detect CD4, CD8, CD3 and HLA-DR, and DQ is potentially useful for prognosis and possibly for the diagnosis of cyclosporine toxicity. Further markers under evaluation may add to the useful information obtained from biopsy and aspiration.

REFERENCES

1. Abouna, G. M., Al-Adnani, M. S., Kremer, G. D., Kumar, S. A., Daddah, S. K., and Kusma, G. (1983): Reversal of diabetic nephropathy in human cadaveric kidneys after transplantation into non diabetic recipients. *Lancet*, 2:1274–1276.
2. Adams, D. O., and Hamilton, T. A. (1987): Molecular transductional mechanisms by which IFNγ and other signals regulate macrophage development. *Immunol. Rev.*, 97:5–27.
3. Ahern, A. T., Artruc, S. B., Della-Pelle, P., Cosimi, A. B., Russell, P. S., Colvin, R. B., and Fuller, T. C. (1982): Hyperacute rejection of HLA-AB identical renal allografts associated with B lymphocyte and endothelial reactive antibodies. *Transplantation*, 33:103–106.
4. Alexandre, G. P. J., Squifflet, J. P., De Bruyere, M., Latinne, D., Moriaci, M., Ikabu, N., Carlier, M., and Pirson, Y. (1985): Splenectomy a prerequisite for successful ABO-incompatible renal transplantation. *Transplant. Proc.*, 17:138–143.
5. Andrade, R., and Sibley R. (1987): Renal allograft biopsies in patients with cytomegalovirus disease. *Lab. Invest.* (Abstr.), 56:2A.
6. ASC/NIH Renal Transplant Registry, (1975): Renal transplantation in congenital and metabolic diseases. A report from the ASC/NIH renal transplant registry. *J.A.M.A.*, 232:148–153.
7. Atkinson, K., Biggs, J. C., Hayes, J., Ralston, M., Dodds, A. J., Concannon, A. J., and Nardoo, D. (1983): Cyclosporin A associated nephrotoxicity in the first 100 days after allogeneic bone marrow transplantation: Three distinct syndromes. *Br. J. Haematol.*, 54:59–67.
8. Auffray, C., and Strominger, J. L. (1986): Molecular genetics of the human major histocompatibility complex. *Adv. Hum. Genet.*, 15.P197–P247.
9. Axelsen, R. A., Seymour, A. E., Mathew, T. H., Fisher, G., Canny, A., and Pascoe, V. (1984): Recurrent focal glomerulosclerosis in renal transplants. *Clin. Nephrol.*, 21:110–114.
10. Axelsen, R. A., Seymour, A. E., Mathew, T. H., Canny, A., and Pascoe, V. (1985): Glomerular transplant rejection: A distinctive pattern of early graft damage. *Clin. Nephrol.*, 23:1–11.
11. Bachman, B. A., Biava, C., Amend, W., Feduska, N., Melzer, J., Salvatierra, O., and Vincenti, F. (1986): The clinical course of IgA nephropathy and Henoch-Schönlein purpura following renal transplantation. *Transplantation*, 42:511–515.
12. Banfi, G., Imbasciati, E., Tarantino, A., and Ponticelli, C. (1981): Prognostic value of renal biopsy in acute rejection of kidney transplantation. *Nephron*, 28:222–226.
13. Bannett, A. D., Bensinger, W. I., Raja, R., Baquero, A., and McAlack, R. F. (1987): Immunoabsorption and renal transplantation in two patients with a major ABO incompatibility. *Transplantation*, 43:909–911.

14. Bariety, J., Oriol, R., Hinglais, N., Zanetti, M., Bretton, R., Daliz, A. M., and Mandet, C. (1980): Distribution of blood group antigen A in normal and pathologic human kidneys. *Kidney Int.*, 17:820–826.

15. Barnes, R. M., Alexander, L. C., and West, C. R. (1984): Beta-2 microglobulin and graft rejection: Relationship to plasma creatinine during stable transplant function and graft rejection. *Transplant. Proc.*, 16:1613–1615.

16. Barrett, M., Milton, A. D., Barrett, J., Taube, D., Bewick, M., Parsons, V. P., and Fabre, J. W. (1987): Evaluation of class II major histocompatibility complex antigen expression for the differential diagnosis of cyclosporine A nephrotoxicity from kidney graft rejection. *Transplant. Proc.*, 19:1769–1771.

17. Beaujean, M. A., and Bouillenne, C. (1977): Glomerulonephritis due to transplant rejection affecting a patient's own kidneys. *Clin. Nephrol.*, 8:487–490.

18. Belitsky, P., Campbell, J., and Gupta, R. (1985): Serial biopsy controlled evaluation of fine needle aspiration in renal allograft rejection. *Lab. Invest.*, 53:580–585.

19. Benacerraf, B. (1981): Role of MHC gene products in immune regulation. *Science*, 212:1229–1238.

20. Berger, J., Noel, L. H., and Nabarra, B. (1984): Recurrence of mesangial IgA nephropathy after renal transplantation. *Contrib. Nephrol.*, 40:195–197.

21. Beschorner, W. E., Burdick, J. F., Williams, G. M., and Solez, K. (1985): Phenotypic identification of intraepithelial lymphocytes (IEL) in acute renal allograft rejection. *Kidney Int.*, 27:206–211.

22. Beschorner, W. E., Burdick, J. F., Williams, G. M., and Solez, L. (1985): The presence of Leu 7 reactive lymphocytes in renal allografts undergoing acute rejection. *Transplant. Proc.*, 17:618–622.

23. Beveridge, T., Krupp, P., McKibbin, C. (1984): Lymphomas and lymphoproliferative lesions under cyclosporin therapy. *Lancet*, 1:788–789.

24. Bhan, A. K., Mihm, M. C., and Dvorak, H. F. (1982): T-cell subsets in allograft rejection. *In situ* characterization of T-cell subsets in human skin allografts by the use of monoclonal antibodies. *J. Immunol.*, 129:1578–1583.

25. Bhathena, D. B., Weiss, J. H., McMorrow, R. G., and Curtis, J. J. (1980): Focal and segmental glomerular sclerosis in reflux nephropathy. *Am. J. Med.*, 68:886–992.

26. Bishop, G. A., Hall, B. M., Duggin, G. G., Horvath, J. S., Sheil, A. G., and Tiller, D. J. (1986): Immunopathology of renal allograft rejection analyzed with monoclonal antibodies to mononuclear cell markers. *Kidney Int.*, 29:708–717.

27. Bishop, G. A., Hall, B. M., Waugh, J., Philips, J., Horvath, J. S., Duggin, G. G., Johnson, J. R., Sheil, A. G., and Tiller, D. J. (1986): Diagnosis of renal allograft rejection by analysis of fine needle aspiration biopsy specimens with immunostains and simple cytology. *Lancet*, 2:645–650.

28. Blackman, M., Yague, J., Kubo, R., Gay, D., Coleclough, C., Palmer, E., Kappler, J., and Marrack, P. (1986): The T cell repertoire may be biased in favor of MHC recognition. *Cell*, 47:349–357.

29. Bohman, S. O., Tyden, G., Wilczek, H., Lundgren, G., Jaremko, G., Gunnarsson, R., Ostman, J., and Groth, C. G. (1985): Prevention of kidney graft diabetic nephropathy by pancreas transplantation in man. *Diabetes*, 34:306–308.

30. Borel, J. F., Feurer, C., Gubler, H. U., and Stahlein, H. (1976): Biological effects of cyclosporin A: A new antilymphocytic agent. *Agents Actions*, 6:468–476.

31. Brando, D., Civati, G., Busnachm, G., Broggi, M. L., Belli, L. S., Brunati, C., Seveso, M., Sommaruga, E., and Minetti, L. (1987): The Leu 2 + 7 + cell subset as a marker of immune activation in renal transplant recipients. *Transplant. Proc.*, 19:1611–1612.

32. Brenner, M. B., McLean, J., Scheft, H., Riberdy, J., Ang, S. L., Seidman, J. G., Devlin, P., and Krangel, M. S. (1987): Two forms of the T cell receptor gamma protein found on peripheral blood cytotoxic T lymphocytes. *Nature*, 325:689–694.

33. Briggs, W. A., Johnson, J. P., Teichman, S., Yeager, H. C., and Wilson, C. B. (1979): Antiglomerular basement membrane antibody mediated glomerulonephritis and Goodpasture's syndrome. *Medicine*, 58:348–361.

34. Broyer, M., Gagnadoux, M. F., Guest, G., Beurton, D., Niaudet, P., Habib, R., and Busson, M. (1987): Kidney transplantation in children: Results of 383 grafts performed at Enfants Malades Hospital from 1973 to 1984. *Adv. Nephrol.*, 16:307–333.

35. Brynger, H., Rydberg, B., Samuelsson, B., and Sandberg, I. (1984): Experience with 14 renal transplants with kidneys from blood group A (subgroup A2) to O recipients. *Transplant. Proc.*, 16:1175–1176.

36. Burdick, J. F., Russell, P. S., Winn, H. J. (1979): Sensitivity of longstanding xenografts of rat hearts to humoral antibodies. *J. Immunol.*, 123:1732–1735.

37. Burdick, J. F., Beschorner, W. E., Smith, W. J., McGraw, D. J., Bender, W. L., Williams, G. M., and Solez, K. (1984): Characteristics of early routine renal allograft biopsies. *Transplantation*, 38:679–684.

38. Busch, G. J., Galvanek, E. G., and Reynolds, E. S., Jr. (1971): Human renal allografts. Analysis of lesions in long-term survivors. *Human Pathol.*, 2:253–298.

39. Busch, G. J., Reynolds, E. S., Galvanek, E. G., Braun, W. E., and Dammin, G. J. (1971): Human renal allografts. The role of vascular injury in early graft failure. *Medicine*, 50:29–83.

40. Cameron, J. S. (1982): Glomerulonephritis in renal transplants. *Transplantation*, 34:237–245.

41. Cardella, C. J., Falk, J. A., Nicholson, M. J., Harding, M., and Cook, G. T. (1982): Successful renal transplantation in patients with T cell reactivity to donor. *Lancet*, 2:1240–1243.

42. Carlsen, E., and Prydz, H. (1987): Enhancement of procoagulant activity in stimulated mononuclear blood cells and monocytes by cyclosporine. *Transplantation*, 43:543–548.

43. Carpenter, C. B., d'Apice, A. J. F., and Abbas, A. K. (1976): The role of antibodies in the rejection and enhancement of organ allografts. *Adv. Immunol.*, 22:1–55.

44. Cerilli, J., Brasile, L., Galouzis, T., Lempert, N., and Clark, J. (1985): The endothelial cell antigen system. *Transplantation*, 39:286–291.

45. Charpentier, B., and Levy, M. (1982): Etude cooperative des glomerulonephrites extra membraneuses *de novo* sur allogreffe renale humaine: rapport de 19 nouveaux cas sur 1550 transplantes renaux du groupe de transplantation de l'Ile de France. *Nephrol.*, 3:158–166.

46. Cher, D. J., and Mosman, T. R. (1987): Two types of murine helper T cell clones. II. Delayed-type hypersensitivity is mediated by T_H1 clones. *J. Immunol.*, 138:3688–3694.

47. Clayman, M. D., Michaud, L., Brentjens, J., Andres, G. A., Kefalides, N. A., and Neilson, E. G. (1986): Isolation of the target antigen of human antitubular basement membrane antibody associated interstitial nephritis. *J. Clin. Invest.*, 77:1143–1147.

48. Cobbold, S., and Waldmann, H. (1986): Skin allograft rejection by L3/T4+ and Lyt 2+ T cell subsets. *Transplantation*, 41:634–639.

49. Collins, T., Lapierre, L. A., Fiers, W., Strominger, J. L., and Pober, J. S. (1986): Recombinant human tumor necrosis factor increases mRNA levels and surface expression of HLA-A,B antigens in vascular endothelial cells and dermal fibroblasts *in vitro. Proc. Natl. Acad. Sci. USA*, 83:446–450.

50. Colvin, R. B., Cosimi, A. B., Burton, R. C., Delmonico, F. L., Jaffers, G., Rubin, R. H., Tolkoff-Rubin, N. E., Giorgi, J. V., McCluskey, R. T., and Russell, P. S. (1983): Circulating T-cell subsets in human renal allograft recipients: the OKT4+/OKT8+ cell ratio correlates with reversibility of graft injury and glomerulopathy. *Transplant. Proc.*, 15:1166–1169.

51. Colvin, R. B., and Dvorak, H. F. (1974): Basophils and mast cells in renal allograft rejection. *Lancet*, 1:212–214.

52. Colvin, R. B., Fuller, T. C., Mackeen, L., King, P. C., Ip, S. H., and Cosimi, A. B. (1987): Plasma interleukin-2 receptor levels in renal allograft recipients. *Clin. Immunol. Immunopathol.*, 43:273–276.

53. Colvin, R. B., Mosesson, M. W., and Dvorak, H. F. (1979): Delayed-type hypersensitivity in congenital afibrinogenemia: Coincident lack of induration and fibrin deposition in delayed skin tests. *J. Clin. Invest.*, 36:1302–1306.

54. Colvin, R. B., and Fang, L. (1988): Interstitial Nephritis. In: *Renal Pathology*, edited by C. C. Tisher, and B. M. Brenner. J.B. Lippincott, Philadelphia (in press).

55. Cosimi, A. B., Burton, R. C., Colvin, R. B., Goldstein, G., Delmonico, F. L., LaQuaglia, M. P., Tolkoff-Rubin, N., Rubin, R., Herrin, J. T., and Russell, P. S. (1981): Treatment of acute renal allograft rejection with OKT3 monoclonal antibody. *Transplantation*, 32:535–539.

56. Cosimi, A. B., Colvin, R. B., Jaffers, G. J., Giorgi, J. V., Delmonico, F. L., Fuller, T. C., and Russell, P. S. (1984): Immunologic monitoring of monoclonal antibody therapy: Comparison of five antibodies as immunosuppressants of renal allograft rejection. *Transplant. Proc.*, 16:1459–1461.

57. Curtis, J. J., Bhathena, D., Lucas, J. A., McRoberts, J. W., and Luke, R. G. (1977): "Hyperacute rejection" due to perfusion injury. *Clin. Nephrol.*, 7:120–124.

58. Curtis, J. J., Wyatt, R. J., Bhathena, D., Lucas, B. A., Holland, N. H., and Luke, R. G. (1979): Renal transplantation for patients with type I and type II membranoproliferative glomerulonephritis: Serial complement and nephritic factor measurements and the problem of recurrence of disease. *Am. J. Med.*, 66:216–225.

59. Daar, A. S., Fuggle, S. V., Fabre, J. W., Ting, A., and Morris, P. J. (1984): The detailed distribution of HLA, A, B, C antigens in normal human organs. *Transplantation*, 38:287–292.

60. Daar, A. S., Fuggle, S. V., Fabre, J. W., Ting, A., and Morris, P. J. (1984): The detailed distribution of MHC class II antigens in normal human organs. *Transplantation*, 38:293–298.

61. Dammin, G. J. (1960): The kidney as a homograft and its host. *U. Mich. Med. Bul.*, 26:278.

62. Dixon, F. J., McPhaul, J. J., Jr., and Lerner, R. (1969): Recurrence of glomerulonephritis in the transplanted kidney. *Arch. Intern. Med.*, 123:554–562.

63. Droz, D., Nabarra, B., Noel, L. H., Leibowitch, J., and Crosnier, J. (1979): Recurrence of dense deposits in transplanted kidneys. I. Sequential survey of the lesions. *Kidney Int.*, 15:386–395.

64. Eddy, A., Sibley, R., Mauer, S. M., and Kim, Y. (1984): Renal allograft failure due to recurrent dense intramembranous deposit disease. *Clin. Nephrol.*, 21:305–313.

65. Evan, A. P., Gattone, V. H., 2d., Filo, R. S., Leapman, S. B., Smith, E. J., and Luft, F. C. (1983): Glomerular endothelial injury related to renal perfusion. A scanning electron microscopic study. *Transplantation*, 35:436–441.

66. Farnsworth, A., Hall, B. M., Ng, A. B. P., Duggin, G. G., Horvath, J. S., Sheil, A. G., and Tiller, D. J. (1984): Renal biopsy morphology in renal transplantation. *Am. J. Surg. Path.*, 8:243–252.

67. Finberg, R., Burakoff, S. J., Cantor, H., and Benacerraf, B. (1978): Biological significance of alloreactivity: T cells stimulated by Sendai virus-coated syngeneic cells specifically lyse allogeneic target cells. *Proc. Natl. Acad. Sci. USA*, 75:5145–5149.

68. Finkelstein, F. O., Seigel, N. J., Bastl, C., Forrest, J. N., Jr., and Kashgarian, M. (1976): Kidney transplant biopsies in the diagnosis and management of acute rejection reactions. *Kidney Int.*, 10:171–178.

69. Finn, W. F., Huffman, K. A., Forman, D. T., and Mandel, S. R. (1984): Value of the serum beta 2 microglo-bulin/serum creatinine ratio following renal transplantation. *Transplant. Proc.*, 16:1609–1612.
70. Finn, O. J., Miceli, M. C., Sanfillipo, F., Bollinger, R. R., and Barry, T. (1987): Analysis of human T cell repertoire in kidney allograft rejection. *Fed. Proc.* (Abstr.), 46:609.
71. Fuggle, S. V., McWhinnie, D. L., Chapman, J. R., Taylor, H. M., and Morris, P. J. (1986): Sequential analysis of HLA class II antigen expression in human renal allografts. Induction of tubular class II antigens and correlation with clinical parameters. *Transplantation*, 42(1)144–150.
72. Fuller, T. C., Forbes, J. B., and Delmonico, F. L. (1985): Renal transplantation with a positive historical donor crossmatch. *Transplant. Proc.*, 17:113–115.
73. Fung, J. J., Zeevi, A., Starzl, T. E., Demetris, J., Iwatsuki S., and Duquesnoy, R. J. (1986): Functional characterization of infiltrating T lymphocytes in human hepatic allografts. *Hum. Immunol.*, 16:182–199.
74. Gay, D., Maddon, P., Sekaly, R., Talle, M. A., Godfrey, M., Long, E., Goldstein, G., Chess, L., Axel, R., Kappler, J., and Marrack, P. (1987): Functional interaction between human T-cell protein CD4 and the major histocompatibility complex HLA-DR. *Nature*, 328:626–629.
75. Glassock, R. J., Feldman, D., Reynolds, E. S., Dammin, G. J., and Merrill, J. P. (1968): Human renal isografts: A clinical and pathologic analysis. *Medicine*, 47:411–454.
76. Gleichmann, H., Gleichmann, E., André-Schwartz, Jr., and Schwartz, R. S. (1972): Chronic allogeneic disease. III. Genetic requirements for the induction of glomerulonephritis. *J. Exp. Med.*, 135:516–532.
77. Gouw, A. S., Houthoff, H. J., Huitema, S., Beelen, J. M., Gips, C. H., and Poppema, S. (1987): Expression of major histocompatibility complex antigens and replacement of donor cells by recipient ones in human liver grafts. *Transplantation*, 43:291–296.
78. Greene, W. C., Depper, J. M., Kronke, M., and Leonard, W. J. (1986): The human interleukin 2 receptor: Analysis of structure and function. *Immunol. Rev.*, 92.P29–P48.
79. Gross, U., Thomas, F., Mathews, C., Thomas, J., Cunningham, P., and Ritter, T. (1987): *In vivo-in vitro* correlates of human rejection using flow cytometry with two-color fluorescence on peripheral blood mono-nuclear cells. *Transplant. Proc.*, 19:1609–1610.
80. Habib, R., Hebert, D., Gagnadoux, M. F., and Broyer, M. (1982): Transplantation in idiopathic nephrosis. *Transplant. Proc.*, 14:489–495.
81. Hall, B. M., Bishop, G. A., Farnsworth, A., Duggin, G. G., Horwath, J. S., Sheil, A. G. R., and Tiller, D. J. (1984): Identification of the cellular subpopulations infiltrating rejecting cadaver renal allografts. Preponderance of the T₄ subset of T cells. *Transplantation*, 37:564–570.
82. Hamburger, J. (1967): A reappraisal of the concept of organ "rejection," based on the study of homotrans-planted kidneys. *Transplantation*, 5:870–884.
83. Hammer, C., Land, W., Stadler, J., Koller, C., and Brendel, W. (1983): Lymphocyte subclasses in re-jecting kidney grafts detected by monoclonal antibodies. *Transplant. Proc.*, 15:356–360.
84. Hancock, W. W., Gee, D., De Moerloose, P., Rickles, F. R., Ewan, V. A., and Atkins, R. C. (1985): Immunohistological analysis of serial biopsies taken during human renal allograft rejection, changing profile of infiltrating cells and activation of the coagulation system. *Transplantation*, 39:430–438.
85. Hancock, W. W., Kraft, N., and Atkins, R. C. (1982): The immunohistochemical demonstration of major histocompatibility antigens in the human kidney using monoclonal antibodies. *Pathology*, 14:409–414.
86. Hancock, W. W., Rickles, F. R., Ewan, V. A., and Atkins, R. C. (1986): Immunohistological studies with A1-3, a monoclonal antibody to activated human monocytes and macrophages. *J. Immunol.*, 136:2416–2420.
87. Hancock, W. W., and Atkins, R. C. (1985): Immunohistological analysis of sequential renal biopsies from patients with acute renal rejection. *Kidney Int.*, 27:341–348.
88. Hanto, D. W., and Simmons, R. L. (1986): Cancer in recipients of organ allografts. In: *Kidney Transplant Rejection: Diagnosis and Treatment*, edited by G. M. Williams, J. F. Burdick, and K. Solez, pp. 459–480. Marcel Dekker, New York.
89. Harlan, W. R., Holden, K. R., Williams, G. M., and Hume, D. M. (1967): Proteinuria and nephrotic syn-drome associated with chronic rejection of kidney transplants. *N. Engl. J. Med.*, 277:769–775.
90. Harry, T. R., Coles, G. A., Davies, M., Bryant, D., Williams, G. T., and Griffin, P. J. (1984): The signifi-cance of monocytes in glomeruli of human renal transplants. *Transplantation*, 37:70–73.
91. Hayashi, R., Sakakibara, I., Suzuki, S., and Amemiya, H. (1987): Two-color flow cytometric techniques as a diagnostic tool for rejection of renal transplantation. *Transplant. Proc.*, 19:1603–1604.
92. Hayes, J. M., Valenzuela, R., Novick, A. C., Steinmuller, D. R., and Williams, G. (1987): Correlation between two-color flow cytometry quantitation of activated T cells and acute rejection. *Transplant. Proc.*, 19:1605–1608.
93. Häyry, P., and von Willebrand, E. (1984): Transplant aspiration cytology. *Transplantation*, 38:7–12.
94. Häyry, P., and von Willebrand, E. (1986): The influence of the pattern of inflammation and administration of steroids on class II MHC antigen expression in renal transplants. *Transplantation*, 42:358–365.
95. Häyry, P. J., and von Willebrand, E. (1986): Aspiration cytology in monitoring human allografts. In: *Kidney Transplant Rejection: Diagnosis and Treatment*, edited by G. M. Williams, J. F. Burdick, and K. Solez, pp. 247–262. Marcel Dekker, New York.

96. Hebert, D., Sibley, R. K., and Mauer, S. M. (1986): Recurrence of hemolytic uremic syndrome in renal transplant recipients. *Kidney Int.* [Suppl.], 19:S51–S58.

97. Helin, H., Pasternack, A., Falck, H., and Kuhlback, B. (1981): Recurrence of renal amyloid and *de novo* membranous glomerulonephritis after transplantation. *Transplantation*, 32:6–9.

98. Helin, H. J., and Edgington, T. S. (1984): Cyclosporin A regulates monocyte/macrophage effector functions by affecting instructor T cells: Inhibition of monocyte procoagulant response to allogeneic stimulation. *J. Immunol.*, 132:1074–1076.

99. Henny, F. C., Weening, J. J., Baldwin, W. M., Oljans, P. J., Tanke, H. J., Van Es, L. A., and Paul, L. C. (1986): Expression of HLA DR antigens on peripheral blood T. lymphocytes and renal graft tubular epithelial cells in association with rejection. *Transplantation*, 42:479–483.

100. Heptinstall, R. H. (1983): *The Pathology of the Kidney*, 3rd Edition. Little, Brown and Co., Boston.

101. Herbertson, B. M., Evans, D. B., Calne, R. Y., and Banerjee, A. K. (1977): Percutaneous needle biopsies of renal allografts: The relationship between morphological changes present in the biopsies and subsequent allograft function. *Histopathology*, 1:161–178.

102. Herrera, G. A., Alexander, R. W., Cooley, C. F., Luke, R. G., Kelly, D. R., Curtis, J. J., and Gockerman, J. P. (1986): Cytomegalovirus glomerulopathy: A controversial lesion. *Kidney Int.*, 29:725–733.

103. Hess, A. D., Colombani, P. M., and Esa, A. H. (1986): Cyclosporine and the immune response: Basic aspects. *CRC Crit. Rev. Immunol.*, 6:123–149.

104. Hiki, Y., Leong, AS-Y, Mathew, T. H., Seymour, A. E., Pascoe, V., and Woodroofe, A. J. (1986): Typing of intraglomerular mononuclear cells associated with transplant glomerular rejection. *Clin. Nephrol.*, 6:244–249.

105. Hill, G. S., Light, J. A., and Perloff, L. J. (1976): Perfusion-related injury in renal transplantation. *Surgery*, 79:440–447.

106. Honkanen, E., Tornroth, T., Pettersson, E., and Kuhlback, B. (1984): Glomerulonephritis in renal allografts: Results of 18 years of transplantations. *Clin. Nephrol.*, 21:210–219.

107. Hosenpud, J., Piering, W. F., Garancis, J. C., and Kauffman, H. M. (1985): Successful second kidney transplantation in a patient with focal glomerulosclerosis. A case report. *Am. J. Nephrol.*, 5:299–304.

108. Hoshinaga, K., Mohanakumar, T., Goldman, M. H., Wolfgang, T. C., Szentpetery, S., Lee, H. M., and Lower, R. R. (1986): Clinical significance of *in situ* detection of T lymphocyte subsets and monocyte/macrophage lineages in heart allografts. *Transplantation*, 38:634–637.

109. Hoy, W. E., Eversole, M., and Sterling, W. A. (1985): Recurrent membranous glomerulonephritis in two renal transplants. *Transplantation*, 40:100–102.

110. Hsu, A. C., Arbus, G. S., Noriega, E., and Huber, J. (1976): Renal allograft biopsy: A satisfactory adjunct for predicting renal function after graft rejection. *Clin. Nephrol.*, 5:260–265.

111. Hsu, H.-C., Suzuki, Y., Churg, J., and Grishman, E. (1980): Ultrastructure of transplant glomerulopathy. *Histopathology*, 4:351–367.

112. Hume, D. M., Sterling, W. A., Weymouth, R. J., Siebel, H. R., Madge, G. E., and Lees, H. M. (1970): Glomerulonephritis in human renal homotransplants. *Transplant. Proc.*, 2:361–363.

113. Jeannet, M., Pinn, V. W., Flax, M. H., Winn, H. J., and Russell, P. S. (1970): Humoral antibodies in renal allotransplantation in man. *N. Engl. J. Med.*, 282:111–117.

114. Johnson, J. P., Moore, J., Jr., Austin, H. A., 3rd, Balow, J. E., Antonovych, T. T., and Wilson, C. B. (1985): Therapy of anti-glomerular basement membrane antibody disease: Analysis of prognostic significance of clinical, pathologic and treatment factors. *Medicine*, 64:219–227.

115. Jonker, M. (1987): Immunosuppressive therapy by monoclonal anti-T lymphocyte subset antibodies. *Leukocyte Typing III*, pp. 923–927, Oxford University Press, Oxford, United Kingdom.

116. Jooste, S. V., Colvin, R. B., and Winn, H. J. (1981): The vascular bed as the primary target in the destruction of skin grafts by antiserum. II. Loss of sensitivity to antiserum in long-term skin grafts. *J. Exp. Med.*, 154:1332–1341.

117. Jordan, S. C., Barkley, S. C., Lemire, J. M., Sakai, R. S., Cohen, A., and Fine, R.N. (1986): Spontaneous anti-tubular basement membrane antibody production by lymphocytes isolated from a rejected allograft. *Transplantation*, 41:173–176.

118. Kanda, H., Kunikata, S., Matsuura, T., Akiyama, T., and Kurita, T. (1987): Spontaneous blastogenesis as a monitor of renal allograft rejection. *Transplant. Proc.*, 19:1592–1594.

119. Kashtan, C., Fish, A. J., Kleppel, M., Yoshioka, K., and Michael, A. F. (1986): Nephritogenic antigen determinants in epidermal and renal basement membranes of kindreds with Alport type familial nephritis. *J. Clin. Invest.*, 78:1035–1044.

120. Kennedy, L. J., and Weissman, I. L. (1971): Dual origin of intimal cells in cardiac allograft arteriosclerosis. *N. Engl. J. Med.*, 285:884.

121. Keown, P. A., Stiller, C. R., and Wallace, A. C. (1986): Nephrotoxicity of cyclosporin A. In: *Kidney Transplant Rejection: Diagnosis and Treatment*, edited by G. M. Williams, J. F. Burdick, and K. Solez, pp. 423–457. Marcel Dekker, New York.

122. Kerman, R. H., Flechner, S. M., Van Buren, C. T., Lorber, M. I., and Kahan, B. D. (1987): Immunoregulatory mechanisms in cyclosporine-treated renal allograft recipients. *Transplantation*, 43:205–210.

123. Kiaer, H., Hansen, H. E., and Olsen, S. (1980): The predictive value of percutaneous biopsies from human renal allografts with early impaired function. *Clin. Nephrol.*, 13:58–63.

124. Kiprov, D. D., Colvin, R. B., and McCluskey, R. T. (1982): Focal and segmental glomerulosclerosis and proteinuria associated with unilateral renal agenesis. *Lab. Invest.*, 46:275–281.

125. Kirkman, R. L., Colvin, R. B., Flye, M. W., Williams, G. M., and Sachs, D. H. (1979): Transplantation in miniature swine. VII. Evidence for cellular immune mechanisms in hyperacute rejection of renal allografts. *Transplantation*, 28:24–30.

126. Kissmeyer-Nielsen, F., Olsen, S., Peterson, V. P., and Fjeldborg, O. (1966): Hyperacute rejection of kidney allografts, associated with pre-existing humoral antibodies against donor cells. *Lancet*, 2:662.

127. Klassen, J., Kano, K., Milgrom, F., Menno, A. B., Anthone, S., Anthone, K., Sepulveda, M., Elwood, C. M., and Andres, G. A. (1973): Tubular lesions produced by autoantibodies to tubular basement membrane in human renal allografts. *Arch. Allergy Appl. Immunol.*, 45:675–682.

128. Klein, J. (1986): *Natural History of the Major Histocompatibility Complex*. John Wiley and Sons, New York.

129. Kolbeck, P. C., Wolfe, J. A., Burchette, J., and Sanfilippo, F. (1987): Immunopathologic patterns of cyclosporine deposition assoc iated witth nephrotoxicity in renal allograft biopsies. *Transplantation*, 3:218–224.

130. Kolbeck, P. C., Scheinman, J. I., and Sanfilippo, F. (1986): Acute cellular rejection and cyclosporine nephrotoxicity monitored by biopsy in a renal allograft recipient. The differentiation of drug nephrotoxicity from rejection by phenotyping of cellular infiltrates. *Arch. Pathol. Lab. Med.*, 110:389–393.

131. Kovarik, J., and Krisch, I. (1986): The histopathologic identification of CMV infected cells in biopsies of human renal allografts. An evaluation of 100 transplant biopsies by *in situ* hybridization. *Pathol. Res. Pract.*, 181:739–745.

132. Kramer, P., Ten, Kate, F. W. J., Bijnen, A. B., Jeekel, J., and Weimar, W. (1984): Recombinant leucocyte interferon A induces steroid resistant acute vascular rejection episodes in renal transplant recipients. *Lancet*, 1:989–990.

133. Krensky, A. M., and Clayberger, C. (1985): Diagnostic and therapeutic implications of T cell surface antigens. *Transplantation*, 39:339–348.

134. Kumano, K., Sakai, T., Mashimo, S., Endo, T., Koshiba, K., Elises, J. S., and Iitaka, K. (1987): A case of recurrent lupus nephritis after renal transplant. *Clin. Nephrol.*, 27:94–98.

135. Kuross, S., Davin, T., and Kjellstrand, C. M. (1981): Wegener's granulomatosis with severe renal failure: Clinical course and results of dialysis and transplantation. *Clin. Nephrol.*, 16:172–180.

136. Lanier, L. L., Lee, A. N., Phillips, J. H., Warner, W. L., and Babcock, G. F. (1983): Subpopulations of human NK cells defined by expression of the Leu 7 (HNK-1) and Leu 11 (NK-15) antigens. *J. Immunol.*, 131:1789–1796.

137. Lazarovits, A. I., Moscicki, R. A., Kurnick, J. T., Camerini, D., Bhan, A. K., Baird, L. G., Erickson, M., and Colvin, R. B. (1984): Lymphocyte activation antigens. I. A monoclonal antibody, anti-Act I, defines a new late lymphocyte activation antigen. *J. Immunol.*, 33:1857–1862.

138. Lawrance, S. K., Smith, C. L., Srivastava, R., Cantor, C. R., and Weissman, S. M. (1987): Megabase-scale mapping of the HLA gene complex by pulsed field gel electrophoresis. *Science*, 235:1387–1390.

139. Legendre, C. M., Guttmann, R. D., Hou, S. K., and Jean, R. (1985): Two color immunofluorescence and flow cytometry analysis of lymphocytes in long term renal allotransplant recipients: Identification of a major Leu 7+/Leu 3+ subpopulation. *J. Immunol.*, 135:1061–1062.

140. Lehman, D. H., Wilson, C. B., and Dixon, F. J. (1970): Extraglomerular immunoglobulin deposits in human nephritis. *Am. J. Med.*, 58:765–796.

141. Leithner, C., Sinzinger, H., Pohanka, E., Schwarz, M., Kretschmer, G., and Syre, G. (1982): Recurrence of haemolytic uraemic syndrome triggered by cyclosporin A after renal transplantation. *Lancet*, 1:1470.

142. Leskinen, R., and Häyry, P. (1986): Topographical distribution of inflammatory leukocyte subsets in acute cellular rejection of a kidney allograft. *Acta Pathol. Microbiol. Immunol. Scand.* [C], 94:69–76.

143. Leumann, E. P., Briner, J., Donckerwolcke, R. A., Kuijten, R., and Largiader, F. (1980): Recurrence of focal segmental glomerulosclerosis in the transplanted kidney. *Nephron*, 25:65–71.

144. Limas, G., Spector, D., and Wright, J. R. (1977): Histologic changes in preserved cadaveric renal transplants. *Am. J. Pathol.*, 88:403–420.

145. Lindquist, R. R., Guttman, R. D., Merrill, J. P., and Dammin, G. J. (1968): Human renal allografts: Interpretation of morphologic and immunohistochemical observations. *Am. J. Pathol.*, 53:851–872.

146. Littman, D. R. (1987): The structure of the CD4 and CD8 genes. *Ann. Rev. Immunol.*, 5:561–584.

147. Lobo, P. I., Sturgill, B. C., and Bolton, W. K. (1984): Cold-reactive alloantibodies and allograft malfunction occurring immediately post transplant. *Transplantation*, 37:76–81.

148. Magil, A., Rubin, J., Ladewig, L., Johnson, M., Goldstein, M. B., and Bear, R. A. (1980): Renal biopsy in acute allograft rejection. Significance of moderate vascular lesions in longterm graft survival. *Nephron*, 26:180–183.

149. Maguire, J. E., Williams, A. H., George, G. L., Gresser, I., and Colvin, R. B. (1987): *In vivo* modulation of major histocompatibility complex (MHC) antigens in the murine kidney by interferon-α/β. *Kidney Int.* (Abstr.), 31:463.

150. Maizel, S. E., Sibley, R. K., Horstman, J. P., Kjellstrand, C. M., and Simmons, R. L. (1981): Incidence and

significance of recurrent focal segmental glomerulosclerosis in renal allograft recipients. *Transplantation*, 32:512–518.

151. Marrack, P., and Kappler, J. (1986): The antigen specific, major histocompatibility complex restricted receptor on T cells. *Adv. Immunol.*, 38:1–30.

152. Martin, S., Short, C. D., Lawler, W., Gokal, R., Johnson, R. W., and Mallick, N. P. (1986): Late cellular rejection in renal transplant recipients. *Transplantation*, 41:262–264.

153. Maryniak, R., First, R. M., and Weiss, M. A. (1985): Transplant glomerulopathy: Evolution of morphologically distinct changes. *Kidney Int.*, 27:799–806.

154. Maryniak, R. K., Mendoza, N., Clyne, D., Balakrishnan, K., and Weiss, M. A. (1985): Recurrence of diabetic nodular glomerulosclerosis in a renal transplant. *Transplantation*, 39:35–38.

155. Mason, D. W., Dallman, M. J., Arthur, R. P., and Morris, P. J. (1984): Mechanisms of allograft rejection: The roles of cytotoxic T-cells and delayed-type hypersensitivity. *Immunol. Rev.*, 77:167–184.

156. Matas, A. J., Tellis, V. A., Sablay, L., Quinn, T., Soberman, R., and Veith, F. J. (1985): The value of needle renal allogrraft biopsy. III. A prospective study. *Surgery*, 98:922–926.

157. Matas, A. J., Scheinman, J. I., Rattazzi, L. C., Mozes, M. F., Simmons, R. L., and Najarian, J. S. (1976): Immunopathological studies of the ruptured human renal allograft. *Transplantation*, 22:420–426.

158. Matas, A. J., Sibley, R., Mauer, M., Sutherland, D. E., Simmons, R. L., and Najarian, J. S. (1983): A retrospective study of biopsies performed during putative rejection episodes. *Ann. Surg.*, 197:226–237.

159. Matis, L. A., Glimcher, L. H., Paul, W. E., and Schwartz, R. H. (1983): Magnitude of response of histocompatibility-restricted T-cell clones is a function of the product of the concentrations of antigen and Ia molecules. *Proc. Nat. Acad. Sci. USA*, 80:6019–6023.

160. Matzinger, P., and Bevan, M. J. (1977): Hypothesis: Why do so many lymphocytes respond to major histocompatibility antigens? *Cell. Immunol.*, 29:1–6.

161. Mauer, S. M., Barbosa, J., Vernier, R. L., Kjellstrand, C. M., Buselmeier, T. J., Simmons, R. L., Najarian, J. S., and Goetz, F. C. (1976): Development of diabetic vascular lesions in normal kidneys transplanted into patients with diabetes mellitus. *N. Engl. J. Med.*, 295:916–920.

162. Mauer, S. M., Hellerstein, S., Cohn, R. A., Sibley, R. K., and Vernier, R. L. (1979): Recurrent steroid-responsive nephrotic syndrome after renal transplantation. *J. Pediatr.*, 95:261–266.

163. Mayer, T. G., Fuller, A. A., Fuller, T. C., Lazarovits, A. I., Boyle, L. A., and Kurnick, J. T. (1985): Characterization of *in vivo* activated allospecific T lymphocytes propagated from human renal allograft biopsies undergoing rejection. *J. Immunol.*, 134:258–264.

164. McCoy, R. C., Johnson, H. K., Stone, W. J., and Wilson, C. B. (1982): Absence of nephritogenic GBM antigen(s) in some patients with hereditary nephritis. *Kidney Int.*, 21:642–647.

165. McKenzie, I. F. C., Colvin, R. B., and Russell, P. S. (1976): Clinical immunopathology of transplantation. In: *Textbook of Immunopathology*, 2nd Edition, edited by P. A. Miescher and H. J. Mueller-Eberhard, pp. 1043–1064. Grune and Stratton, New York.

166. McKenzie, I. F. C., and Whittingham, S. (1968): Deposits of immunoglobulin and fibrin in human renal allografted kidneys. *Lancet*, 2:1313–1315.

167. McPhaul, J. J., Jr., Dixon, F. J., Brettscheider, L., and Starzl, T. E. (1970): Immunofluorescent examination of biopsies from long-term renal allografts. *N. Engl. J. Med.*, 282:412.

168. McWhinnie, D. L., Thompson, J. F., Taylor, H. M., Chapman, J. R., Bolton, E. M., Carter, N. P., Wood, R. F., and Morris, P. J. (1986): Morphometric analysis of cellular infiltration assessed by monoclonal antibody labeling in sequential human renal allograft biopsies. *Transplantation*, 2:352–358.

169. Mejia, G., Zimmerman, S. W., Glass, N. R., Miller, D. T., Sollinger, H. W., and Belzer, F. O. (1983): Renal transplantation in patients with systemic lupus erythematosus. *Arch. Intern. Med.*, 143:2089–2092.

170. Metzgar, R. S., Seigler, H. F., Ward, F. E., and rowlands, D. T., Jr. (1972): Immunological studies on elutes from human renal allografts. *Transplantation*, 13:131–137.

171. Mihatsch, M. J., Theil, G., Spichtin, H. P., Oberholzer, M., Brunner, F. P., Harder, F., Olivieri, V., Bremer, R., Ryffel, B., Stocklin, E., Torhorst, J., Gudat, F., Zollinger, H. U., and Loershter, R. (1983): Morphological findings in kidney transplants after treatment with cyclosporine. *Transplant. Proc.*, 15 [Suppl 1]:2821–2835.

172. Mihatsch, M. J., Thiel, G., and Ryffel, B. (1986): Cyclosporin nephropathy. A tubulo-interstitial and vascular disease. In: *Drugs and Kidney*, edited by T. Bertani, G. Remuzzi, and S. Garattini, pp. 153–170. Serono Symposia, Raven Press, New York.

173. Milliner, D. S., Pierdes, A. M., and Holley, K. E. (1982): Renal transplantation in Alport's syndrome. Anti-glomerular basement membrane glomerulonephritis in the allograft. *Mayo Clin. Proc.*, 57:35–42.

174. Miyajima, T., Higuchi, H., Kashiwabara, H., Yokoyama, T., and Fujimoto, S. (1980): Anti-idiotypic antibodies in patients with a functioning renal allograft. *Nature*, 283:306–308.

175. Mohanakumar, T., Ellis, T. M., Reinitz, E. R., Page, S. D., Medez-Picon, G., Goldman, M. H., Lower, R., and Lee, H. M. (1984): Daily monitoring of T cell populations in renal allograft recipients: High resolution measurement of T cell kinetics and their relevance to clinical course. *Transplant. Proc.*, 16:1490–1494.

176. Moreau, J. F., Bonneville, M., Peyrat, M. A., Godard, A., Jacques, Y., Desgranges, C., and Soulillou, J. P. (1986): T lymphocyte cloning from rejected human kidney allografts. Growth frequency and functional/phenotypic analysis. *J. Clin. Invest.*, 78:874–879.

177. Morzycka, M., Croker, B. P., Jr., Siegler, H. F., and Tisher, C. C. (1982): Evaluation of recurrent glomerulonephritis in kidney allografts. *Am. J. Med.*, 72:588–598.
178. Myburgh, J. A., Cohen, I., Gecelter, L., Meyers, A. M., Abrahams, C., Furman, K. I., Goldberg, B., and van Blerk, P. J. P. (1969): Hyperacute rejection in human-kidney allografts—Shwartzman or Arthus reaction? *N. Engl. J. Med.*, 281:131–135.
179. Myers, B. D., Ross, J., Newton, L., Luetscher, J., and Perlroth, M. (1984): Cyclosporine-associated chronic nephropathy. *N. Engl. J. Med.*, 311:699–705.
180. Nabarra, B., and Descamps, B. (1976): Ultrastructure of cells infiltrating human kidney allografts. *Clin. Exp. Immunol.*, 24:300–309.
181. Nast, C. C., Ward, H. J., Koyle, M. A., and Cohen, A. H. (1987): Recurrent Henoch-Schönlein purpura following renal transplantation. *Am. J. Kidney Dis.*, 9:39–43.
182. Nathan, C. F., Prendergast, T. J., Wiebe, M. E., Stanley, E. R., Platzer, E., Remold, H. G., Welte, K., Rubin, B. Y., and Murray, H. W. (1984): Activation of human macrophages. Comparison of other cytokines with interferon gamma. *J. Exp. Med.*, 160:600–605.
183. Neild, G. H., Rueben, R., Hartley, R. B., and Cameron, J. S. (1985): Glomerular thrombi in renal allografts associated with cyclosporine treatment. *J. Clin. Path.*, 38:253–258.
184. Neild, G. H., Rocchi, G., Imberti, L., Fumagalli, F., Brown, Z., Remussi, G., and Williams, D. G. (1983): Effect of Cyclosporin A on prostacyclin synthesis by vascular tissue. *Thromb. Res.*, 32:373–379.
185. Nemlander, A., Saksela, E., and Häyry, P. (1983): Are "natural killer" cells involved in allograft rejection? *Eur. J. Immunol.*, 13:348–350.
186. Oakes, D. D., Spees, E. K., McAllister, H. A., and Saddler, W. (1981): Arterial injury during perfusion preservation: A possible cause of posttransplantation renal artery stenosis. *Surgery*, 89:210–215.
187. Obermiller, L. E., Hoy, W. E., Eversole, M., and Sterling, W. A. (1985): Recurrent membranous glomerulonephritis in two renal transplants. *Transplantation*, 40:100–102.
188. Olsen, S., Bohman, S-O., and Petersen, V. P. (1974): Ultrastructure of the glomerular basement membrane in long term renal allografts with transplant glomerular disease. *Lab. Invest.*, 30:176–189.
189. Olsen, T. S. (1986): Pathology of allograft rejection. In: *Kidney Transplant Rejection: Diagnosis and Treatment*, edited by G. M. Williams, J. F. Burdick, and K. Solez, pp. 173–206. Marcel-Dekker, New York.
190. Om, A., Baquero, A., Raja, R., Kim, P., and Bannett, A. D. (1987): The prognostic significance of the presence of monocytes in glomeruli or renal transplant allografts. *Transplant. Proc.*, 19:1618–1622.
191. Orfilo, C., Rakotoarivony, J., Durand, D., and Suc, J. M. (1979): A correlative study of immunofluorescence, electron, and light microscopy in immunologically mediated renal tubular disease in man. *Nephron*, 23:14–22.
192. Ortho, Multicenter Transplant Study Group. (1985): A randomized clinical trial of OKT3 monoclonal antibody for acute rejection of cadaveric renal transplants. *N. Engl. J. Med.*, 313:337–342.
193. Pasternack, A. (1970): Fine-needle aspiration biopsy of human renal homografts. *Lancet*, 2:82–84.
194. Penn, I. (1985): Risk of cancer in the transplant patient. In: *Principles of Organ Transplantation*, edited by M. W. Flye. W.B. Saunders, Philadelphia.
195. Penn, I. (1987): Cancers following cyclosporine therapy. *Transplantation*, 43:32–35.
196. Perkins, J. D., Wiesner, R. H., Banks, P. M., LaRusso, N. F., Ludwig, J., and Krom, R. A. (1987): Immunohistologic labeling as an indicator of liver allograft rejection. *Transplantation*, 43:105–108.
197. Petersen, V. P., Olsen, T. S., Kissmeyer-Nielsen, F., Bohman, S., Hansen, H. E., Hansen, E. S., Skov, P. E., and Solling, K. (1975): Late failure of human renal transplants. An analysis of transplant disease and graft failure among 125 recipients surviving for one to eight years. *Medicine*, 54:45–71.
198. Phillips, J. H., Lanier, L. L. (1986): Lectin-dependent and anti-CD3 induced cytotoxicity are preferentially mediated by peripheral blood cytotoxic T lymphocyytes expressing Leu 7 antigen. *J. Immunol.*, 136:1579–1585.
199. Pinto, J., Lacerda, G., Cameron, J. S., Turner, D. R., Bewick, M., and Ogg, C. S. (1981): Recurrence of focal segmental glomerulosclerosis in renal allografts. *Transplantation*, 32:83–89.
200. Platt, J. L., LeBien, T. W., and Michael, A. F. (1982): Interstitial mononuclear cell populations in renal graft rejection. Identification by monoclonal antibodies in tissue sections. *J. Exp. Med.*, 155:17–30.
201. Platt, J. L., Sibley, R. K., and Michael, A. F. (1985): Interstitial nephritis associated with cytomegalovirus infection. *Kidney Int.*, 28:550–552.
202. Platt, J. L., Ferguson, R. M., Sibley, R. K., Gajl-Pecza, K. J., and Michael, A. F. (1983): Renal interstitial cell populations in cyclosporine nephrotoxicity. Identification using monoclonal antibodies. *Transplantation*, 36:343–346.
203. Pober, J. S., Collins, T., Gimbrone, M. A., Jr., Libby, P., and Reiss, C. S. (1986): Inducible expression of class II major histocompatibility complex antigens and the immunogenicity of vascular endothelium. *Transplantation*, 41:141–146.
204. Porter, K. A., Andres, G. A., Calder, M. W., Dossetor, J. B., Hsu, K. C., Rendall, J. M., Seegal, B. C., and Starzl, T. E. (1968): Human renal transplants. II. Immunofluorescence and immunoferritin studies. *Lab. Invest.*, 18:159–175.
205. Porter, K. A., Dossetor, J. B., Marchioro, T. L., Peart, W. S., Rendall, J. M., Starzl, T. E., and Terasaki, P. I. (1967): Human renal transplants. I. Glomerular changes. *Lab. Invest.*, 16:153–181.

206. Porter, K.A. (1983): Renal transplantation. In: *The Pathology of the Kidney*, 3rd Edition, edited by R. H. Heptinstall, pp. 1455–1547. Little, Brown and Company, Boston.

207. Porter, K. A., Owen, K., Mowbray, J. F., Thompson, W. B., Kenyon, J. R., and Peart, W. S. (1963): Obliterative vascular changes in four human kidney homotransplants. *Br. Med. J.*, 2:639–643.

208. Powles, R. L., Barrett, A. J., Clink, H., Kay, H. E., Sloane, J., McElwain, T. J. (1978): Cyclosporin A for the treatment of graft versus host disease in man. *Lancet*, 2:1327–1331.

209. Preffer, F. I., Colvin, R. B., Leary, C. P., Boyle, L. A., Tuazon, T. A., Lazarovits, A. I., Cosimi, A. B., and Kurnick, J. T. (1986): Two color flow cytometry and functional analysis of lymphocytes cultured from human renal allografts: Identification of a Leu 2^+3^+ subpopulation. *J. Immunol.*, 137:2823–2830.

210. Querin, S., Noel, L. H., Grunfeld, J. P., Droz, D., Mahieu, P., Berger, J., and Kreis, H. (1986): Linear glomerular IgG fixation in renal allografts: Incidence and significance in Alport's syndrome. *Clin. Nephrol.*, 25:134–140.

211. Rammensee, H. G., Robinson, P. J., Crisanti, A., and Bevan, M. J. (1986): Restricted recognition of beta 2 microglobulin by cytotoxic T lymphocytes. *Nature*, 319:502–504.

212. Remuzzi, G., Marchesi, D., Misiani, R., Mecca, G., DeGaetano, G., and Donati, M. B. (1978): Haemolytic-uremic syndrome: Deficiency of plasma factor(s) regulating prostacyclin activity. *Lancet*, 2:871–872.

213. Richardson, W. P., Colvin, R. B., Cheeseman, S. H., Tolkoff-Rubin, N. E., Herrin, J. T., Cosimi, A. B., Collins, A. B., Hirsch, M. S., McCluskey, R. T., Russell, P. S., and Rubin, R. H. (1981): Glomerulopathy associated with cytomegalovirus viremia in renal allografts. *N. Engl. J. Med.*, 305:57–63.

214. Rosenberg, A. S., Mizuochi, T., and Singer, A. (1986): Analysis of T-cell subsets in rejection of K^b mutant skin allografts differing at class I MHC. *Nature*, 322:829–831.

215. Rosenberg, A. S., Mizuochi, T., Sharrow, S. O., and Singer, A. (1987): Phenotype, specificity, and function of T cell subsets and T cell interactions involved in skin allograft rejection. *J. Exp. Med.*, 65:1296–1315.

216. Rotellar, C., Noel, L. H., Droz, D., Kreis, H., and Berger, J. (1986): Role of antibodies directed against tubular basement membranes in human renal transplant. *Am. J. Kidney*, 7:157–161.

217. Rowlands, D. T., Jr., Burkholder, P. M., Bossen, E. H., and Lin, H. H. (1970): Renal allografts in HL-A matched recipients. Light, immunofluorescence and electron microscopic studies. *Am. J. Pathol.*, 61:177–210.

218. Rubin, L. A., Jay, G., and Nelson, D. L. (1986): The released interleukin 2 receptor binds interleukin 2 efficiently. *J. Immunol.*, 137:3841–3844.

219. Russell, P. S., Chase, C. M., Colvin, R. B., and Plate, J. M. D. (1978): Kidney transplants in mice. An analysis of the immune status of mice bearing long-term, H-2 incompatible transplants. *J. Exp. Med.*, 147:1449–1468.

220. Russell, P. S., Colvin, R. B., and Cosimi, A. B. (1984): Monoclonal antibodies for the diagnosis and treatment of transplant rejection. *Ann. Rev. Int. Med.*, 35:63–81.

221. Ryffel, B., Siegel, H., Thiel, G., and Mihatsch, M. J. (1986): Experimental cyclosporine nephrotoxicity. In: *Kidney Transplant Rejection: Diagnosis and Treatment*, edited by G. M. Williams, J. F. Burdick, and K. Solez, pp. 383–410. Marcel Dekker, New York.

222. Sachs, D. H. (1984): The major histocompatibility complex. In: *Fundamental Immunology*, edited by W. E. Paul, pp. 303–346. Raven Press, New York.

223. Salomon, R. N., Kurnick, J. T., Preffer, F. I., Stamenkovic, I., Stegagno, M., and Colvin, R. B. (1987): Southern blot analysis of T lymphocyte clonality in rejecting human allografts. *Fed. Proc.* (Abstr.), 46:731.

224. Sanfilippo, F., Croker, B. P., and Bollinger, R. R. (1982): Fate of four cadaveric donor renal allografts with mesangial IgA deposits. *Transplantation*, 33:370–372.

225. Sanfilippo, F., Kolbeck, P. C., Vaughn, W. K., and Bollinger, R. R. (1985): Renal allograft cell infiltrates associated with irreversible rejection. *Transplantation*, 40:679–685.

226. Schooley, R. T., Hirsch, M. S., Colvin, R. B., Cosimi, A. B., Tolkoff-Rubin, N. E., McCluskey, R. T., Burton, R. C., Russell, P. S., Herrin, J. T., Delmonico, F. L., Giorgi, J. V., Henle, W., and Rubin, R. H. (1983): Association of herpes virus infection with T-lymphocyte subset alterations, glomerulopathy, and opportunistic infections after renal transplantation. *N. Engl. J. Med.*, 308:307–313.

227. Schwartz, R. H. (1984): The role of the major histocompatibility complex in T cell activation and cellular interactions. In: *Fundamental Immunology*, edited by W. E. Paul, pp. 379–438. Raven Press, New York.

228. Schweitzer, R. T., Bartus, S. A., Perkins, H. A., and Belzer, F. O. (1982): Renal allograft failure and cold red blood cell autoagglutinins. *Transplantation*, 33:77–79.

229. Shen, S. Y., Weir, M. R., Kosenko, A., Revie, D. R., Ordonez, J. V., Dagher, F. J., Chretien, P., and Sadler, J. H. (1985): Reevaluation of T cell subset monitoring in cyclosporine treated renal allograft recipients. *Transplantation*, 40:620–623.

230. Shimokado, K., Raines, E. W., Madtes, D. K., Barrett, T. B., Benditt, E. P., and Ross, R. (1985): A significant part of macrophage derived growth factor consists of at least two forms of PDGF. *Cell*, 43:277–286.

231. Shinohara, N., Bluestone, J. A., and Sachs, D. H. (1986): Cloned cytotoxic T lymphocytes that recognize an I A region product in the context of a class I antigen. *J. Exp. Med.*, 163:972–980.

232. Shulman, H., Striker, G., Deeg, H. J., Kennedy, M., Storb, R., and Thomas, E. D. (1981): Nephrotoxicity of cyclosporin A after allogeneic marrow transplantation. Glomerular thromboses and tubular injury. *N. Engl. J. Med.*, 305:1392–1395.

233. Sibley, R. K., Olivari, M. T., Ring, W. S., and Bolman, R. M. (1986): Endomyocardial biopsy in the cardiac allograft recipient. A review of 570 biopsies. *Ann. Surg.*, 203:177–187.
234. Sibley, R. K., Rynasiewicz, J. J., Ferguson, R. M., Fryd, D., Sutherland, D. E. R., Simmons, R. L., and Najarian, J. S. (1983): Morphology of cyclosporine nephrotoxicity and acute rejection in patients immunosuppressed with cyclosporine and prednisone. *Surgery*, 94:245–254.
235. Silva, F. G., Chandler, P., Pirani, C. L., and Hardy, M. A. (1982): Disappearance of glomerular mesangial IgA deposits after renal allograft transplantation. *Transplantation*, 33:214–216.
236. Simonson, M., Buemann, J., Gammeltoft, A., Jensen, F., and Jorgensen, K. (1953): Biological incompatibility in kidney transplantation in dogs. I. Experimental and morphological investigations. *Acta Pathol. Microbiol. Immunol. Scand.*, 32:1–23.
237. Simpson, E. (1983): Immunology of H-Y antigen and its role in sex determination. *Proc. R. Soc. Lond.*, 220:31–46.
238. Skoskievicz, M. J., Colvin, R. B., Schneeberger, E. E., and Russell, P. S. (1985): Widespread and selective induction of MHC-determined antigens *in vivo* by interferon-γ. *J. Exp. Med.*, 162:1645–1664.
239. Smith, S. H., Kirklin, J. K., Geer, J. C., Caulfield, J. B., and McGiffin, D. C. (1987): Arteritis in cardiac rejection after transplantation. *Am. J. Cardiol.*, 59:1171–1173.
240. Smith, W. J. (1987): Monitoring the components of the immune system. In: *Kidney Transplant Rejection: Diagnosis and Treatment*, edited by G. M. Williams, J. F. Burdick, and K. Solez, pp. 264–282. Marcel Dekker, New York.
241. Snover, D. C., Freese, D. K., Sharp, H. L., Bloomer, J. R., Najarian, J. S., and Ascher, N. L. (1987): Liver allograft rejection. An analysis of the use of biopsy in determining outcome of rejection. *Am. J. Surg. Pathol.*, 11:1–10.
242. Solez, K., McGraw, D. J., Beschorner, W. E., Kone, B. C., Racusen, L. C., Whelton, A., and Burdick, J. K. (1985): Reflections on use of the renal biopsy as the "gold standard" in distinguishing transplant rejection from cyclosporine nephrotoxicity. *Transplant. Proc.*, 17 [Suppl. 1]:123–133.
243. Sommer, B. G., Innes, J. T., Whitehurst, R. M., Sharma, H. M., and Ferguson, R. M. (1985): Cyclosporine associated renal arteriopathy resulting in loss of allograft function. *Am. J. Surg.*, 149:756–764.
244. Southern, J. F., Fallon, J. T., Brown, M. C., Kung, P. C., and Colvin, R. B. (1987): Serum IL-2 receptor in the diagnosis of cardiac allograft transplant rejection. *Lab. Invest.* (Abstr.), 56:75A.
245. Soulillou, J. P., DeMougon-Cambon, A., Duboid, C., Blanc, M., Peyrat, M. A., and Mahieu, P. (1981): Immunological studies of eluates of 83 rejected kidneys. *Transplantation*, 32:368–374.
246. Soulillou, J. P., Peyronnet, P., Le Mauff, B., Hourmant, M., Olive, D., Mawas, C., Delaage, M., Hirn, M., and Jacques, Y. (1987): Prevention of rejection of kidney transplants by monoclonal antibody directed against interleukin 2. *Lancet*, 1:1339–1342.
247. Spector, D., Limas, C., Frost, J. L., Zachary, J. B., Sterioff, S., Williams, G. M., Rolley, R. T., and Sadler, J. H. (1976): Perfusion nephropathy in human transplants. *N. Engl. J. Med.*, 295:1217–1219.
248. Sprent, J., Schaefer, M., Lo, D., and Korngold, R. (1986): Properties of purified T cell subsets. II. *In vivo* responses to class I vs. class II H-2 differences. *J. Exp. Med.*, 163:998–1011.
249. Starzl, T. E., Lerner, R. A., Dixon, F. J., and Groth, C. G. (1968): Shwartman reaction after human renal homotransplantation. *N. Engl. J. Med.*, 278:642–646.
250. Steinmuller, D. (1985): Which T cells mediate allograft rejection? *Transplantation*, 40:229–233.
251. Stegagno, M., Boyle, L., Preffer, F. I., Leary, C. P., Colvin, R. B., Cosimi, A. B., and Kurnick, J. T. (1987): Functional analysis of lymphocyte subsets and clones in human renal allografts. *Transplant. Proc.*, 19:394–397.
252. Stelzer, G. T., McLeish, K. R., Lorden, R. E., and Watson, S. L. (1984): Alterations in T lymphocyte subpopulations associated with renal allograft rejection. *Transplantation*, 37:261–264.
253. Stiller, C. R., Sinclair, N. R. S., Abrahams, S., McGirr, D., Singh, H., Howson, W. T., and Ulan, R. A. (1976): Anti-donor immune responses in the prediction of transplant rejection. *N. Engl. J. Med.*, 294:978–982.
254. Striegel, J. E., Sibley, R. K., Fryd, D. S., and Mauer, S. M. (1986): Recurrence of focal segmental sclerosis in children following renal transplantation. *Kidney Int.* [Suppl.], 19:S44–S50.
255. Strom, T. B., and Colvin, R. B. (1988): Case records of the Massachusetts General Hospital. *N. Engl. J. Med.*, 318:31–40.
256. Sturgill, B. C., Lobo, P. I., and Bolton W. K. (1984): Cold-reacting IgM antibody-induced renal allograft failure. Similarity to hyperacute rejection. *Nephron*, 36:125–127.
257. Suzuki, T., Furusato, M., Takasaki, S., and Ischikava, E. (1975): Giant mitochondria in the epithelial cells of the proximal convoluted tubules of diseased human kidneys. *Lab. Invest.*, 33:578–590.
258. Swain, S. L. (1983): T cell subsets and the recognition of MHC class. *Immunol. Rev.*, 74:129–142.
259. Taube, D., Welsh, K., Hobby, P., and Williams, D. G. (1984): Human renal allograft and peripheral blood T lymphocyte subpopulations during the onset and treatment of rejection. *Clin. Nephrol.*, 22:127–132.
260. Taube, D. H., Neild, G. H., Williams, D. G., Cameron, J. S., Hartley, B., Ogg, C. S., Rudge, C. J., and Welsh, K. I. (1985): Differentiation between allograft rejection and cyclosporine nephrotoxicity in renal transplant recipients. *Lancet*, 2:171–174.
261. Thoenes, G. H., Pielsticker, K., and Schubert, G. (1979): Transplantation-induced immune complex kidney disease in rats with unilateral manifestations in the allografted kidney. *Lab. Invest.*, 41:321–329.

262. Tilney, N. L., Garovoy, M. R., Busch, G. J., Strom, T. B., Graves, M. J., and Carpenter, C. B. (1979): Rejected human renal allografts: Recovery and characteristics of infiltrating cells and antibody. *Transplantation*, 28:421–426.

263. Tisher, C. C., and Brenner, B. M. (1988): *Renal Pathology*. J.B. Lippincott, Philadelphia.

264. Tolkoff-Rubin, N., Cosimi, A. B., Fuller, T. L., Rubin, R. H., and Colvin, R. B. (1978): IgA nephropathy (Berger's disease) in H-LA identical siblings of B-35 phenotype: Potential source of apparent "recurrence" in transplanted kidneys. *Transplantation*, 26:430–433.

265. Tolkoff-Rubin, N. E., Cosimi, A. B., Delmonico, F. L., Russell, P. S., Thompson, R. E., Piper, D. J., Hansen, W. P., Bander, N. H., Finstad, C. L., and Cordon Cardo, C. (1986): Diagnosis of tubular injury in renal transplant patients by a urinary assay for a proximal tubular antigen, the adenosine deaminase binding protein. *Transplantation*, 41:593–597.

266. Tuazon, T. V., Schneeberger, E. E., Bhan, A. K., McCluskey, R. T., Cosimi, A. B., Schooley, R. T., Rubin, R. H., and Colvin, R. B. (1987): Mononuclear cells in acute allograft glomerulopathy. *Am. J. Pathol.*,

267. Unanue, E. R., and Allen, P. M. (1987): The basis for the immunoregulatory role of macrophages and other accessory cells. *Science*, 236:551–557.

268. Van Buren, D., Van Buren, C. T., Flechner, S. M., Maddox, A. M., Verani, R., and Kahan, B. D. (1985): *De novo* hemolytic uremic syndrome in renal transplant recipients immunosuppressed with cyclosporine. *Surgery*, 98:54–62.

269. Van Es, A., Myer, C. J., Oljans, P. J., Tanke, H. J., and Van Es, L. A. (1984): Mononuclear cells in renal allografts. Correlation with peripheral blood T lymphocyte populations and graft prognosis. *Transplantation*, 37:134–139.

270. Verani, R., and Dan, M. (1982): Membranous glomerulonephritis in renal transplant. A case report and review of the literature. *Am. J. Nephrol.*, 31:20–28.

271. Verani, R. R., Flechner, S. M., Van Buren, C. T., and Kahan, B. D. (1984): Acute cellular rejection or Cyclosporine A nephrotoxicity? A review of transplant renal biopsies. *Am. J. Kidney Dis.*, 4:185–191.

272. Verani, R. R., and Hawkins, E. P. (1986): Recurrent focal segmental glomerulosclerosis. A pathological study of the early lesion. *Am. J. Nephrol.*, 6:263–270.

273. von Willebrand, E., and Häyry, P. (1983): Cyclosporin A deposits in renal allografts. *Lancet*, 2:189–192.

274. von Willebrand, E. (1983): OKT4/8 ratio in the blood and in the graft during episodes of human renal allografts rejection. *Cell. Immunol.*, 77:196–201.

275. Waltzer, W. C., Miller, F., Arnold, A., Anaise, D., and Rapaport, F. T. (1987): Immunohistologic analysis of human renal allograft dysfunction. *Transplantation*, 43:100–105.

276. Weir, M. R., Hall-Craggs, M., Shen. S. Y., Posner, J. N., Alongi, S. V., Dagher, F. J., and Sadler, J. H. (1986): The prognostic value of the eosinophil in acute renal allograft rejection. *Transplantation*, 41:709–712.

277. White, D. J. G., Blatchford, N. R., and Cauwenbergh, G. (1984): Cyclosporine and ketoconazole. *Transplantation*, 37:214–215.

278. Wiener, J., Spiro, D., and Russell, P. S. (1964): An electron microscopic study of the homograft rejection. *Am. J. Pathol.*, 44:319–332.

279. Williams, K. A., Hart, D. N. S., Fabre, J. W., and Morris, P. J. (1980): Distribution and quantitation of HLA-ABC and Dr. (Ia) antigens on human kidney and other tissues. *Transplantation*, 29:274–279.

280. Williams, G. M., Hume, D. M., Huson, R. P., Jr., Morris, P. J., Kano, K., and Milgrom, F. (1968): "Hyperacute" renal-homograft rejection in man. *N. Engl. J. Med.*, 279:611–615.

281. Wilson, C. B., Lehman, D. H., McCoy, R. C., Guinness, J. C., and Stickel, D. L. (1974): Antitubular basement membrane antibodies after renal transplantation. *Transplantation*, 18:447–452.

282. Winn, H. J. (1986): Antibody mediated rejection. In: *Kidney Transplant Rejection: Diagnosis and Treatment*, edited by G. M. Williams, J. F. Burdick, and K. Solez, pp. 17–27. Marcel Dekker, New York.

283. Yoshioka, K., Morimoto, Y., Iseki, T., and Maki, S. (1986): Characterization of tubular basement membrane antigens in human kidney. *J. Immunol.*, 136:1654–1660.

284. Zimmerman, S. W. (1985): Plasmapheresis and dipyridamole for recurrent focal glomerular sclerosis. *Nephron*, 40:241–245.

285. Zimmerman, C. E. (1980): Renal transplantation for focal segmental glomerulosclerosis. *Transplantation*, 29:172.

286. Zoja, C., Furci, L., Ghilardi, F., Zilio, P., Benigni, A., and Remuzzi, G. (1986): Cyclosporin induced endothelial cell injury. *Lab. Invest.*, 55:455–462.

287. Zollinger, H. U., and Mihatsch, M. J. (1978): *Renal Pathology in Biopsy*, p. 581, Springer-Verlag, Berlin.

288. Zollinger, H. U., Moppert, J., Thiel, G., and Rohr H-P. (1973): Morphology and pathogenesis of glomerulopathy in cadaver kidney allografts treated with antilymphocyte globulin. *Curr. Top. Pathol.*, 57:1–48.

289. Mahan, J. D., Maver, S. M., Sibley, R. K., and Vernier, R. L. (1984): Congenital nephrotic syndrome: evolution of medical management and results of transplantation. *J. Pediatr.*, 105:549–557.

Diagnostic Immunopathology,
edited by R.B. Colvin,
A.K. Bhan, and R.T. McCluskey.
Raven Press, New York © 1988.

8 / Differentiation Antigens and Strategies in Tumor Diagnosis

Atul K. Bhan

Immunopathology Unit, Department of Pathology, Massachusetts General Hospital,
Harvard Medical School, Boston, Massachusetts 02114

This chapter presents an overview of immunohistochemical techniques in tumor diagnosis and a description of the most useful markers in diagnostic pathology. The strategies in selecting the most instructive immunostaining panels in commonly encountered problems in surgical pathology are emphasized. Specific applications are discussed in individual chapters: cytoskeletal proteins and neuronal tumors (Chapter 9), leukemias (Chapter 10), lymphomas (Chapter 11), endocrine tumors (Chapter 12), gynecological and genitourinary tumors (Chapter 13) and soft tissue tumors (Chapter 14).

Traditional morphologic criteria are usually adequate for the diagnosis and classification of well-differentiated tumors. However, these criteria do not always suffice for poorly differentiated tumors. Pathologists have relied on histochemical techniques for decades to prove the nature of tumor cells by the detection of various tissue components (lipids, glycoproteins, enzymes, glycogen, mucin, reticulin). Immunohistochemical techniques (18,37,61,74,221,222) have provided a new generation of "special" stains that detect specific molecules, based on the ability of antibodies to bind specific antigens. Hybridoma technology allowed generation of monoclonal antibodies against a wide variety of antigens, many previously unrecognized with conventional polyclonal antisera (100,119). Monoclonal antibodies have exquisite specificity and are available in perpetuity so that batch variation is minimized. Certain problems arise with monoclonal antibodies, and better results can be obtained with polyclonal antisera in some situations (discussed in Chapter 17).

Enzyme conjugates are superior to fluorescent labels in paraffin-embedded sections. Although most antigens are better preserved by quick freezing, frozen blocks are frequently not available in surgical pathology units. Highly sensitive immunoenzyme techniques must be used in order to detect antigens that survive routine tissue fixation and processing. Most diagnostic laboratories use horseradish peroxidase conjugated reagents (immunoperoxidase techniques) for the detection of antigens in tissue sections (215) (see Chapter 17 for technical details).

ANTIGENS AS MARKERS OF CELLULAR DIFFERENTIATION

That cells of different types can be distinguished by immunophenotyping presumes that each cell type possesses a distinctive set of antigens (differentiation molecules). The ex-

TABLE 1. *Commonly used markers of tumor cell differentiation*[a]

Antigens (Markers)	Important Diagnostic Applications
Actin (present in a wide variety of cells but abundant in smooth muscle and myoepithelial cells.)	Tumors showing myogenic differentiation
Alpha-1 antichymotrypsin	Tumors showing histocytic differentiation; malignant fibrous histiocytoma
Alpha-1 antitrypsin	Hepatocellular carcinoma; ovarian and testicular germ cell tumors; tumors showing histiocytic differentiation; malignant fibrous histiocytoma.
Alpha-lactalbumin	Breast carcinoma
Alpha-fetoprotein	Hepatocellular carcinoma; ovarian and testicular germ cell tumors (endodemal sinus tumor and tumors showing hepatoid differentiation)
Blood group antigens	State of differentiation of tumors (transitional cell carcinoma of the bladder)
Carcinoembryonic antigen	Marker of epithelial differentiation; adenocarcinomas and certain squamous cell carcinomas; medullary thyroid carcinoma; distinguishes adenocarcinomas from mesothelioma
Epithelial membrane antigen (EMA) (an antigen related to milk fat globule protein)	Distinguishes tumors showing epithelial differentiation from sarcomas and lymphomas (some epithelial tumors may be negative and some nonepithelial tumors such as plasmacytomas may stain for EMA)
Factor VIII-related antigen (present in endothelial cells and megakaryocytes)	Neoplasms of endothelial cells (Binding of lectin Ulex europaeus agglutinin 1 to the tumor cells is a more sensitive but less specific marker of neoplastic endothelial cells)
Hormones and related proteins	
Chromogranin proteins	Endocrine secretory granules; neuroendocrine tumors
Calcitonin	Medullary carcinoma of thyroid; C-cell hyperplasia
Thyroglobulin	Neoplasms of thyroid origin
Pituitary Hormones (adrenocorticotropin, growth hormone, prolactin, thyroid stimulating hormone)	Characterization of pituitary tumor cells; ectopic hormone production by tumors
Hormones related to pancreatic islet cells and gastrointestinal hormones (insulin, glucagon, somatostatin, gastrin, pancreatic polypeptide, vasoactive intestinal peptide, bombesin, substance P) and serotonin	Characterization of islet cell tumors; gastrointestinal endocrine tumors including carcinoids; ectopic hormone production by tumors
Testosterone	Testicular and ovarian tumors
Chorionic gonadotropin and Placental lactogen	Classification of germ cell tumors of the testes and ovary; trophoblastic neoplasms

Hormonal receptors

Estrogen receptor

Estrogen receptor status of tumors (breast carcinoma)

Intermediate filament proteins

Keratins (contains a family of proteins of various molecular weights)

Tumors showing epithelial differentiation; distinguishes carcinomas from malignant melanoma, chordoma from chondrosarcoma, thymoma from lymphoma, synovial sarcoma and epithelioid sarcoma from other sarcomas

Desmin

Myogenic (smooth and skeletal muscle) tumors

Glial fibrillary acidic protein (GFAP)

Gliomas; distinguishes gliomas from other brain tumors including metastatic tumors

Vimentin

Tumors of mesenchymal origin; lymphomas, some poorly differentiated carcinomas (also present in cultured epithelial cells)

Neurofilament

Tumors of neuronal origin; peochromocytoma; ganglioneuroblastoma, Merkel cell tumor; small cell carcinoma of lung

Leukocyte markers

Common leukocyte antigen (LCA,T200)

Distinguishes hematopoietic malignancies from non-hematopoietic tumors

Immunoglobulins (IgM, IgG, IgD, IgA, kappa and lambda light chains)

Malignant lymphomas and leukemias of B-cell origin; multiple myeloma.

Lymphocyte, monocyte and myeloid associated antigens as defined by monoclonal antibodies

Malignant lymphomas and leukemias; multiple myeloma; Hodgkin's disease; histiocytosis-X

Terminal deoxynucleotidyl transferase

Lymphoblastic lymphoma; leukemias

Lysozyme (muramidase)

Tumors of histiocytes and monocytes; myeloid tumors

Myoglobin

Neoplasms showing skeletal muscle (rhabdomyoblastic) differentiation

Myosin

Tumors showing myogenic differentiation.

Neuron-specific enolase

Neuroendocrine tumors including Merkel cell tumor and neuroblastoma

Prostatic acid phosphatase

Prostatic carcinoma

Prostate specific antigen

Prostatic carcinoma

S-100 protein

Distinguishes nerve sheath tumors from other mesenchymal tumors and malignant melanoma from carcinomas; histiocytosis-X; mixed tumors of salivary glands (myoepithelial cells); breast tumors; chondroid tumors; liposarcoma

---

[a]The table lists antigens which are routinely used in surgical pathology. Other antigens which may also be useful in the characterization of tumors are referred to in the text and in Chapters 9,10,11, 12,13 and 14. All the antigens listed in the table with the notable exception of many lymphocyte, monocyte and myeloid associated cell surface antigens and terminal deoxynucleotidyl transferase can be demonstrated in routinely processed paraffin-embedded sections by immunoperoxidase techniques (Chapter 17). However, in many instances better results may be obtained by using frozen tissue sections or fixatives other than formalin (Chapter 17).

pression of many cellular components is dependent on the stage of differentiation as well as the functional state of the cells. Well-differentiated tumor cells should express molecules most similar to those in corresponding normal cells, whereas poorly differentiated tumors would not be expected to retain such fidelity. "Ectopic" hormones are classic examples of aberrant differentiation in neoplastic cells. Most of the commonly used tumor markers (Table 1) belong to the group of differentiation antigens and include cell structural proteins (cytoskeletal proteins), enzymes, secretory products (hormones, immunoglobulins) or cell surface antigens associated with special functions (54,100).

The fact that it is possible to generate an immune response to certain syngeneic tumors in experimental animals suggests that some tumors may express antigens that are not expressed by normal cells (tumor-associated antigens) (159). The development of hybridoma technology has generated a new wave of interest in the identification of the tumor-associated antigens (119,192). Intact tumor cell lines, fresh tumors, selected fractions of tumor cells and synthesized peptide antigens have been used to immunize mice (100,119, 192,229). Early claims that certain antibodies were restricted in their reactivity to tumor cells were found to be false when more sensitive techniques and a larger spectrum of normal adult tissues, fetal tissues, and tumors were used to screen the reactivity of the antibodies. In some instances, antigens that are expressed on tumor cells but are masked in normal cells, can be revealed by treating sections with appropriate enzymes (50). Nevertheless, hybridoma technology has allowed recognition of a large number of cell surface and cytoplasmic antigens, many of which can be helpful in defining the phenotype of the tumor cells (18). Furthermore, some monoclonal antibodies against tumor cells have been found to be useful in monitoring the course of tumor in a patient by detecting shed antigens in the blood (7,8,58).

An attractive approach is to use human antibodies. It has been difficult, however, to demonstrate antibodies with reactivity restricted to tumor cells in tumor-bearing patients (159), even though inflammatory mononuclear cells are often present in the tumors (16, 19,99,185). Attempts are being made to use lymphocytes obtained from peripheral blood, draining lymph nodes or tumor infiltrates from tumor-bearing patients to develop human monoclonal antibodies against tumor cells (48,191).

Selection of Antigens

Immunohistochemical studies can reveal microheterogeneity of tumor cells, as in many instances, only a small proportion of the tumor cells express a given antigen. This may be due to the presence of several different clones of tumor cells or to the presence of tumor cells in various states of differentiation and function. Because of the marked microheterogeneity in tumors and because many antigens are shared by different types of tumors, it is essential that a carefully selected panel of antibodies be used for a reliable diagnosis.

In the following sections some of the important applications of commonly used markers (antigens) in tumor diagnosis will be briefly discussed (Table 1). It is important to note that with the exception of a few markers (immunoglobulin light chains), staining for most antigens is not helpful in differentiating malignant from benign neoplasms or even from normal tissues.

Epithelial Markers

Keratin, carcinoembryonic antigen (CEA) and epithelial membrane antigen (EMA) are the most commonly used markers of epithelial differentiation. Of these, keratin is the most reliable (172,223). Recently, *involucrin* (187,189,243) and *desmosomal proteins* (138) have also been used for the characterization of epithelial tumors.

Keratin

Keratin is a member of intermediate-sized filaments (about 10 nm diameter), which are part of the cytoskeleton of eukaryocytic cells. They differ in size and structure from actin filaments, microtubules and myosin (56,70,78). Biochemically, five types of intermediate filament proteins have been isolated, namely keratin, vimentin, desmin, neurofilament triplet proteins and glial fibrillary acidic protein (GFAP). Although these proteins share antigenic determinants, polyclonal and monoclonal antibodies specific for each of the intermediate filament proteins have been developed (56,70,78,79).

The demonstration of intermediate filament proteins in tumor cells is useful in defining their state of differentiation (56,70,166). Keratin is restricted to epithelial cells, desmin to myogenic cells (smooth and skeletal), GFAP to glial cells and neurofilament to cells showing neuronal differentiation. Vimentin is a characteristic protein of mesenchymal cells, but can also be demonstrated in epithelial cells in culture and in tumor cells showing epithelial differentiation (5,131). (For further discussion of intermediate filament proteins, in particular neurofilament triplet proteins, see also Chapter 9.)

Keratins have long been recognized as markers of epithelial cells because of their association with stratified squamous epithelium and because keratins were recognized as tonofilaments in certain epithelial cells by electron microscopy (64). Gel electrophoresis of keratins extracted from cells has demonstrated that keratin contains a family of 19 polypeptides, ranging in molecular weights from 40 kd to 68 kd (43,139,217). Keratin proteins have been divided into acidic and basic subfamilies. Members of basic subfamilies have a corresponding member in acidic subfamilies and are usually expressed in the cells as "keratin pairs" (45,217). Several studies have indicated that the keratin profile of cells may vary, depending on the tissue type and the stage of differentiation of the cells (43,217).

The usefulness of defining the keratin profile of tumor cells is related to the premise that keratins are conserved in neoplastic analogues of normal cells (43,52,122). In general, high molecular weight keratins are present in stratified squamous epithelia and in epithelia showing keratinization (epidermis), whereas keratins of low molecular weight are present in simpler and glandular epithelia (45,217). Keratin proteins within cells are often referred to as cytokeratins, as opposed to keratins present in the acellular layer of stratified squamous epithelium. This distinction is inaccurate, as there is overlap in the distribution of keratins between cornified and noncornified epithelia (45).

Although a large number of polyclonal and monoclonal antibodies that recognize different types of keratin have been produced (111,117,199,223), it is impossible to recognize all types of keratins by commercially available antibodies. In our experience, polyclonal antibodies generally lack reactivity to low molecular weight keratins. It is difficult to select an appropriate panel of monoclonal antibodies for keratin typing of tumor. Depending on the reactivity of the antibodies to simple, ductal or squamous epithelia, Gown and Vogel

(77) have divided selected groups of monoclonal antibodies to keratin into four classes. Class 1 antibodies react with all carcinomas; class 2 antibodies react with squamous cell carcinomas but not with tumor of ductal or simple epithelium; class 3 antibodies react with nonsquamous epithelial tumors, and class 4 antibodies react with both squamous and ductal neoplasms (77). For reliable evaluation of the presence of keratin in the tumor cells, it is essential that antibodies capable of reacting with all types of epithelia be used. A broad range of reactivity can be obtained by preparing a cocktail of monoclonal antibodies with different specificities. As expected, however, the commercially available mixture of monoclonal antibodies do not react with all types of keratins (117). Fixation and tissue processing can lead to a selective loss of staining of certain keratin types. It is often necessary to treat formalin-fixed, paraffin-embedded sections with proteolytic enzymes (trypsin) to obtain optimal staining for keratin (discussed in Chapter 17).

In addition to defining the epithelial nature of the tumor cells (26,183,199,207), the demonstration of various keratins in the tumor cells may help to differentiate certain histologic types of epithelial neoplasms (43,45,156,165,170,193,199,225,249). In one study, variation in the expression of keratin in normal and neoplastic colonic epithelium was observed (36). The presence of keratin in embryonal carcinoma can help differentiate it from seminoma, which usually does not stain for keratin (10). By using antikeratin antibodies of different specificities, Fischer et al. (67) were able to discriminate cholangiocarcinomas from hepatocellular carcinomas. Studies carried out by Said et al. (186) indicate that adenocarcinomas of the lung show variable staining for 45, 46 and 55 kd keratin proteins but not for the 63 kd protein, whereas mesotheliomas and reactive mesothelial cells stain for 63 kd protein as well as for keratins of lower molecular weights. Thus, antibodies to 63 kd keratin should allow differentiation of mesotheliomas from adenocarcinomas, a differential diagnosis often faced in diagnostic pathology. It may also be possible to differentiate adenocarcinomas from mesothelioma by observing the type of keratin staining present in the tumor cells (38,47). In mesotheliomas, the cytoplasmic staining appears to be predominantly around the nucleus, whereas the staining in adenocarcinomas often appears to be in the periphery along the cell membrane. Interestingly, epithelial tumors with neuroendocrine differentiation show punctuate (ball-like) cytoplasmic staining for keratin (11). Squamous differentiation in lung tumors can be evaluated by demonstrating involucrin, a precursor of the envelope protein present in stratum corneum, in the tumor cells (187). Demonstration of involucrin has also been helpful in evaluating squamous differentiation in other tumors (189,243).

The presence of keratin in a cell does not indicate the germ layer origin of the cell but rather the state of differentiation of the cell. For example, mesothelial cells and proximal tubular cells of the kidney, although of mesenchymal origin, contain keratin (45). Myoepithelial cells, which show features of myogenic cells, stain for keratin (45). Therefore, it is not surprising that many tumors considered to be sarcomas and of mesenchymal origin, such as synovial sarcoma, epithelioid sarcoma, and meningioma, have been found to contain cells that stain for keratin (35,46,68,132).

Carcinoembryonic antigen (CEA)

A glycoprotein that was first considered to be specific for colonic carcinoma, CEA was later found to be present in fetal and to a lesser extent in adult colonic mucosa (1,221). Other epithelial tumors, especially those arising in tissues derived from the endoderm (lung, pancreas) and breast may also show reactivity for CEA (2,75,90,91,158,169,180,216).

Nevertheless, staining for CEA can be helpful in the differential diagnosis of certain carcinomas (9,38). In most studies performed on paraffin-embedded sections, adenocarcinomas of the lung usually stain intensely for CEA, whereas mesotheliomas either do not stain or stain faintly (9,38,47,92,126,188). Similarly, CEA has been reported to be present in most cases of mucinous carcinomas of the ovary but not in serous carcinomas (34); however, variable results have been obtained with different anti-CEA antisera. The differences obtained in various studies may be related to the presence of antibodies in the polyclonal antisera to CEA that cross-react with substances closely related to CEA. These substances are referred to as nonspecific cross-reacting antigens (NCA) and are widely distributed in tissues (31,221). Granulocytes provide a good marker for the presence of antibodies reactive with NCA. The reactivity with granulocytes can be abolished by absorbing the anti-CEA antisera with spleen powder (38). The development of monoclonal antibodies against CEA promises to provide reagents specific for CEA (98,108,146,179,240). Recently, by using anti-CEA monoclonal antibodies with restricted reactivity, CEA was found to be absent in the normal colonic tissue but present in abnormal or neoplastic colonic epithelium (98,146). In a study using polyclonal and monoclonal antibodies, Schroeder and Kloppel (194) demonstrated that cross-reacting antigens can be demonstrated in all types of thyroid carcinoma, while CEA is present only in medullary thyroid carcinomas and hyperplastic C-cell nodules. A monoclonal anti-CEA antibody has been found to react with carcinomas of the gastrointestinal tract but not with ovarian carcinomas (228).

Epithelial membrane antigen (EMA)

Milk fat globules are surrounded by apical membrane portions of the secretory mammary cells, and antisera raised against milk fat globules have been found to be reactive with breast epithelium. The antibodies recognize a group of closely related high molecular weight molecules with a high carbohydrate content (epithelial membrane antigen) (3). However, epithelial membrane antigen (EMA) is not restricted to human breast epithelium; many exocrine glands and different types of epithelial tumors express this antigen (90, 173). As the antigen is preserved in paraffin-embedded tissue sections, EMA has been widely used as an epithelial marker in diagnostic pathology. In a study performed with commercially available monoclonal antibodies to EMA, Pinkus and Kurtin (173) reported that carcinomas of various sites, including breast, lung, stomach, intestine, prostate, kidney, and thyroid showed reactivity for EMA. In contrast, many endocrine tumors (carcinoid, medullary carcinoma of thyroid, adrenocortical carcinoma, and pheochromocytoma), germ cell tumors and soft tissue tumors lacked reactivity for EMA. Like keratin, EMA is expressed by epithelioid sarcomas, synovial sarcomas, and chordomas (173,250). Although normal or reactive mesothelial cells show little or no staining for EMA, intense staining for EMA is observed in mesotheliomas (38). In one study using an antibody to human fat globule protein (HMFG-2), Battifora and Kopinski (9) demonstrated that malignant mesotheliomas did not stain for HMFG-2, whereas most adenocarcinomas stained for the antigen; however, this difference in staining for HMGF-2 has not been confirmed by others (38). Studies carried out by many investigators have demonstrated that EMA is not restricted to cells that show an epithelial differentiation (55,173). Plasma cells, Reed-Sternberg cells, T-cell lymphomas, malignant histiocytes and plasmacytomas have been found to be reactive with antibodies to EMA (55,173). Furthermore, antibodies to EMA are less likely to be reactive with different types of epithelial tumors than anti-keratin antibodies (223). In some instances (small cell anaplastic carcinomas and some cases of renal cell carcinoma and pulmonary adenocarcinoma), however, EMA has been reported to better define the epithelial nature of the tumor cells, as keratin may not be demonstrable in some of these tumors (172). Therefore, EMA alone cannot be considered as a reliable marker of epithelial cell differentiation, but can be a useful complementary marker along with keratin (172,223).

Nonepithelial Markers

Intermediate filament proteins

Mesenchymal cells (fibroblasts, muscle cells, endothelial cells, lymphoid cells, Schwann cells, ependymal cells, melanocytes) characteristically express the intermediate filament protein *vimentin* (135). However, as vimentin can be expressed also by certain epithelial cells (glomerular epithelial cells) and by many epithelial tumors (5,131,235), vimentin by itself is not a useful diagnostic marker. In the absence of epithelial-associated antigens, vimentin can be a useful indicator of mesenchymal cells, especially if the cells also express other antigens (desmin, myosin, myoglobin, factor VIII-related antigen) characteristically present in differentiated mesenchymal cells.

Closely related to vimentin, *desmin* is found in all muscle cells (cardiac, skeletal and smooth muscle) and is an excellent marker of myogenic differentiation of tumor cells (56,135,137,166). Desmin and vimentin can be demonstrated in both leiomyosarcomas and rhabdomyosarcomas; in poorly differentiated tumor cells only vimentin is seen (56). These two tumors often show distinct histological appearances and can be further differentiated either by electron microscopy or by the demonstration of *myoglobin*, which supports the diagnosis of rhabdomyosarcoma (27,53). Recently, Osborn et al. (164) have shown that antibodies to *titin* can help discriminate rhabdomyosarcomas (titin +) from leiomyosarcomas (titin −). Desmin-like vimentin can be demonstrated best in frozen tissue sections or tissues fixed in Carnoy's fixative (78,79). Antibodies capable of reacting with desmin and vimentin in formalin-fixed and paraffin-embedded tissue sections have become available. Actin, myosin, and isoenzymes BB and MM of creatine kinase and Z-protein have also been used as markers of myogenic differentiation (53,66,142,144).

The intermediate filament proteins, *glial fibrillary acidic protein (GFAP)* and *neurofilament triplet proteins* are associated with distinct cell populations in the nervous system. An excellent marker of astrocytes, GFAP (52 kd) is also present in ependymal cells and can be demonstrated in gliomas (astrocytoma, glioblastoma multiforme, ependymoma) and focally in medulloblastomas (125,220,242). Unexpectedly, reactivity for GFAP has been demonstrated in pleomorphic adenomas of the salivary gland (154) and nerve sheath tumors (209). Neurofilament triplet proteins, which are excellent markers of neuronal differentiation (232), are discussed in detail in Chapter 9.

S-100 protein

An acidic protein containing two polypeptide chains (alpha and beta) S-100 protein was originally isolated from bovine brain. This protein has acquired its name because of the unique characteristic of remaining soluble in a 100% solution of ammonium sulfate at a neutral pH (150). Widely distributed throughout the body, S-100 protein is found in the neural tissue (glial cells, satellite cells, Schwann cells), chondrocytes, adipose tissue, melanocytes, interdigitating reticulum cells of lymphoid tissue, Langerhans cells, and certain epithelial cells (myoepithelial cells, some ductular epithelial cells in breast, salivary glands, sweat glands in skin, serous acini in bronchial glands) (150,236). Therefore, it is not surprising that S-100 protein has been demonstrated in various tumors, including malignant melanoma, neurogenic tumors, chondrosarcoma, chordoma, liposarcoma, meningioma, and tumors of the breast and salivary gland (88,150,152,212). Despite this wide distribution, demonstration of S-100 protein in tumor cells in certain situations can be of great diagnostic help (102), especially if the tumor is also stained for intermediate filament proteins. The S-100 protein is present in all benign nerve sheath tumors (schwannomas) and in about 50% of malignant schwannomas but not in other spindle cell tumors such as leiomyosarcoma and fibrosarcoma (247). Virtually all malignant melanomas stain for S-100 protein (94,150), and there appears to be an inverse relationship between the intensity of staining for this protein and melanin content in the neoplastic melanocytes (151). The demonstration of S-100 protein and vimentin (181) in the tumor cells with an absence of staining for keratin is extremely helpful in establishing the diagnosis of malignant melanoma in cases where the melanoma cannot be differentiated histologically from poorly differentiated carcinomas. Demonstration of S-100 protein in granular cell myoblastomas and in many tumors considered to be myogenic tumors on the basis of morphologic features, has helped provide evidence for neurogenic (Schwann cell) differentiation of these tumors (128,143,153). Antibodies to *myelin basic protein* (39.168) and anti-Leu 7 (an antibody capable of reacting with a wide variety of cells including natural killer cells and neuroendocrine cells) (29) have also been used in the diagnosis of peripheral nerve sheath tumors (218). (See Chapter 14 for further details).

Factor VIII-related antigen

Factor VIII-related antigen is commonly used to identify neoplasms showing endothelial differentiation (17,30,82,130,250). However, the antigen has not been very useful in the diagnosis of poorly differentiated endothelial tumors. Recent studies indicate that lectin *Ulex europaeus agglutinin 1 (UEA-1)*, which binds to endothelial cells, is a more sensitive marker of poorly differentiated endothelial tumor cells than factor VIII-related antigen (112,118,161). Nevertheless, the reactivity of UEA-1 is not restricted to endothelial cells; normal epithelial cells, carcinomas and nonvascular tumor cells may also bind UEA-1 (112,250).

Alpha-1 antitrypsin and alpha-1 antichymotrypsin

Antibodies to *alpha-1 antitrypsin* and *alpha-1 antichymotrypsin* (enzymes often present in macrophages) have been used to determine the histiocytic nature of tumor cells in spindle cell tumors, such as malignant fibrous histiocytomas (51). As these serum proteins can also be demonstrated in epithelial tumors (162,254), it is important to evaluate the significance of these antigens in the light of findings obtained with other relevant markers such as keratin, desmin, and S-100 protein. Although the tumor cells in malignant fibrous histiocytoma have been reported not to stain for most macrophage markers by some investigators (182,255), others have described staining of the spindle cells in malignant fibrous histiocytoma with monoclonal antibodies against antigens associated with monocytes/macrophages (214). Whether malignant fibrous histiocytoma is a distinct entity or a poorly differentiated variant of other spindle cell tumors is yet to be determined (28).

Leukocyte Markers

One of the areas of diagnostic pathology where application of monoclonal antibodies has already made a great impact is in the diagnosis and classification of tumors of the hematopoietic system (20). Their use has allowed a comparison of antigenic phenotype of tumor cells with morphologic classification and characterization of the lymphoid tumors according to their state of differentiation relative to the stages of normal lymphoid differentiation (69,85,86,149). More importantly from a diagnostic point of view, leukocyte markers have helped in the differentiation of lymphoid neoplasms from reactive lymphoid tissue and from nonlymphoid neoplasms (20,84). As the usefulness of leukocyte markers in the diagnosis and classification of leukemias and malignant lymphomas is described in detail in Chapters 10 and 11, only the most frequently used markers in diagnostic pathology will be briefly discussed.

Generally, the most useful markers in the diagnosis of lymphomas are the leukocyte common antigen (LCA,T200) and the immunoglobulin light chains. A marker of hematopoietic cells, LCA can be detected in frozen as well as paraffin-embedded tissue sections and is extremely useful in differentiating lymphoid neoplasms from non hematopoietic tumors (12,107,244). However, as certain lymphoid tumors, in particular tumor cells showing plasmacytoid differentiation may not stain for LCA (85,107), absence of staining for this antigen does not rule out hematopoietic neoplasms. Immunoglobulins are the most reliable markers of B cells, and they are expressed by B cells (on the surface and/or in the cytoplasm) in almost all stages of B cell differentiation (21,149). Since each B cell expresses kappa or lambda immunoglobulin light chains, the staining for one type of light chain by a vast majority of cells in a lymphoproliferative lesion indicates the presence of a monoclonal population of B cells and supports the diagnosis of lymphoma.

Unlike B cells, there is no marker like immunoglobulin light chains currently available to determine monoclonality of T cells by immunohistochemical techniques. Nevertheless, molecular biological techniques (Southern blot technique) similar to those being used to detect rearrangements of immunoglobulin genes, have been used to determine rearrangements of T-cell receptor genes and to provide evidence for the presence of a monoclonal T cell population (106). It is possible that when antibodies reactive to most of the specific variable regions of the T-cell receptor chain genes become available, determination of the presence of clonal T-cell population by immunohistochemical techniques may become a reality (171). At this time, the monoclonal antibodies to T-cell associated antigens are useful in defining the T-cell nature of lymphoproliferative disorders and relating the immunophenotype of the tumor cells to the stages of T-cell differentiation (22,149). It is of interest that the tumor cells (T or B cell type) can express antigens different from those of their putative normal counterparts, either by acquisition of antigens not expressed by their normal counterparts or by the loss of antigens or both (127). This apparent abnormal pattern of antigen expression (antigenic infidelity) may be of a considerable diagnostic value, especially in the diagnosis of T-cell lymphomas (171).

Antibodies against lysozyme and myeloid or monocyte-associated antigens, have also been used for the characterization of leukemias and lymphomas (81,133). One of the granulocyte-associated antigens, Leu-M1, can be helpful in the identification of Reed-Sternberg cells in Hodgkin's disease (93). Because Leu-M1 is not a specific marker (196), the absence of staining for Leu-M1 does not rule out Hodgkin's disease. An antibody to Leu-M1 has been reported to be helpful in differentiating adenocarcinoma (Leu-M1[+])

from mesothelioma (Leu-M1⁻) (195). Antibodies to hemoglobin have been found useful in the detection of erythroid cells (174).

One of the important observations made during the characterization of lymphoid tissue with monoclonal antibodies to T-cell associated antigens was that the antibody anti-T6 (CD1), which reacts with a majority of cortical thymocytes but not with peripheral T cells, also reacts with Langerhans cells in skin, lymph nodes, and other tissues (18,20,147,175). This has provided confirmatory evidence that histocytosis-X cells represent abnormal Langerhans cells (87). Langerhans cells and histiocytosis-X cells share other antigens such as S-100 protein, HLA-DR and Leu-M3 (13). Histiocytosis-X cells also stain for CD4 (87). This T cell associated antigen is also expressed by monocytes/macrophages and by some normal Langerhans cells (256).

Tumor Associated Antigens

Despite the generation of numerous monoclonal antibodies against a wide variety of tumors (44,89,119,204,257,258), only a few monoclonal antibodies against tumor-associated antigens have found use in diagnostic pathology. None of the antibodies have been specific for tumor cells. Certain antibodies, such as those against prostate specific antigen (148,180,213), have been very useful in differentiating prostatic carcinoma from carcinomas arising in other organs. These antibodies, however, are incapable of differentiating normal or benign prostatic epithelium from malignant epithelial cells.

Monoclonal antibodies reactive with serous or mucinous ovarian tumors have been produced (7,8,24,49). One of these antibodies, OC125, was found to react with all benign and borderline serous ovarian tumors, with most cases of serous cystadenocarcinoma and endometroid carcinoma, and with about 40% of clear cell carcinomas, but not with mucinous tumors of the ovary (11). In a recent study, however, OC125 was reported to react with mucinous tumors, following pronase digestion of paraffin-embedded sections (202). So far, this antibody has been used primarily in the sera of patients with ovarian tumors to detect the antigen (CA 125) and to monitor the course of the tumor progression (7,8,58).

Numerous monoclonal antibodies against breast cancer have been reported (32,42, 119,191). These antibodies, in general, have been specific for epithelial cells rather than for breast cancer. Schlom and his associates (96,97,219,227) have found one of these antibodies, B72.3, (reactive with a high molecular weight mucin) to be useful in differentiating carcinoma cells, including breast and lung cancer from mesenchymal tumors (lymphomas, sarcomas) or from benign and malignant mesothelial cells. Monoclonal antibodies against estrogen receptors have made it possible to detect estrogen receptors in breast cancer by immunohistochemical methods, both in frozen and paraffin-embedded sections (177,200). This is of clinical importance, since the prognosis of breast cancer is related to the expression of estrogen receptors by cancer cells (57,129).

Monoclonal antibodies against lung tumor cells hold the promise of being useful in the differentiation of various histological subtypes of lung cancer and the detection of metastatis (15,114,145,206,210). The monoclonal antibody, SM-1, which is reactive with small cell carcinoma of the lung (15), was found to be helpful in detecting bone marrow metastasis in patients with small cell carcinoma (211). Monoclonal antibodies against colonic carcinomas that have been reported to be of diagnostic importance include antibodies against CA 19-9 (4,34,58), CEA, and CEA-like antigens (146,228). Recently, a monoclonal antibody (RC 38) was reported by Oosterwijk et al. (160) to react with 46 of 47 renal cell carcinomas and 8 of 13 metastatic renal cell carcinomas but not with 179 tumors of various origins.

Numerous investigators have developed monoclonal antibodies against malignant melanomas, but as expected, reactivity of the antibodies has not been restricted to malignant nevomelanocytic cells (71,80,155,184). In one immunohistochemical study, two monoclonal antibodies were found to be stain dysplastic nevus cells and melanomas but not normal skin melanocytes (226). One of the antibodies, however, was reactive with HLA-DR, which has a wide tissue distribution. Esclamado et al. (63) have described three monoclonal antibodies that are highly specific for malignant melanoma and are reactive with 97% of melanomas in paraffin-embedded sections. In another study, monoclonal antibodies against melanosomal proteins were used to detect neoplastic melanocytes in formalin-fixed tissues (123).

Recently, monoclonal antibodies have been used to detect a new class of markers which may be expressed on tumor cells due to activation of proto-oncogenes (cellular oncogenes) (95). These normal cell genes, when activated, lead to transformation of the cell as well as expression of gene products (95). Although many oncogenes have been described, most of the immunohistochemical studies have been performed with the ras family of cellular oncogenes, in particular with antibodies reactive with a protein with a molecular weight of 21 kd (p21). Increased expression of ras p21 protein as compared to normal tissue has been reported in a broad range of tumors, including cancers of the breast (228), prostate (238), stomach (167), and urinary bladder (239) by immunohistochemical analyses of formalin-fixed, paraffin-embedded tissues. These results indicate that transformation of the cells from the benign to malignant phenotype is associated with an increase in ras p21 expression (239). It is likely that alteration in the expression of proto-oncogenes leads to changes in biological function of the cells including cellular proliferation; this alteration, however, may not be necessarily related to the development of malignancy, since expression of proto-oncogenes may be regulated as a function of cell growth and differentiation (95). As new antibodies against various gene products, in particular oncogene products, become available, it may be possible to classify tumors in a way that is based on their biological behavior, which may identify groups of tumors that are responsive to a particular therapy (95).

DIAGNOSTIC PROBLEMS IN SURGICAL PATHOLOGY

In the following sections, strategies in the immunohistochemical analysis of the common diagnostic problems encountered in surgical pathology will be discussed. These are based largely on personal experience and also on the growing literature. As stated above, in those cases where a precise diagnosis cannot be made on the basis of morphologic features, a differential diagnosis should be carefully considered before selecting the immunohistologic stains (Tables 1 and 2).

Metastatic Epithelial Tumors

To determine the primary site of a metastatic epithelial tumor is a challenge faced routinely in surgical pathology (72,73). If the histological features clearly indicate that the tumor cells are epithelial in nature, there is no need to perform a battery of stains for

TABLE 2. *An immunohistochemical staining panel for the characterization of poorly differentiated malignant tumors*

Tumor	Keratin	EMA	LCA	S-100 Protein	Vimentin	Desmin
Carcinoma[a]	+	+	−	−/+	−/+	−
Malignant melanoma	−	−	−	+	+	−
Malignant lymphoma[b]	−	−	+	−	−/+	−
Sarcoma[c]	−/+	−/+	−	−/+	+	−/+

[a]Some epithelial tumors, especially breast and salivary gland tumors, may also stain for S-100 protein. Vimentin has been detected in a wide variety of epithelial tumors. Staining for CEA may help discriminate adenocarcinomas (CEA+) from mesotheliomas (CEA). Specific markers (prostate specific antigen, thyroglobulin) may help determine the primary site. Neuroendocrine differentiation of the tumor can be evaluated by staining for markers such as chromogranin, neuron-specific enolase and neurofilament (see Chapter 12).

[b]Plasmacytomas may also stain for EMA and cells showing plasmacytoid differentiation may not stain for LCA. Moreover, the staining for LCA in paraffin-embedded sections is not as reliable as in frozen tissue sections. Further characterization of the tumor can be carried out by staining for lymphoid markers (see Chapters 10 and 11).

[c]Staining for keratin and EMA is observed in synovial sarcoma and epithelioid sarcoma. Nerve sheath tumors and liposarcomas can be S-100+. Staining of tumor cells for desmin indicates myogenic differentiation. In the absence of staining for keratin, S-100 protein, desmin and endothelial markers (factor VIII-related antigen and binding of lectin Ulex europaeus agglutinin I), presence of reactivity for alpha-1 antitrypin and alpha-1 antichymotrypsin is consistent with a diagnosis of malignant fibrous histiocytoma (see Chapter 14).

epithelial markers. In this situation, it is important to demonstrate a tissue-specific antigen in the tumor cells that may be unique to a given organ site (65). Currently, there are only a limited number of antigens available for this purpose. These include thyroglobulin (carcinoma of thyroid), calcitonin (medullary carcinoma of the thyroid), prostatic acid phosphatase, and prostate specific antigen (carcinoma of prostate), and lactalbumin (carcinoma of breast) (6,25,113,124,198,241). Even with these markers, unexpected immunoreactivity has been observed. For example, prostatic acid phosphatase has been demonstrated in some cases of adenocarcinoma of the urinary bladder (60), carcinoids (40,104,205), islet cell tumors (40), and breast cancer (115) (see Chapter 13).

Demonstration of two or more nonrestricted antigens in the tumor cells, reflecting a distinctive antigenic phenotype, can also be helpful in defining the nature of the tumor cells in a given situation. As discussed above, the presence of keratin and CEA can help differentiate adenocarcinomas from mesotheliomas, which stains intensely for keratin but not for CEA. The presence of keratin, EMA, and S-100 protein in a bone tumor suggests a diagnosis of chordoma (41,134,136). Reactivity for keratin and S-100 protein may also be observed in tumors of the salivary gland, breast, and sweat glands of the skin. In contrast, malignant melanomas stain for S-100 protein but not for keratin. The presence of alpha fetoprotein and alpha-1 antitrypsin in the tumor cells can help support a diagnosis of hepatocellular carcinoma (105,162,254) or of a germ cell tumor of the ovary or testis (109,178,254), depending on the site and presentation of the tumor. Although placental alkaline phosphatase can be demonstrated in various tumors, the presence of this enzyme in the tumor cells in seminomas can help differentiate seminomas from other testicular tumors (234).

Neuroendocrine differentiation of epithelial tumors can be evaluated by staining for neuron-specific enolase (14,120,197,203,208,237,251), chromogranin (121,253), neurofilament (141,203,231), synaptophysin (76) and neuropeptides (245,246) (discussed in detail in Chapter 12). In a study of lung tumors by Said et al. (190), the staining with a monoclonal antibody to chromogranin appeared to correlate with the density of neuroendo-crine granules in the tumor cells. Carcinoid tumors were stained for serotonin and showed a greater density of cytoplasmic neuroendocrine granules than found in small cell carci-nomas. A ball-like staining for keratins, which can be observed in most cases of Merkel cell tumors and some carcinoids, but not in oat cell carcinomas and malignant lymphomas, can be helpful in the diagnosis of neuroendocrine carcinomas (11). Great caution needs to be exercised while interpreting staining for neuron-specific enolase (NSE), as non-neuroen-docrine tumors may also show reactivity for NSE (83,223,237). A monoclonal antibody against NSE has been developed and may provide a more specific reagent for the demon-stration of NSE in tissue sections (224). The monoclonal antibody, Leu-7 (HNK-1), may be helpful in defining the neurendocrine differentiation of the tumor cells (29,116, Chapter 12).

Poorly Differentiated Malignant Tumors (Table 2)

It can often be difficult to distinguish large cell lymphomas from nonlymphoid tumors, such as poorly differentiated carcinomas (nasopharyngeal carcinoma and small cell carci-noma), Merkel cell tumors, and round cell tumors of childhood (neuroblastoma, Ewing's sarcoma, rhabdomyosarcoma) (72,73). Characterization of lymphoid neoplasms can be best performed on frozen tissue sections, using monoclonal antibodies directed against lymphoid differentiation antigens (discussed in detail in Chapter 11). More recently, antibodies capable of reacting with lymphoid cells in paraffin-embedded sections have become available (59,107,157,176,248). Of these markers, leukocyte common antigen (LCA), is the most commonly used marker for differentiating malignant lymphomas from nonhematopoietic neoplasms (23,107). A lack of staining for leukocyte common antigen does not rule out a lymphoid neoplasm, unless studies are carried out for other lymphoid markers in frozen tissue sections, or nonlymphoid markers are demonstrated in the tumor cells. As EMA can be expressed in plasmacytomas (173), it is more reliable to use antibod-ies to keratin in the initial panel to rule out a possibility of poorly differentiated epithelial neoplasm.

A selected panel of antibodies can be helpful in discriminating different types of round cell tumors of childhood (163,230,233, Chapter 14). Neuroblastomas generally stain for NSE and neurofilament; neurofilament is more often present in ganglioneuroblastomas than in poorly differentiated neuroblastomas (163). Staining for chromogranin, if present, is usually focal. Neuroblastomas do not stain for keratin or S-100 protein. Presence of the S-100 positive cells in ganglioneuroblastomas reflects differentiation of a component of the tumor to Schwann cells (201). Rhabdomyosarcomas, as stated above, stain for vimentin and depending on the state of differentiation, the tumor cells also stain for desmin (137) and less frequently for myoglobin (27,53). Ewing's sarcomas stain for vimentin but do not express desmin, S-100 protein, or leukocyte common antigens. Some cases of Ewing's sarcoma, however, do not stain for vimentin (A.K. Bhan and A.E. Rosenberg, *unpublished observations*), and in a few cases tumor cells have been reported to stain for antigens such as neuron-specific enolase, Leu-7, and synaptophysin which are associated with neuroec-todermal tumors (103). In a recent study, 9 out of 11 cases of Ewing's sarcoma were demonstrated to contain scattered or clustered cells expressing simple epithelial type keratins (140). This raises the possibility that Ewing's sarcoma includes a heterogenous group of tumors, with the tumor cells capable of differentiating along different pathways (33,140).

Spindle Cell Malignant Tumors

The differential diagnosis of spindle cell malignant tumor includes sarcomas as well as poorly differentiated carcinomas (110). Immunohistologic findings in these tumors are discussed in great detail in Chapter 14 and briefly under the section entitled "Nonepithelial Markers." The panel of immunohistochemical stains should include keratin, S-100 protein, desmin, factor VIII-related antigen, Ulex europaeus agglutinin 1 and vimentin (Tables 1 and 2). Although staining for S-100 protein is present in both malignant schwannomas and malignant melanomas (212), Isobe et al. (94) have reported the presence of an alpha subunit of S-100 protein in malignant melanomas but not in schwannomas. Electron microscopy may be needed to differentiate between these two tumors. Since there can be overlap between the antigenic phenotype of various soft tissue sarcomas, it is essential that multiple markers be used to assess the state of differentiation of the tumor cells (252) (Chapter 14).

CONCLUSIONS

The application of immunohistologic techniques in diagnostic pathology has allowed characterization of normal and tumor cells, not only by their morphologic features, but also by the presence of distinctive molecular markers. In many situations, immunohistochemical studies allow a more precise diagnosis to be made, and in certain situations the primary site of a metastatic tumor can be accurately determined. The usefulness of the technique is restricted to a large extent by the availability of antibodies that can recognize tissue-specific antigens or antigens associated with the specialized function of the cells. Most of the antigens currently used in diagnostic pathology are not restricted to one type of tumor and often the antigenic phenotype of tumor cells, as delineated by the immunohistochemical studies, is not specific enough to render a precise diagnosis. Moreover, the lack of optimally preserved tissue in surgical pathology, restricts the use of many valuable antibodies. The presence of nonspecific reactivities in the antibodies used and the inexperience of the investigator to appreciate problems associated with immunohistochemical studies can lead to an erroneous diagnosis.

One of the important applications of immunohistochemical studies is in the characterization of undifferentiated malignant tumors. The lack of differentiation as reflected by the morphologic appearance of the tumors is often associated with absence of antigens which are present in differentiated normal cells (62). Therefore, immunophenotyping of poorly differentiated tumors in many instances may not provide any clue to the exact nature of the tumor cells. Furthermore, tumor cells may not maintain the same scheme of expression of antigens as present in the normal cellular counterpart and may express a different set of antigens. This "antigenic infidelity" may prevent exact determination of the nature of the tumor cells; however, in some instances this may help discriminate normal cells or benign tumor cells from malignant tumor cells. Another potential problem may arise when metastatic tumors differ from primary tumors in the type and amount of antigen present in the primary tumor.

Despite the limitations of immunophenotyping of tumor cells (61), immunohistochemical techniques have become essential tools in diagnostic pathology, and to a large extent, immunoperoxidase stains have replaced conventional special stains. The interpretation of the staining should be done with caution by pathologists who are familiar with histological features of the case and who are aware of the pitfalls and limitations of the immunohisto-chemical techniques. The development of monoclonal antibodies has contributed greatly to increasing the specificity of immunoperoxidase stains and has allowed identification of antigens that could not be demonstrated by conventional antisera. This is best exemplified by the large number of monoclonal antibodies available for the characterization of normal and neoplastic lymphoid cells.

Although attempts to produce monoclonal antibodies against "tumor-specific" antigens have generally been disappointing, some antibodies raised against tumor cells have been helpful in detecting antigens shed from tumor cells in blood. An increase in the serum level of these antigens appears to occur with growth and spread of the tumor. Demonstration of these antigens in the tumor specimen will be necessary if the serum levels of the antigens are going to be used to monitor the course of the disease.

With a better understanding of the antigens associated with normal and tumor cells and the availability of a larger spectrum of antibodies, immunohistologic techniques are likely to become extremely useful in diagnosis and classification of tumors.

REFERENCES

1. Ahen, D. J., Nakane, P. K., and Brown, W. R. (1982): Ultrastructural localization of carcinoembryonic antigen in normal intestine and colon cancer: Abnormal distribution of CEA on the surfaces of colon cancer cells. *Cancer*, 49:2077–2090.
2. Albores-Saavedra, J., Nadji, M., Morales, A. R., and Henson, D. E. (1983): Carcinoembryonic antigen in normal, preneoplastic and neoplastic gallbladder epithelium. *Cancer*, 52:1069–1072.
3. Arklie, J., Taylor-Papadimitriou, J., Bodmar, W., Egan, M., and Millis, R. (1981): Differentiation antigens expressed by epithelial cells in the lactating breast are also detectable in breast cancer. *Int. J. Cancer*, 28:23–29.
4. Atkinson, B. F., Ernst, C. S., Herlyn, M., Steplewski, Z., Sears, H. F., and Koprowski, H. (1982): Gastro-intestinal cancer-associated antigen in immunoperoxidase assay. *Cancer Res.*, 42:4820–4823.
5. Azumi, N., and Battifora, H. (1987): The distribution of vimentin and keratin in epithelial and non-epithelial neoplasms. A comprehensive immunohistochemical study on formalin- and alcohol-fixed tumors. *Am. J. Clin. Pathol.*, 88:286–296.
6. Bailey, A. J., Sloane, J. P., Trickey, B. S., and Ormerod, M. G. (1982): An immunocytochemical study of alpha-lactalbumin in human breast tissue. *J. Pathol.*, 137:13–23.
7. Bast, R. C., Jr., Klug, T. L., St. John, E., Jenison, E., Nilfoff, J. M., Lazarus, H., Berkowitz, R. S., Leavitt, T. L., Griffiths, T. C., Parker, L., Zurawski, V. R., Jr., and Knapp, R. C. (1983): A radioimmuno-assay using a monoclonal antibody to monitor the course of epithelial ovarian cancer. *N. Engl. J. Med.*, 309:883–887.
8. Bast, R. C., Jr., and Knapp, R. C. (1987): The emerging role of monoclonal antibodies in the clinical management of epithelial ovarian carcinoma. In: *Important Advances in Oncology*, edited by V. T. DeVita, Jr., S. Hellman, and S. A. Rosenberg, pp. 39–53. J. B. Lippincott Company, Philadelphia.
9. Battifora, H., and Kopinski, M. I. (1985): Distinction of mesothelioma from adenocarcinoma. An immuno-histochemical approach. *Cancer*, 55:1679–1685.
10. Battifora, H., Sheibani, K., Tubbs, R. R., Kopinski, M., and Sun, T. T. (1984): Antikeratin antibodies in tumor diagnosis. Distinction between seminoma and embryonal carcinoma. *Cancer*, 54:843–848.
11. Battifora, H., and Silva, E. G. (1986): The use of antikeratin antibodies in the immunohistochemical dis-tinction between neuroendocrine (Merkle cell) carcinoma of the skin, lymphoma and oat cell carcinoma. *Cancer*, 58:1040–1046.
12. Battifora, H., and Trowbridge, I. S. (1983): A monoclonal antibody useful for the differential diagnosis between malignant lymphomas and non-hematopoietic neoplasms. *Cancer*, 51:816–821.
13. Beckstead, J. H., Wood, G. S., and Turner, R. R. (1984): Histiocytosis X cells and Langerhans cells: En-zyme histochemical and immunologic similarities. *Hum. Pathol.*, 15:826–833.
14. Bergh, J., Thomas, E., Steinholtz, L., Nilsson, K., and Pahlman, S. (1985): Immunocytochemical demon-stration of neuron-specific enolase (NSE) in human lung cancer. *Am. J. Clin. Pathol.*, 84:1–7.

15. Bernal, S. D., and Speak, J. A. (1984): Membrane antigen in small cell carcinoma of the lung defined by monoclonal antibody SM1. *Cancer Res.*, 44:265–270.
16. Bell, D. A., Flotte, T. J., and Bhan, A. K. (1987): Immunohistochemical characterization of seminoma and its inflammatory cell infiltrate. *Hum. Pathol.*, 18:511–520.
17. Bhagavan, B. S., Dorfman, H. D., Murthy, M. S., and Eggleston, J. C. (1982): Intravascular bronchiolo-alveolar tumor (IVBAT): A low-grade sclerosing epithelioid angiosarcoma of the lung. *Am. J. Surg. Pathol.*, 6:41–52.
18. Bhan, A. K. (1984): Application of monoclonal antibodies to tissue diagnosis. In: *Advances in Immunohisto-chemistry*, edited by R. A. DeLellis, pp. 1–29. Masson Publishing USA Inc., New York.
19. Bhan, A. K., and DesMarais, C. L. (1983): Immunohistologic characterization of major histocompatibility antigens and inflammatory cellular infiltrate in human breast cancer. *JNCI*, 71:507–516.
20. Bhan, A. K., and Harris, N. L. (1986): The immunohistology of normal and neoplastic lymphoid tissue. In: *Lymphoproliferative Disorders of the Skin*, edited by G. F. Murphy and M. C. Mihm, Jr., pp. 31–72. Butterworth, Boston.
21. Bhan, A. K., Nadler, L. M., Stashenko, P., McCluskey, R. T., and Schlossman, S. F. (1981): Stages of B-cell differentiation in human lymphoid tissues. *J. Exp. Med.*, 154:737–749.
22. Bhan, A. K., Reinherz, E. L., Poppema, S., McCluskey, R. T., and Schlossman, S. F. (1980): Location of T cell and major histocompatibility complex antigens in the human thymus. *J. Exp. Med.*, 152:771–782.
23. Bhawan, J., Wolff, S. M., Ucci, A. A., and Bhan, A. K. (1985): Malignant lymphoma and malignant angio-endotheliomatosis: One disease. *Cancer*, 55:570–576.
24. Bhattacharya, M., Chatterjee, S. K., Barlow, J. J., and Hiroshi, F. J. (1982): Monoclonal antibodies recognizing tumor-associated antigen in human ovarian mucinous cystadenocarcinomas. *Cancer Res.*, 42:1650–1660.
25. Bocker, W., Dralle, H., and Dorn, G. (1981): Thyroglobulin: An immunohistochemical marker in thyroid disease. In: *Diagnostic Immunochemistry*, edited by R. A. DeLellis, pp. 37–59. Masson Publishing USA Inc., New York.
26. Broers, J., Huysmans, A., Moesker, O., Vooijs, P., Ramaekers, F., and Wegenaar, S. (1985): Small cell lung cancers contain intermediate filament of the cytokeratin type. *Lab. Invest.*, 52:113–115.
27. Brooks, J. J. (1982): Immunohistochemistry of soft tissue tumors. Myoglobin as a tumor marker for rhabdomyosarcoma. *Cancer*, 50:1757–1763.
28. Brooks, J. J. (1986): The significance of double phenotypic patterns and markers in human sarcomas: A new model of mesenchymal differentiation. *Am. J. Pathol.*, 125:113–123.
29. Bunn, P. A., Jr., Linnoila, I., Minna, J. D., Carney, D., and Gazdar, A. F. (1985): Small cell lung cancer, endocrine cells of the fetal bronchus, and other neuroendocrine cells express the Leu-7 antigenic determinant present on natural killer cells. *Blood*, 65:764–768.
30. Burgdorf, W. H., Mukai, K., Rosai, J. (1981): Immunohistochemical identification of factor VIII-related antigen in endothelial cells of cutaneous lesions of alleged vascular nature. *Am. J. Clin. Pathol.*, 75:167–171.
31. Burtin, P., Calmettes, C., and Fondaneche, M. C. (1979): CEA and nonspecific cross-reacting antigen (NCA) in medullary carcinomas of the thyroid. *Int. J. Cancer*, 23:741–745.
32. Cardiff, R. D., Taylor, C. R., Weldings, S. R., and Colcher, D., and Schlom, J. (1983): Monoclonal antibodies in immunoenzyme studies of breast cancer. *Ann. N.Y. Acad. Sci.*, 420:140–146.
33. Cavazzana, A., Miser, J. S., Jefferson, J., and Triche, T. J. (1987): Experimental evidence for a neural origin of Ewings sarcoma. *Am. J. Pathol.*, 127:507–518.
34. Charpin, C., Bhan, A. K., Zurawski, V. R., Jr., and Scully, R. E. (1982): Carcinoembryonic antigen (CEA) and carbohydrate determinant 19-9 (CA 19-9) localization in 121 primary and metastatic ovarian tumors: An immunohistochemical study with the use of monoclonal antibodies. *Int. J. Gynecol. Pathol.*, 1:231–245.
35. Chase, D. R., Enzinger, F. M., Weiss, S. W., and Langloss, J. M. (1984): Keratin in epithelioid sarcoma. An immunohistochemical study. *Am. J. Surg. Pathol.*, 8:435–441.
36. Chesa, P. G., Rettig, W. J., and Melamed, M. R. (1986): Expression of cytokeratins in normal and neoplastic colonic epithelial cells. *Am. J. Surg. Pathol.*, 10:829–835.
37. Chess, Q., and Hadju, S. (1986): The role of immunoperoxidase staining in diagnostic cytology. *Acta Cytol.*, 30:1–7.
38. Cibas, E. S., Corson, J. M., and Pinkus, G. S. (1987): The distinction of adenocarcinoma from malignant mesothelioma in cell blocks of effusions: The role of routine mucin histochemistry and immunohistochemical assessment of carcinoembryonic antigen, keratin proteins, epithelial membrane antigen and milk fat globule-derived antigen. *Hum. Pathol.*, 18:67–74.
39. Clark, H. B., Minesky, J. J., Agarwal, D., and Agarwal, H. C. (1985): Myelin basic protein and P2 protein are not immunohistochemical markers for Schwann cell neoplasms. *Am. J. Pathol.*, 121:96–101.
40. Cohen, C., Bentz, M. S., and Budgeon, L. R. (1983): Prostatic acid phosphatase in carcinoid and islet cell tumors (letter). *Arch. Pathol. Lab. Med.*, 107:277.
41. Coindre, J. M., Rivel, J., Trojani, M., De-Mascarl, I., and DeMascarl, A. (1986): Immunohistological study in chordomas. *J. Pathol.*, 150:61–63.

42. Colcher, D., Hand, P.H., Nuti, M., and Schlom, J. (1981): A spectrum of monoclonal antibodies reactive with human mammary tumor cells. *Proc. Natl. Acad. Sci. U.S.A.*, 78:3199–3203.

43. Cooper, D., Schermer, A., and Sun, T. T. (1985): Classification of human epithelial and their neoplasms using monoclonal antibodies to keratins. Strategies, application and limitations. *Lab. Invest.*, 52:243–256.

44. Cordon-Cardo, C. (1985): Monoclonal antibodies in the diagnosis of solid tumors. Studies on renal carcinomas, transitional cell carcinomas and melanoma. In: *Immunohistochemistry in Tumor Diagnosis*, edited by J. Russo, pp. 281–292. Martinus Nijhoff Publishers, Boston.

45. Corson, J. M. (1986): Keratin protein immunohistochemistry in surgical pathology practice. In: *Pathology Annual*, Part 2, edited by S. C. Sommers, P. P. Rosen, and R. E. Fechner, pp. 47–81. Appleton-Century-Crofts, Norwalk, CT.

46. Corson, J. M., Weiss, L. M., Banks-Schlegel, S. P., and Pinkus, G. S. (1984): Keratin proteins and carcinoembryonic antigen in synovial sarcomas. An immunohistochemical study of 24 cases. *Hum. Pathol.*, 15:615–621.

47. Corson, J. M., and Pinkus, G. S. (1982): Mesothelioma: Profile of keratin proteins and carcinoembryonic antigen: An immunoperoxidase study of 20 cases and comparison with pulmonary adenocarcinomas. *Am. J. Pathol.*, 108:80–87.

48. Cote, R. J., Morrissey, D. M., Houghton, A. N., Beattie, E. J., Jr., Oettgen, H. F., and Old, L. J. (1983): Generation of human monoclonal antibodies reactive with cellular antigens. *Proc. Natl. Acad. Sci. USA*, 80:2026–2030.

49. Croghan, G. A., Wingate, M. B., Gamarra, M., Johnson, E., Chu, T. M., Allen, H., Valenzuela, L., Tsukada, Y., and Papsielero, L. D. (1984): Reactivity of monoclonal antibody F36/22 with human ovarian adenocarcinomas. *Cancer Res.*, 44:1954–1962.

50. Damajanov, I., and Knowles, B. B. (1983): Biology of disease, monoclonal antibodies and tumor-associated antigens. *Lab. Invest.*, 48:510–525.

51. de Boulery, C. E. H. (1982): Demonstration of alpha-1-antitrypsin and alpha-1-antichymotrypsin in fibrous histiocytomas using the immunoperoxidase technique. *Am. J. Surg. Pathol.*, 6:559–564.

52. Debus, E., Moll, R., Franke, W., Webber, K., and Osborn, M. (1984): Immunohistochemical distinction of human carcinomas by cytokeratin typing with monoclonal antibodies. *Am. J. Pathol.*, 114:121–130.

53. de Jong, A. S. H., Van Vark, M., Albus-Lutter, C. E., Van Raamsdonk, and Voute, P. A. (1984): Myosin and myoglobin as tumor markers in the diagnosis of rhabdomyosarcoma. A comparative study. *Am. J. Surg. Pathol.*, 8:521–528.

54. DeLellis, R. A. (1981): Diagnostic immunohistochemistry in tumor pathology. An overview. In: *Diagnostic Immunohistochemistry*, edited by R. A. DeLellis, pp. 1–5. Masson Publishing USA, Inc., New York.

55. Delsol, G., Gatter, K. C., Stein, H., Erber, W. N., Pupford, K. A. F., Zinne, K., and Mason, D. Y. (1984): Human lymphoid cells express epithelial membrane antigen. Implications for diagnosis of human neoplasms. *Lancet*, 2:1124–1128.

56. Denk, H., Krepler, R., Artlieb, U., Gabbiani, G., Rungger-Brandle, E., Leoncini, P., and Franke, W. W. (1983): Proteins of intermediate filaments: An immunohistochemical and biochemical approach to the classification of soft tissue tumors. *Am. J. Pathol.*, 110:193–208.

57. DeSombre, E. R., Thorpe, S. M., Rose, C., Blough, R., Anderson, K. W., Remussen, B. B., Kling, W. J. (1986): Prognostic usefulness of estrogen receptor immunohistochemical assays for human breast cancer. *Cancer Res.*, 46:4256s–4264s.

58. Dietel, M., Arps, H., Klapdor, R., Muller-Hagen, S., Sieck, M., and Hoffman, L. (1986): Antigen detection by the monoclonal antibodies CA 19-9 and CA 125 in normal and tumor tissue and patients sera. *J. Cancer Research Oncol.*, 111:527–565.

59. Epstein, A. L., Marder, R. J., and Winter, J. N., and Fox, R. I. (1984): Two new monoclonal antibodies (LN-1, LN-2) reactive in B5 formalin-fixed, paraffin-embedded tissues with follicular center and mantle zone human B lymphocytes and derived tumors. *J. Immunol.*, 133:1028–1036.

60. Epstein, J. I., Kuhajda, F. P., and Lieberman, P. H. (1986): Prostate-specific acid phosphatase immunoreactivity in adenocarcinomas of the urinary bladder. *Hum. Pathol.*, 17:939–942.

61. Erlandson, R.A. (1984): Diagnostic immunohistochemistry of human tumors: An interim evaluation. *Am. J. Surg. Pathol.*, 8:615–624.

62. Ernst, C., Thurin, J., Atkinson, B., Wurzel, H., Herlyn, M., Stromberg, N., Civin, C., and Kaprowski, H. (1984): Monoclonal antibody localization of A and B isoantigens in normal and malignant fixed human tissues. *Am. J. Pathol.*, 117:451–461.

63. Esclamado, R. M., Gown, A. M., and Vogel, A. M. (1986): Unique protein defined by monoclonal antibodies specific for human melanoma. Some potential clinical application. *Am. J. Surg.*, 152:376–385.

64. Espinoza, C. G., and Azar, H. A. (1982): Immunohistochemical localization of keratin-type proteins in epithelial neoplasm. Correlation with electron microscopic findings. *Am. J. Clin. Pathol.*, 78:500–507.

65. Espinoza, C. G., Balis, J. U., Saba, S. R., Piciga, J. T., and Shelley, S. A. (1984): Ultrastructural and immunohistochemical studies of bronchiolo-alveolar carcinoma. *Cancer*, 54:2182–2189.

66. Eusebi, V., Rilke, F., Ceccarelli, C., Fedel, F., Schiaffino, S., and Bussolati, G. (1986): Fetal heavy chain skeletal muscle myosin. An oncofetal antigen expressed by rhabdomyosarcoma. *Am. J. Surg. Pathol.*, 10:680–686.

67. Fischer, H. P., Altmannsbergery, M., Weber, K., and Osborn, M. (1987): Keratin polypeptides in malignant epithelial liver tumors. Differential diagnosis and histogenetic aspects. *Am. J. Pathol.*, 127:530–537.

68. Fisher, C. (1986): Synovial sarcoma: Ultrastructural and immunochemical features of epithelial differentiation in monophasic and biphasic tumors. *Hum. Pathol.*, 10:996–1008.

69. Foon, K. A., Schroff, R. W., and Gale, R. P. (1982): Surface markers on leukemia and lymphoma cells: Recent advances. *Blood*, 60:1–19.

70. Gabbiani, G., Kapanci, Y., Barazzone, P., and Franke, W. W. (1981): Immunochemical identification of intermediate-sized filaments in human neoplastic cells: A diagnostic aid for the surgical pathologist. *Am. J. Pathol.*, 104:206–216.

71. Garrigues, H. J., Tilgen, W., Hellstrom, I., Franke, W., and Hallstrom, K. E. (1982): Detection of human melanoma-associated antigen, P97, in histologic sections of primary human melanomas. *Int. J. Cancer*, 29:511–515.

72. Gatter, K. C., Alcock, C., Heryet, A., Pufford, K. A., Hyderman, E., Taylor-Papadimitriou, J., Stein, H., and Mason, D. Y. (1984): The differential diagnosis of routinely processed anaplastic tumors using monoclonal antibodies. *Am. J. Clin. Pathol.*, 82:33–43.

73. Gatter, K. C., Alcock, C., Heryet, A., and Mason, D. Y. (1985): Clinical importance of analyzing malignant tumors of uncertain origin with immunohistological techniques. *Lancet*, 1:1302–1305.

74. Ghosh, A. K., Spriggs, A. L., Taylor-Papadimitriou, J., and Mason, D. Y. (1983): Immunocytochemical staining of cells in pleural and peritoneal effusions with a panel of monoclonal antibodies. *J. Clin. Pathol.*, 36:1154–1169.

75. Goslin, R. H., O'Brien, M. J., Skarin, A. T., and Zamcheck, N. (1983): Immunocytochemical staining for CEA in small cell carcinoma of lung predicts clinical usefulness of the plasma assay. *Cancer*, 52:301–306.

76. Gould, V. E., Lee, I., Wiedermann, B., Moll, R., Chejfee, G., and Franke, W. W. (1986): A novel marker for neurons, certain neuroendocrine cells and their neoplasms. *Hum. Pathol.*, 17:979–983.

77. Gown, A. M., and Vogel, A. M. (1985): Monoclonal antibodies to human intermediate filament proteins. III. Analysis of tumors. *Am. J. Clin. Pathol.*, 84:413–424.

78. Gown, A. M., and Gabbiani, G. (1984): Intermediate sized filaments in human tumors. In: *Advances in Immunohistochemistry*, edited by R. A. DeLellis, pp. 89–110. Masson Publishing Inc., USA, New York.

79. Gown, A. M., and Vogel, A. M. (1984): Monoclonal antibodies to human intermediate filament proteins. II. Distribution of filament proteins in normal human tissues. *Am. J. Pathol.*, 114:309–314.

80. Gown, A. M., Vogel, A. M., Oak, D., Gough, F., and McNutt, M. (1986): Monoclonal antibodies specific for melanocytic tumors distinguish subpopulations of melanocytes. *Am. J. Pathol.*, 123:195–203.

81. Griffin, J. D., Ritz, J., Nadler, L. M., and Schlossman, S. F. (1982): Expression of myeloid differentiation antigens on normal and malignant myeloid cells. *J. Clin, Invest.*, 68:932–941.

82. Guarda, L. G., Ordonez, N. G., Smith, J. L., Jr., and Hansen, G. (1982): Immunoperoxidase localization of factor VIII in angiosarcomas. *Arch. Pathol. Lab. Med.*, 106:515–516.

83. Haimoto, H., Takahashi, Y., Koshikawa, T., Nagura, H., and Kato, K. (1985): Immunohistochemical localization of gamma enolase in normal human tissues other than nervous and neuroendocrinic tissue. *Lab. Invest.*, 52:257–263.

84. Harris, N. L., Pilch, B. Z., Bhan, A. K., and Goodman, M. L. (1984): Immunohistologic diagnosis of orbital lymphoid infiltrates. *Am. J. Surg. Pathol.*, 8:83–90.

85. Harris, N. L., and Bhan, A. K. (1985): B cell neoplasia of lymphocytic, lymphoplasmacytoid, and plasma cell type: Immunohistologic analysis and clinical correlation. *Human Pathol.*, 16:829–837.

86. Harris, N. L., Nadler, L. M., and Bhan, A. K. (1984): Immunohistological characterization of two malignant lymphomas of germinal center type (centroblastic/centrocytic and centrocytic) with monoclonal antibodies. Follicular and diffuse lymphomas of small cleaved cell type are related but distinct entities. *Am. J. Pathol.*, 117:262–272.

87. Harrist, T. J., Bhan, A. K., Murphy, G. F., Sato, S., Berman, R. S., Gellis, S. E., Freedman, S., and Mihm, M. C., Jr. (1983): Histiocytosis X: *In situ* characterization of cutaneous infiltrates with monoclonal antibodies. *Am. J. Clin. Pathol.*, 79:294–300.

88. Hashimoto, H., Daimaru, Y., Enjoji, M. (1984): S100 protein distribution in liposarcoma. An immunoperoxidase study with special reference to the distinction of liposarcoma from myxoid malignant fibrous histiocytoma. *Virchows (A). Pathol. Anat.*, 405:1–10.

89. Hellstrom, I., Horn, D., Linsley, P., Brown, J. P., Brankoran, V., and Hellstrom, K. E. (1986): Monoclonal mouse antibodies raised against human lung carcinoma. *Cancer Res.*, 46:3917–3923.

90. Heyderman, E., Graham, R. M., Chapman, D. V., Richardson, T. C., and McKee, P. H. (1984): Epithelial markers in primary skin cancer: An immunoperoxidase study of the distribution of epithelial membrane antigen (EMA) and carcinoembryonic antigen (CEA) in 65 primary skin carcinomas. *Histopathology*, 8: 423–434.

91. Hockey, M. S., Stokes, H. J., Thomson, H., Woodhouse, C. S., Macdonald, T., Fielding, S W. L., and Ford, G. H. J. (1984): Carcinoembryonic antigen (CEA) expression and heterogeneity in primary and autologous metastatic gastric tumours demonstrated by a monoclonal antibody. *Br. J. Cancer*, 49:129–133.

92. Holden, J., and Churg, A. (1984): Immunohistochemical staining for keratin and carcinoembryonic antigen in the diagnosis of malignant mesothelioma. *Am. J. Surg. Pathol.*, 8:277–279.

93. Hsu, S. M., Yang, K., and Jaffe, E. S. (1985): Phenotypic expression of Hodgkin's and Reed-Sternberg cells in Hodgkin's disease. *Am. J. Pathol.*, 118:209–217.

94. Isobe, T., Ichimori, K., Nakajima, T., and Okuyama, T. (1984): The alpha subunit of S100 protein is present in tumor cells of human malignant melanoma, but not in Schwannoma. *Brain Res.*, 294:381–384.

95. Israel, M. A., Helman, L. J., and Miser, J. (1987): Patterns of proto-oncogene expression: A novel approach to the developmeent of tumor markers. In: *Important Advances in Oncology*, edited by V. T. DeVita, Jr., S. Hellman, and S. A. Rosenberg, pp. 87–103. J.B. Lippincott Company, Philadelphia.

96. Johnston, W. W., Szpak, C. A., Lottich, S. C., Thor, A., and Schlom, J. (1985): Use of monoclonal antibody (B72.3) as an immunocytochemical adjunct to diagnosis of adenocarcinoma in human effusions. *Cancer Res.*, 45:1894–1900.

97. Johnston, W. W., Szpak, C. A., Thor, A., and Schlom, J. (1986): Phenotype characterization of lung cancers in fine needle aspiration biopsies using monoclonal antibody B72.3. *Cancer Res.*, 46:6462–6470.

98. Jothy, S., Brazinsky, S. A., Chin-A-Loy, M., Haggarty, A., Krantz, M. J., Cheung, M., and Fuks, A. (1986): Characterization of monoclonal antibodies to carcinoembryonic antigen with increased tumor specificity. *Lab. Invest.*, 54:108–117.

99. Kabawat, S. E., Bast, R. C., Jr., Welch, W. R., Knapp, R. C., and Bhan, A. K. (1983): Expression of major histocompatibility antigens and nature of inflammatory cellular infiltrate in ovarian neoplasms. *Int. J. Cancer*, 32:547–554.

100. Kabawat, S. E., Preffer, F. I., and Bhan, A. K. (1985): Monoclonal antibodies in diagnostic pathology. In: *Handbook of Monoclonal Antibodies, Application in Biology and Medicine*, edited by S. Ferrone and M. P. Dierich, pp. 293–298. Noyes Publications, Park Ridge, New Jersey.

101. Kabawat, S. E., Bast, R. C., Jr., Bhan, A. K., Welch, W. R., Knapp, R. C., and Colvin, R. G. (1983): Tissue distribution of a coelomic epithelium-related antigen recognized by the monoclonal antibody OC125. *Int. J. Gynecol. Pathol.*, 2:275–285.

102. Kahn, H. J., Marks, A., Thom, H., and Baumal, R. (1983): Role of antibody to S100 protein in diagnostic pathology. *Am. J. Clin. Pathol.*, 79:341.

103. Kawaguchi, K., and Koike, M. (1986): Neuron-specific enolase and leu-7 immunoreactive small round cell neoplasm. The relationship to Ewing's sarcoma in bone and soft tissue. *Am. J. Clin. Pathol.*, 86:79–93.

104. Kimura, N., and Sasano, N. (1986): Prostate-specific acid phosphatase in carcinoid tumors. *Virchows Arch.*, (A) 410:247–251.

105. Kojiro, M., Kawano, Y., Isomura, T., and Nakashima, T. (1981): Distribution of albumin- and/or alpha-fetoprotein-positive cells in hepatocellullar carcinoma. *Lab. Invest.*, 44:221–226.

106. Korsmeyer, S. J. (1987): Immunoglobulin and T-cell receptor genes reveal the clonality, lineage and translocations of lymphoid neoplasm. In: *Important Advances in Oncology*, edited by V. T. DeVita, Jr., S. Hellman, and S. A. Rosenberg, pp. 3–38. J.B. Lippincott Company, Philadelphia.

107. Kurtin, P. J., and Pinkus, G. S. (1985): Leukocyte common antigen is a diagnostic discriminant between hematopoietic and nonhematopoietic neoplasms in paraffin sections using monoclonal antibodies. *Hum. Pathol.*, 16:353–363.

108. Kupchik, H. Z., Zurawski, V. R., Jr., Hurrell, J. G. R., Zamcheck, N., and Black, P. H. (1981): Monoclonal antibodies to carcinoembryonic antigen produced by somatic cell fusion. *Cancer Res.*, 41:3306–3310.

109. Kurman, R. J., and Scardino, P. T. (1981): Alpha-fetoproteins and human chronic gonadotropin in ovarian and testicular germ cell tumors. In: *Diagnostic Immunocytochemistry*, edited by R. A. DeLellis, pp. 277–298. Masson Publishing USA Inc., New York.

110. Kuwano, H., Hashimoto, H., and Enjoji, M. (1985): Atypical fibroxanthoma distinguishable from spindle cell carcinoma in sarcoma-like skin lesions. A clinicopathologic and immunohistochemical study of 21 cases. *Cancer*, 55:172–180.

111. Leader, M., Patel, J., Makin, C., and Henry, K. (1986): An analysis of the sensitivity and specificity of the cytokeratin marker CAM 5.2 for epithelial tumors. Results of 203 sarcomas, 50 carcinomas and 28 malignant melanomas. *Histopathology*, 10:1315–1324.

112. Leader, M., Collins, M., Patel, J., and Henry, K. (1986): Staining for factor VIII related antigen and Ulex europaeus agglutinin (UEA-1) in 230 tumors. An assessment of their specificity for angiosarcomas and Kaposi's sarcoma. *Histopathology*, 10:1153–1162.

113. Lee, A. K., DeLellis, R. A., Rosen, P. P., Herbert-Stanton, T., Tallberg, K., Garcia, C., and Wolfe, H. J. (1984): Alpha-lactalbumin as an immunohistochemical marker for metastatic breast carcinomas. *Am. J. Surg. Pathol.*, 8:93–100.

114. Lee, I., Radosevich, J. A., Chejfee, G., Ma, Y-K., Warren, W. H., Rosen, S. T., and Gould, V. E. (1986): Malignant mesotheliomas: Improved differential diagnosis from lung adenocarcinomas using monoclonal antibodies 44-3AG and 624A12. *Am. J. Pathol.*, 123:497–507.

115. Li, C. Y., Lam, W. K., and Yam, L. T. (1980): Immunohistochemical diagnosis of prostatic cancer with metastasis. *Cancer*, 46:706–712.

116. Lipinski, M., Braham, K., Caillaud, J. M., Carlu, C., and Tursz, T. (1983): HNK-1 antibody detects an antigen expressed on neuroectodermal cells. *J. Exp. Med.*, 158:1775–1780.

117. Listrom, M. B., and Dalton, L. W. (1987): Comparison of keratin monoclonal antibodies MAK-6, AE 1:AE 3, and CAM-51.2. *Am. J. Clin. Pathol.*, 88:297–301.

118. Little, D., Said, J. W., Siegel, R. J., Fealey, M., and Fishbein, M. C. (1986): Endothelial cell markers in

vascular neoplasms: An immunohistochemical study comparing factor VIII-related antigen, blood group specific antigen, 6-Keto-PGF1 alpha and Ulex europaeus 1 lectin. *J. Pathol.*, 149:89–95.

119. Lloyd, K. O. (1983): Human tumor antigens: Detection and characterization with monoclonal antibodies. In: *Basic and Clinical Tumor Immunology*, edited by R. B. Herberman, pp. 159–214. Martinus Nijhoff Publishers, Boston.

120. Lloyd, R. V., and Warner, T. F. (1984): Immunohistochemistry of neuron-specific enolase. In: *Advances in Immunohistochemistry*, edited by R. A. DeLellis, pp. 127–140. Masson Publishing USA Inc., New York.

121. Lloyd, R. V., and Wilson, B. S. (1983): Specific endocrine tissue marker defined by a monoclonal antibody. *Science*, 222:628–635.

122. Madri, J. A., and Barwick, K. W. (1982): An immunohistochemical study of nasopharyngeal neoplasms using Keratin antibodies: Epithelial versus nonepithelial neoplasms. *Am. J. Surg. Pathol.*, 6:143–149.

123. Maeda, K., and Jimbow, K. (1987): Development of MoA6 HMSA-2 for melanosomes of human melanoma and its application to immunohistopathologic diagnosis of neoplastic melanocytes. *Cancer*, 59:415–423.

124. Manley, P. N., Mahan, D. E., Bruce, A. W., and Franchi, L. (1981): Prostate specific acid phosphatase. In: *Diagnostic Immunohistochemistry*, edited by R. A. DeLellis, pp. 313–324. Masson Publishing USA, Inc., New York.

125. Mannoji, H., Takeshita, I., Fukui, M., Ohta, M., and Kitamura, K. (1981): Glial fibrillary acidic protein in medulloblastoma. *Acta Neuropathol.*, (Berl.), 55:63–69.

126. Marshall, R. J., Herbert, A., Braye, S. G., and Jones, D. B. (1984): Use of antibodies to carcinoembryonic antigen and human milk fat globule to distinguish carcinoma, mesothelioma and reactive mesothelium. *J. Clin. Pathol.*, 37:1215–1221.

127. Mason, D. Y. (1987): A new look at lymphoma immunohistology. (Editorial) *Am. J. Pathol.*, 128:1–4.

128. Mazur, M. T., and Clark, H. B. (1983): Gastric stromal tumors: Reappraisal of histogenesis. *Am. J. Surg. Pathol.*, 7:507–519.

129. McClelland, R. A., Berger, U., Miller, L. S., Powles, T. J., Jensen, E. V., and Coombes, R. C. (1986): Immunocytochemical assay for estrogen receptor. Relationship to outcome of therapy in patient with advanced breast cancer. *Cancer Res.*, 46:4241S–4243S.

130. Mccomb, R. D., Jones, T. R., Pizzo, S. V., and Bigner, D. D. (1982): Specificity and sensitivity of immunohistochemical detection of factor VIII/von Willebrand factor antigen in formalin-fixed paraffin-embedded tissue. *J. Histochem. Cytochem.*, 30:371–377.

131. McNutt, M. A., Bolen, J. W., Crown, A. M., Hammar, S. P., and Vogel, A. M. (1985): Coexpression of intermediate filaments on human epithelial neoplasms. *Ultrastr. Pathol.*, 9:31–43.

132. Meis, J. M., Ordonez, N. G., and Bruner, J. M. (1986): Meningiomas. An immunohistochemical study of 50 cases. *Arch. Pathol. Lab. Med.*, 110:934–937.

133. Mendelsohn, G., Eggleston, J. C., and Mann, R. B. (1980): Relationship of lysozyme (muramidase) to histiocytic differentiation in malignant histiocytosis. An immunohistochemical study. *Cancer*, 45:273–279.

134. Miettinen, M. (1984): Chordoma. Antibodies to epithelial membrane antigen and carcinoembryonic antigen in differential diagnosis. *Arch. Pathol. Lab. Med.*, 108:891–892.

135. Miettinen, M., Lehto, V. P., Badley, R. A., and Virtanen, I. (1982): Expression of intermediate filaments in soft-tissue sarcomas. *Int. J. Cancer*, 30:541–546.

136. Miettinen, M., Lehto, V. P., Dahl, D., and Virtanen, I. (1983): Differential diagnosis of chordoma, chondroid, and ependymal tumors as aided by anti-intermediate filament antibodies. *Am. J. Pathol.*, 112:160–169.

137. Molenaar, W. M., Osterhuis, J. W., Osterhuis, A. M., and Ramaekers, C. S. (1984): Mesenchymal and muscle specific intermediate filaments (vimentin and desmin) in relation to differentiation in childhood rhabdomyosarcoma. *Hum. Pathol.*, 16:838–843.

138. Moll, R., Cowin, P., Kapprell, H. P., and Franke, W. V. (1986): Desmosomal proteins: New markers for identification and classification of tumors. *Lab. Invest.*, 54:4–25.

139. Moll, R., Franke, W. W., Schiller, P. L., Geiger, B., and Krepler, R. (1982): The catalog of human cytokeratins: Patterns of expression in normal epithelia, tumors and cultured cells. *Cell*, 31:11–24.

140. Moll, R., Lee, I., Gould, V. E., Brendt, R., Roessner, A., and Franke, W. W. (1987): Immunohistochemical analysis of Ewing's tumors: Patterns of expression of intermediate filaments and desmosomal proteins indicate cell type heterogeneity and plurpotential differentiation. *Am. J. Pathol.*, 127:288–304.

141. Muijen, G. N. P., Ruiter, D. J., Leeuwen, C. V., Prins, F. A., Rietsema, K., and Warnaar, S. O. (1984): Cytokeratin and neurofilament in lung carcinomas. *Am. J. Pathol.*, 116:363–369.

142. Mukai, K., Schollmeyer, J. V., and Rosai, J. (1981): Immunohistochemical localization of actin: Applications in surgical pathology. *Am. J. Surg. Pathol.*, 5:91–97.

143. Mukai, M. (1983): Immunohistochemical localization of S-100 protein and peripheral nerve myelin proteins (P2 protein, PO protein) in granular cell tumors. *Am. J. Pathol.*, 112:139–146.

144. Mukai, M., Iri, M., Torikata, C., Kageyama, K., Morikawa, Y., Shimizu, K. (1984): Immunoperoxidase demonstration of a new muscle protein (Z-protein) in myogenic tumors as a diagnostic aid. *Am. J. Pathol.*, 114:164–170.

145. Mulshine, J. L., Cuttitta, F., Bibro, M., Fedorko, J., Fargion, S., Little, C., Carney, D. N., Gazdar, A. F.,

and Minna, J. D. (1983): Monoclonal antibodies that distinguish non-small cell from small cell lung cancer. *J. Immunol.*, 131:497–502.

146. Muraro, R., Wunderlich, D., Thor, A., Lundy, J., Noguchi, P., Cunningham, R., and Schlom, J. (1985): Definition by monoclonal antibodies of a repertoire of epitopes on carcinoembryonic antigen differentially expressed in human colon carcinomas versus normal adult tissues. *Cancer Res.*, 45:5769–5780.

147. Murphy, G. F., Bhan, A. K., Soto, S., Harrist, T. J., and Mihm, M. C., Jr. (1981): Characterization of Langerhans cells by the use of monoclonal antibodies. *Lab. Invest.*, 95:465–468.

148. Nadji, M., Tabei, Z., Castro, A., Chu, T. M., Murphy, G. P., Wang, M. C., and Morales, A. R. (1981): Prostate specific antigen: An immunohistologic marker for prostatic neoplasms. *Cancer*, 48:1229–1230.

149. Nadler, L. M., Ritz, J., Griffin, J. D., Todd, R. F., III, Reinherz, E. L., and Schlossman, S. F. (1981): Diagnosis and treatment of human leukemias and lymphomas utilizing monoclonal antibodies. *Prog. Haematol.*, 12:187–225.

150. Nakajima, T., Kameya, T., Watanabe, S., Hirota, T., Shimosato, Y., and Isobe, T. (1984): S100 protein distribution in normal and neoplastic tissues. In: *Advances in Immunohistochemistry*, edited by R. A. DeLellis, pp. 141–158. Masson Publishing USA Inc., New York.

151. Nakajima, T., Watanabe, S., Sato, Y., Kameya, T., Shimosato, Y., and Ishihara, K. (1982): Immunohistochemical demonstration of S-100 protein in malignant melanoma and pigmented nevus, and its diagnostic application. *Cancer*, 50:912–918.

152. Nakamura, Y., Beckar, L. E., and Marks, A. (1983): S-100 protein in tumors of cartilage and bone. An immunohistological study. *Cancer*, 512:1920–1924.

153. Nakazato, Y., Ishizeki, J., Takahasi, K., and Yamaguchi, H. (1982): Immunohistochemical localization of S-100 protein in granular cell myoblastoma. *Cancer*, 49:1624–1628.

154. Nakazato, Y., Ishizeki, J., Takahasi, K., Yamaguchi, H., Kamei, T., and Mori, T. (1982): Localization of S-100 protein and glial fibrillary acidic protein related antigen in pleomorphic adenoma of the salivary glands. *Lab. Invest.*, 46:621–626.

155. Natali, P. G., Bigotti, A., Cavaliere, R., Nicotra, M. R., and Ferrone, S. (1984): Phenotyping of lesions of melanocytic origin with monoclonal antibodies to melanoma associated antigens and to HLA antigens. *JNCI*, 73:13–24.

156. Nelson, W. G., Battifora, H., Santana, H., and Sun, T. T. (1984): Specific keratins as molecular markers for neoplasms with a stratified epithelial origin. *Cancer Res.*, 44:1600–1603.

157. Norton, A. J., Ramsay, A. D., Smith, S. H., Beverly, P. C. L., and Isaacson, P. G. (1986): Monoclonal antibody (UCHL1) that recognizes normal and neoplastic T cells in routinely fixed tissues. *J. Clin. Pathol.*, 39:399–405.

158. O'Brien, M. J., Zamcheck, N., Burke, B., Kirkham, S. E., Saravis, C. A., and Gottlieb, L. S. (1981): Immunocytochemical localization of carcinoembryonic antigen in benign and malignant colorectal tissues. Assessment of diagnostic value. *Am. J. Clin. Pathol.*, 75:283–290.

159. Old, L. J. (1981): Cancer immunology. The search for specificity. *Cancer Res.*, 41:361–375.

160. Oosterwijk, E., Wakka, J. C., Huistkens, J. W., Meij, V. D., Jonas, U., Fleuren, G. J., Zwartendsjk, J., Hoedemaeker, P. H., and Warnaar, S. O. (1986): Immunohistochemical analysis of monoclonal antibodies to renal antigens: Application in the diagnosis of renal cell carcinoma. *Am. J. Pathol.*, 123:301–309.

161. Ordonez, N. G., and Batsakis, J. G. (1984): Comparison of Ulex europaeus 1 lectin with factor VIII-related antigen in vascular lesions. *Arch. Pathol. Lab. Med.*, 108:129–132.

162. Ordonez, N. G., and Manning, J. T., Jr. (1984): Comparison of alpha-1-antitrypsin and alpha-1-antichymotrypsin in hepatocellular carcinoma: An immunoperoxidase study. *Am. J. Gastroenterol.*, 79:959–963.

163. Osborn, M., Dirk, T., Kaser, H., Weber, K., and Altmannsberger, M. (1986): Immunohistochemical localization of neurofilaments and neuron-specific enolase in 29 cases of neuroblastoma. *Am. J. Pathol.*, 122:433–442.

164. Osborn, M., Hill, C., Altmannsberger, M., and Weber, K. (1986): Monoclonal antibodies to titin in conjunction with antibodies to desmin separate rhabdomyosarcoma from other tumor types. *Lab. Invest.*, 55:101–108.

165. Osborn, M., Van-Lessen, G., Webber, K., Kloppel, G, and Altmannsberger, M. (1986): Differential diagnosis of gastrointestinal carcinoma by using monoclonal antibodies specific for individual keratin polypeptides. *Lab. Invest.*, 55:497–504.

166. Osborn, M., and Weber, K. (1983): Biology of disease. Tumor diagnosis by intermediate filament typing: a novel tool for surgical pathology. *Lab. Invest.*, 48:372–394.

167. Ouchi, N., Horan-Hand, P., Merlo, G., Fujita, I., Mariani-Constantini, R., Thor, A., Nose, M., Callahan, R., and Schlom, J. (1987): Enhanced expression of C-Ha-ras p. 21 in human stomach adenocarcinomas defined by immunoassays using monoclonal antibodies and *in situ* hybridization. *Cancer Res.*, 147:1413–1420.

168. Penneys, N. S., Mogollan, R., Kowalczyk, A., Nadji, M., and Adachi, K. (1984): A survey of cutaneous neural lesions for the presence of myelin basic protein. An immunohistochemical study. *Arch. Dermatol.*, 120:210–213.

169. Penneys, N. S., Nadji, M., Ziegels-Weissman, J., Ketabachi, M., and Morales, A. R. (1982): Carcinoembryonic antigen in sweat-gland carcinomas. *Cancer*, 50:1608–1611.

170. Permanetter, W., Nathrath, W. B., and Lohrs, U. (1982): Immunohistochemical analysis of thyroglobulin and keratin in benign and malignant thyroid tumours. *Virchows Arch. (A)*, 398:221–228.

171. Picker, L. J., Weiss, L. M., Medeiros, L. J., Wood, G. S., and Warnke, R. A. (1987): Immunophenotypic criteria for the diagnosis of non-Hodgkin's lymphoma. *Am. J. Pathol.*, 128:181–201.

172. Pinkus, G. S., Etheridge, C. L., and O'Connor, E. M. (1986): Are keratin proteins a better marker than epithelial membrane antigen? A comparative immunohistochemical study of various paraffin-embedded neoplasms using monoclonal and polyclonal antibodies. *Am. J. Clin. Pathol.*, 85:269–277.

173. Pinkus, G. S., and Kurtin, P. J. (1985): Epithelial membrane antigen. A diagnostic discriminant in surgical pathology. Immunohistochemical profile in epithelial, mesenchymal, hematopoietic neoplasms using paraffin sections and monoclonal antibodies. *Hum. Pathol.*, 16:929–940.

174. Pinkus, G. S., and Said, J. W. (1981): Intracellular hemoglobin-specific marker of erythroid cells in paraffin sections. An immunoperoxidase study of normal, megaloblastic, and dysplastic erythropoiesis, including erythroleukemia and other myeloproliferative disorders. *Am. J. Pathol.*, 102:308–313.

175. Poppema, S., Bhan, A. K., Reinherz, E. L., McCluskey, R. T., and Schlossman, S. F. (1981): Distribution of T cell subsets in human nodes. *J. Exp. Med.*, 153:30–41.

176. Poppema, S., Hollema, H., Visser, L., and Vos, H. (1987): Monoclonal antibodies (MT1, MT2, MB1, MB2, MB3) reactive with leukocyte subsets in paraffin-embedded tissue sections. *Am. J. Pathol.*, 127:418–429.

177. Poulsen, H. S., Ozzello, L., King, W. J., and Greene, G. L. (1985): The use of monoclonal antibodies to estrogen receptors (ER) for immunoperoxidase detection of ER in paraffin sections of human breast cancer tissue. *J. Histochem. Cytochem.*, 33:87–92.

178. Prat, J., Bhan, A. K., Dickersin, G. R., Robboy, S. J., and Scully, R. E. (1982): Hepatoid yolk sac tumor of the ovary (endodermal sinus tumor with hepatoid differentiation). *Cancer*, 50:2344–2368.

179. Primus, F. J., Kuhns, J. K., and Goldenberg, D. M. (1983): Immunological heterogeneity of carcinoembryonic antigen determinants in colonic tumors with monoclonal antibodies. *Cancer Res.*, 43:693–701.

180. Purnell, D. M., Heatfield, B. M., and Trump, B. F. (1984): Immunocytochemical evaluation of human prostatic carcinomas for carcinoembryonic antigen, nonspecific cross-reacting antigen, beta-chorionic gonadotrophin, and prostate-specific antigen. *Cancer Res.*, 44:285–292.

181. Ramaekers, F. C. S., Puts, J. J. G., Moesker, O., Kant, A., Vooijs, G. P., and Jap, P. H. K. (1983): Intermediate filaments in malignant melanomas. Identification and use as marker in surgical pathology. *J. Clin. Invest.*, 71:635–643.

182. Roholl, P. J. M., Kleyne, J., and Van Unnik, J. A. M. (1985): Characterization of tumor cells in malignant fibrous histiocytoma and other soft tissue tumors in comparison with malignant histiocytes. Immunoperoxides study on cryostat sections. *Am. J. Pathol.*, 121:269–274.

183. Rosai, J., and Pinkus, G. S. (1982): Immunohistochemical demonstration of epithelial differentiation in adamantinoma of the tibia. *Am. J. Surg. Pathol.*, 6:427–434.

184. Ruiter, D. J., Dingjan, G. M., Steijen, R. M., Beveren-Hooyer, M. V., De Groaf-Reitsma, C. B., Bergman, W., Van Muijen, G. N. P., and Warnaar, S. O. (1985): Monoclonal antibodies selected to discriminate between malignant melanomas and nevocellular nevi. *J. Invest. Dermatol.*, 85:4–8.

185. Ruiter, D. J., Bhan, A. K., Harrist, T. J., Sober, A. J., and Mihm, M. C., Jr. (1982): Major histocompatibility antigens and mononuclear inflammatory infiltrates in benign nevomelanoctyic proliferation and malignant melanoma. *J. Immunol.*, 129:2808–2815.

186. Said, J. W., Nash, G., Banks-Schlegel, S., Sassoon, A. F., Murakami, S., and Shintaku, I. P. (1983): Keratin human lung tumors. Patterns of localization of different-molecular weight keratin proteins. *Am. J. Pathol.*, 113:27–32.

187. Said, J. W., Nash, G., Sassoon, A. F., Shintaku, I. P., and Banks-Schlegel, S. (1985): Involucrin in lung tumors. A specific marker for squamous differentiation. *Lab. Invest.*, 49:563–568.

188. Said, J. W., Nash, G., Tepper, G., and Banks-Schlegel, S. (1983): Keratin proteins and carcinoembryonic antigen in lung carcinoma: An immunoperoxidase study of over fifty-four cases, with ultrastructural correlations. *Hum. Pathol.*, 14:70–76.

189. Said, J. W., Sassoon, A. F., Shintaku, I. P., and Banks-Schlegel, S. (1984): Involucrin in squamous and basal cell carcinomas of the skin: An immunohistochemical study. *J. Invest. Dermatol.*, 82:449–452.

190. Said, J. W., Vimadalal, S., Nash, G., Shintaku, I. P., Heusser, R. C., Sassoon, A. F., and Lloyd, R. V. (1985): Immunoreactive neuron-specific enolase, bombesin and chromogranin as markers for neuroendocrine lung tumors. *Hum. Pathol.*, 16:236–240.

191. Schlom, J., Wunderlich, D., and Teramoto, Y. A. (1980): Generation of human monoclonal antibodies reactive with human mammary carcinoma cells. *Proc. Natl. Acad. Sci. USA*, 77:6841–6845.

192. Schlom, J. (1986): Basic principles and application of monoclonal antibodies in the management of carcinomas. Richard and Hinda Rosenthal Award Lecture. *Cancer Res.*, 46:3225–3228.

193. Schroder, S., Dockhorn-Dworniczak, B., Kastenidieck, H., Bocker, W., and Franke, W. W. (1986): Intermediate filament expression in thyroid gland carcinomas. *Virchows Arch. (A)*, 409:751–766.

194. Schroeder, S., and Kloppel, G. (1987): Carcinoembryonic antigen and nonspecific cross reacting antigens in thyroid cancer. An immunohistochemical study using polyclonal and monoclonal antibodies. *Am. J. Surg. Pathol.*, 112:100–108.

195. Sheibani, K., Battifora, H., and Burke, J. S. (1986): Antigenic phenotype of malignant mesotheliomas and pulmonary adenocarcinomas. An immunohistologic analysis demonstrating the value of Leu-M1 antigen. *Am. J. Pathol.*, 123:212–219.

196. Sheibani, K., Battifora, H., Burke, J. S., and Rappaport, H. (1986): Leu-M1 antigen in human neoplasm. An immunohistologic study of 400 cases. *Am. J. Surg. Pathol.*, 10:227–236.

197. Sheppard, M. N., Corrin, B., Bennett, M. H., Marangos, P. J., Bloom, S. R., and Polak, J. M. (1984): Immunocytochemical localization of neuron specific enolase in small cell carcinomas and carcinoid tumours of the lung. *Histopathology*, 8:171–181.

198. Shevchuk, M. M., Romas, Ng, P. Y., Ying, N. G., Tannenbaum, M., and Olsson, C. A. (1983): Acid phosphatase localization in prostatic carcinoma. A comparison of monoclonal antibody to heteroantisera. *Cancer*, 52:1642–1646.

199. Shi, S. R., Goodman, M. L., Bhan, A. K., Pilch, B. Z., Chen, L. B., and Sun, T-T. (1984): Immunohistochemical study of nasopharyngeal carcinoma using monoclonal keratin antibodies. *Am. J. Pathol.*, 117:53–63.

200. Shimada, A., Kimura, S., Abe, K., Nagasaki, K., Adachi, I., Yamaguchi, K. Suzuki, M., Nakajima, T., and Miller, L. S. (1985): Immunocytochemical staining of estrogen receptor in paraffin sections of human breast cancer by use of monoclonal antibody comparison with that in frozen sections. *Proc. Natl. Acad. Sci. USA*, 82:4803–4807.

201. Shimada, H., Aoyama, C., Chiba, T., and Newton, W. A. (1985): Prognostic subgroups for undifferentiated neuroblastoma: Immunohistochemical study with anti-S-100 protein antibody. *Hum. Pathol.*, 16:471–476.

202. Shishi, J., Ghaizadeh, M., Oguro, T., Aihara, K., and Araki, T. (1986): Immunohistochemical localization of CA 125 antigen in formalin-fixed paraffin sections of ovarian tumors with the use of pronase. *Am. J. Clin. Pathol.*, 85:595–598.

203. Sibley, R. K., and Dahl, D. (1985): Primary neuroendocrine (Merkel cell?) carcinoma of the skin. II. An immunohistochemical study of 21 cases. *Am. J. Surg. Pathol.*, 9:109–116.

204. Sikora, K., and Wright, R. (1981): Human monoclonal antibodies to lung cancer antigens. *Br. J. Cancer*, 43:696–700.

205. Sobin, L. H., Hjermstad, B. M., Sesterhenn, I. A., and Helwig, E. B. (1986): Prostatic acid phosphatase activity in carcinoid tumor. *Cancer*, 58:136–138.

206. Sobol, R. E., Peters, R. E., Astarita, R. W., Hofeditz, C., Masui, H., Burton, D., Handley, H. H., Glassy, M. C., Fairshter, R., Carlo, D. J., and Royston, I. (1986): A novel monoclonal antibody-defined antigen which distinguishes human non-small cell lung carcinomas. *Cancer Res.*, 46:4746–4750.

207. Spagnolo, D. V., Michie, S. A., Crabtree, G. S., Warnke, R. A., and Rouse, R. V. (1985): Monoclonal anti-keratin (AEI) reactivity in routinely processed tissue from 166 neoplasms. *Am. J. Clin. Pathol.*, 84:697–704.

208. Springall, D. R., Lackie, P., Levene, M. N., Marangos, P. J., and Polak, J. M. (1984): Immunostaining of neuron-specific enolase is a valuable aid to the cytological diagnosis of neuroendocrine tumours of the lung. *J. Pathol.*, 143:259–265.

209. Stanton, C., Perentes, E., Collins, V. P., and Rubinstein, L. J. (1987): GFA protein reactivity in nerve sheath tumors: A polyvalent and monoclonal antibody study. *J. Neuropathol. Exp. Neurol.*, 46:634–643.

210. Statiel, R. A., Speak, J. A., and Bernal, S. D. (1985): Murine monoclonal antibody LAM2 defines cell membrane determinant with preferential expression on human lung small-cell carcinoma and squamous cell carcinoma. *Int. J. Cancer*, 35:11–17.

211. Statiel, R. A., Mabry, M., Skanu, A. T., Speak, J., and Bernal, S. D. (1985): Detection of bone marrow metastatis in small cell lung cancer by monoclonal antibody. *J. Clin. Oncol.*, 3:455–461.

212. Stefansson, K., Wollmann, R., and Jerkovic, M. (1982): S-100 protein in soft-tissue tumors derived from Schwann cells and melanocytes. *Am. J. Pathol.*, 106:261–268.

213. Stein, B. S., Petersen, R. O., Vangore, S., and Kendall, A. R. (1982): Immunoperoxidase localization of prostate-specific antigen. *Am. J. Surg. Pathol.*, 6:553–557.

214. Strauchen, J. A., and Dimitriu-Bona, A. (1986): Malignant fibrous histiocytoma. Expression of monocytes/macrophage differentiation antigens detected with monoclonal antibodies. *Am. J. Pathol.*, 124:303–309.

215. Sternberger, L. A. (1979): *Immunocytochemistry*, 2nd Ed. John Wiley and Sons, New York.

216. Sun, N. C., Edgington, T. D., Carpentier, C. L., McAfee, W., Terry, R., and Bateman, J. (1983): Immunohistochemical localization of carcinoembryonic antigen (CEA), CEA-S and nonspecific cross-reacting antigen (NCA) in carcinomas of lung. *Cancer*, 52:1632–1641.

217. Sun, T-T., Eichner, R., Nelson, W. G., Tseng, S. C. G., Weiss, R. A., Jarvinen, M., and Woodcock-Mitchell, J. (1983): Keratin classes: Molecular markers for different types of epithelial differentiation. *J. Invest. Dermatol.*, 81:190s–115s.

218. Swanson, P. E., Manivel, J. C., Wick, M. R. (1987): Immunoreactivity for Leu-7 in neurofibrosarcoma and other spindle cell sarcomas of soft tissue. *Am. J. Pathol.*, 126:546–560.

219. Szpak, C. A., Johnston, W. W., Roggli, V., Kolbeck, J., Lottich, S. C., Vollmer, R., Thor, A., and Schlom, J. (1986): The diagnostic distinction between malignant mesothelioma of the pleura and adenocarcinomas of the lung as defined by a monoclonal antibody (B72.3). *Am. J. Pathol.*, 122:252–260.

220. Tascos, N. A., Parr, J., and Gonata, N. K. (1982): Immunocytochemical study of the glial fibrillary acidic protein in human neoplasms of the central nervous system. *Hum. Pathol.*, 13:454–458.
221. Taylor, C. R. (1986): *Immunomicroscopy: A Diagnostic Tool for the Surgical Pathologist.* W.B. Saunders, Philadelphia.
222. Taylor, C. R., and Kledzik, G. (1981): Immunohistologic techniques in surgical pathology, a spectrum of "new" special stains. *Hum. Pathol.*, 12:590–596.
223. Thomas, P., and Battifora, H. (1987): Keratin versus epithelial membrane antigen in tumor diagnosis. An immunohistochemical comparison of five monoclonal antibodies. *Hum. Pathol.*, 18:728–734.
224. Thomas, P., Battifora, H., Manderino, G. L., and Patrick, J. (1987): A monoclonal antibody against neuron-specific enolase. Immunohistochemical comparison with a polyclonal antiserum. *Am. J. Clin. Pathol.*, 88:146–152.
225. Thomas, P., Said, J. W., Nash, G., and Banks-Schlegel, S. (1982): Profiles of keratin proteins in basal and squamous cell carcinomas of the skin. An immunohistochemical study. *Lab. Invest.*, 50:36–41.
226. Thompson, J. J., Herlyn, M. F., Elder, D. E., Clark, W. H., Steplewski, Z., and Koprowski, H. (1982): Use of monoclonal antibodies in detection of melanoma-associated antigens in intact human tumors. *Am. J. Pathol.*, 107:357–361.
227. Thor, A., Ohuchi, N., Szpak, C. A., Johnston, W. W., and Schlom, J. (1986). The distribution of oncofetal antigen TAG-72 defined by monoclonal antibody B72.3. *Cancer Res.*, 46:3118–3124.
228. Thor, A., Muraro, R., Gorstein, F., Ohuchi, N., Viglione, M., Szpak, C. A., Johnston, W.W., and Schlom, J. (1987): Adjunct to the diagnostic distinction between adenocarcinomas of the ovary and the colon utilizing a monoclonal antibody (COL-4) with restricted carcinoembryonic antigen reactivity. *Cancer Res.*, 47:505–512.
229. Thor, A., Ohuchi, N., Horand-Hand, P., Callahan, R., Weeks, M. P., Theillet, C., Tidereau, R., Escot, C., Page, D. L., Vilas, V., and Schlom, J. (1986): ras gene alterations and enhanced levels of ras gene alterations and enhanced levels of ras p21 expression in a spectrum of benign and malignant human mammary tissues. *Lab. Invest.*, 55:603–615.
230. Triche, T. J., Askin, F. B. (1983): Neuroblastoma and the differential diagnosis of small, round, blue-cell tumors. *Hum. Pathol.*, 15:569–595.
231. Trojanowski, J. Q., Lee, V., Pillsbury, N., and Lee, S. (1982): Neuronal origin of human esthesioneuroblastoma demonstrated with anti-neurofilament monoclonal antibodies. *N. Engl. J. Med.*, 307:159–161.
232. Trojanowski, J. Q., Lee, V., and Schlaepfer, W. W. (1984): An immunohistochemical study of human central and peripheral nervous system tumors, using monoclonal antibodies against neurofilaments and glial filaments. *Hum. Pathol.*, 15:248–257.
233. Tsokos, M., Linnoila, R. I., Chandra, R. S., and Triche, T. J. (1984): Neuron-specific enolase in the diagnosis of neuroblastoma and other small, round-cell tumors in children. *Hum. Pathol.*, 15:575–584.
234. Uchida, T., Shikata, T., and Iino, S. (1984): Immunohistochemical localization of placental and intestinal alkaline phosphatases. In: *Advances in Immunohistochemistry*, edited by R. A. DeLellis, pp. 185–199. Masson Publishing, Inc., New York.
235. Upton, M. P., Hirohashi, A., Tome, Y., Miyazawa, N., Suemasku, K., and Shimosato, Y. (1986): Expression of vimentin in surgically resected adenocarcinomas and large cell carcinomas of lung. *Am. J. Surg. Pathol.*, 10:560–567.
236. Vanstapel, M. J., Gatter, K. C., de Wolfe-Peeters, C., Mason, D. Y., and Desmet, V. D. (1986): New sites of S-100 immunoreactivity directed with monoclonal antibodies. *Am. J. Clin. Pathol.*, 85:160–168.
237. Vinores, S. A., Bonnin, J. M., Rubinstein, L. J., Marangos, P. J. (1984): Immunohistochemical demonstration of neuron-specific enolase in neoplasms of the CNS and other tissues. *Arch. Pathol. Lab. Med.*, 108:536–540.
238. Viola, M. V., Fromowitz, F., Oravez, S., Deb. S., Finkel, G., Lundy, J., Hand, P., Thor, A., and Schlom, J. (1986): Expression of ras oncogene p21 in prostate cancer. *N. Engl. J. Med.*, 314:133–137.
239. Viola, M. V., Fromowitz, F., Oravez, S., Deb, S., and Schlom, J. (1985): ras oncogene p21 expression is increased in premalignant lesions and high grade bladder carcinoma. *J. Exp. Med.*, 161:1213–1218.
240. Wagener, C., Petzold, P., and Kohler, W., Totovic, V. (1984): Binding of five monoclonal anti-CEA antibodies with different epitope specificities to various carcinoma tissues. *Int. J. Cancer*, 33:469–475.
241. Walker, R. A. (1984): Immunohistochemistry of biological marker of breast carcinoma. In: *Advances in Immunohistochemistry*, edited by R. A. DeLellis, pp. 223–242. Masson Publishing, USA Inc., New York.
242. Wang, E., Cairncross, J. G., and Liem, R. K. H. (1984): Identification of glial filament protein and vimentin in the same intermediate filament system in human glioma cells. *Proc. Natl. Acad. Sci. USA*, 81:2102–2106.
243. Warhol, M. J., Rice, R. H., Pinkus, G. S., and Robboy, S. J (1984): Evaluation of squamous epithelium in adenoacanthoma and adenosquamous carcinoma of the endometrium: Immunoperoxidase analysis of involucrin and keratin localization. *Int. J. Gynecol. Pathol.*, 3:82–91.
244. Warnke, R. A., Gatter, K. C., Falini, B., Hildreth, P., Woolston, R-E., Pulford, K., Cordell, J. L., Cohen, B., De Wolf-Peeters, C., and Mason, D. Y. (1983): Diagnosis of human lymphoma with monoclonal anti-leukocyte antibodies. *N. Engl. J. Med.*, 309:1275–1281.

245. Warren, W. H., Memoli, V. A., Kittle, C. F., Jensik, R. J., Faber, L. P., and Gould, V. E. (1984): The biologic implication of bronchial tumors. *J. Thorac. Cardiovasc. Surg.*, 87:274–282.

246. Warren, W. H., Memoli, V. A., and Gould, V. E. (1984): Immunohistochemical and ultra-structural analysis of bronchopulmonary neuroendocrine neoplasms. I. Carcinoids. *Ultrastruct. Pathol.*, 6:15–28.

247. Weiss, S. W., Langloss, J. M., and Enzinger, F. M. (1983): Value of S-100 protein in the diagnosis of soft tissue tumors with particular reference to benign and malignant Schwann cell tumors. *Lab. Invest.*, 49: 299–308.

248. West, K. P., Warford, A., Fray, L., Allen, M., Campbell, A. C., and Lauder, I. (1986): The demonstration of B-cell, T-cell and myeloid antigens in paraffin sections. *J. Pathol.*, 150:89–101.

249. Wick, M. R., Cherwitz, D. L., McGlennen, R. C., and Dehner, L. P. (1986): Adrenocortical carcinoma: An immunohistochemical comparison with renal cell carcinoma. *Am. J. Pathol.*, 122:343–352.

250. Wick, M. R., and Manivel, J. C. (1987): Epithelioid sarcoma and epithelioid hemangioendothelioma: An immunohistochemical and lectin-histochemical comparison. *Virchows Arch. (A)*, 410:309–316.

251. Wick, M. R., Scheithauer, B. W., and Kovacs, K. (1983): Neuron-specific enolase in neuroendocrine tumors of the thymus, bronchus, and skin. *Am. J. Clin. Pathol.*, 79:703–707.

252. Wick, M. R., Swanson, P. E., Scheihauer, B. W., and Manivel, J. C. (1987): Malignant peripheral nerve sheath tumor. An immunohistochemical study of 62 cases. *Am. J. Clin. Pathol.*, 87:425–433.

253. Wilson, B. S., and Lloyd, R. V. (1984): Detection of chromogranin in neuroendocrine cells with a monoclonal antibody. *Am. J. Pathol.*, 115:458–468.

254. Wolfe, H. J., and Palmer, P. E. (1981): Alpha-1-antrypsin: Its immunohistochemical localization and significance in diagnostic pathology. In: *Diagnostic Immunohistochemistry*, edited by R. A. DeLellis, pp. 227–238. Masson Publishing USA Inc., New York.

255. Wood, G. S., Beckstead, J. H., Turner, R. R., Hendrickson, M. R., Kempson, R. L., Warnke, R. A. (1986): Malignant fibrous histiocytoma tumor cells resemble fibroblasts. *Am. J. Surg. Pathol.*, 10:323–335.

256. Wood, G. S., Warner, N. L., and Warnke, R. A. (1983): Anti-Leu-3/T4 antibodies react with cells of monocytes/macrophages and Langerhans lineage. *J. Immunol.*, 131–212.

257. Woods, J. C., Spriggs, A. I., Harris, H., and McGee, J. O'D. (1982): A new marker for human cancer cells. 3. Immunocytochemical detection of malignant cells in serous fluids with the Cal antibody. *Lancet*, 2:512–514.

258. Wright, G. L., Beckett, M., Starling, J. J., Schellhammer, P. F., Sieg, S. M., Ladaga, L. E., and Poleski, S. (1983): Immunohistochemical localization of prostate carcinoma-associated antigens. *Cancer Res.*, 43: 5509–5516.

Diagnostic Immunopathology,
edited by R.B. Colvin,
A.K. Bhan, and R.T. McCluskey.
Raven Press, New York © 1988.

9 / Cytoskeletal Proteins and Neuronal Tumors

John Q. Trojanowski

*Division of Neuropathology, Department of Pathology and Laboratory Medicine,
The University of Pennsylvania School of Medicine,
Philadelphia, Pennsylvania 19104*

Molecules that program normal neurons and glial cell interactions during ontogeny and in maturity are beginning to be identified, as are the mechanisms whereby such complex interactions are governed. This knowledge is a keystone to a full understanding of the complexity of normal nervous system development, architecture, and function. Some of the insights have diagnostic applications.

Progress in elucidating the highly orchestrated molecular signals in the nervous system has been fostered by rapid technical advances in immunology and neurobiology. A large array of macromolecules now are known to be expressed by restricted populations of nervous system cell types (24,69,86), and some of these peptides and polypeptides may play a role in intercellular communication, in the differentiation of functionally distinct cell types, or in mediating the specialized activities assigned to specific subclasses of mature nervous system cells. Table 1 shows representative examples of some of the more well-characterized molecules that are selectively expressed by different classes of cells found in the mature central nervous system (CNS). It is possible now to exploit such molecules for the recognition of subclasses of neurons and to characterize different stages in their maturation. This is especially important, as it becomes increasingly apparent that morphologic criteria for the enumeration of functionally distinct classes of neurons are severely limited.

Neoplasia largely results from various perturbations of the genome, such as chromosomal translocations, amplifications, deletions, point mutations and retroviruses (5,7,43,67). The information encoded by a normal or aberrant gene in a tumor cell is transcribed and translated into peptides or macromolecules that may foster or hinder the process of oncogenesis. Oncogenes are a group of normal cellular genes, the expression of which is regulated in an aberrant manner in tumors because of several different mechanisms (43).

The chromosomal abnormalities associated with different kinds of nervous system tumors are being characterized and catalogued (5), and models are being developed that provide a molecular understanding of nervous system malignancies, such as the infiltration of normal brain by tumor cells (5,41,42). A full understanding of the cell biology of oncogene products and neuron and glial specific molecules should help elucidate the multistep process of oncogenesis and contribute to the diagnosis of human neuronal and glial

TABLE 1. *Selected marker molecules of central nervous system cells*

Cell type	Specific marker or antigen
Neurons	Chromogranins
	Microtubule-associated proteins
	Neurofilament proteins
	Neuron-specific enolase
	Synaptophysin
	Neurotransmitters and peptide hormones
Glia	
Astrocytes	Glial filament protein
	Non-neuronal enolase
	Carbonic anhydrase II
Oligodendroglia	Myelin basic protein and related proteins
	Carbonic anhydrase II
	Galactocerebroside
Epithelial cells	Keratin filament proteins
Lymphoid cells	Vimentin filament protein
	B and T cell markers
Vascular cells	Desmin and vimentin filament proteins
	Factor VIII

Selected examples of some of the more well-characterized cell type specific proteins of the mature, mammalian nervous system. Intermediate filament (IF) proteins are discussed later in this chapter.

tumors (5,8,37,41,42). Efforts to elucidate these events will also have an impact on the development of strategies to diagnose and treat tumors of the nervous system.

This chapter reviews the use of monoclonal antibodies to analyze and treat neuronal tumors of the CNS and peripheral (PNS) nervous system. Studies of human neuronal tumors using monoclonal antibodies to neuron specific cytoskeletal proteins, especially intermediate filament (IF) proteins are worth consideration here for two reasons: (a) neuronal tumors comprise one of the most common groups of childhood neoplasms, yet they remain poorly understood and are difficult to treat (10,18,74–77); and (b) monoclonal antibodies to IF proteins are extremely useful in addressing questions such as tumor differentiation, histogenesis, classification, and tumor progression (1,3,4,6,11,14–22,52–54, 58–60,62,68,90–92,94–98,104,105). Other neuron-specific proteins, including components of the neuronal cytoskeleton, have a similar potential once the precise molecular identity and distribution of such polypeptides are more completely established. For example, microtubule associated proteins (MAPs), chromogranins, and synaptophysin appear to be restricted in their expression to neurons and neuroendocrine cells, and antibodies to these proteins appear to be useful for the diagnosis of tumors derived from such cell types (2,30,35,57,81,101,106) (see Chapter 12).

The cell-type-specific IF macromolecules emphasized in this chapter and the triplet of neurofilament (NF) polypeptides that comprise the IFs of normal neurons are cytoplasmic proteins. As constitutively expressed gene products restricted to neurons (79,84), they appear to be potentially useful for improving the diagnosis and classification of putative neuronal tumors. For example, NF proteins (or posttranslationally modified variants or isoforms thereof) appear to be expressed by all or nearly all classes of human CNS and PNS neurons. If the same applies to tumors derived from neurons, NF proteins could be exploited as markers for tumors derived from neurons in diagnostic studies. Since other IF proteins have been shown to be expressed by some tumors that also express NF proteins, it is important at this point to survey briefly other IF polypeptides before considering NF proteins of normal and neoplastic neurons.

INTERMEDIATE FILAMENTS

Relationships of Intermediate Filaments

Intermediate filaments are a family of five different classes of biochemically related cytoskeletal fibrous elements (Chapter 8) (89). The protein subunits comprising each class of IFs are listed in Table 2. By electron microscopy, IFs are approximately 10 nm in diameter filamentous structures. The diameter of an IF is larger than that of an actin filament (4 to 6 nm in diameter), but smaller than that of a microtubule (22 to 24 nm in diameter). Actin filaments and microtubules are the two other major, fibrous cytoskeletal components of cells.

IFs form part of the cytoskeleton of nearly all nucleated mammalian cells, but some exceptions to this rule are well known. For example, mature oligodendrocytes, the myelin-forming glial cells of the CNS, are one of the few cell types that lack IFs by ultrastructural criteria. In contrast, the PNS counterparts of oligodendrocytes, myelin-forming Schwann cells, do contain IFs (1,17,36). The precise function of IFs in cells that contain them is unknown, and it is unclear why different cell types require IFs that differ biochemically.

The five different classes of hetero- and homopolymeric IFs are distinguished by biochemical and immunochemical criteria. By these criteria, about 26 different IF subunits are now recognized, and each one is presumably encoded by a separate gene. Recent studies suggest, however, that the nuclear lamins also should be included in this family of proteins (26,61). By transmission electron microscopy, IFs are nearly indistinguishable, except that NFs have distinctive, projecting sidearms (34). Each class of IFs, excluding vimentin, is

TABLE 2. *Polypeptide subunits of mammalian intermediate filaments[a]*

IF Class	Polypeptide composition	Normal distribution
Neurofilaments	70kd, 170kd, and 195kd protein subunits	CNS and PNS neurons, axons and dendrites
Glial filaments	51kd protein	Astroglia, some extra-CNS cells
Vimentin filaments	57kd protein	Mesenchymal cells, may be co-expressed with all other IF classes
Desmin filaments	53kd protein	Smooth, striated and cardiac muscle
Keratin filaments	A family of 20 different polypeptides ranging from 40kd to 68kd	Keratinizing and nonkeratinizing epithelial cells

[a]Proteins encoded by the approximately 26 different IF genes. The apparent molecular weight (M_r) in kilodaltons (kd) of these proteins, and the distribution of these proteins in differentiated or mature cell types are also listed here. As discussed in the text, estimates of M_r by SDS PAGE may not be accurate for all IF proteins, especially those that are heavily phosphorylated as is the case with the two high M_r NF proteins. Nuclear lamins are not included in this table although they may well comprise a sixth class of IF proteins based on their biochemical and immunochemical properties[61].

restricted to limited cell types in the mature organism; that is, IFs can be regarded as cell-type-specific gene products (31,32,89).

Although NF proteins and glial filament (GF) protein or glial fibrillary acidic protein (GFAP) are the major IF proteins of neurons and glia, respectively, all five classes of IFs can be found in other cell types in the CNS (21–24,29,32,36,78–80,83,84,89). The two other cell-type-specific IF classes present in the nervous system are restricted to vascular smooth muscle (desmin) or epithelial cells (keratins), for example, choroid plexus (32,58, 89). Vimentin filament (VF) protein is present in many cell types, including fibroblasts, neurons, and astrocytes (31,32,89). It is the only IF protein that clearly is not cell type specific. In fact, it can coexist with each of the other four classes of IFs in cultured cells and in some normal mature cell types *in situ*. For example, both VF and GF are expressed by fibrous astrocytes (21), and both NF and VF coexist in some neurons (89). Further, the expression of different IF genes may be turned on and off in a sequential programmatic manner that correlates with the progressive differentiation of a cell. This has been demonstrated, for example, in neuroblasts of the developing nervous system; they first express VF and later, after becoming committed neurons, express only NF (88).

In the past, work on the immunochemistry and distribution of IF proteins was limited by the extensive homologies among the different IF polypeptides (89). Indeed, monoclonal antibodies that recognize more than one or even all five classes of IFs have been reported by a number of laboratories (49,50,70). For this reason, antisera are of limited utility for probing IF proteins. However, monoclonal antibodies specific for each of the five classes of IFs have been developed (29,31,32,45–50,68,83,84,86,87,104,105).

The biochemical properties of IF proteins and their distribution in different tissues and cell types have been extensively studied, but only limited information is available on the IF protein isoforms that result from the posttranslational modification of these proteins. Further, only a few IF genes have been cloned, including some expressed in neurons and astrocytes (55,56,64,72). In fact, there still is a considerable paucity of information concerning a number of important aspects of the cell biology of IF proteins. Intermediate filament proteins differ across species and can be modified after translation (e.g., partial proteolysis, phosphorylation) under normal circumstances and as a result of disease (12,46, 47,65,66,79,84,87,89). Further, the recently described homologies between lamins, the nuclear envelope proteins, and IF proteins (26,61) raises intriguing questions about the exact nature of the IF family of polypeptides.

Neurofilament Proteins and Neurofilament Protein Isoforms

The NFs are heteropolymers distinct from all other IFs because they are composed of three different subunits with apparent molecular weights (M_r) (in cytoskeletal extracts of human spinal cord) of about 70 kilodalton (kd), 170 kd, and 195 kd (48,78,79,84,87). Because of small variations in the M_r of these proteins among mammals, the NF subunits of mammals are often referred to as the low (NF-L), middle (NF-M), and high (NF-H) M_r NF subunits. The polypeptides which comprise the other IFs (see Table 2) have an M_r in the 40 to 70 kd range (89). The antigenic determinants of each of these NF subunits may be either unique or shared (48), and it is recognized that each NF protein is a separate gene product. In fact, the NF-L and NF-M genes have been cloned (56,64,72).

Prior to the use of NF subunit specific monoclonal antibodies, the co-expression of each NF subunit in populations of CNS (e.g., cerebellar Purkinje neurons) and PNS (e.g., neurons of dorsal root ganglia) neurons was fraught with controversy. Using NF subunit specific monoclonal antibodies, it subsequently was shown that Purkinje neurons of the cerebellum express all three NF subunits (100). All three NF subunits can be detected in other populations of CNS and PNS neurons as well (80,101,103). This suggests that NF-L, NF-M, and NF-H genes are expressed constitutively by nearly all neurons of the CNS and PNS, especially those with long, projecting axons. A well-documented and notable exception is the bipolar neuron of olfactory epithelium, which sends its axons into the olfactory bulb. These neurons contain IFs that are comprised solely of VF proteins even in their axons (82). Olfactory sensory neurons are unique among neurons for another reason; they are the only neurons of mature mammals that die and are replenished throughout the life span of the organism. With the exception of an unconfirmed report that avian NF-L is present in chicken erythrocytes (33), NF proteins have not been detected so far in normal non-neuronal mammalian cells in a convincing manner. Further, NF gene expression appears to be coupled with other cellular events that correlate with the differentiation of blast cells into committed neurons (13,88).

It is important to emphasize that antibodies are used most commonly to detect NF subunits in individual neurons and that the failure to detect individual NF subunits in certain populations of neurons (e.g., Purkinje cells) or portions (e.g., axons, dendrites, perikarya) of highly asymmetrical neurons may reflect technical limitations in the use of antibodies as molecular probes. For example, tissue preparative methods significantly affect the immunoreactivity of NF antigens. Fixation-dependent effects on NF subunit immunoreactivity in different neuronal domains can alter the apparent distribution of NF subunits (91,93,97–103). Further, biochemical and immunological microheterogeneity of NF subunits in different portions of a neuron may also explain the apparent absence of NF proteins in certain locations (11,29,46,47,79,80,86,87). Whether or not this is due to posttranslational modifications, such as phosphorylation (12,13,46,47,66,80,86,87), partial proteolysis (65) or other factors, remains to be determined.

Based on recent studies of NF protein immunoreactivity and NF protein phosphorylation states, it is highly likely that newly synthesized forms of NF subunits (NF mRNA translation products that have not yet undergone posttranslational modifications) are not detected readily by most antibodies raised to NF proteins extracted from white matter (brain tissue enriched in axonal or posttranslationally modified NFs). This was demonstrated most effectively by Lee et al. who raised monoclonal antibodies specific for poorly phosphorylated or non-phosphorylated NF-H, only after using enzymatically de-phosphorylated NF proteins as immunogens (46,47). These points should be kept in mind when studies of CNS and PNS neoplasms are conducted, using monoclonal antibodies as molecular probes.

Interpretation of Studies of Nervous System Tumors
Probed with Monoclonal Antibodies to IF Proteins

Before considering the use of monoclonal antibodies to NF proteins for studies of neuronal tumors, it is worth examining the assumptions upon which studies of tumors conducted with monoclonal antibodies to different IF proteins, including NF proteins, are based. Antibodies to IF proteins were first introduced into pathology for the diagnostic evaluation of human tumors about 10 years ago by Deck and Duffy and their collaborators, who used antiserum raised to GFAP by Eng and co-workers (15,19–23). These and other pioneering studies led to the development of important hypotheses concerning the expression of these antigens in normal and neoplastic cells. These hypotheses are that: (a) IFs are composed of immunochemically distinct protein subunits; (b) IF genes (except VF) are expressed in a cell-type-specific manner; and (c) neoplastic cells, with some exceptions, express the same IF genes as their presumed progenitor cells.

These ground rules for the expression of IF genes are the basis for the use of these markers in diagnostic pathology. Thus far, with some qualifications, these hypotheses appear to be substantiated. Examples of primary and metastatic brain tumors that were probed with monoclonal antibody to GF protein are shown in Figure 1. Intracranial tumors known to contain cells that express NF and/or GF proteins are listed in Table 3, and extra-CNS tumors known to express either or both of these antigens are listed in Table 4.

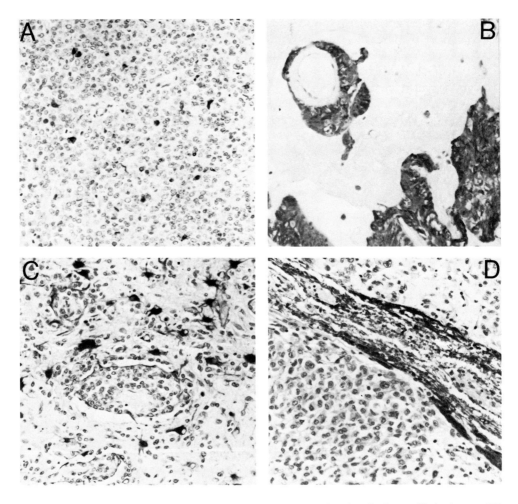

FIG. 1. Primary and metastatic CNS tumors probed with a monoclonal antibody specific for human GF protein (2.2B10) by immunohistochemistry. An oligodendroglioma contains scattered GF positive cells (**A**). The myxopapillary ependymoma in **B** exhibits GF immunoreactivity in the majority of cells. In **C**, a primary CNS lymphoma infiltrates brain, especially around blood vessels (center of photomicrograph). The neoplastic lymphoid cells are devoid of GFAP but numerous reactive astrocytes are present within the area infiltrated by the tumor cells. The metastatic carcinoma cells in E are GFAP negative, but a tongue of GFAP positive reactive astrocytes extends into the metastasis.

TABLE 3. *Intrancranial tumors with NF and/or GF protein positivity*

Tumor	NF Positive	GF Positive
Astroblastoma	−	+
Astrocytoma (grades I-IV)	−	+
Cerebral neuroblastoma*	+	+
Choroid plexus papilloma	−	+
Ependymoma	−	+
Ganglioglioma	+	+
Gemistocytic astrocytoma	−	+
Hemangioblastoma	−	+
Medulloblastoma*	+	+
Mixed glioma	−	+
Oligodendrcglioma	−	+
Pineal parenchymal tumor*	+	+
Pituitary adenoma	−	+
Retinoblastoma*	−	+
Subependymal giant cell astrocytoma	−	+
Subependymoma	−	+

*Common primary intra- and extracranial tumors that express either or both NF and GF proteins are listed in Table 3 and 4, respectively. These tables do not include information on the NF subunit(s) expressed by each of the tumors listed here since this important information is not available for most of them. Tumors identified with an asterisk in Table 3 and 4 are also referred to as primitive neuro-ectodermal neoplasms (PNETs)[74,75]. The term pineal parenchymal tumor includes only pineocytomas and pineoblastomas. It does not include germ cell tumors (formerly termed "pinealomas"); a much more common group of pineal tumors.

TABLE 4. *Extracranial tumors with NF and/or GF positivity*

Tumor	NF Positive	GF Positive
Carcinoid#	+	−
Esthesioneuroblastoma*	+	−
Ganglioneuroblastoma	+	−
Ganglioneuroma	+	−
"Merkel cell" tumor of skin#	+	−
Neuroblastoma*	+	−
Oat cell carcinoma#	+	−
Paraganglioma	+	−
Pheochromocytoma	+	−
Pleomorphic adenoma	−	+
Teratoma	+	+

The # symbol in Table 4 identifies tumors that co-express NF and keratin proteins in the same cell; these tumors presumably arise from neuroendocrine cells of the diffuse neuroendocrine system. Teratomas also are capable of expressing multiple IF proteins, but teratomas are known to be composed of cells derived from different germ layers. The asterisks indicate PNETs (see footnote Table 3).

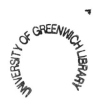

Soon after the introduction of anti-GFAP antibodies for tumor diagnosis in neuropathology, antibodies to desmin and keratin proteins were used for diagnostic studies of other classes of tumors (1,3,6,15,18,39,53,54,58–60,62,68,104,107,109). Anti-NF protein antibodies were the last to be introduced into pathology for the diagnosis of neuron-derived tumors (9,15,39,40,52,53,62,68,90–92,95–98,108). Examples of CNS, PNS, and metastatic brain tumors that were examined with monoclonal antibodies specific for human NF and GF proteins are shown in Figures 2 and 3. Further, it is evident that IF proteins are implicated in the pathogenesis of certain non-neoplastic conditions (79,86). Thus antibodies specific for different IF polypeptides are being used successfully not only for the assessment of neoplastic lesions, but also to probe numerous different non-neoplastic conditions.

The interpretation of immunohistochemical studies based on the use of anti-IF specific antibodies is not always straightforward. For example, metastatic tumors are capable of including residual brain deep within the mass of the metastasis, and such brain cells may be positive when probed with anti-NF and anti-GF monoclonal antibodies (see Figs. 1 and 2). Lack of appreciation of this aspect of the behavior of metastases may lead to erroneous conclusions regarding the nature of a tumor. Obviously, primary brain tumors may behave in a similar manner when they insidiously infiltrate adjacent brain. Since monoclonal antibodies to IF proteins do not discriminate between normal and neoplastic cells, cytological or other criteria still must be applied to determine whether or not the labeled cells indeed are neoplastic. The mere presence of a neuron in a tumor, as identified with probes to NF proteins, does not mean the cell is a neoplastic neuron. However, it is possible that the abnormal appearance or composition of the IF proteins of neoplastic cells may aid in the differentiation of reactive from neoplastic cells. For example, aggregates of immunoreactive NF proteins that correspond to abnormal whorls of IFs have thus far only been seen in diseased and not in normal neurons (15,44,51,52,62,92,95,97,98).

The detection of IF proteins in cells within a tumor is a significant step forward in the evaluation of the cell types comprising different tumors, because this approach introduces molecular criteria into the diagnostic evaluation of human neoplasms, which may be more objective than morphological criteria alone. There is a need, however, for a more thorough understanding of IF protein biology if diagnostic studies of human tumors with monoclonal antibodies to IF proteins (or any other cell-type-specific antigen) are to be properly interpreted. For example, not all tumors that regularly express GFAP are astrocytomas. Ependymomas, choroid plexus papillomas, medulloblastomas, and oligodendrogliomas all have been shown to contain GFAP positive cells to a variable extent, but each of these tumors has a morphology, epidemiology, and clinical outcome that distinguishes them from astrocytomas (10,77). If these latter tumors do not represent different manifestations of a transformed astrocyte, how does one explain the high incidence of GFAP positive cells within some of them? Do the GFAP positive cells represent tumor cells modified by their environment to express this protein as appears to occur under different tissue culture conditions (38,71)? Does this represent a form of metaplasia or aberrant differentiation in a tumor (107,108)? In many instances, the GF positive cells in non-astrocytic brain tumors such as ependymomas or oligodendrogliomas appear neoplastic rather than entrapped, reactive astrocytes; however, little is known at present concerning the response of neurons and astrocytes, as well as their respective IF proteins, to an infiltrating neoplasm.

Similar interpretive problems arise when monoclonal antibodies to IF proteins are used to evaluate PNS tumors. For example, NF antigens have been detected in small cell tumors of skin, pheochromocytomas and carcinoids (15,51–54,60,62,68,96–98). Small cell tumors of skin are termed Merkel cell tumors, because they are believed to arise from

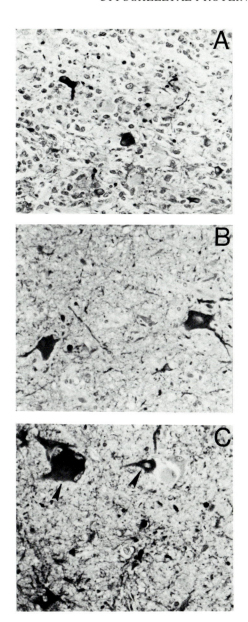

FIG. 2. A CNS lymphoma (**A**) and a ganglioglioma (**B** and **C**) were probed with monoclonal antibodies specific for human GFAP (2.2B10) or for phosphorylated isoforms of human NF-H (TA51) by immunohistochemistry. Lymphoid cells of the CNS lymphoma are NF negative, but NF positive degenerating neurons and axons are trapped within the area infiltrated by the lymphoma. The tumor in **B** and **C** is a ganglioglioma; within the tumor, NF immunoreactivity is seen in a number of cells (**B**) with a bizzare morphology. In an adjacent section (**C**) GFAP positive cells assume morphological profiles similar to reactive or neoplastic astrocytes (*left arrowhead*) and neurons (*right arrowhead*). Double immunofluorescence staining of this tumor failed to demonstrate the co-localization of NF and GF immunoreactivity in the same cells.

normal Merkel cells in the skin. However, the morphological evidence for this is not supported by studies of the IF proteins of Merkel cells and small cell tumors of the skin, since the IF proteins of normal Merkel cells belong to the keratin family. Thus, the histogenesis of so-called Merkel cell tumors remains unresolved, and it is further complicated by the observation that Merkel cell tumors may express both NF and keratin proteins. Studies of pheochromocytomas with anti-IF monoclonal antibodies have resulted in a different outcome. Normal human adrenal chromaffin cells and pheochromocytomas express NF proteins and no other cell-type-specific IF proteins. This suggests a histogenetic relationship between adrenal chromaffin cells and pheochromocytomas.

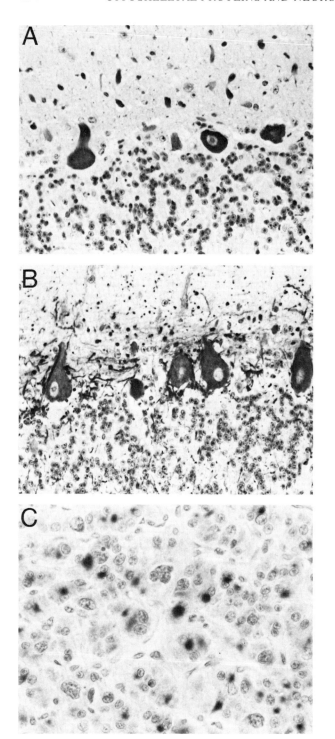

FIG. 3. Sections of autopsy-derived normal human cerebellum (**A** and **B**), and a biopsy specimen of a lung carcinoid were probed with a monoclonal antibody (DP1) specific for poorly phosphorylated isoforms of human NF-M and NF-H (**C**). The section in **A** shows the limited distribution of DP1 staining (i.e., principally confined to the perikarya of Purkinje neurons) in sections treated with buffer that did not contain E. coli alkaline phosphatase prior to immunohistochemistry. In contrast, when an adjacent section was enzymatically dephosphorylated with alkaline phosphatase prior to immunohistochemistry, DP1 is seen to stain many process (i.e., basket cell axon collaterals in the vicinity of the Purkinje cells) that failed to stain with this monoclonal antibody in **A**. The DP1 immunoreactivity in the carcinoid tumor (**C**) is aggregated in ball-like profiles near the nucleus, and enzymatic dephosphorylation did not alter this pattern of staining (from Christen et al., ref. 15, with permission).

Recent studies indicate that bronchial carcinoids, in addition to other putative neuroendocrine tumors, express both NF and keratin polypeptides, although no normal mature cells contain both of these IF proteins. This may be evidence against the hypothesis that tumor cells express the same IF proteins as their progenitor cells. Alternatively, perhaps these tumors arise from stem cells that normally express both of these classes of IF polypeptides. This is plausible, since keratins are the first IF proteins to appear during ontogeny (89). A similar explanation has been offered to explain the appearance of gamma enolase in tumors that arise from tissues that express this antigen in development, but not in maturity (85). However, from careful and detailed work such as that recently published by Achstatter et al. (1), which provided strong evidence for the co-expression of GF and keratin proteins in normal and neoplastic parotid gland cells, it is evident that the simultaneous expression of two different classes of putatively cell-type-specific IF proteins may not be as novel or uncommon as currently assumed.

The foregoing discussion of IF protein expression in CNS and PNS tumors suggests advantages and limitations to the use of monoclonal antibodies to IF proteins for the diagnostic and prognostic study of these tumors.

Medulloblastomas: Their Histogenesis, Differentiation, and Cell Biology

Recent studies of a complex group of neoplasms, i.e., medulloblastomas, are considered in depth. These childhood neoplasms, regarded by some as primitive neuroectodermal tumors, may provide insights into strategies that can be used to overcome some of the limitations discussed earlier.

Medulloblastomas are small cell CNS tumors that are distinguished from other CNS tumors by their apparent lack of differentiated features. They are the most common of childhood brain tumors, but they respond variably to current treatment modalities and may well represent a biologically heterogeneous class of morphologically similar neoplasms (10,18,25,74–77). Nevertheless, medulloblastomas are morphologically similar to a number of other intra- and extracranial, small cell, undifferentiated tumors that occur with high frequency in childhood such as neuroblastomas, pineoblastomas, retinoblastomas, etc.

Little is known regarding how medulloblastomas (and other brain tumors for that matter) undergo initiation, promotion, and progression (8,25,37,41,42), nor is there agreement on how to classify these and other morphologically similar primitive childhood brain tumors (10,18,74–77). In fact, the major cell types that comprise medulloblastomas have not yet been identified. This hinders efforts to subtype these tumors in order to devise more effective therapeutic strategies for treating them. Rorke and co-workers have operationally defined these poorly differentiated tumors as primitive neuroectodermal neoplasms, and have subdivided them further on the basis of their location and evidence of focal neuronal or glial differentiation (74,75). Other schemes for classifying medulloblastomas and morphologically similar primitive brain tumors have been proposed as well (18,76,77), but a consensus on this issue has not yet emerged. This is due in part to the lack of information on the cellular components in these tumors and their biologic properties. Although morphologic criteria form the basis upon which current classification schemes have been developed, in the normal developing CNS, precursor cells which differentiate into neurons, astrocytes, or oligodendroglia are not readily distinguished on the basis of their morphologic features. Further, it is difficult to distinguish by morphologic criteria pre-existing or trapped, normal, or reactive brain cells in a tumor from those that may differentiate from primitive neuroectodermal tumor cells and indeed represent neoplastic cells.

Molecular markers of neuronal or glial differentiation have been used to address these problems, but it has been impossible thus far to resolve these controversies by probing biopsy or autopsy specimens of medulloblastomas and other primitive brain tumors with antibodies to cell-type-specific molecules. Although monoclonal antibodies to different IF proteins have been used successfully to enumerate the classes of cells present in many different types of neoplasms (54,68,91,104,105), they have been less helpful in determining the cell types present in medulloblastomas (see Tables 3 and 4).

A recent study of a large series of medulloblastomas and other primitive brain tumors reported the presence of NF positive cells using antiserum to NF-L (73). Our studies of a similar group of tumors, using monoclonal antibodies specific for NF-L, NF-M, NF-H, GF or VF (90), indicated that GF protein is the most commonly expressed IF protein in these tumors, while NF and VF subunits are rather uncommon. Thus, the major cell types present in medulloblastomas, based on studies of the type just described, remain to be identified. Examples of NF positive and GF positive cells within a medulloblastoma biopsy specimen are shown in Figure 4.

In contrast to immunochemical and immunohistochemical studies of surgically derived specimens of human medulloblastomas, a human medulloblastoma cell line, recently isolated by Friedman et al. (25), now has been shown to express all three NF subunits and no other cell-type-specific IF proteins (92). However, similar to other normal and neoplastic cells grown in culture, this cell line (designated D283 MED) also expressed VF protein. Further, while over 90% of the cells contained NF-H and NF-M immunoreactivity, less than 10% of the D283 MED cells contained NF-L immunoreactivity. It was concluded, on the basis of these studies, that NF proteins were the major IF proteins expressed in this cell line. These two studies have provided the first strong molecular evidence that medulloblastomas contain a population of neoplastic cells capable of expressing the same IF gene products that are present in mature, nondividing neurons. Mork et al. (63) have also provided similar data on another human medulloblastoma cell line. Further, although GF protein positive cells were present in the initial brain biopsy specimen of the tumor from whence the D283 MED cell line was derived, GF protein positive cells were not seen in an abdominal metastasis from the same tumor. In additional experiments conducted with the cell line, xenografts to nude mouse brain did contain GF positive tumor cells, but subcutaneous xenografts did not (25). Since the monoclonal antibodies (2.2B10) to GF protein (49) used in these experiments is not species specific, it could not be determined whether the GF positive cells in the nude mouse brain xenografts were of mouse origin or whether they arose from the human D283 MED medulloblastoma cells. These interesting results obtained with the monoclonal antibody to GF protein raise the possibility that the GF protein positive cells so commonly seen in biopsy specimens of medulloblastomas arise from nonneoplastic glial cells trapped within the tumor rather than from neoplastic components of the tumor. Representative immunohistochemical and immunoblot data from the D283 MED cell line are shown in Figure 5.

Because IFs may form a linkage system extending from the plasma membrane to the nucleus and appear to play a role in determining cell shape, cell motility, and cell-cell interactions (3,4,11,14,26–28,89), monoclonal antibodies to IF proteins may help elucidate the role these cytoskeletal components play in the molecular events that lead to tumor promotion and tumor progression, in addition to their use in tumor nosology and diagnosis.

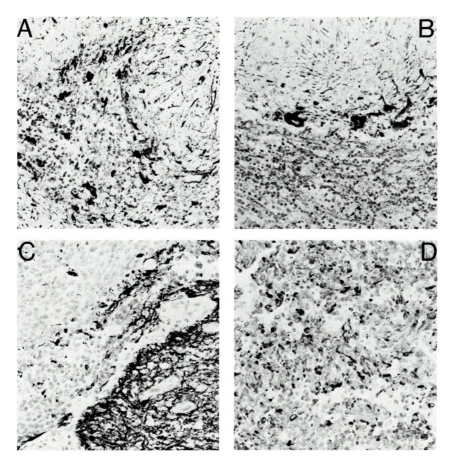

FIG. 4. Sections from a biopsy of a medulloblastoma that infiltrates cerebellum were probed with mono-clonal antibodies to human GFAP (**A** and **C**) or to phosphorylated isoforms of human NF-H and NF-M (**B** and **D**). Reactive and degenerating GFAP positive astrocytic (**A**, lower right in **C**) and NF positive neuro-nal elements (**B**) are evident in cerebellum near the tumor. The tumor itself contains rare GFAP positive cells (upper left in **C**). The numerous NF positive cells in D do not resemble normal or reactive cerebellar neurons; most likely they are tumor cells that contain immunoreactive NF proteins.

Indeed, data on the NF proteins of the D283 MED cells (92) suggests that the NF proteins in this cell line are abnormal compared with their counterparts in normal neurons for the following reasons: (a) NF immunoreactivity in the D283 MED cells is arranged primarily in abnormal perinuclear aggregates that are not seen in normal neurons; (b) the majority of D283 MED cells lack immunoreactive NF-L and at the same time express NF-M and NF-H; and (c) electron microscopic studies of D283 MED xenografts and cultured cells reveal few IFs in most cells, or those IFs that can be recognized are frequently abnormal. That is, they are collapsed together into perinuclear bundles, and they generally lack the projecting side arms, so characteristic of the NFs of normal neurons (34).

These observations regarding the IFs of the D283 MED cells provide strong evidence in support of the hypothesis that at least some of the cells within a medulloblastoma bear a phenotypic resemblance to neurons. That is, some populations of medulloblastoma cells express the same class of IF proteins that are constitutively expressed by nearly all mature

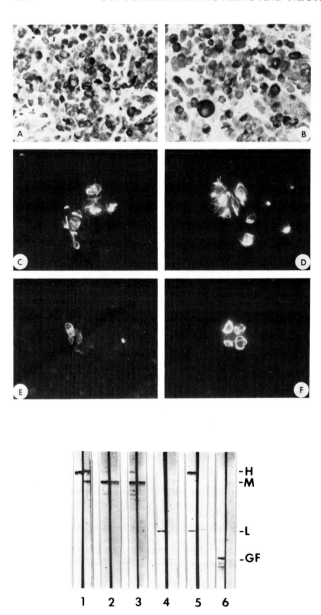

FIG. 5. A human medulloblastoma cell line (D283 MED) examined with diverse monoclonal antibodies to human GFAP and NF subunits using immunocytochemical (upper montage) and immunoblot (lower montage) methods. In the upper montage, immunoperoxidase (**A** and **B**) and immunofluorescence (**C**–**F**) procedures were used to demonstrate the presence of NF-H, NF-M and NF-L in this cell line. NF-H and NF-M were present in numerous cells (**A**–**D**, and **F**), while NF-L was expressed only by rare cells (**E**). The immunoblot strips to the left in each of the pairs of strips numbered 1–6 in the lower montage demonstrate the specificity of the monoclonal antibodies used in this study for normal human NF-H, NF-M, NF-L and GFAP (designated H, M, L, and GF, respectively in this figure). The right hand strip in each pair of strips contains whole homogenates of the D283 MED cells probed with the same monoclonal antibodies. NF-H and NF-M immunobands are dark, while the NF-L immunobands are faint and no GFAP immunoband is seen in the tumor. (From Trojanowski, ref. 92, with permission.)

neurons. At the same time, these studies raise a number of intriguing questions about the biology of the cellular components of human medulloblastomas. Do the GF protein positive cells, frequently observed in medulloblastomas studied as surgical specimens, represent trapped, reactive astrocytes pre-existing in the area infiltrated by these tumors, or does the CNS milieu provide an environment in which glial differentiation from primitive neuroectodermal tumor cells is possible? Although some cells derived from a medulloblastoma express neuron-specific gene products (e.g., NF polypeptides) and at the same time retain important phenotypic properties of neoplastic cells (e.g., ability to undergo cell division indefinitely, chromosomal abnormalities, growth as an invasive tumor in experimental animals), why do so few cells in biopsies of medulloblastomas contain detectable NF proteins? It should now be possible to evaluate whether differences in the complement of IF proteins found in medulloblastomas, as compared with normal mature or developing neurons, result from tumor-specific alterations of these cytoskeletal proteins, tissue-processing factors, limitations in the use of monoclonal antibodies raised against IF proteins from experimental animals to probe human tissues, or other factors.

Human medulloblastoma cell lines may thus provide interesting model systems in which to probe aspects of the cell biology of these tumors that are difficult to examine *in vivo.* At present, two medulloblastoma cell lines have been shown to express at least one of the three subunit polypeptides that form NFs (25,63,92), but only the D283 MED cell line was found to be capable of expressing all three NF proteins. Neither cell line expresses GF protein. Although these two cell lines provide tentative evidence for a close relationship between medulloblastoma cells and normal mature neurons, or primitive neuronal stem cells that retain the ability to undergo neuron-like differentiation, other medulloblastoma cell lines must be examined in the same manner discussed here in order to come to a more informed understanding of the cells of origin of this important group of childhood neoplasms and their ability to give rise to other more differentiated cell types. Ultimately, it may be possible to determine if the spectrum of cell types in medulloblastomas result from genetic and molecular aberrations in the normal sequence of maturational events associated with the ontogeny of neurons (i.e., the step-wise progression of stem cells to neuroblasts, followed by the transition of these cells to committed or immature neurons and then to differentiated neurons). This information should lead to a more detailed understanding of the cell biology of these tumors, and it can then be exploited to classify and treat these tumors in a more effective manner. The strategies described here for unraveling the complex cell biology of medulloblastomas also provide an outline for analyzing other classes of human neoplasms, using molecular probes to cytoskeletal proteins.

ACKNOWLEDGMENTS

Appreciation is expressed to Drs. V.M.-Y. Lee and W.W. Schlaepfer for advice and helpful collaboration in the studies discussed here. Ms. T. Schuck, Ms. C. Page, and Mr. M. Memmo contributed invaluably to all aspects of this work. Dr. V. LiVolsi of the Hospital of the University of Pennsylvania, and Drs. J. Chatten, R. Packer, and L. Rorke kindly contributed tissue from Children's Hospital of Philadelphia for some of the studies described herein. Drs. D. Bigner and H. Friedman kindly made the D283 MED cell line available for collaboration and study. Work discussed here conducted by the author and his colleagues was supported primarily by CA-36245, NS-18616, and Teacher Investigator Development Award KO7 NS-00762.

REFERENCES

1. Achstatter, T., Moll, R., Anderson, A., Kuhn, C., Pitz, S., Schwechheimer, K., and Franke, W. W. (1986): Expression of glial filament protein (GFP) in nerve sheaths and non-neuronal cells re-examined using monoclonal antibodies, with special emphasis on the co-expression of GFP and cytokeratins in epithelial cells of human salivary gland and pleomorphic adenomas. *Differentiation*, 31:206–227.
2. Artleib, U., Krepler, R., and Wiche, G. (1985): Expression of microtubule associated proteins, Map-1 and Map-2, in human neuroblastomas and differential diagnosis of immature neuroblastomas. *Lab Invest.*, 53:684–691.

3. Asch, B. B., and Asch, L. A. (1986): A keratin epitope that is exposed in a subpopulation of preneoplastic and neoplastic mouse mammary epithelial cells but not in normal cells. *Cancer Res.*, 46:1255–1262.

4. Ben-Ze'ev, A., Zoller, M., and Raz, A. (1986): Differential expression of intermediate filament proteins in metastatic and nonmetastatic variants of the BSp73 tumor. *Cancer Res.*, 46:785–790.

5. Bigner, S. H., Bjerkvig, R., and Laerum, O. D. (1985): DNA content and chromosomal composition of malignant human gliomas. *Neurol. Clin.*, 3:769–784.

6. Bonnin, J. M., and Rubinstein, L. J. (1984): Immunohistochemistry of central nervous system tumors. Its contributions to neurosurgical diagnosis. *J. Neurosurg.*, 60:1121–1133.

7. Boutwell, R. K. (1984): On the role of tumor promotion in chemical carcinogenesis. In: *Models, Mechanisms and Etiology of Tumor Promotion*, edited by M. Borzsonyi, K. Lapis, N. E. Day, and H. Yamasaki, pp. 3–11. IARC Scientific Publications, Lyon.

8. Bressler, J. P., and Kornblith, P. L. (1986): Some thoughts on the ontogeny of gliomas. *Prog. Neuropathol.*, 6:189–198.

9. Brooks, J. S. J., LiVolsi, V., and Trojanowski, J. Q. (1987): Do chondroid chordomas exist? *Acta Neuropathol.*, 72:229–235.

10. Burger, P. C., and Vogel, F. S. (1982): *Surgical Pathology of the Nervous System and Its Coverings*, 2nd Ed. Baltimore, Williams & Wilkins.

11. Bunn, C. L., White, F. A., O'Guin, W. M., Sawyer, R. H., and Knapp, L. W. (1985): Intermediate filament expression and lifespan potential in human somatic cell hybrids. *In Vitro Cell Devel. Biol.*, 21:716–720.

12. Carden, M. J., Schlaepfer, W. W., and Lee, V. M.-Y. (1985): The structure, biochemical properties, and immunogenicity of neurofilament peripheral regions are determined by phosphorylation state. *J. Biol. Chem.*, 260:9805–9817.

13. Carden, M. J., Trojanowski, J. Q., Schlaepfer, W. W., Lee, V. M.-Y. (1987): Two-stage expression of neurofilament polypeptides during rat neuro-genesis with early establishment of adult phosphorylation patterns. *J. Neurosci.*, 7:3489–3504.

14. Cellis, J. E., Fey, S. J., Larsen, P. M., and Celis, A. (1985): Preferential phosphorylation of keratins and vimentin during mitosis in normal and transformed human amnion cells. *Ann. N.Y. Acad. Sci.*, 455:268–281.

15. Christen, B., Trojanowski, J. Q., Pietra, G. G. (1987): Immunohistochemical demonstration of phosphorylated and non-phosphorylated forms of the largest neurofilament subunit in human pulmonary carcinoids. *Hum. Pathol.*, 18:997–1001.

16. Coakham, H. B., Garson, J. A., Brownell, B., and Kemshead, J. T. (1985): Diagnosis of cerebral neoplasms using monoclonal antibodies. *Prog. Exp. Tumor Res.*, 29:57–77.

17. Deck, J. H. N., Eng, L. F., Bigbee, J., and Woodcock, S. M. (1978): The role of glial fibrillary acidic protein in the diagnosis of central nervous system tumors. *Acta Neuropathol.*, 42:183–190.

18. Dehner, L. P. (1986): Peripheral and central primitive neuroectodermal tumors: A nosologic concept seeking a consensus. *Arch. Pathol. Lab. Med.*, 110:997–1005.

19. Duffy, P. E., Graf, L., Huang, Y. Y., and Rapport, M. M. (1979): Glial fibrillary acidic protein in ependymomas and other brain tumors. Distribution, diagnostic criteria, and relation to formation of processes. *J. Neurol. Sci.*, 40:133–146.

20. Duffy, P. E., Graf, L., and Rapport, M. M. (1977): Identification of glial fibrillary acidic protein by the immunoperoxidase method in human brain tumors. *J. Neuropathol. Exp. Neurol.*, 36:645–652.

21. Eng, L. F. (1985): Glial fibrillary acidic protein (GFAP): The major protein of glial intermediate filaments in differentiated astrocytes. *J. Neuroimmunol.*, 8:203–214.

22. Eng, L. F., and DeArmond, S. J. (1982): Immunocytochemical studies of astrocytes in normal development and disease. *Adv. Cell. Neurobiol.*, 3:145–171.

23. Eng, L. J., Vanderhaeghen, J. J., Bignami, A., and Gerstel, B. (1971): An acidic protein isolated from fibrous astrocytes. *Brain Res.*, 28:351–354.

24. Fields, K. L. (1985): Neuronal and glial surface antigens on cells in culture. In: *Cell Culture and Neuroscience*, edited by J. E. Bottenstein and G. Sato, pp. 44–93. Plenum Press, New York.

25. Friedman, H. S., Burger, P. C., Bigner, S. H., Trojanowski, J. Q., Wikstrand, C. J., Halperin, E. C., and Bigner, D. D. (1985): Establishment and characterization of the human medulloblastoma cell line and transplantable xenograft D283 MED. *J. Neuropathol. Exp. Neurol.*, 44:592–605.

26. Gerace, L. (1987): Nuclear lamina and organization of nuclear architecture. *TIBS*, 11:443–446.

27. Georgatos, S. D., and Blobel, G. (1987): Two distinct attachment sites for vimentin along the plasma membrane and the nuclear envelope in avian erythrocytes: A basis for a vectorial assembly of intermediate filaments. *J. Cell Biol.*, 105:105–115.

28. Georgatos, S. D., Blobel, G. (1987): Lamin B constitutes an intermediate filament attachment site at the nuclear envelope. *J. Cell Biol.*, 105:117–125.

29. Goldstein, M. E., Sternberger, L. A., and Sternberger, N. H. (1983): Microheterogeneity ("neurotypy") of neurofilament proteins. *Proc. Natl. Acad. Sci. U.S.A.*, 80:3101–3105.

30. Gould, V. E., Wiedenmann, B., Lee, I., Schwechheimer, K., Dockhorn-Dworniczak, B., Radosevich, J. A., Moll, R., and Franker, W. (1987): Synaptophysin expression in neuroendocrine neoplasms as determined by immunocytochemistry. *Am. J. Pathol.*, 126:243–257.

31. Gown, A., and Vogel, A. (1982): Monoclonal antibodies to intermediate filament proteins of human cells: Unique and cross-reacting antibodies. *J. Cell Biol.*, 95:414–424.

32. Gown, A. M., and Vogel, A. M. (1984): Monoclonal antibodies to human intermediate filament proteins. II. Distribution of filament proteins in normal human tissues. *Am. J. Pathol.*, 114:309–321.

33. Granger, B. L., and Lazarides, E. (1983): Expression of the major neurofilament subunit in chicken erythrocytes. *Science*, 221:553–556.

34. Hirokawa, N., Glicksman, M. A., and Willard, M. B. (1984): Organization of mammalian neurofilament polypeptides within the neuronal cytoskeleton. *J. Cell Biol.*, 98:1523–1536.

35. Hogue-Angeletti, R. A. (1986): Chromogranins and neuroendocrine secretion. *Lab. Invest.*, 55:387–390.

36. Jessen, K. R., Thorpe, R., and Mirsky, R. (1984): Molecular identity, distribution and heterogeneity of GFAP: An immunoblotting and immunohistochemical study of Schwann cells, satellite cells, enteric glia and astrocytes. *J. Neurocytol.*, 13:187–200.

37. Katz, D. A., and Liotta, L. A. (1986): Tumor invasion and metastasis in the central nervous system. *Prog. Neuropathol.*, 6:119–131.

38. Kim, S. U., Moretto, G., Shin, D. H., and Lee, V. M.-Y. (1985): Modulation of antigenic expression in cultured adult human oligodendrocytes by derivatives of adenosine 3′,5′ cyclic monophosphate. *J. Neurol. Sci.*, 69:81–91.

39. Kivela, T., Tarkkanen, A., and Virtanen, I. (1986): Intermediate filaments in the human retina and retinoblastoma: An immunohistochemical study of vimentin, glial fibrillary acidic protein and neurofilaments. *Invest. Ophthalmol. Vis. Sci.*, 27:1075–1084.

40. Korat, O., Trojanowski, J. Q., LiVolsi, V., and Merino, M. (1988): Antigen expression in normal paraganglia and paragangliomas. *Surg. Pathol.*, 1:33–40.

41. Laerum, O. D., Bjerkvig, R., Steinsvag, S. K., and de Ridder, L. (1984): Invasiveness of primary brain tumors. *Cancer Metastasis Rev.*, 3:223–236.

42. Laerum, O. D., Steinsvag, S., and Bjerkvig, R. (1985): Cell and tissue culture of the central nervous system: Recent developments and current applications. *Acta Neurol. Scand.*, 72:529–549.

43. Lebovitz, R. M. (1986): Oncogenes as mediators of cell growth and differentiation. *Lab. Invest.*, 55:249–251.

44. Lee, V. M.-Y. (1985): Neurofilament protein abnormalities in PC12 cells: Comparison with neurofilament proteins of normal cultured rat sympathetic neurons. *J. Neurosci.*, 5:3039–3046.

45. Lee, V. M.-Y., and Andrews, P. W. (1986): Differentiation of NTERA-2 clonal human embryonal carcinoma cells into neurons involves the induction of all three neurofilament proteins. *J. Neurosci.*, 6:514–521.

46. Lee, V. M.-Y., Carden, M. J., Schlaepfer, W. W., and Trojanowski, J. Q. (1987): Monoclonal antibodies distinguish several differentially phosphorylated states of the two largest rat neurofilament subunits (NF-H and NF-M) and demonstrate their existence in the normal nervous system of adult rats. *J. Neurosci.*, 7:3474–3488.

47. Lee, V. M.-Y., Carden, M. J., and Trojanowski, J. Q. (1986): Novel monoclonal antibodies provide evidence for the *in situ* existence of a non-phosphorylated form of the largest neurofilament subunit. *J. Neurosci.*, 6:850–858.

48. Lee, V. M.-Y., Carden, M. J., and Schlaepfer, W. W. (1986): Structural similarities and differences between neurofilament proteins from five different species as revealed using monoclonal antibodies. *J. Neurosci.*, 6:2177–2186.

49. Lee, V. M.-Y., Page, C., Wu, H.-L., and Schlaepfer, W. W. (1984): Monoclonal antibodies against gel excised glial filament proteins and their reactivity with other intermediate filament proteins. *J. Neurochem.*, 42:25–32.

50. Lee, V. M.-Y., Wu, H.-L., and Schlaepfer, W. W. (1982): Monoclonal antibodies recognize individual neurofilament triplet proteins. *Proc. Natl. Acad. Sci. U.S.A.*, 70:6089–6092.

51. Lee, V. M.-Y., Trojanowski, J. Q., and Schaepfer, W. W. (1982): Induction of neurofilament triplet proteins in PC12 cells by nerve growth factor. *Brain Res.*, 238:169–180.

52. Leff, E. L., Brooks, J. S. J., and Trojanowski, J. Q. (1985): Expression of neurofilament and neuron-specific enolase in small cell tumors of skin using immunohistochemistry. *Cancer*, 56:625–631.

53. Lehto, V.-P., Miettinen, M., and Virtanen, I. (1986): Antibodies to intermediate filaments in surgical pathology. *Arch. Geschwulstforsch*, 56:283–298.

54. Lehto, V.-P., Bergh, J., and Virtanen, I. (1986): Immunohistology in the classification of lung cancer. In: *Lung Cancer: Basic and Clinical Aspects*, edited by H. H. Hansen, pp. 1-30. Martinus Nijhoff Publishers, Boston.

55. Lewis, S. A., Balcarek, J. M., Krek, V., Shelenski, M., and Cowan, N. J. (1984): Sequence of a cDNA clone encoding mouse glial fibrillary acidic protein: Structural conservation of intermediate filaments. *Proc. Natl. Acad. Sci. U.S.A.*, 81:2743–2746.

56. Lewis, S. A., and Cowan, N. J. (1985): Genetics, evolution, and expression of the 68,000 mol wt neurofilament protein: Isolation of a cloned cDNA probe. *J. Cell Biol.*, 100:843–850.

57. Matus, A. (1987): Putting together the neuronal cytoskeleton. *T.I.N.S.*, 10:186–188.

58. Miettinen, M., Clark, R., and Virtanen, I. (1986): Intermediate filament proteins in choroid plexus and ependyma and their tumors. *Am. J. Pathol.*, 123:231–240.

59. Miettinen, M., Lehto, V. P., Dahl, D., and Virtanen, J. (1983): Differential diagnosis of chordoma, chondroid, and ependymal tumors as aided by anti-intermediate filament antibodies. *Am. J. Pathol.*, 112:160–169.

60. Miettinen, M., Lehto, V.-P., and Virtanen, I. (1985): Immunofluorescence microscopic evaluation of the intermediate filament expression of the adrenal cortex and medulla and their tumors. *Am. J. Pathol.*, 118:360–366.

61. McKeon, F. D., Kirschner, M. W., and Caput, D. (1986): Homologies in both primary and secondary structure between nuclear envelope and intermediate filament proteins. *Nature*, 319:463–468.

62. McNutt, M. A., Bolen, J. W., Gown, A. M., Hammar, S. P., and Vogel, A. M. (1985): Coexpression of intermediate filaments in human epithelial neoplasms. *Ultrastruct. Pathol.*, 9:31–43.

63. Mork, S. J., May, E. E., Papasozomenos, S. C., and Vinores, S. A. (1986): Characteristics of human medulloblastoma cell line TE-671 under different growth conditions *in vitro*: A morphological and immunohistochemical study. *Neuropathol. Applied Neurobiol.*, 12:277–289.

64. Myers, M. W., Lazzarini, R. A., Lee, V. M.-Y., Schlaepfer, W. W., and Nelson, D. L. (1987): The human mid-size neurofilament subunit: A repeated protein sequence and the relationship of its gene to the intermediate filament gene family. *E.M.B.O. J.*, 6:1617–1626.

65. Nixon, R. A., Brown, B. A., and Marotta, C. A. (1982): Posttranslational modification of neurofilament protein during axoplasmic transport: Implications for regional specialization of CNS axons. *J. Cell Biol.*, 94:150–158.

66. Nixon, R. A., Lewis, S. E., and Marotta, C. A. (1987): Posttranslational modification of neurofilament proteins by phosphate during axoplasmic transport in retinal ganglion cell neurons. *J. Neurosci.*, 7:1145–1158.

67. Nowell, P. C., and Croce, C. M. (1986): Chromosomes, genes and cancer. *Am. J. Pathol.*, 125:8–15.

68. Osborn, M., Altmannsberger, M., Debus, E., and Weber, K. (1985): Differentiation of the major tumor groups using conventional and monoclonal antibodies specific for individual intermediate filament proteins. *Ann. N.Y. Acad. Sci.*, 455:649–668.

69. Polak, J. M., and Van Noorden, S. (1986): *Immunocytochemistry: Modern Methods and Applications*, 2nd Ed. John Wright & Sons, Bristol.

70. Pruss, R. M., Mirsky, R., and Raff, M. C. (1981): All classes of intermediate filaments share a common antigenic determinant defined by a monoclonal antibody. *Cell*, 27:419–428.

71. Raff, M. C., Miller, R. H., and Noble, M. (1980): A glial progenitor cell that develops *in vitro* into an astrocyte or an oligodendrocyte depending on culture medium. *Nature*, 303:390–396.

72. Robinson, P. A., Wion, D., and Anderton, B. H. (1986): Isolation of a cDNA for the rat heavy neurofilament polypeptide (NF-H). *FEBS*, 209:203–205.

73. Roessmann, U., Velasco, M. E., Gambetti, P., and Autilio-Gambetti, L. (1983): Neuronal and astrocytic differentiation in human neuroepithelial neoplasms: An immunohistochemical study. *J. Neuropath. Exp. Neurol.*, 42:113–121.

74. Rorke, L. B. (1983): The cerebellar medulloblastoma and its relationship to primitive neuroectodermal tumors. *J. Neuropathol. Exp. Neurol.*, 42:1–15.

75. Rorke, L. B., Gilles, F. H., Davis, F. L., and Becker, L. E. (1985): A revision of the World Health Organization classification of brain tumors for childhood brain tumors. *Cancer*, 56:1866–1868.

76. Rubinstein, L. J. (1986): A commentary on the proposed revision of the World Health Organization classification of brain tumors for childhood brain tumors. *Cancer*, 56:1869–1886.

77. Russell, D. S., and Rubinstein, L. J. (1977): *Pathology of Tumors of the Nervous System*, 4th Ed. Williams & Wilkins Co., Baltimore.

78. Schlaepfer, W. W., and Freeman, L. A. (1978): Neurofilament proteins of rat peripheral nerve and spinal cord. *J. Cell Biol.*, 78:653–662.

79. Schlaepfer, W. W. (1987): Neurofilaments: Structure, metabolism and implications in disease. *J. Neuropathol. Exp. Neurol.*, 46:117–129.

80. Schmidt, L. M., Carden, M. J., Lee, V. M.-Y., and Trojanowski, J. Q. (1987): Phosphate dependent and independent neurofilament epitopes in the axonal swellings of patients with motor neuron disease and controls. *Lab. Invest.*, 56:282–294.

81. Schwechheimer, B., Wiedenmann, B., and Franke, W. W. (1987): Synaptophysin: A reliable marker for medulloblastomas. *Virchows Arch (A)*, 411:53–59.

82. Schwob, J. E., Farber, N. B., and Gottlieb, D. I. (1986): Neurons of the olfactory epithelium in adult rats contain vimentin. *J. Neurosci.*, 6:208–217.

83. Shaw, G., Weber, K. (1984): The intermediate filament complement of the brain: A comparison between different mammalian species. *Eur. J. Cell Biol.*, 33:95–104.

84. Shaw, G. (1986): Neurofilaments: Abundant but mysterious neuronal structures. *Bio. Essays*, 4:161–166.

85. Shinohara, H., Semba, R., Kato, K., Kashiwamata, S., and Tanaka, O. (1986): Immunohistochemical localization of gamma-enolase in early human embryos. *Brain Res.*, 382:33–38.

86. Sternberger, L. A. (1986): Immunocytochemistry, 3rd Ed. John Wiley & Sons, New York.

87. Sternberger, L. A., and Sternberger, N. H. (1983): Monoclonal antibodies distinguish phosphorylated and nonphosphorylated forms of neurofilaments *in situ*. *Proc. Natl. Acad. Sci. U.S.A.*, 80:6126–6130.

88. Tapscott, S. J., Bennett, G. S., Toyama, Y., Kleinbart, F., and Holzer, H. (1981): Intermediate filament proteins in the developing chick spinal cord. *Dev. Biol.*, 86:40–54.

89. Traub, P. (1985): *Intermediate Filaments*. Springer-Verlag, New York.

90. Tremblay, G. F., Lee, V. M.-Y., and Trojanowski, J. Q. (1985): Expression of vimentin, glial filament, and neurofilament proteins in primitive childhood brain tumors: A comparative immunoblot and immunoperoxidase study. *Acta Neuropathol.*, 68:239–244.

91. Trojanowski, J. Q. (1986): Neurofilaments and glial filaments in neuropathology. In: *Immunocytochemistry: Modern Methods and Applications*, edited by J. Polak and S. Van Norden, pp. 413–424. John Wright & Sons, Bristol.

92. Trojanowski, J. Q., Friedman, H. S., Burger, P. C., and Bigner, D. D. (1987): A rapidly dividing human medulloblastoma cell line (D283 MED) expresses all three neurofilament subunits. *Am. J. Pathol.*, 126: 358–363.

93. Trojanowski, J. Q., Gordon, D., Obrocka, M. A., and Lee, V. M.-Y. (1984): Developmental expression of neurofilament and glial filament proteins in the developing human pituitary gland. *Devel. Brain Res.*, 13:229–239.

94. Trojanowski, J. Q., and Hickey, W. F. (1984): Human teratomas express differentiated neural antigens: An immunohistochemical study with monoclonal antibodies against neurofilaments, glial filaments and myelin basic protein. *Am. J. Pathol.*, 115:383–389.

95. Trojanowski, J. Q., Lee, V., Pillsbury, N., and Lee, S. (1982): Neuronal origin of human esthesioneuroblastoma demonstrated with anti-neurofilament monoclonal antibodies. *New Engl. J. Med.*, 307:159–161.

96. Trojanowski, J. Q., and Lee, V. M.-Y. (1983): Anti-neurofilament monoclonal antibodies: Reagents for the evaluation of human neoplasms. *Acta Neuropathol.*, 59:155–158.

97. Trojanowski, J. Q., Lee, V. M.-Y., and Schlaepfer, W. W. (1984): An immunohistochemical study of central and peripheral nervous system tumors with monoclonal antibodies against neurofilaments and glial filaments. *Hum. Pathol.*, 15:248–257.

98. Trojanowski, J. Q., and Lee, V. M.-Y. (1985): Expression of neurofilament antigens by normal and neoplastic human adrenal chromaffin cells. *New Engl. J. Med.*, 313:101–104.

99. Trojanowski, J. Q., Lee, V. M.-Y., and Schlaepfer, W. W. (1985): Neurofilament breakdown products in degenerating rat and human peripheral nerves. *Ann. Neurol.*, 16:349–355.

100. Trojanowski, J. Q., Obrocka, M. A., and Lee, V. M.-Y. (1985): Distribution of neurofilament subunits in neurons and neuronal processes: Immunohistochemical studies of bovine cerebellum with subunit-specific monoclonal antibodies. *J. Histochem. Cytochem.*, 33:557–563.

101. Trojanowski, J. Q., Schuck, T., and Lee, V. M.-Y. (1988): The distribution and prolonged postmortem immunological stability of neurofilament subunits and two microtubule associated proteins (MAP), tau and MAP2, in bovine hippocampus: Implications for studies of normal and diseased human hippocampus. (In press.)

102. Trojanowski, J. Q., Stone, R. A., and Lee, V. M.-Y. (1985): Presence of an alpha-MSH-like epitope in the 150,000 Dalton neurofilament subunit from diverse regions of the CNS: An immunohistochemical and immuno-blot study in guinea pig. *J. Histochem. Cytochem.*, 33:900–904.

103. Trojanowski, J. Q., Walkenstein, N., and Lee, V. M.-Y. (1986): Expression of neurofilament subunits in neurons of the central and peripheral nervous system: An immunohistochemical study with monoclonal antibodies. *J. Neurosci.*, 6:650–660.

104. Virtanen, I., Miettinin, M., Lehto, L.-P., Kariniemi, A.-L., and Paasivuo, R. (1985): Diagnostic application of monoclonal antibodies to intermediate filaments. *Ann. N.Y. Acad. Sci.*, 455:635–648.

105. Vogel, A. M., and Gown, A. M. (1984): Monoclonal antibodies to intermediate filament proteins: Use in diagnostic surgical pathology. In: *Cell and Muscle Motility*, edited by J. W. Shay, Vol. 5, pp. 379–402. Plenum Publishing Corp., New York.

106. Weidenmann, B., Franke, W. W., Kuhn, C., Moll, R., and Gould, V. E. (1986): Synaptophysin: A marker for neuroendocrine cells and neoplasms. *Proc. Natl. Acad. Sci. U.S.A.*, 83:3500–3504.

107. Weston, J. A. (1985): Phenotypic diversification in neural crest-derived cells: The time and stability of commitment during early development. *Curr. Topics Devel. Biol.*, 20:195–210.

108. Yachnis, A. Y., Trojanowski, J. Q., Memmo, M., and Schlaepfer, W. W. (1988): Expression of neurofilament proteins in the hypertrophic granule cells of Lhermitte Duclos disease: An explanation for the mass effect and the myelination of parallel fibers in the disease state. *J. Neuropathol. Exp. Neurol.*, 47:206–214.

109. Zarbo, R. J., Regezi, J. A., Hatfield, J. S., Maisel, H., Trojanowski, J. Q., Batsakis, J. G., and Crissman, J. D. (1988): Immunoreactive glial fibrillary acidic protein in normal and neoplastic salivary gland. *Surg. Pathol.*, 1:55–63.

Diagnostic Immunopathology,
edited by R.B. Colvin,
A.K. Bhan, and R.T. McCluskey.
Raven Press, New York © 1988.

10 / *Leukemias and the Ontogeny of Leukocytes*

Arnold S. Freedman, James D. Griffin, and Lee M. Nadler

Division of Tumor Immunology, Dana-Farber Cancer Institute, and the Department of Medicine, Harvard Medical School, Boston, Massachusetts 02115

The acute and chronic leukemias have long been recognized for being morphologically and clinically heterogeneous. Leukemic cells are thought to be derived from hematopoietic precursor cells that are "frozen" at distinct stages of lymphoid or myeloid differentiation. While morphology and cytochemistry serve to distinguish myeloid and lymphoid leukemias in the majority of patients, approximately 25% of cases remain in which there is either insufficient or conflicting information about leukemic cell lineage. Although the assignment of lineage may be difficult for some patients, the identification of leukemic cell lineage has become increasingly important in predicting clinical course as well as in determining therapeutic approach.

Until the advent of monoclonal antibodies directed against lineage-restricted surface antigens, the assignment of lymphoid and myeloid cellular derivation often proved ambiguous. The B cells traditionally were defined as cells that expressed surface immunoglobulins (Ig) or could be induced to secrete immunoglobulin. Although morphologically indistinguishable from B cells, T cells were classically defined by the expression of sheep red blood cell receptors (E rosette receptors). In contrast, myeloid cells did not express integral sIg or E rosette receptors but did express nonlineage-restricted markers, like HLA class II (Ia) antigens, receptors for the C3 components of complement, and the Fc portion of IgG. In the past decade with the development of monoclonal antibodies directed against lymphoid and myeloid antigens, significant advances have been made in the characterization of lymphoid and myeloid cells. The application of these markers to the study of leukemias has begun to advance our understanding of tumor cell heterogeneity as well as the biologic and clinical behavior of these tumors. It is now possible to assign a lineage derivation to a neoplastic hematopoietic cell in virtually all cases by the expression of lineage-restricted intracellular (cytoplasmic) and cell surface antigens. Moreover, by using markers that define stages of T, B, and myeloid differentiation, it is now possible to begin to identify subsets of patients within histologically defined subgroups of leukemias that demonstrate unique clinical presentations and disease courses. Furthermore, immunophenotyping has led to the identification of several new subtypes of leukemia and has become essential in the diagnosis and characterization of "mixed lineage" or biphenotypic leukemias.

Through the efforts of hundreds of laboratories worldwide to produce and characterize monoclonal antibodies directed against lymphoid and myeloid antigens, several hundred of such antibodies are now available with which to investigate both normal and neoplastic hematopoietic differentiation. These monoclonal antibodies have been extensively characterized over the past 6 years in the Paris, Boston, and Oxford Congresses on the Human Leukocyte Differentiation Antigens in an effort to simplify classification (18,81,116,133). Monoclonal antibodies defining unique cell surface antigens expressed on lymphoid and myeloid cells have been segregated into cluster designation (CD) groups according to antigen expression and molecular weight in an effort to facilitate the classification of both the monoclonal antibodies and antigens (see Table 2, Chapter 18) (18,81,116, 133). It is within the context of a biological understanding of lymphoid and myeloid ontogeny that an attempt will be made to review the expression of lymphoid and myeloid antigens on the acute and chronic leukemias. For each lineage, normal ontogeny and then the expression of lineage-restricted and associated antigens on leukemic B, T, and myeloid cells will be reviewed in an attempt to relate the malignant cell to its normal cellular counterpart. Finally, the heterogeneity of antigen expression within histologically defined subgroups will be examined.

METHODS FOR DETECTING CELL SURFACE ANTIGENS

The majority of antibodies under consideration here have been generated by immunizing mice with human leukemic cells or leukemic cell membranes. There is no clear evidence at this time that any "leukemic-specific" antigens have been identified. All antilymphoid and antimyeloid monoclonal antibodies also react with subsets of normal lymphoid or myeloid cells, and some also react with subsets of other hematopoietic or non-hematopoietic cells. The function of only a small number of these cell surface structures are known at this time (see Table 2, Chapter 18). However, it is likely that over the next few years the function of the majority of these structures will be discovered. These functions will certainly be diverse and will include structures involved in activation and differentiation signals, migration signals, adhesion antigens, cell surface receptors for growth factors, and other regulatory molecules.

At the current time, immunofluorescence is most commonly used to detect binding of monoclonal antibodies, either by an immunofluorescence microscope (see Chapter 16) or a flow cytometer (see Chapter 18). The flow cytometer has numerous advantages over the fluorescent microscope, but also some disadvantages. The flow cytometer is more sensitive and newer instruments can detect 1000 to 5000 molecules per cell. The degree of reproducibility is higher, and it is simple to produce an objective record of the assay. More importantly, a considerable amount of additional information can be generated, including an indication of the size of the cells relative to fluorescence intensity and the distribution of cells by fluorescence intensity (a direct measure of antigen density). Thus, the flow cytometer can reveal subpopulations of cells that differ in antigen density within a population of leukemic cells. Flow cytometers can be equipped with multiple lasers, and the ability to detect two, three, or even four different determinants simultaneously has been developed (see Chapter 18). A disadvantage of the flow cytometer is the inability to examine the distribution of antigen expression on individual cells. Moreover, the machines are expensive, the cost of maintenance is substantial, and flow cytometer operators require substantial training. The investment, however, is likely to be worthwhile for most hospital laboratories involved in phenotyping myeloid and lymphoid leukemias.

Immunochemical techniques to identify cell surface antigens have become increasingly popular in the analysis of solid tumors but have not been extensively applied to cells in the blood (see Chapter 17). This has been partially due to difficulties in distinguishing the enzymatic label from endogenous enzyme activity, since peroxidase and alkaline phosphatase activities are high in normal and malignant myeloid cells. However, many of these problems have been solved by identifying ways to inhibit endogenous enzyme activities (see Chapter 16). For example, endogenous peroxidase can be inhibited by hydrogen peroxide (0.3% in methanol for 30 minutes). Alkaline phosphatase can be inhibited by levamasole (1 mM). Also, it has been shown that endogenous human alkaline phosphatase has little activity at high pH (8.5 to 9.0), while calf intestinal alkaline phosphatase activity remains optimal. Mason and colleagues have described a particularly useful technique in which antibody binding is identified by the addition of rabbit anti-mouse Ig followed by the addition of alkaline phosphatase-anti-alkaline phosphatase complexes (42, 122). In our laboratory, this technique has been used with success for many of the myeloid, erythroid, and lymphoid antibodies described below.

B CELLS

Normal B Cell Ontogeny

By definition, a B lymphocyte is capable of differentiating into an antibody-producing cell. The essential characteristic is the expression of cytoplasmic and/or integral cell surface immunoglobulin (sIg) (62,146). Ontogeny of the B cell has been operationally divided into stages: pre-B cell, resting B cell, activated B cell, proliferating B cell, differentiating B cell and plasma cell (Fig. 1). These stages can be defined by the expression of unique cytoplasmic and cell surface markers. Human B cell antigens can be grouped into broad categories that include antigens that span ontogeny (the so-called pan B cell antigens), antigens of the resting B cell that are lost with activation, antigens that first appear following activation, and antigens that first appear at the terminal stages of differentiation (Fig. 1) (Table 1).

The earliest pre-B cells have been defined by their expression of cell surface antigens including Ia antigens (HLA-DR) and CD19 (B4) and rearrangements of immunoglobulin μ heavy chain genes (Fig. 2) (102). By its B lineage restriction, the CD19 antigen is the most reliable cell surface marker of B lineage at the pre-B cell level. Whether there are Ia^+, μ chain rearranged, $CD19^-$ pre-B cells is presently unknown. Hokland and his colleagues were able to identify discrete stages of human pre-B cell differentiation by isolating pre-B cells from fetal hematopoietic tissues and adult bone marrow (85–87). In those experiments a sequence of pre-B cell differentiation was established by isolating distinct populations of pre-B cells and then inducing them to differentiate *in vitro*. Following the appearance of the CD19 antigen, cells express the CD10 common acute lymphoblastic leukemia antigen (CALLA) (63,153), and finally they express the pan-B cell CD20 (B1) antigen (132,165). The expression of these antigens define stages of B cell differentiation (Fig. 2) based on cell surface antigens, which include $Ia^+CD19^+CALLA^-CD20^-$, $Ia^+CD19^+CALLA^+CD20^-$, and $Ia^+CD19^+CALLA^+CD20^+$ (86). In addition to these cell surface antigens, cytoplasmic μ chains and cytoplasmic CD22 (HD39/B3) (46) antigen also are useful in defining pre-B cell differentiative stages (Fig. 2). Recent studies have demonstrated that CD22, B-cell-restricted molecules appear in the cytoplasm at the earliest stages of pre-B cell differentiation but are not exported to the cell surface until the resting mature B cell stage (Fig. 2). Finally, the last stage of pre-B cell

STAGES OF HUMAN B-CELL ONTOGENY

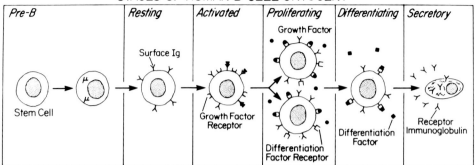

CELL SURFACE ANTIGEN EXPRESSION

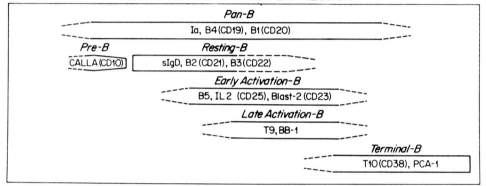

FIG. 1. Stages of normal B cell differentiation. Several groups of antigens characterize these stages including: pan-B cell antigens which span differentiation; antigens expressed on pre-B cells, antigens on mature B cells which are lost following activation; antigens expressed on activated but not resting B cells; and antigens expressed at the plasma cell stage.

TABLE 1. *Cell surface antigen expression in B cell ontogeny*

Antigen	CD No.	MW(kD)	Expression in B cell ontogeny
CALLA	10	100	Pre-B
J2	9	26	Pre-B
Ia		29/34	Pan-B
B4	19	95	Pan-B
B1	20	35	Pan-B
BA-1	24	42	Pan-B
sIg		M(900)	Resting B lost with activation
		G(150)	
		D(150)	
B2	21	140	Resting B lost with activation
HD39/B3*	22	130/140	Resting B lost with activation
Blast-2	23	45	Activation antigen
B5		75	Activation antigen
BB1		37	Activation antigen
Blast-1		45	Activation antigen
IL-2R	25	55	Activation antigen
T9		90	Activation antigen
T10	38	45	Terminally differentiated B
PCA-1		26	Terminally differentiated B

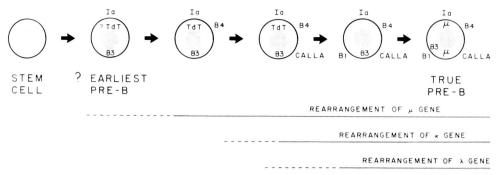

FIG. 2. Expression of cell surface antigens during pre-B cell differentiation, and relationship to Ig gene rearrangements.

ontogeny appears with the expression of μ heavy chains in the cytoplasm (cmu) without the expression of light chains. The expression of cmu further divides the Ia^+CD19^+ $CALLA^+CD20^+$ stage into the cmu^- and cmu^+ stages (Fig. 2).

In the adult, pre-B cell ontogeny appears to take place in the bone marrow. As pre-B cells mature to resting B cells, they are exported to the peripheral blood and lymphoid tissues, where they reside until activated by antigen (Fig. 2). At the present time, the definition of the true resting B cell is controversial. Traditionally, this cell was considered to be a dense small cell which expressed sIgM/D. These cells continue to express Ia, CD19, CD20 and in addition, express cell surface CD22 and the CD21 antigen (B2) which is the receptor for the C3d component of complement (C3d-R) and for Epstein-Barr Virus (EBV-R) (54,89,128,131). However, this population has recently been shown to be heterogeneous by virtue of metabolic, genetic, and cell surface markers of activation. As early as minutes following binding of antigen or mitogen, resting B cells demonstrate one or more events of activation. These include increases in both intracellular Ca^{++} concentration and inositol phospholipid metabolism, expression of myc, synthesis of RNA, increases in size, and entrance into the G_1 phase of the cell cycle (139). In this context, the resting B cell is a dense small cell that expresses sIgM/D, is in the G_0 stage of the cell cycle, and has not yet begun to undergo any of the above-mentioned events of activation.

Following triggering with antigen or various mitogens, resting B cells are activated and then proliferate (Fig. 2). *In vitro*, DNA synthesis begins between 30 and 48 hours and peaks at 72 hours. From both *in vitro, in vivo*, and *in situ* studies, the activation of resting B cells is accompanied by a distinct sequence of cell surface antigenic changes (27,95, 166–168). Within 24 hours of activation, resting B cells begin to lose cell surface IgD, CD21, and CD22, and this process is virtually complete by 72 to 96 hours. As these antigens are lost, a number of B cell associated and restricted activation antigens sequentially appear (Fig. 2). These activation antigens are excellent candidates for those molecules that are growth factor receptors and other important regulatory structures. These activation antigens can be divided into those that are B cell associated transferrin receptor (T9) (174), 4F2 (80), CD25 (IL-2R) (28,184) and those that are B cell restricted B5 (59), Blast-1 (176), CD23 (Blast-2) (175), BB1 (196), AB-1 (91), Ba (98), and Bac-1 (171). Most of these antigens demonstrate peak expression by 72 hours and are lost by 120 hours. At the activation/proliferation stage, there appear to be at least four growth factors (99,107, 111,197), including a low and high molecular weight B cell growth factor (BCGF), gamma interferon, and IL-2 for B cells.

Proliferating B cells then interact with additional lymphokines, which halt cell division and induce these cells to differentiate into immunoglobulin-producing cells (Fig. 2). Several lymphokines have been associated with this function, including IL-2, gamma interferon, and B cell differentiation factor (99). Accompanying this differentiating stage is the gradual loss of the above mentioned cell surface activation antigens, as well as the pan B cell antigens Ia, CD19, CD20, and CD24. This stage is also characterized by the appearance of several other antigens, including CD38 (T10) and PCA-1, which are expressed on plasma cells (Fig. 2).

B Cell Leukemias

Non-T Cell Acute Lymphoblastic Leukemia (ALL)

Leukemic cells from approximately 80% of patients with ALL lack sIg and T cell antigens and therefore are considered to be of non-B, non-T cell derivation. Although the expression of a number of cell surface antigens, including Ia, CD10 (CALLA), CD9 (J2/BA2) (96), CD24 (BA1) (1) and the transferrin receptor (T9) identify most non-B, non-T cell ALLs, these do not define lineage. Several lines of evidence have subsequently supported the conclusion that these leukemias are derived from stages of pre-B cell differentiation. Initially, cmu were noted in the tumor cells from approximately 20% of patients (31,65,191). Further studies demonstrated that 50% of these leukemias expressed the B-cell-restricted CD20, and further suggested that these ALLs were of B cell origin (100, 104,132). Finally, the observation that greater than 95% of non-B, non-T cell ALLs expressed the B-cell-restricted CD19 suggested that these ALLs were derived from pre-B cells (1,55,129).

The expression of Ia, CD19, CALLA (CD10), and CD20 has led to the definition of four subgroups of ALL that correspond to the stages of normal pre-B cell ontogeny (Fig. 3). Nadler et al. examined 138 cases of non-T cell ALL and noted that tumor cells could

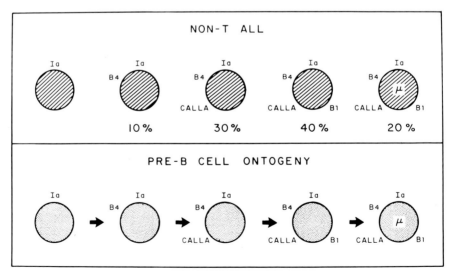

FIG. 3. Stages of normal pre-B ontogeny (bottom) with corresponding subgroups of non-T cell ALL.

be assigned to one of these four subgroups: Ia alone (4%); Ia,CD19 (14%); Ia,CD19, CALLA (33%); and Ia,CD19,CALLA,CD20 (49%) (129). The observation that subgroups of non-T cell ALL existed, coupled with the evidence that these leukemias could be induced *in vitro* with phorbol ester or T-cell-conditioned medium has led to the ordering of the appearance of these antigens (94,130). The subgroup Ia appears very early on B cell precursors, followed by CD19 and CALLA, CD20, and finally cytoplasmic μ is detected. Recent studies have suggested that CD22 (B3) is detected in the cytoplasm of most non-T cell ALLs, and it has been suggested that cytoplasmic CD22 may appear in ontogeny as early as CD19 (Fig. 3) (47). The identification of subgroups of pre-B cell ALL has not yet had an impact on either prognosis or therapy, however, it is suggested that cell surface phenotype may correlate with age at presentation. Most very young children (less than 2 years) appear to develop ALL from the earliest pre-B cells (Ia,CD19) (129). In contrast, the commonest pre-B ALL in adults express the most mature phenotype (Ia,CD19, CALLA,CD20). This hypothesis is consistent with the hypothesis that the neoplastic event affects the major pre-B cell population found at each level of development. For example, a large proportion of cells in the fetal bone marrow express Ia and CD19, whereas the most common pre-B cell population in adults express Ia,CD19,CALLA,CD20.

Chronic B Cell Leukemias (CLL)

Approximately 95% of CLLs are of B cell origin (5,105). Whereas 80% of CLLs express monoclonal sIg, the remaining sIg⁻, non-T cell CLLs expressed B-cell-associated determinants, including receptors for mouse red blood cells (MRBC) and complement components, suggesting that these were also of B cell derivation. More recent demonstration that CLLs express B-cell-restricted antigens and have rearranged Ig heavy and light chain genes provides definitive evidence for a B cell origin of 95% of CLLs (10). Although the lineage of CLLs has been defined, the state of differentiation of B-CLL is unclear. Morphologically and by conventional cell surface markers, B-CLL resembles the small peripheral blood B cell. This conclusion was based on the observation that B-CLLs express sIgM/D, C3d receptors (CD21), as well as Ia, CD19, CD20, and CD24. However, in contrast to peripheral blood B cells, B-CLLs generally do not express CD35 (C3b receptors) and only 25% of cases express CD22 (5). Moreover, virtually all B-CLLs express CD5 (T1), which is expressed on mature T cells, but is not detectable on normal unstimulated B cells (26,92,105,144). These studies suggested that B-CLL cells were not derived from small resting B cells. More recently, CLLs have been shown to express several antigens that are not detected on resting B cells but appear with activation. These include the B-cell-restricted activation antigens B5, Blast-1, and Blast-2 as well as CD25 (IL-2R) (60).

Several studies have demonstrated that cells which phenotypically resemble B-CLL cells can be detected in normal lymphoid populations (11,23,33,74). Caligaris-Cappio and colleagues have observed small numbers of cells that coexpress CD5 and weak sIg and form MRBC rosettes in normal adult lymph node (33). In addition, CD5⁺ B cells have been observed at the periphery of the germinal center of lymph nodes. Very small numbers of CD20⁺CD5⁺ cells have also been isolated from adult peripheral blood and tonsil, but not from bone marrow (61). Further studies have shown that CD5⁺ B cells are a major subset of fetal B cells and that they closely resemble most B-CLLs by virtue of their expression of Ia, CD19, CD20, CD21, weak sIg, CD5, but lack of C3b R(CD35) (61).

The demonstration of expression of activation antigens on B-CLL cells has led our laboratory and others (120) to examine normal, *in vitro*, activated B cells for a normal, cellular counterpart of B-CLL. Whereas anti-immunoglobulin activated B cells express a variety of B-cell-restricted and associated activation antigens, including B5, Blast-1, CD23, Bac-1, and CD25, they do not express CD5. However, a subset of B cells stimulated with phorbol ester, which directly activates cells via protein kinase C, express CD5, B5, and CD25. These studies suggest that B-CLLs phenotypically resemble a subset of normal *in vitro* activated B cells.

Prolymphocytic Leukemia (PLL)

Although considered to be a chronic leukemia of predominantly B cell origin, PLL differs from B-CLL both morphologically and clinically. Similar to most B-CLLs, prolymphocytic leukemia cells express Ia, CD19, CD20, and CD22. In contrast to most CLLs, however, PLL cells express sIg more intensely and generally lack MRBC receptors and CD5 (36). The FMC7 monoclonal antibody, which defines a subset of normal B cells, is reactive with most PLLs but largely unreactive with CLLs (30,35). In a preliminary study from our laboratory, where PLLs were examined with a panel of monoclonal antibodies that define B cell activation markers, similar to B-CLLs, most PLLs (4/5 cases) expressed B5 and Blast-1 (5/5), with less frequent expression of IL-2R and CD23 (2/5). The expression of these activation antigens is therefore quite similar to that seen with B-CLL; however, by virtue of other differences in cell surface antigens, the normal cellular counterpart of PLL is different than CLL.

Hairy Cell Leukemia

Hairy cell leukemias (HCLs) are of B lineage derivation as judged by the expression of sIg (37) and the demonstration of rearranged immunoglobulin genes (103). However, the normal B cell(s) from which HCL is derived is controversial. Generally HCLs express the pan B cell Ags Ia, CD19, CD20, CD24, as well as antigens more limited in their expression on B cells, including CD22 and sIg (7,45). Although lineage has been clarified by the expression of these antigens, insight into the state of differentiation has come about by studies with addition reagents. The expression on most cases of HCL of several B cell activation antigens, including B5, CD25, CD23, Bac-1 (171), and HC2 (145), would lead to the hypothesis that HCL corresponds to a subset of activated B cells. However, the demonstration that most HCLs express the monocyte-associated antigen CD11 (Mol/SHCL3) (159) and CD38 and PCA-I suggests that HCL corresponds to a unique minor subpopulation of B cells (7). Of recent interest is the observation that although HCLs express CD25 (103), they do not respond *in vitro* to IL-2, implying that these are low affinity receptors or are down regulated by some other mechanism (154). However, the same cells will proliferate in response to B cell growth factor, and they may in fact produce autostimulatory BCGF (57).

T CELLS

Normal T Cell Ontogeny

A large number of monoclonal antibodies have been developed that define cell surface structures expressed on human T cells (81). These antibodies have been used to characterize the stages of T cell ontogeny and differentiation, identify subsets of functionally distinct T cells, and elucidate the function of some of these cell surface antigens (see Chapter 1).

During embryonic and early postnatal life, bone marrow precursor cells migrate to the thymus. The thymic microenvironment provides a setting for the processing and eventual development of functionally competent T cells. These cells are subsequently exported into peripheral lymphoid tissues and the circulation (123,134,135,170). A sequence of changes in cell surface antigens are observed to accompany intrathymic differentiation (150) (Table 2). The cells in the earliest stage (I) of intrathymic differentiation, which constitute 10% of the thymic lymphocytes, express T-cell-restricted antigens, CD2 (T11, E rosette receptor) (88), and 3 nonlineage-restricted antigens, the transferrin receptor (T9) (78,174), CD38 (T10), and CD7 (3A1) (79,191). Cells subsequently lose T9, acquire T6 (CD1) (174), and coexpress T4 (CD4) and T8 (CD8). This population, coexpressing CD4, CD1, CD8, CD38, CD2, and CD7, constitutes 70% of thymoctyes (stage II). With further maturation, cells lose CD1 and acquire mature T cell antigens T1 (CD5), T3 (CD3), and T12 (CD6) (stage III). Subsequently, these cells are further subdivided into two populations identified by the expression of either CD4 (helper/inducer) or CD8 (cytotoxic/suppressor). In parallel with the expression of CD3, cells express the T cell receptor for antigen Ti in association with CD3 and therefore are immunocompetent (2). When cells leave the thymus, they no

TABLE 2. *Cell surface antigen expression in T cell ontogeny*

Antigen	CD No.	MW(kD)	Prothymocyte Stage I	Thymocyte Stage II	Thymocyte Stage III	Mature T	Activated T
				Expression in T Cell Ontogeny			
T11	2	50	X	X	X	X	X
3A1	7	40	X	X	X	X	X
T9		90	X				
T10	38	45	X	X	X		
T6	1	49		X			
T4	4	62		X	X	X	X
T8	8	30/32		X	X	X	X
T1	5	67			X	X	X
T3	3	25			X	X	X
Ti		90			X	X	X
T12	6	120			X	X	X
Ta1	—	105			X	X	X
IL-2R	25	55					X
J2	9	26					X
Ia		29/34					X

Abbreviations: CD, cluster designation; MW, molecular weight longer express T10 and are segregated into cells expressing CD4 or CD8, constituting 60% to 70% and 30% to 40% of peripheral blood T cells, respectively. More recently, a series of monoclonal antibodies has been developed which further subdivide CD4 helper cells into inducers of help 2H4 (CD45R) and the inducers of suppression 4B4 (CDW29) (124, 125). Peripheral T cells, when activated by antigen, mitogen, anti-CD2, anti-CD3, or anti-Ti monoclonal antibodies, undergo additional changes in cell surface structures. During the first 2 days after activation, T cells express the IL-2 receptor (CD25) (185) and a T-cell-restricted activation antigen Tal (58). The transferrin receptor and CD9, a T cell associated activation antigen (83), as well as CD38 (T10) reappear by 4 days of *in vitro* culture and Ia antigens are present by 6 to 8 days.

Monoclonal antibodies directed against T cell antigens have also been used to assign a functional role for several of these cell surface molecules. For example, the 50kD CD2 glycoprotein which is expressed throughout T cell ontogeny has been shown to be involved in an antigen independent alternative pathway of T cell activation. Peripheral blood T cells can be induced to proliferate by the binding of antibodies directed against two different epitopes of the CD2 molecule (119). This triggers T cell activation, IL-2 production, and CD25 expression (autocrine regulation). Similarly, stage I and II thymocytes can be induced to express CD25 by the CD2 (T11) pathway, however, they only proliferate in response to exogenous IL-2. This pathway may therefore serve as an amplification mechanism for both resting peripheral T cells and thymocytes.

The CD3/Ti structure expressed on stage III thymocytes and mature peripheral T cells represents the T cell receptor for antigen and MHC. It consists of the 90kd Ti heterodimer (alpha, beta) noncovalently associated with the 3 chain (20 to 25kd) CD3 molecule (3, 156). The Ti structure, with its similarity to the antigen receptor of B cells, sIg, is involved in antigen recognition, whereas CD3 appears to be involved in membrane signal transduction, as evidenced by changes in both calcium flux and phosphotidylinositol (2). More recently, a CD3 associated complex has been described on a subpopulation of T cells, which appears to be a second T cell receptor (29).

T Cell Leukemias

Studies of cell surface molecules have demonstrated that a minority of acute and chronic leukemias are of T cell lineage. With the definition of a series of differentiation antigens, T cell malignancies generally correspond to distinct stages of normal T cell ontogeny (Table 2).

T Cell Acute Lymphoblastic Leukemias

The T cell acute lymphoblastic leukemias (ALLs) constitute 15% to 20% of all cases of ALL. The initial demonstration that certain cases of ALL were of T lineage was by the observation that cells from certain cases formed rosettes with sheep red blood cells (48,97). More recently, through the use of heterantisera and subsequently monoclonal antibodies, lineage can be clearly assigned for essentially all cases of ALL. Several antibodies that define a 40kD pan-T cell antigen, CD7 (3A1) WT-1, and Leu-9 have demonstrated highly specific and sensitive detection of T cell ALLs (24). Monoclonal antibodies to CD7 (190) react with 100% of T ALLs and 75% of Ia⁻, E-rosette- ALLs, which also lack a variety of T cell antigens (CD2, CD3, CD4, CD5, CD8). However, a small number of AMLs

(6%) and CML blast crisis of myeloid type were also CD7$^+$. This antigen, although highly conserved in T cell ontogeny from early thymocytes to and including mature T cells does not identify heterogeneity of T cell ALLs. Another pan-T cell antigen CD6 (T12) (OKT17), identifies approximately half of the cases of T cell ALL (115). In a study that compared various T cell markers with OKT17, the CD6$^-$ cases expressed CD7. Studies with a panel of antibodies defining T cell differentiation antigens have demonstrated that generally T-ALL cells correspond phenotypically to cells in early stages of intrathymic differentiation. Reinherz et al. (149) examined cells from 21 patients with T-ALL and found that the majority correspond to stage I thymocytes (CD38$^+$ with or without the transferrin receptor) (Table 2). Only 20% express the phenotype of stage II thymocytes (CD1$^+$, CD4$^+$, CD8$^+$). One case resembled stage III thymocytes by the expression of CD3. Others have observed T-ALL to be more heterogeneous with additional cases expressing the phenotypes of mature thymocytes. Link et al. (109) recently demonstrated in 10 cases of T-ALL, that all were essentially CD5$^+$, CD7$^+$ and CD38$^+$ with 4 cases expressing CD3. Interestingly, all of the CD3$^-$ cases had intracytoplasmic CD3, suggesting that cytoplasmic expression may occur early in T cell ontogeny. As previously discussed, the CD3 molecules are not expressed on thymocutes in the early stages of differentiation. Similarly, on both early thymocytes and the T cell ALLs which are CD3$^-$, the 90dK T cell receptor, Ti, is not detected. In contrast, T cell ALL cell lines which expressed CD3, also co-express the noncovalently associated Ti structure.

Adult T Cell Leukemia/Lymphoma

Adult T cell leukemia/lymphoma (ATL) has been shown to be associated with the human T cell leukemia virus I (HTLV I), with a cluster of cases in southern Japan, southeastern United States, and the Caribbean (187). An initial examination of cell surface markers found 3 cases to express the phenotype of mature, activated T helper cells (CD5$^+$, CD3$^+$, CD4$^+$, CD38$^+$) (77). The expression of the CD25 (IL-2R) has been variable in some reports, often less intense or absent on freshly isolated cells, and increasing during culture (186,192). These cells are generally transferrin receptor positive and Ia$^+$ (both expressed on activated T cells) and CD6$^+$ (T12) (marker of mature peripheral T cells) but CD1$^-$ (T6). Atypical cases have been described that co-express CD4 and CD8 as well (194,195). Functional studies of ATL cells have demonstrated that in spite of CD25 expression by these cells, most are of low affinity; these cells do not proliferate in response to exogenous IL-2, whereas a case of T-CLL which expressed CD25 responded to IL-2, and the receptor was modulated by IL-2 (183,192). In contrast, although ATL cells express CD4, they lack helper activity in a pokeweed mitogen driven system of Ig production by normal B lymphocytes. A consistent observation has been that ATL cells actuallyy mediate suppression of normal Ig production and appear to correspond to the normal subset of CD4$^+$ peripheral blood T cells, which are inducers of suppression (126).

Chronic T Cell Leukemias

Chronic lymphocytic leukemias are generally of B cell derivation, whereas less than 5% of CLLs and about 20% of PLLs are of T cell origin. Most cases of T-CLL (12,25, 101,137,138,148,160,164) and T-PLL (38,182,193) have mature T helper cell phenotypes (CD2$^+$, CD3$^+$, CD4$^+$, CD5$^+$, CD7$^+$), with occasional reported cases of cells coexpressing CD4 and CD8. Both T-CLL and T-PLL have been recently shown to express CD25; T CLL required PHA stimulation to induce the IL-2R. The proliferative response to mitogens of T-CLL/T-PLL cells are generally diminished. Occasional cases have intact helper function, with either pokeweed mitogen or IL-2-driven Ig synthesis.

Several cases have been described of T-CLL which lack CD5 and CD4 and express CD8 or CD11b (Mo1) (172,173). These cases generally express CD3 and receptors for the Fc portion of IgG (CD16) and are probably part of the T-gamma lymphoproliferative disorder (117,151,157). Morphologically these cells often resemble normal large granular lymphocytes (53). These populations resemble natural killer cells, which express CD16, CD2, often CD38, CD8 (dim), and CD11b. The neoplastic cells also generally express CD2 with certain populations expressing CD3. *In vitro* assays of functional activity have demonstrated that cells from certain cases of Fc gamma-positive T-CLL and T gamma lymphoproliferative disease can function as natural killer and/or suppressor cells (as measured by suppression of Ig production by normal B cells in a pokeweed mitogen driven system) (136). The recent characterization of discrete subpopulations of peripheral blood lymphocytes with NK activity (82) may provide further understanding of this disorder and certain of its manifestations, including anemia, neutropenia, and hypogammaglobulinemia.

MYELOID CELLS

Normal Myeloid Ontogeny

In normal bone marrow, pluripotent stem cells with both self regenerating and differentiating properties give rise to all mature myeloid cells. As the progeny of these pluripotent stem cells differentiate, they become committed to a single hematopoietic lineage (Fig. 4). Colony assays have been developed for committed progenitor cells of the erythroid lineage (BFU-E, CFU-E), granulocyte/monocyte lineage (CFU-GM), and platelet lineage (CFU-mega). In addition, multipotent, colony-forming cells can be assayed (CFU-GEMM), but no *in vitro* assay has been discovered for pluripotent human stem cells. In all stages of normal myelopoiesis, proliferation is tightly coupled to differentiation, where each maturing cell stage has less proliferative potential. This in contrast to acute myelogenous leukemia (AML), in which proliferation proceeds in the absence of terminal differentiation. Therefore, analysis of cell surface antigens and functional capacity of normal myeloid progenitors may provide insight into aberrant differentiation of myeloid leukemias.

Various techniques have been employed to isolate myeloid progenitor cells in order to examine the cell surface phenotype of these cells and the patterns of expression of a variety of antigens during normal myeloid differentiation (Table 3, Fig. 4). Cells at an immature

TABLE 3. *Cell surface antigen expression in myeloid cell ontogeny*

Stages of myeloid differentiation	Antigen	MW	CD
CFU-GEMM, CFU-GM, granulocyte, monocyte	MY7 (MCS-2)	160	13
CFU-GEMM, CFU-GM, promyelocyte, monocyte	MY9	67	33
CFU-GEMM, CFU-GM, myeloblast, monocyte	Ia	29,34	
CFU-GEMM, CFU-GM, monocyte	S3-13	29	
CFU-GEMM, CFU-GM, myeloblast	3C5, MY10	115	34
CFU-GEMM, CFU-GM, myelocyte, monocyte	S16-144		
CFU-GM, granulocyte, monocyte	AHN-7, PM-81, AML-2-23	28-65	
myeloblast, granulocyte, monocyte	Mo1, E11, MY8	155/94	11
promyelocyte, granulocytes, monocyte	Tg1		
promonocytes, monocytes	Mo2, MY4, UCHM1	55	14

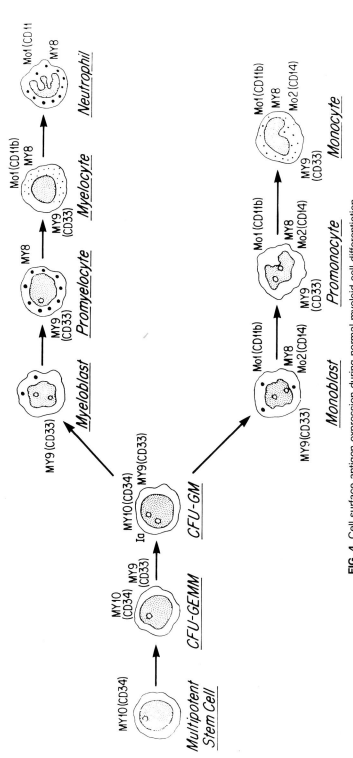

FIG. 4. Cell surface antigen expression during normal myeloid cell differentiation.

level of differentiation, CFU-GM, express Ia antigens, CD13 (MY7) (70), CD33 (MY9) (67), as well as antigens identified by monoclonal antibodies AHN-7 (p28-65) (169), S3-13 (p29), S8-6 (p61) and S16-144 (106). These immature cells lack CD11 (Mo1), MY8, and CD14 (MY4) (71,180). With differentiation along the granulocyte pathway PM-81, AML-2-23 (13), CD14 and CD11 are acquired, and cells are no longer reactive with S8-6 and S16-144. As granulocyte maturation continues, cells lose Ia at the promyelocyte level and CD11 increases in antigen density. Initially, monocyte maturation from the CFU-GM is characterized by acquisition of PM-81, AML-2-23, similar to granulocyte differentiation. Further maturation is characterized by the acquisition of CD11 followed by CD14. In contrast to granulocyte precursors and granulocytes, wherein Ia and CD33 are lost, the monocyte pathway is characterized by the persistent expression of Ia and CD33 through to and including differentiated monocytes.

As previously discussed, monoclonal antibodies directed against cell surface antigens on T and B lymphocytes has aided the functional characterization of several of these cell surface antigens and functionally distinct subsets of cells. Studies involving myeloid antigens have demonstrated, for example, that CD11b (Mo1), which consists of 2 polypeptide chains of 94 and 155 kd, is the receptor for the C3bi cleavage fragment of the third component of complement (10). Moreover, anti-Mo1 inhibits phagocytosis of opsinized particles. As previously discussed, CD13 is present on CFU-GM cells. Griffin et al. (70) have observed that this antigen identifies a subset of CFU-GM cells that are most actively proliferating. Therefore, CD13$^-$ contains few cells which are actively synthesizing DNA.

Myeloid Leukemias

Acute Myelogenous Leukemia (AML)

Although most acute leukemias can be classified by morphology and cytochemical staining as being of lymphoid or myeloid lineage, a small number are unclassifiable. As in the case of B and T cell derived leukemias, in which expression of a series of cell surface antigens have defined subgroups of non-T cell and T-cell ALLs, anti-myeloid (monoclonal antibodies) have been useful in defining the lineages of acute leukemias, identifying subgroups of AML with different prognoses, and correlating myeloid leukemias with normal myeloid progenitor cells (50,69,93,158,177,189).

Despite the generation of a large number of monoclonal antibodies, which identify myeloid cells, many of these reagents have not been tested on large numbers of patients. The reactivity of these antibodies must be shown to be restricted to cells of myeloid lineage. For example, Ia antigens are present on essentially all cases of AML, but are also expressed on nearly 100% of non-T cell ALLs. Several antibodies have been extensively screened and have excellent ability to distinguish AML from ALL. These antibodies include antibodies to CD13 (anti-MY7, MCS-2), CD33 (anti-MY9), and PM-81, which are myeloid restricted. All three have been noted to identify over 80% of AMLs (except FAB classification M6). Another antibody termed VIM-2 (112) identifies over 90% of AMLs of M1–5 FAB classification. A recently described monoclonal antibody termed 3C5 (CD34) reacts with normal myeloid and mixed colony forming cells in 85% of M1 AMLs; however, the antigen is also expressed by some ALLs and cells from patients with CML in lymphoid blast crisis (93,177).

The immunologic phenotyping of AML cells can distinguish essentially all cases of

AML from ALL. However, a small number of leukemias are reported to be of dual lineage. Many of these cases consist of two different populations of leukemic cells, for example, CALLA$^+$ lymphoblasts intermingled with blasts expressing myeloid antigens. There have also been cases of lymphoid and myeloid markers on the same cell. These include a patient with acute leukemia whose cells co-expressed Ia, CALLA, and also CD13 (147). Another case of CML in blast crisis revealed cells reported to co-express T cell antigens CD3, CD11, and CD13 (72). In a recent study of 74 cases of adult ALL, 31% of cases were found to co-express lymphoid and myeloid cell surface antigens (163). These biphenotypic cases tended to be older (45 years versus 34 years) and had a statistically significant poorer response to therapy (CR 30% versus 73%, $p > 0.01$) and shorter survival.

The definition of lineage of acute leukemias has become a major use of monoclonal antibodies as diagnostic reagents. Further studies have identified subgroups of AML and attempted to correlate cell surface phenotype with the FAB classification. Ball and Fanger (13) examined cells from 28 patients with AML using 3 monoclonal antibodies, PMN-6, and PMN-29, both of which are granulocyte specific, and AML-2-23, which is granulocyte and monocyte specific. They observed that less differentiated AMLs of M1 and M2 FAB classification lacked all 3 antigens, whereas M4 (myelomonocytic) AMLs express all 3 antigens. The monocytic leukemias (M5) were reactive with AML-2-23. This study therefore demonstrated that subsets defined by these 3 monoclonal antibodies correlated highly with FAB classification. Linch et al. (108) examined 70 cases of AML and found that the reactivity of a series of monoclonal antibodies that define antigens on monocytes (CD14, UCH-ALF, and E11) correlated well with FAB subgroups M4 and M5. These antibodies were essentially unreactive with M1 and M2 leukemias. They also observed that TG1, which reacts with monocytes and granulocyte precursors, also specifically identified monocytic involvement. A recent study of 191 cases of AML revealed that VIM-D5 (CD15) was generally very weakly or unreactive with promyelocytic leukemias (M3), whereas most myeloid leukemias of FAB classifications M2, M4, and M5 were reactive with VIM-D5 (20). Griffin et al. (69) have examined 70 cases of AML with a panel of monoclonal antibodies including anti-Ia, MY4, MY7, MY8, MY9, and Mo1, which had previously been used to characterize stages of normal myeloid differentiation. Four phenotypes characteristic of normal immature myeloid cells have been characterized. The cell surface phenotyes of 62 of the 70 patients were identical to one of these four groups: the most immature, group I (13 patients) corresponding to the CFU-GM expressed Ia, CD13, CD33. The majority (79%) of these patients were classified as M1 or M2 subtypes. Group II included 16 cases, expressing Ia, CD13, CD33, and detectable levels of CD11, phenotypically resembling normal myeloblasts. Similar to group I, 73% were considered to have M1 or M2 leukemias, while 27% were of the M4 subtype. The third group (III, promyelocytes) characterized by loss of Ia included all cases of acute promyelocytic leukemia and some patients with AML or AMML. The largest group (IV, promonocyte), expressing antigens acquired by cells destined to be monocytes CD11, CD14, as well as CD13, CD33, and Ia, included 28 cases. The vast majority (81%) of these had monocyte morphology (M4/M5), and 19% were considered to have AML. Although cell surface phenotype is related to the FAB classification in this study, phenotypic groups did contain patients of differing morphologies. This study related surface antigen expression to stages of normal myeloid differentiation and, as will be discussed, the use of this antibody panel may provide important clinical correlations.

The identification of subgroups with poor prognosis AML has been difficult. Although in certain studies, factors such as a history of prior myelodysplastic syndrome, prior chemotherapy or radiotherapy, and monocytic features within the FAB classification have identified patients with a poor prognosis, these are controversial (32,94). With the observation of heterogeneity of myeloid antigen expression on AML, attempts have been made to identify clinically relevant subgroups by surface antigen expression. Civin et al. (41) examined 33 patients for expression of MY1 (CD15, X hapten) and MY10 (CD34). They observed that the expression of CD15 and the lack of CD34 identified patients with a greater likelihood of obtaining a complete remission. A recent investigation (66) examined the surface antigen expression of 196 patients with AML, with a panel of 16 antibodies. All patients were uniformly treated in this study. It was observed that the expression of 2 antigens, CD13 and CD14, predicted a low rate of complete remission. As previously discussed, CD14 is expressed by cells with monocytic feature, whereas CD13 is expressed on multipotent stem cells as well as more mature myeloid cells (granulocytes and monocytes). Cases of CD14[+] had a complete remission (CR) rate of 53%, while CD14[−] cases had a CR rate of 69% (p = 0.03). Cases that were CD13[+] had CR rates of 55%, while 73% of CD13[−] cases had a CR (p = 0.01). The absence of both markers was associated with a CR rate of 82%, while the CR rate for all other cases was 54%. Two other groups, identified by the expression of Ia, CD11a and b, and CD11a alone, were associated with decreased continuous CR rate in 1 year and a lower 1 year survival rate respectively. These studies suggest that immunologically defined subgroups may have clinical significance beyond that predicted by standard criteria, such as the FAB classification.

Chronic Myelogenous Leukemia (CML)

Chronic myelogenous leukemia in chronic phase is characterized by the proliferation of mature granulocytes and their relatively mature precursors. After a variable period of time, most patients enter a terminal phase resembling acute blastic leukemia. Morphologically, about ⅓ of these blast crisis leukemias resemble lymphoblasts and express CALLA. The majority of cases, however, are heterogeneous and felt to be related to AML. The clarification of lineage of CML in blast crisis is clinically relevant, as the subgroup of patients with lymphoid blast crisis frequently respond to therapy with vincristine and prednisone. Outside of the characterization of the lymphoid blast crisis with reactivity with anti-CALLA, the remaining cases have until recently only been characterized by their lack of lymphoid markers. Using a panel of antibodies reactive with myeloid, erythroid, lymphoid, or megakaryocyte lineage cells, Griffin et al. (73) determined the cell surface phenotypes of 30 patients with CML blast crisis. Eleven cases were phenotypically similar to ALL cells, expressing Ia and CALLA, with 5 of the cases being CD20[+]. One-third of the cases were CD13[+], Ia[+] with variable expression of CD11a, CD11b, and CD14. This group resembled early myeloid cells, commonly seen in AML. One patient had an erythroleukemia phenotype (expressing glycophorin), and one expressed Plt-1, representing a megakaryoblastic phenotype. One case had a mixed population of CD13[+]/CALLA[+] cells, and 6 cases were termed undifferentiated, as they did not express markers characteristic of any lineage. Another study by Bettelheim et al. (21) examined 45 cases of CML blast crisis and observed that the majority (28 patients) were of myeloid derivation (Ia[+], CD13[+], and VIM-2[+]). Similar to the study by Griffin, about ⅓ were lymphoid (Ia[+], CALLA[+], VIBC-5[+]). Two other cases were of mixed myeloid and lymphoid cells and one was unclassifiable. Although CML blast crisis cells of T lineage were not observed in these studies, several cases have been reported of lymphoid blast crisis with T cell markers

(4,72). In most cases, these studies have demonstrated that a dominant population of cells could be identified of only one lineage. Moreover, CML blast crisis cells represent limited differentiation of the pluripotent stem cell, believed to be the target of leukemic transformation.

MIXED OR BIPHENOTYPIC LEUKEMIAS

As noted above, in many initial studies of leukemia phenotyping, small numbers of cases were identified in which markers of more than one lineage were expressed either on the same leukemic cell or on distinct populations of leukemic cells (67,68). In the former situation, terms such as "lineage-infidelity" (69) or "lineage-promiscuity" (70) have been applied to describe the phenomenon, and the concept of biphenotypic leukemia is now generally accepted. The clinical significance of such acute leukemias has remained unclear as the number of reported cases has been small, and in most instances, these patients were not evaluable for chemotherapy response or survival. In a recent study by Sobol (162), 76 adult patients with acute leukemia (morphologically lymphoid) were prospectively studied with an antibody panel identifying B cells (CD19, CD20, CD24), T cells (CD2, CD5), and myeloid (CD13, CD33) antigens. Unexpectedly, myeloid antigen expression was identified in 33% of cases, usually in conjunction with B and T cell antigens. The most common of the mixed phenotypes was myeloid/B, and 6 of 6 tested cases were found to have rearranged immunoglobulin genes. In 8 other cases that expressed myeloid antigens, there was no expression of B cell or T cell antigens, and these cases did not have rearrangements of Ig or T cell receptor genes. Such cases should be classified as AML, despite morphology. Importantly, the myeloid antigen positive patients as a group had a significantly lower incidence of complete remissions that did myeloid antigen negative patients (35% versus 76%, p < 0.01). None of the patients with pure myeloid phenotypes achieved complete remission, and these cases had a median survival of only 1.5 months. Those cases which co-expressed myeloid and B cell antigens had a complete remission rate of only 29%. These findings were interpreted as indicating that myeloid antigen expression identifies a type of biphenotypic leukemia with extremely poor response rate to standard ALL therapy. Similar findings were reported by Mirro (72) in children with ANLL expressing lymphoid markers. Identification of these patients is critical and can only be realistically done by surface marker analysis (Table 4). Other prospective phenotyping studies of both morphological ALL patients and morphological AML patients are warranted.

TABLE 4. *Discriminating AML and ALL with monoclonal antibodies*

| Monoclonal Antibody | | Myeloid Leukemia | | Lymphoid Leukemia | |
| | | AML | CML-BC (My) | ALL | CML-BC (Ly) |
		% + (N)	% + (N)	% + (N)	% + (N)
MY7	CD13	63 (293)	92 (13)	1 (109)	0 (13)
MY8		53 (267)	7 (15)	0 (82)	0 (11)
MY9	CD33	79 (369)	95 (21)	1 (185)	0 (18)
MCS-2	CD13	92 (294)			
VIM-D5	CD15	68 (116)	88 (8)	2 (88)	
Mol	CD11	60 (421)	57 (23)	0 (82)	0 (11)
B4	CD19	2 (196)		96 (138)	45 (11)
J5 (CALLA)	CD10	1 (100)	0 (13)	82 (138)	100 (11)

ACKNOWLEDGMENTS

Supported by The National Institutes of Health Grants No. CA25369, CA34183, CA 40216. PHS Grant No. 5K08CA01105-01 awarded by the National Cancer Institute, DHHS.

REFERENCES

1. Abramson, C., Kersey, J. H., and LeBien, T. W. (1981): A monoclonal antibody (BA-1) primarily reactive with cells of human B lymphocyte lineage. *J. Immunol.*, 126:83–88.
2. Acuto, O., and Reinherz, E. L. (1985): The human T-cell receptor: Structure and function. *N. Engl. J. Med.*, 312:1100–1111.
3. Acuto, O., Hussey, R. E., Fitzgerald, K. A., Protentis, J. P., Meuer, S. C., Schlossman, S. F., and Reinherz, E. L. (1983): The human T cell receptor: Appearance in ontogeny and biochemical relationship of alpha and beta subunits on IL-2 dependent clones and T cell tumors. *Cell*, 34:717–726.
4. Allouche, M., Bourinbaiar, A., Georgoulias, V., Consolini, R., Salvatore, A., Auclair, H., and Jasmin, C. (1985): T cell lineage involvement in lymphoid blast crisis of chronic myeloid leukemia. *Blood*, 66:1155–1161.
5. Anderson, K. C., Bates, M. P., Slaughenhoupt, B. L., Pinkus, G. S., O'Hara, C., Schlossman, S. F., and Nadler, L. M. (1984): Expression of human B cell associated antigens on leukemias and lymphomas: A model of B cell differentiation. *Blood*, 63:1424–1431.
6. Anderson, K. C., Park, K., Bates, M., Leonard, R. C. F., Hardy, M., Schlossman, S. F., and Nadler, L. M. (1983): Antigens on human plasma cells identified by monoclonal antibodies. *J. Immunol.*, 130:1132–1138.
7. Anderson, K. C., Boyd, A. W., Fisher, D. C., Leslie, D., Schlossman, S. F., and Nadler, L. M. (1985): Hairy cell leukemia: A tumor of pre-plasma cells. *Blood*, 65:620–629.
8. Andrews, R. G., Brentnall, T. A., Torok-Storb, B., and Bernstein, I. D. (1984): Stages of myeloid differentiation identified by monoclonal antibodies. In: *Leucocyte Typing*, edited by A. Bernard, L. Boumsell, J. Dausset, C. Milstein, and S. F. Schlossman, pp. 395–404. Springer-Verlag, New York.
9. Andrews, R. G., Torok-Storb, B., and Bernstein, I. D. (1983): Myeloid-associated differentiation antigens on stem cells and their progeny identified by monoclonal antibodies. *Blood*, 62:124–132.
10. Arnaout, M. A., Todd, R. F., Dana, N., Melamed, J., Schlossman, S. F., and Colten, H. R. (1983): Inhibition of phagocytes of complement C3 or IgG coated particles and of C3Gi binding by monoclonal antibodies to a monocyte-granulocyte membrane glycoprotein (Mo1). *J. Clin. Invest.*, 72:171–179.
11. Arnold, A., Cossman, J., Bakhshi, A., Jaffe, E. S., Waldmann, T. A., and Korsmeyer, S. J. (1983): Immunoglobulin-gene rearrangements as unique clonal markers in human lymphoid neoplasms. *N. Engl. J. Med.*, 309:1593–1599.
12. Baldini, L., DiPadova, F., Cortelezzi, A., et al. (1985): Functional and multimarker analysis of T cell chronic lymphocytic leukemia. *Scand. J. Haematol.*, 34:88–96.
13. Ball, E. D., and Fanger, M. W. (1983): The expression of myeloid-specific antigens on myeloid leukemia cells: Correlations with leukemia subclasses and implications for normal myeloid differentiation. *Blood*, 61:456–463.
14. Ball, E. D., Graziano, R. F., Fanger, M. W. (1983): A unique antigen expressed on myeloid cells and acute leukemia blast cells defined by a monoclonal antibody. *J. Immunol.*, 130:2937–2945.
15. Ball, E. D., Graziano, R. F., Shen, L., and Fanger, M. W. (1982): Monoclonal antibodies to novel myeloid antigens reveal human neutrophil heterogeneity. *Proc. Natl. Acad. Sci. U.S.A.*, 79:5374–5379.
16. Bernard, A., Boumsell, L., Reinherz, E. L., Nadler, L. M., Ritz, J., Coppin, H., Richard, Y., Valensi, F., Dausett, J., Flandrin, G., Lemerle, J., and Schlossman, S. F. (1981): Cell surface characterization of malignant T cells from lymphoblastic lymphoma using monoclonal antibodies: Evidence for phenotypic differences between malignant T cells from patients with acute lymphoblastic leukemia and lymphoblastic lymphoma. *Blood*, 57:1105–1110.
17. Bernstein, I. D., Andrews, R. G., Cohen, S. F., McMaster, B. E. (1982): Normal and malignant human myelocytic and monocytic cells identified by monoclonal antibodies. *J. Immunol.*, 128:876–882.
18. Bernstein, I. D., Self, S. (1986): Joint report of the myeloid section of the Second International Workshop and Conference on Human Leukocyte Differentiation Antigens. In: *Leukocyte Typing II*, edited by E. L. Reinherz, B. F. Haynes, L. M. Nadler, and I. D. Bernstein, Vol. 3, pp. 1–26. Springer-Verlag, New York.
19. Bettelheim, P., Paietta, E., Majdic, O., Gadner, H., Schwarzmeier, J., and Knapp, W. (1982): Expression of a myeloid marker on TdT-positive acute lymphocytic leukemia cells: Evidence by double fluorescence staining. *Blood*, 60:1392–1396.
20. Bettelheim, P., Panzer, S., Majdic, P., Stockinger, H., Roithner, A., Köller, U., Meryn, S., Lechner, K., and Knapp, W. (1985): Unexpected absence of a myeloid surface antigen (3-fucosyl-n-acetyllactosamine) in promyelocytic leukemia. *Leuk. Res.*, 9:1323–1327.

21. Bettelheim, P., Lutz, D., Majdic, O., Paietta, E., Haas, O., Linkesch, W., Neumann, E., Lechner, K., and Knapp, W. (1985): Cell lineage heterogeneity in blast crisis of chronic myeloid leukaemia. *Br. J. Haematol.*, 59:395–409.

22. Bhan, A. K., Nadler, L. M., Stashenko, P., McCluskey, R. T., and Schlossman, S. F. (1981): States of B cell differentiation in human lymphoid tissues. *J. Exp. Med.*, 154:737–749.

23. Bofill, M., Janossy, G., Janossa, M., Burford, G. D., Seymour, G. J., Wernet, P., Kelemen, E. (1985): Human B cell development. II. Subpopulations in the human fetus. *J. Immunol.*, 134:1531–1538.

24. Borowitz, M. J., Dowell, B. L., Boyett, J. M., Falletta, J. M., Pullen, D. J., Crist, W. M., Humphrey, G. B., and Metzgar, R. S. (1985): Monoclonal antibody definition of T cell acute leukemia: A pediatric oncology group study. *Blood*, 65:785–788.

25. Boumsell, L., Bernard, A., Reinherz, E. L., Nadler, L. M., Ritz, J., Coppi, H., Richard, Y., Dubertret, L., Valensi, F., Degos, L., Lemerle, J., Flandrin, G., Dausset, J., Schlossman, S. F. (1981): Surface antigens on malignant Sezary and T-CLL cells correspond to those of mature T cells. *Blood*, 57:526–530.

26. Boumsell, L., Coppin, H., Pham, D., Raynal, B., Lemerle, J., Dausset, J., and Bernard, A. (1980): An antigen shared by a human T cell subset and B cell chronic lymphocytic leukemic cells. *J. Exp. Med.*, 152:229–234.

27. Boyd, A. W., Anderson, K. C., Freedman, A. S., Fisher, D. C., Slaughenhoupt, B. L., Schlossman, S. F., and Nadler, L. M. (1985): Studies of *in vitro* activation and differentiation of human B lymphocytes. I. Phenotypic and functional characterization of the B cell population responding to anti-Ig antibody. *J. Immunol.*, 134:1516–1523.

28. Boyd, A. W., Fisher, D. C., Fox, D., Schlossman, S. F., and Nadler, L. M. (1985): Structural and functional characterization of IL-2 receptors on activated B cells. *J. Immunol.*, 134:2387–2392.

29. Brenner, M. B., McLean, J., Dialynas, D. P., Strominger, J. L., Smith, J. A., Owen, F. L., Seidman, J. G., Ip, S., Rosen, F., and Krangel, M. S. (1986): Identification of a putative second T-cell receptor. *Nature*, 322:145–149.

30. Brooks, D. A., Beckman, I. G. R., Bradley, J., McNamara, P. J., Thomas, M. E., and Zola, H. (1981): Human lymphocyte markers defined by antibodies derived from somatic cell hybrids. IV. A monoclonal antibody reacting specifically with a subpopulation of human B lymphocytes. *J. Immunol.*, 126:1373–1377.

31. Brouet, J. C., Preud'homme, J. L., Penit, C., Valensi, F., Rouget, P., and Seligmann, M. (1979): Acute lymphoblastic leukemia with pre-B cell characteristics. *Blood*, 54:269–273.

32. Cadman, E. C., Capizzi, R. L., Bertino, J. R. (1977): Acute nonlymphocytic leukemia. A delayed complication of Hodgkin's disease therapy. Analysis of 109 cases. *Cancer*, 40:1280–1296.

33. Caligaris-Cappio, F., Gobbi, M., Bofill, M., and Janossy, G. (1982): Infrequent normal B lymphocytes express features of B chronic lymphocytic leukemia. *J. Exp. Med.*, 155:623–627.

34. Cannistra, S. A., Herrmann, F., Davis, R., and Griffin, J. D. (1986): Relationship between HLA-DR expression by normal myeloid progenitor cells and inhibition of colony growth by prostaglandin E. *J. Clin. Invest.*, 77:13–20.

35. Catovsky, D., Cherchi, M., Brooks, D., Bradley, J., and Zola, H. (1981): Heterogeneity of B-cell leukemias demonstrated by the monoclonal antibody FMC7. *Blood*, 58:406–408.

36. Catovsky, D., Cherchi, M., Okos, A., Hedge, U., and Galton, D. A. G. (1976): Mouse red blood cell rosettes in B lymphoproliferative disorders. *Br. J. Haematol.*, 33:173–177.

37. Catovsky, D., Pettit, J. E., Galetto, J., Okos, A., Galton, D. A. G. (1974): The B-lymphocyte nature of the hairy cell of leukemic reticuloendotheliosis. *Br. J. Haematol.*, 26:29–37.

38. Catovsky, D., Wechsler, A., and Matutes, E. et al. (1982): The membrane phenotype of T-prolymphocytic leukemia. *Scand. J. Haematol.*, 29:398–404.

39. Chan, L. C., Pegram, S. M., Greaves, M. F. (1985): Contribution of immunophenotype to the classification and differential diagnosis of acute leukemia. *Lancet*, 1:475.

40. Civin, C. I., Strauss, L. C., Brovall, C., Fackler, M. J., Schwartz, J. F., and Shaper, J. H. (1984): Antigenic analysis of hematopoiesis. III. A hematopoiesis progenitor cell surface antigen defined by a monoclonal antibody raised KG-1a cells. *J. Immunol.*, 133:157.

41. Civin, C. I., Vanghan, W. P., Strauss, L. C., Schwartz, J. F., Karp, J. E., and Burke, P. J. (1983): Diagnostic and prognostic utility of cell surface markers in acute non-lymphocytic leukemia (ANLL). *Exp. Hematol.*, 11 [Suppl. 14]: 152a.

42. Cordell, J. L., Falini, B., Erber, W. N., Glosh, A. K., Abdulaziz, Z., MacDonald, S., Pulford, K. A. F., Stein, H., and Mason, D. Y. (1984): Immunoenzymatic labelling of monoclonal antibodies using immune complexes of alkaline phosphatase and monoclonal anti-alkaline phosphatase (APAAP complexes). *J. Histochem. Cytochem.*, 32:219.

43. Cossman, J., and Jaffe, E. S. (1981): Distribution of complement receptor subtypes in non-Hodgkins lymphomas of B cell origin. *Blood*, 58:20–26.

44. Cossman, J., Neckers, L. M., Arnold, A., and Korsmeyer, S. J. (1982): Induction of differentiation in a case of common acute lymphoblastic leukemia. *N. Engl. J. Med.*, 307:1251–1254.

45. Divine, M., Farcet, J. P., Gourdin, M. F., Tabilio, A., Vasconcelos, A., Andre, C., Jouault, A., Bouguet, J., Reyes, F. (1984): Phenotype study of fresh and cultured hairy cells with the use of immunologic markers and electron microscopy. *Blood*, 64:547–552.

46. Dorken, B., Moldenhauer, G., Pezzutto, A., Schwartz, R., Feller, A., Kiesel, S., and Nadler, L. M. (1986): HD39 (B3), a B lineage-restricted antigen whose cell surface expression is limited to resting and activated human B lymphocytes. *J. Immunol.*, 136:4470–4479.

47. Dorken, B., Pezzutto, A., and Hunstein, W. (1988): Expression of cytoplasmic CD22 in B cell ontogeny. *Leukocyte Typing III*, Oxford Press, New York (in press).

48. Dow, L. W., Borella, A., and Sen L., Aur, R. J. A., George, S. L., Mauer, A. M., and Simone, J. V. (1977): Initial prognostic factors and lymphoblast-erythrocyte rosette formation in 109 children with acute lympho-blastic leukemia. *Blood*, 50:671–682.

49. Drexler, H. G., and Minowada, J. (1986): The use of monoclonal antibodies for the identification and classi-fication of acute myeloid leukemias. *Leuk. Res.*, 10:279.

50. Drexler, H. G., Sagawa, K., Menon, M., and Minowada, J. (1986): Reactivity pattern of "myeloid mono-clonal antibodies" with emphasis on MCS-2. *Leuk. Res.*, 10:17–23.

51. Ellegaard, J., Kucharska-Pulczynska, M., and Hokland, P. Analysis of leukocyte differentiation antigens in blood and bone marrow from patients with Waldenstrom's macroglobulinemia. *Leukocyte Typing III*, Ox-ford Press, New York (*in press*).

52. Hokland, P., Kucharska-Pulezynska, M., and Ellegaard, J. (1987): Analysis of leukocyte differentiation antigens in blood and bone marrow from patients with Waldenstrom's microglobulinemia. *Leukocyte Typing III*, edited by A. J. McMichael, pp. 512–515. Oxford University Press, Oxford.

53. Ferrarini, M., Romagnani, S., and Montesoro, E., et al. (1983): A lymphoproliferative disorder of the large granular lymphocytes with natural killer activity. *J. Clin. Immunol.*, 3:30–41.

54. Fingeroth, J. D., Weis, J., Tedder, T. F., Strominger, J. L., Biro, P. A., and Fearon, D. T. (1984): Epstein-Barr virus receptor of human B lymphocytes is the C3d receptor CR2. *Proc. Natl. Acad. Sci. U.S.A.*, 81:4510–4514.

55. Flug, F., Dodson, L., Wolff, J., Guarini, L., Rausen, A., Wang, C. Y., and Knowles, D. M. (1985): B-lymphocyte associated antigen expression by non-B, non-T acute lymphoblastic leukemia. *Leuk. Res.*, 9:1051–1058.

56. Foon, K. A., and Todd, R. F. (1986): Immunologic classification of leukemia and lymphoma. *Blood*, 68:1.

57. Ford, R. J., Yoshimura, L., Morgan, J., Quesada, J., Montagna, R., and Maizel, A. (1985): Growth factor-mediated tumor cell proliferation in hairy cell leukemia. *J. Exp. Med.*, 162:1093–1098.

58. Fox, D. A., Hussey, R. E., Figzgerald, K. A., Acuto, O., Poole, C., Palley, L., Daley, J. F., Schlossman, S. F., and Reinherz, E. L. (1984): Tal, a novel 105 kd human T cell activation antigen defined by a mono-clonal antibody. *J. Immunol.*, 133:1250–1256.

59. Freedman, A. S., Boyd, A. W., Anderson, K. C., Fisher, D. C., Schlossman, S. F., and Nadler, L. M.: (1985): B5, a new B cell restricted activation antigen. *J. Immunol.*, 134:2228–2235.

60. Freedman, A. S., Boyd, A. W., Berrebi, A., Horowitz, J. C., Rosen, K. J., Slaughenhoupt, B., Levy, D., Daley, J., Levine, H., Nadler, L. M. (1987): Expression of B cell activation antigens on normal and malig-nant B cells. *Leukemia*, 1:9–15.

61. Freedman, A. S., Boyd, A. W., Bieber, F. R., Dailey, J., Rosen, K., Horowitz, J. C., Levy, D., and Nadler, L. M. (1987): Normal cellular counterparts of B cell chronic lymphocytic leukemia. *Blood*, 70:418–427.

62. Gathings, W. E., Lawton, A. R., and Cooper, M. D. (1977): Immunofluorescent studies on the development of pre-B cells, B lymphocytes and immunoglobulin isotype diversity in humans. *Eur. J. Immunol.*, 7:804–810.

63. Greaves, M. F., Hariri, G., Newman, R. A., Sutherland, D. R., Ritter, M. A., and Ritz, J. (1983): Selective expression of the common acute lymphoblastic leukemia (gp100) antigen on immature lymphoid cells and their malignant counterparts. *Blood*, 61:628–630.

64. Greaves, M. F., Sieff, C., and Edwards, P. A. W. (1983): Monoclonal antiglycophorin as a probe for eryth-roleukemias. *Blood*, 61:645–652.

65. Greaves, M. F., Verbi, W., Vogler, L.B., Cooper, M., Ellis, R., Ganeshguru, K., Hoffbrand, V., Janossy, G., and Bollum, F. J. (1980): Antigenic and enzymatic phenotypes of the pre-B subclass of acute leukemia. *Leuk. Res.*, 3:353–362.

66. Griffin, J. D., Davis, R., Nelson, D. A., Davey, F. R., Mayer, R. J., Schiffer, C., McIntyre, O. R., and Bloomfield, C. D. (1986): Use of surface marker analysis to predict outcome of adult acute myeloblastic leukemia. *Blood*, 68:1232–1241.

67. Griffin, J. D., Linch, D., Sabbath, K. D., Larcom, P., and Schlossman, S. F. (1984): A monoclonal antibody reactive with normal and leukemic human myeloid progenitor cells. *Leuk. Res.*, 8:521–534.

68. Griffin, J. D., and Löwenberg, B. (1986): Clonogenic cells in acute myeloblastic leukemia. *Blood*, 68: 1182–1195.

69. Griffin, J. D., Mayer, R. J., Weinstein, H. J., Rosenthal, D. S., Coral, F. S., Beveridge, R. P., and Schloss-man, S. F. (1983): Surface marker analysis of acute myeloblastic leukemia: Identification of differentiation-associated phenotypes. *Blood*, 62:557–563.

70. Griffin, J. D., Ritz, J., Beveridge, R. P., Lipton, J. M., Daley, J. F., and Schlossman, S. F. (1983): Expres-sion of MY7 antigen on myeloid progenitor cells. *Int. J. Cell. Cloning*, 1:33–48.

71. Griffin, J. D., Ritz, J., Nadler, L. M., and Schlossman, S. F. (1981): Expression of myeloid differentiation antigens in normal and malignant myeloid cells. *J. Clin. Invest.*, 69:932–939.

72. Griffin, J. D., Tantravahi, R., Canellos, G. P., Wisch, J. S., Reinherz, E. L., Sherwood, G., Beveridge, R. P., Daley, J. F., Lane, H., and Schlossman, S. F. (1983): T cell surface antigens in a patient with blast crisis of chronic myeloid leukemia. *Blood*, 61:640–644.
73. Griffin, J. D., Todd, R. F., Ritz, J., Nadler, L. M., Canellos, G. P., Rosenthal, D., Gallivan, M., Beveridge, R. P., Weinstein, H., Karp, D., and Schlossman, S. F. (1983): Differentiation patterns in the blastic phase of chronic myeloid leukemia. *Blood*, 61:85–91.
74. Griffin, J. D., and Nadler, L. M. (1985): Immunobiology of chronic leukemias. In: *Neoplastic Diseases of the Blood*, edited by P. H. Wiernik, G. P. Canellos, R. A. Kyle, and C. A. Schiffer, pp. 51–80. Churchill Livingstone, New York.
75. Griffin, J. D., Ritz, J., Nadler, L. M., and Schlossman, S. F. (1981): Expression of myeloid differentiation antigens on normal and malignant myeloid cells. *J. Clin. Invest.*, 68:932–941.
76. Hast, R., Dowding, C., Robak, T., and Goldman, J. M. (1988): Immune phenotype of leukaemic cells and clonogenic cells in acute myeloid leukemia. *Leuk. Res. (in press)*.
77. Hattori, T., Uchiyama, T., Toibana, T., Takatsuki, K., and Uchino, H. (1981): Surface phenotype of Japanese adult T-cell leukemia cells characterized by monoclonal antibodies. *Blood*, 58:645–647.
78. Haynes, B., Hemler, B. F., Cotner, T., Mann, D. L., Eisenberth, G. S., Strominger, J. L., and Fauci, A. S. (1981): Characterization of a monoclonal antibody (5E9) that defines a human cell surface antigen of cell activation. *J. Immunol.*, 127:347–351.
79. Haynes, B. F., Eisenberth, G. S., and Fauci, A. S. (1979): Human lymphocyte antigens: Production of a monoclonal antibody that defines functional thymus derived lymphocyte subsets. *Proc. Natl. Acad. Sci. U.S.A.*, 76:5829–5833.
80. Haynes, B. F., Hemler, M. E., Mann, D. L., Eisenberth, G. S., Shelhamer, J., Mostowski, H. S., Thomas, C. A., Strominger, J. L., and Fauci, A. S. (1981): Characterization of a monoclonal antibody (4F2) that binds to human monocytes and to a subset of activated lymphocytes. *J. Immunol.*, 126:1409–1420.
81. Haynes, B. F. (1986): Summary of T cell studies performed during the Second International Workshop and Conference on Human Leukocyte Differentiation Antigens. In: *Leukocyte Typing II*, edited by E. L. Reinherz, B. F. Haynes, L. M. Nadler, and I. D. Bernstein, Vol. 1, p. 1. Springer-Verlag, New York.
82. Hercend, T., Griffin, J. D., Bensussan, A., Schmidt, R. E., Edson, M. A., Brennan, A., Murray, C., Daley, J. F., Schlossman, S. F., and Ritz, J. (1985): Generation of monoclonal antibodies to a human natural killer clone: Characterization of two natural killer cell-associated antigens, $NKH1_A$ and NKH2, expressed on subsets of large granular lymphocytes. *J. Clin. Invest.*, 75:932–943.
83. Hercend, T., Nadler, L. M., Pesando, J. M., Reinherz, E. L., Schlossman, S. F., and Ritz, J. (1981): Expression of a 26,000 dalton glycoprotein on activated human T cells. *Cell. Immunol.*, 64:192–199.
84. Herrmann, F., Komischke, B., Odenwald, E., and Ludwig, W. D. (1983): Use of monoclonal antibodies as a diagnostic tool in human leukemia. I. Acute myeloid leukemia and acute phase of chronic myeloid leukemia. *Blut*, 47:157.
85. Hokland, P., Nadler, L. M., Griffin, J. D., Schlossman, S. F., and Ritz, J. (1984): Purification of the common acute lymphoblastic leukemia antigen (CALLA) positive cells from normal bone marrow. *Blood*, 64:662–666.
86. Hokland, P., Ritz, J., Schlossman, S. F., and Nadler, L. M. (1985): Orderly expression of B cell antigens during the *in vitro* differentiation of non-malignant human pre-B cell. *J. Immunol.*, 135:1746–1751.
87. Hokland, P., Rosenthal, P., Griffin, J. D., Nadler, L. M., Daley, J. F., Hokland, M., Schlossman, S. F., and Ritz, J. (1983): Purification and characterization of fetal hematopoietic cells that express the common acute lymphoblastic leukemia antigen (CALLA). *J. Exp. Med.*, 157:114–129.
88. Howard, F. D., Ledbetter, J. A., Wong, J., Bieber, C. P., Stinson, E. B., and Herzenberg, L. A. (1981): A human T lymphocyte differentiation marker defined by monoclonal antibodies that block E-rosette formation. *J. Immunol.*, 126:2117–2122.
89. Iida, K., Nadler, L. M., and Nussenzweig, V. (1983): The identification of the membrane receptor for the complement fragment C3d by means of a monoclonal antibody. *J. Exp. Med.*, 158:1021–1033.
90. Janowska-Wieczorek, A., Mannoni, P., Turner, A. R., McGann, L. E., Shaw, A. R. E., and Turc, J.-M. (1984): Monoclonal antibody specific for granulocytic lineage cells and reactive with human pluripotent and committed haematopoietic progenitor cells. *Br. J. Haematol.*, 58:159.
91. Jung, L. K., and Fu, S. M. (1984): Selective inhibition of growth factor-dependent human B cell proliferation by monoclonal antibody AB1 to an antigen expressed by activated B cells. *J. Exp. Med.*, 160:1919–1924.
92. Kamoun, M., Kadin, M. F., Martin, P. J., Nettleton, J., and Hansen, J. A. (1981): A novel human T cell antigen preferentially expressed on mature T cells and also on (B type) chronic lymphatic leukemic cells. *J. Immunol.*, 127:987–996.
93. Katz, F. E., Tindle, R., Sutherland, D. R., and Greaves, M. F. (1985): Identification of a membrane glycoprotein associated with haemopoietic progenitor cells. *Leuk. Res.*, 9:191–198.
94. Keating, M. J. (1982): Early identification of potentially cured patients with acute myelogenous leukemia —A recent challenge. In: *Adult Leukemias 1*, edited by C. D. Bloomfield, pp. 237–263. Martinus Nijhoff, Boston.
95. Kehrl, J. H., Muraguchi, A., and Fauci, A. S. (1984): Differential expression of cell activation markers after stimulation of resting human B lymphocytes. *J. Immunol.*, 132:2857–2861.

96. Kersey, J. H., LeBien, T. W., Abramson, C. S., Newman R., Sutherland, R., and Greaves, M. (1981): p24: A human hemopoietic progenitor and acute lymphoblastic leukemia-associated celll surface structure identified with a monoclonal antibody. *J. Exp. Med.*, 153:726–731.

97. Kersey, J. H., Sabad, A., Gajl-Peczalska, F., Nesbit, M., Hallgren, H., and Yunis, E. (1973): Acute lymphoblastic leukemic cells with T (thymus-derived) lymphoma markers. *Science*, 182:1355–1356.

98. Kikutani, H., Kimura, R., Nakamura, H., Sato, R., Muraguchi, A., Kawamura, N., Hardy, R. R., and Kishimoto, T. (1986): Expression and function of an early activation marker restricted to human B cells. *J. Immunol.*, 136:4019–4036.

99. Kishimoto, T. (1985): Factors affecting B cell growth and differentiation. *Ann. Rev. Immunol.*, 3:133–152.

100. Knapp, W., Bettelheim, P., Majdic, O., Liszka, K., Schmidmeier, W., Lutz, D. (1984): Diagnostic value of monoclonal antibodies to leucocyte differentiation antigens in lymphoid and nonlymphoid leukemias. In: *Leucocyyte Typing*, edited by A. Bernard, L. Boumsell, J. Dausset, C. Milstein, and S. F. Schlossman, p. 564. Springer-Verlag, New York.

101. Knowles, D. M., II, Halper, J. P., Machin, G. A., Byeff, P., Mertelsman, R., and Chess, L. (1982): Phenotypic heterogeneity of human T cell malignancies: Demonstration by monoclonal antibodies and cytochemical markers. *Am. J. Hematol.*, 12:233–241.

102. Korsemeyer, J. S., Arnold, A., Bakhshi, A., Ravetch, J. V., Siebenlist, V., Hieter, P. A., Sharrow, S. O., LeBien, T. W., Kersey, J. H., Poplack D. G., Leder, P., and Waldman, T. A. (1983): Immunoglobulin gene rearrangement and cell surface antigen expression in acute lymphocytic leukemias of T cell and B cell precursor origins. *J. Clin. Invest.*, 71:301–313.

103. Korsmeyer, S. J., Greene, W. C., Cossman, J., Hsu, S.-M., Jensen, J. P., Neckers, L. M., Marshall, S. L., Bakhshi, A., Depper, J. M., Leonard, W. J., Jaffe, E. S., and Waldmann, T. A. (1983): Rearrangement and expression of immunoglobulin genes and expression of Tac antigen in hairy cell leukemia. *Proc. Natl. Acad. Sci. U.S.A.*, 80:4522–4526.

104. Korsmeyer, S. J., Hieter, P. A., Ravetch, J. V., Poplack, D. G., Waldmann, T. A., and Leder, P. (1981): Developmental hierarchy of immunoglobulin gene rearrangements in human leukemic pre-B cells. *Proc. Natl. Acad. Sci. U.S.A.*, 78:301–313.

105. Koziner, B., Gebhard, D., Denny, T., and Evans, R. L. (1982): Characterization of B cell type chronic lymphocytic leukemia cells by surface markers and a monoclonal antibody. *Am. J. Med.*, 73:802–807.

106. Lange, B., Ferrero, D., Pessano, S., Palumbo, A., Faust, J., Meo, P., and Rovera, G. (1984): Surface phenotype of clonogenic cells in acute myeloid leukemia defined by monoclonal antibodies. *Blood*, 64:693–700.

107. Leanderson, T., Lundgren, E., Ruuth, E., Borg, H., Persson, H., and Countinho, A. (1982): B cell growth factor and B cell maturation factor. *Proc. Natl. Acad. Sci. U.S.A.*, 79:7455–7459.

108. Linch, D. C., Allen, C., Beverley, P. C. L., Bynoe, A. G., Scott, C. S., and Hogg, N. (1984): Monoclonal antibodies differentiating between monocytic and nonmonocytic variants of AML. *Blood*, 63:566–573.

109. Link, M. P., Stewart, S. J., Warnke, R. A., and Levy, R. (1985): Discordance between surface and cytoplasmic expression of the Leu-4 (T3) antigen in thymocytes and in blast cells from childhood T lymphoblastic malignancies. *J. Clin. Invest.*, 76:248–253.

110. Löwenberg, B., and Bauman, J. G. J. (1985): Further results in understanding the subpopulation structure in AML: Clonogenic cells and their progeny identified by differentiation markers. *Blood*, 66:1225–1232.

111. Maizel, A., Sahasrubuddhe, C., Mehta, S., Morgan, J., Lachman, L., and Ford, R. (1982): Biochemical separation of human B cell mitogenic factor. *Proc. Natl. Acad. Sci. U.S.A.*, 79:5998–6002.

112. Majdic, O., Bettelheim, P., Stockinger, H., Aberer, W., Liszka, K., Lutz, D., and Knapp, W. (1984): M2, a novel myelomonocytic cell surface antigen and its distribution on leukemic cells. *Int. J. Cancer*, 33:617–623.

113. Majdic, O., Liszka, K., Lutz, D., and Knapp, W. (1981): Myeloid differentiation antigen defined by a monoclonal antibody. *Blood*, 58:1127–1133.

114. Martin, P. J., Hansen, J. A., Nowinski, R. C., and Brown, M. A. (1980): A new human T cell differentiation antigen: Unexpected expression on chronic lymphocytic leukemia cells. *Immunogenetics*, 11:429–439.

115. Matutes, E., Parreira, A., Foa, R., and Catovsky, D. (1985): Monoclonal antibody OKT17 recognizes most cases of T-cell malignancy. *Br. J. Haematol.*, 61:649–656.

116. McMichael, A. (1988): *Leuckocyte Typing III*, Oxford University Press, Oxford.

117. Meidema, F., and Melief, J. M. (1986): Immunobiology of the expanded T cells in T-cell leukemia and T-gamma lymphocytosis. *Leuk. Res.*, 10:469–474.

118. Mertelsmann, R., Koziner, B., Ralph, P., Filippa, D., McKenzie, S., Arlin, Z. A., Gee, T. S., Moore, M. A. S., and Clarkson, B. D. (1978): Evidence for distinct lymphocytic and monocytic populations in a patient with terminal transferase-positive acute leukemia. *Blood*, 51:1051.

119. Meuer, S. C., Hussey, R. E., Fabbi, M., Fox, D., Acuto, O., Fitzgerald, K. A., Hodgdon, J. C., Protentis, J. P., Schlossman, S. F., and Reinherz, E. L. (1984): An alternative pathway of T cell activation: A functional role for the 50kd T11 sheep erythrocyte receptor protein. *Cell*, 36:897–906.

120. Miller, R. A., and Gralow, J. (1984): The induction of Leu-1 antigen expression in human malignant and normal B cells by phorbol myristic acetate (PMA). *J. Immunol.*, 133:3408–3414.

121. Mirro, J., Zipf, T. F., Ching-Hon, P., Kutchingman, G., Williams, D., Melvin, S., Murphy, S. B., and

Stass, S. (1985): Acute mixed lineage leukemia: Clinicopathologic correlations and prognostic significance. *Blood*, 66:1115–1123.

122. Moir, D. J., Glosh, A. R., Abdulaziz, Z., Knight, P. M., and Mason, D. Y. (1983): Immunoenzymatic staining of hematologic samples with monoclonal antibodies. *Br. J. Haematol.*, 55:395.

123. Moore, M. A. S., and Owen, J. T. (1967): Experimental studies on the development of the thymus. *J. Exp. Med.*, 126:715–725.

124. Morimoto, C., Letvin, N. L., Boyd, A. W., Hagan, M., Brown, H. M., Kornacki, M. M., and Schlossman, S. F. (1985): The isolation and characterization of the human helper inducer T cell subset. *J. Immunol.*, 134:3762–3769.

125. Morimoto, C., Letvin, N. L., Distaso, J. A., Aldrich, W. R., and Schlossman, S. F. (1985): The isolation and characterization of the human suppressor inducer T cell subset. *J. Immunol.*, 134:1508–1515.

126. Morimoto, C., Matsuyama, T., Oshige, C., Tanaka, H., Hercend, T., Reinherz, E. L., and Schlossman, S. F. (1985): Functional and phenotypic studies of Japanese adult T cell leukemia cells. *J. Clin. Invest.*, 75:836–843.

127. Nadler, L. M., Anderson, K. C., Marti, G., Bates, M. P., Park, E. K., Daley, J. F., and Schlossman, S. F. (1983): B4, a human B cell associated antigen expressed on normal, mitogen activated, and malignant B lymphocytes. *J. Immunol.*, 131:244–250.

128. Nadler, L. M., Boyd, A. W., Park, E., Anderson, K. C., Fisher, D., Slaughenhaupt, B., Thorley-Lawson, D. A., and Schlossman, S. F. (1986): The B cell-restricted glycoprotein (B2) is the receptor for Epstein-Barr virus. In: *Leukocyte Typing II*, edited by E. L. Reinherz, B. F. Haynes, L. M. Nadler, I. D. Bernstein, p. 509. Springer-Verlag, New York.

129. Nadler, L. M., Korsmeyer, S. J., Anderson, K. C., Boyd, A. W., Slaughenhoupt, B., Park, E., Jensen, J., Coral, F., Mayer, R. J., Sallan, S. E., Ritz, J., and Schlossman, S. F. (1984): B cell origin of non-T cell acute lymphoblastic leukemia. A model for discrete stages of neoplastic and normal pre-B cell differentiation. *J. Clin. Invest.*, 74:332–340.

130. Nadler, L. M., Ritz, J., Bates, M. P., Park, E. K., Anderson, K. C., Sallan, S. E., and Schlossman, S. F. (1982): Induction of human B cell antigens in non-T cells acute lymphoblastic leukemia. *J. Clin. Invest.*, 70:433–442.

131. Nadler, L. M., Stashenko, P., Hardy, R., van Agthoven, A., Terhorst, C., and Schlossman, S. F. (1981): Characterization of a B cell specific (B2) distinct from B1. *J. Immunol.*, 126:1941–1947.

132. Nadler, L. M., Stashenko, P., Ritz, J., Hardy, R., Pesando, J. M., Schlossman, S. F. (1981): A unique cell surface antigen identifying lymphoid malignancies of B cell origin. *J. Clin. Invest.*, 67:134–140.

133. Nadler, L. M. (1986): B cell/leukemia panel workshop: Summary and comments. In: *Leucocyte Typing II*, edited by E. L. Reinherz, B. F. Haynes, L. M. Nadler, and I. D. Bernstein. Vol. 2, p. 3. Springer-Verlag, New York.

134. Owen, J. J. T., and Raff, M. C. (1970): Studies on the differentiation of thymus-derived lymphocytes. *J. Exp. Med.*, 132:1216–1232.

135. Owen, J. J. T., and Ritter, M. A. (1969): Tissue interactions in the development of thymus lymphocytes. *J. Exp. Med.*, 129:431–437.

136. Palutke, M., Eisenberg, L., Kaplan, J., Hussain, M., Kithier, K., Tabaczka, P., Mirchandani, I., and Tenenbaum, D. (1983): Natural killer suppressor T cell chronic lymphocytic leukemia. *Blood*, 62:627–634.

137. Pandolfi, F., De Rossi, G., Ranucci, A., Bonomo, G., Pasqualetti, D., Napolitano, M., and Manzari, V. (1985): Tac-positive, HTLV-negative, T helper phenotype chronic lymphocytic leukemia cells. *Blood*, 65:1531–1537.

138. Pandolfi, F., Rossi, G. D., Semenzato, G., Quinti, I., Ranucci, A., De Sanctis, G., Lopez, M., Gasparotto, G., and Aiuti, F. (1982): Immunologic evaluation of T chronic lymphocyte leukemia cells: Correlations among phenotype, functional activities, and morphology. *Blood*, 59:688–695.

139. Paul, W. E., Mizuguchi, J., Brown, M., Nakanishi, K., Hornbeck, P., Rabin, E., and Ohara, J. (1986): Regulation of a B-lymphocyte activation, proliferation, and immunoglobulin secretion. *Cell Immunol.*, 99:7–13.

140. Pelus, L. M., Saletan, S., Silver, R., and Moore, M. A. (1982): Expression of Ia antigens on normal and chronic myeloid leukemia human granulocyte-macrophage colony forming cells is associated with the regulation of cell proliferation by prostaglandin E. *Blood*, 59:284.

141. Perussia, B., Trinchieri, G., Leibman, D., Jankiewicz, L., Lang, B., and Rovera, G. (1982): Monoclonal antibodies that detect differentiation surface antigens on human myelomonocytic cells. *Blood*, 59:382.

142. Pessano, S., Ferrero, D., Palumbo, A., Bottero, L., Faust, J., Lange, B., and Rovera, G. (1983): Differentiation antigens of normal and leukemic myelomonocytic cells. In: *UCLA Symposia on Molecular and Cellular Biology*, New Series, edited by D. N. Golde, and P. A. Marks, p. 197. Liss, New York.

143. Pessano, S., Palumbo, A., Ferrero, D., Pagliardi, G. L., Bottero, L., Lai, S. K., Meo, P., Carter, C., Hubbell, H., Lange, B., and Rovera, G. (1984): Subpopulation heterogeneity in human acute myeloid leukemia determined by monoclonal antibodies. *Blood*, 64:275.

144. Pilarski, L. M., Mant, M. J., and Reuther, B. A. (1985): Pre-B cells in peripheral blood of multiple myeloma patients. *Blood*, 66:416–422.

145. Posnett, D. N., Wang, C. Y., Chiorazzi, N., Crow, M. K., and Kunkel, H. G. (1985): An antigen charac-

teristic of hairy cell leukemia cells is expressed on certain activated B cells. *J. Immunol.*, 133:1635–1640.

146. Preud'homme, J. L., and Seligman, M. (1972): Surface bound immunoglobulins as a cell marker in human lymphoproliferative diseases. *Blood*, 40:777–791.

147. Pui, C. H., Dahl, G. V., Melvin, S., Williams, D. L., Peiper, S., Mirro, J., Murphy, S. B., and Stass, S. (1984): Acute leukaemia with mixed lymphoid and myeloid phenotype. *Br. J. Haematol.*, 56:121–130.

148. Reinherz, E. L., Nadler, L. M., Rosenthal, D. A., Molony, W. C., and Schlossman, S. F. (1979): T cell subset characterization of human T-CLL. *Blood*, 53:1066–1075.

149. Reinherz, E. L., Nadler, L. M., Sallen, S. E., and Schlossman, S. F. (1979): Subset derivation of T-cell acute lymphoblastic leukemia in man. *J. Clin. Invest.*, 64:392–397.

150. Reinherz, E. L., and Schlossman, S. F. (1980): The differentiation and functions of human T lymphocytes: A review. *Cell*, 19:821–827.

151. Reynolds, C. W., and Foon, K. A. (1984): Ty-lymphoproliferative disease and related disorders in man and experimental animals: A review of the clinical, cellular and functional characteristics. *Blood*, 64:1146–1158.

152. Ritz, J., Nadler, L. M., Bhan, A. K., Notis-McConarty, J., Pesando, J., and Schlossman, S. F. (1981): Expression of common acute lymphoblastic leukemia antigen (CALLA) by lymphomas of B cell and T cell lineage. *Blood*, 58:648–652.

153. Ritz, J., Pesando, M., Notis-McConarty, J., Lazarus, H., and Schlossman, S. F. (1980): A monoclonal antibody to human acute lymphoblastic leukemia antigen. *Nature*, 283:583–585.

154. Robb, R. J., Greene, W. C., and Rusk, C. M. (1984): Low and high affinity cellular receptors for interleukin-2. *J. Exp. Med.*, 160:1126–1146.

155. Rosenthal, D., Griffin, J. D., Todd, R. F., Ritz, J., Nadler, L. M., Canellos, G. P., Gallivan, M., Beveridge, R. P., Weinstein, H., Karp, D., and Schlossman, S. F. (1983): Differentiation patterns in the blastic phase of chronic myeloid leukemia. *Blood*, 61:85.

156. Royer, H. D., Acuto, O., Fabbi, M., Tizard, R., Ramachandran, K., Smart, J. E., and Reinherz, E. L. (1984): Genes encoding the Ti beta subunit of the antigen/MHC receptor undergo rearrangement during intrathymic ontogeny prior to surface T3-Ti expression. *Cell*, 39:261–266.

157. Rümke, H., Miedema, F., Berge, I. J. M., Terpstra, F., van der Reijden, H. J., van de Griend, R. J., de Bruin, H. G., von dem Borne, A. E. G., Smit, J. W., Zeijlemaker, W. P., and Melief, C. J. M. (1982): Functional properties of T cells in patients with chronic T gamma lymphocytosis and chronic T cell neoplasia. *J. Immunol.*, 129:419–426.

158. Sabbath, K. D., Ball, E. D., Larcom, P., Davis, R. B., and Griffin, J. D. (1985): Heterogeneity of clonogenic cells in acute myeloblastic leukemia. *J. Clin. Invest.*, 75:746–753.

159. Schwarting, R., Stein, H., and Wang, C. Y. (1985): The monoclonal antibodies alpha-S-HCL1 (alpha-Leu-14) and alpha-S-HCL3 (alpha-Leu-M5) allow the diagnosis of hairy cell leukemia. *Blood*, 65:974–983.

160. Simpkins, H., Kiprov, D. D., Davis, J. L., Morand, P., Puri, S., and Grahn, E. P. (1985): T cell chronic lymphocytic leukemia with lymphocytes of unusual immunologic phenotype and function. *Blood*, 65:127–133.

161. Smith, L. J., Curtis, J. E., Messner, H. A., Senn, J. S., Furthmayr, H., and McCulloch, E. A. (1983): Lineage infidelity in acute leukemia. *Blood*, 61:1138.

162. Sobol, R. E., Mick, R., Royston, I., Davey, F., Ellison, R. R., Newman, R., Cuttner, J., Griffin, J. D., Collins, H., Nelson, D. A., and Bloomfield, C. D. (1987): Clinical significance of myeloid antigen expression in adult acute lymphoblastic leukemia. *New Engl. J. Med.*, 316:1111–1117.

163. Sobol, R. E., Royston, I., LeBien, T., Minowada, J., Anderson, K., Davey, F. R., Cuttner, J., Schiffer, C., Ellison, R. R., and Bloomfield, C. D. (1985): Adult acute lymphoblastic leukemia phenotypes defined by monoclonal antibodies. *Blood*, 65:730–735.

164. Spiers, A. S. D., Davis, M. P., and Levine M., et al. (1985): T-cell chronic lymphocytic leukemia: Anomalous cell markers, variable morphology and marker responsiveness to pentostatin (2'-deoxycoformycin). *Scand. J. Haematol.*, 34:57–67.

165. Stashenko, P., Nadler, L. M., Hardy, R., and Schlossman, S. F. (1980): Characterization of a new B lymphocyte specific antigen in man. *J. Immunol.*, 125:1678–1685.

166. Stashenko, P., Nadler, L. M., Hardy, R., and Schlossman, S. F. (1981): Expression of cell surface markers following human B cell activation. *Proc. Natl. Acad. Sci. U.S.A.*, 78:3848–3852.

167. Stein, H., Gerdes, J., and Mason, D. Y. (1982): The normal and malignant germinal centre. *Clin. Haematol.*, 11:531–539.

168. Stein, H., Siemssen, V., and Lennert, K. (1978): Complement receptor subtypes C3b and C3d in lymphocytic tissue and follicular lymphoma. *Br. J. Cancer*, 37:520–532.

169. Strauss, L. C., Skubitz, K. M., August, J. T., and Civin, C. I. (1984): Antigenic analysis of hematopoiesis: II. Expression of human neutrophil antigens on normal and leukemic marrow cells. *Blood*, 63:574–578.

170. Stutman, O., and Good, R. A. (1971): Immunocompetence of embryonic hematopoietic cells after traffic to thymus. *Transplant. Proc.*, 3:923–925.

171. Suzuki, T., Sanders, S. K., Butler, J. L., Gartland, G. L., Komiyama, K., and Cooper, M. D. (1986): Identification of an early activation antigen (Bac-1) on human B cells. *J. Immunol.*, 137:1208–1213.

172. Tagawa, S., Konishi, I., Kuratune, H., Katagiri, S., Taniguchi, N., Tamaki, T., Inoue, R., Kanayama, Y.,

Tsubakio, T., Machii, T., Yonezawa, T., and Kitani, T. (1983): A case of T cell chronic lymphocytic leukemia (T-CLL) expressing a peculiar phenotype (E$^+$, OKM1$^+$, Leu 1$^+$, OKT3$^-$, and IgG EA$^-$). *Cancer*, 52:1378–1384.

173. Tagawa, S., Taniguchi, N., Tokumine, Y., Tamaki, T., Konishi, I., Kanayama, Y., Inoue, R., Machii, T., and Kitani, T. (1986): OKM1-positive T-cell leukemias: Relationships among morphologic features, phenotype, and functional activities. *Cancer*, 57:1507–1514.

174. Terhorst, C., van Agthoven, A., Le Clair, K., Reinherz, E. L., and Schlossman, S. F. (1981): Biochemical studies in the human thymocyte antigens T6, T9, and T10. *Cell*, 23:771–780.

175. Thorley-Lawson, D. A., Nadler, L. M., Bhan, A. K., and Schooley, R. T. (1985): Blast-2 (EBVCS) an early cell surface marker of human B cell activation, is superinduced by Epstein-Barr virus. *J. Immunol.*, 134:3007–3012.

176. Thorley-Lawson, D. A., Schooley, R. T., Bhan, A. K., and Nadler, L. M. (1982): Epstein-Barr virus superinduces a new human B cell differentiation antigen (B-LAST-1) expressed on transformed lymphoblasts. *Cell*, 30:415–425.

177. Tindle, R. W., Nichols, R. A. B., Chan, L., Campana, D., Catovsky, D., and Birnie, G. D. (1985): A novel monoclonal antibody BI-3C5 recognizes myeloblasts and non-B non-T lymphoblasts in acute leukaemias and CGL blast crises, and reactis with immature cells in normal bone marrow. *Leuk. Res.*, 9:1–9.

178. Todd, R. F., III, Roach, J. A., and Arnaout, M. A. (1985): The modulated expression of Mo5, a human myelomonocytic plasma membrane antigen. *Blood*, 65:964-973.

179. Todd, R. F. III, and Schlossman, S. F. (1984): Differentiation antigens on human monocytes and macrophages defined by monoclonal antibodies. In: *Mononuclear Phagocyte Biology*, edited by A. Volkman, p. 129. Marcel Dekker, New York.

180. Todd, R. F., Nadler, L. M., and Schlossman, S. F. (1981): Antigens on human monocytes identified by monoclonal antibodies. *J. Immunol.*, 126:1435–1442.

181. Todd, R. F., Schlossman, S. F. (1982): Analysis of antigenic determinants on human monocytes and macrophages. *Blood*, 59:775–786.

182. Tsai, L. C., Tsai, C. C., Hyde, T. P., Thomas L. A., and Broun, G. O. (1984): T cell prolymphocytic leukemia with helper-cell phenotype and a review of the literature. *Cancer*, 54:463–470.

183. Tsudo, M., Uchiyama, T., Uchino, H., and Yodoi, J. (1983): Failure of regulation of Tac antigen/TCGF receptor on adult T-cell leukemia cells by anti-Tac monoclonal antibody. *Blood*, 61:1014–1016.

184. Tsudo, M., Uchiyama, T., and Uchino, H. (1984): Expression of TAC antigen on activated normal human B cells. *J. Exp. Med.*, 160:612–617.

185. Uchiyama, T., Broder, S., and Waldmann, T. A. (1981): A monoclonal antibody (anti-TAC) reactive with activated and functionally mature T cells. I. Production of anti-TAC monoclonal antibody and distribution of Tac (+) cells. *J. Immunol.*, 126:1393–1403.

186. Uchiyama, T., Hori, T., Tsudo, M., Wano, Y., Umadome, H., Tamori, S., Yodoi, J., Maeda, M., Sawami, H., and Uchino, H. (1985): Interleukin-2 receptor (Tac antigen) expressed on adult T cell leukemia cells. *J. Clin. Invest.*, 76:446–453.

187. Uchiyama, T., Yodoi, J., Sagawa, K., Takatsuki, K., and Uchino, H. (1977): Adult T-cell leukemia: Clinical and hematologic features of 16 cases. *Blood*, 50:481–492.

188. Vainchenker, W., Deschamps, J. F., Bastin, J. M., Guichard, J., Titeux, M., Breton-Gorius, J., and Mc-Michael, A. J. (1982): Two monoclonal antiplatelet antibodies as markers of human megakaryocyte maturation: Immunofluorescent staining and platelet peroxidase detection in megakaryocyte colonies and *in vivo* cells from normal and leukemic patients. *Blood*, 59:514.

189. Van der Reijden, H. J., van Rhenen, D. J., Lansdorp, P. M., van't Veer, M. B., Langenhuijsen, M. M. A. C., Engelfriet, C. P., and Kr. von dem Borne, A. E. G. (1983): A comparison of surface marker analysis and FAB classification in acute myeloid leukemia. *Blood*, 61:443–448.

190. Van der Valk, P., van den Besselaar-Dingjan, G., Daha, M. R., and Meijer, C. J. L. M. (1983): Analysis of large cell lymphomas using monoclonal and heterologous antibodies. *J. Clin. Pathol.*, 36:44–50.

191. Vodinelich, L., Tax, W., Bai, Y., Pegram, S., Capel, P., and Greaves, M. F. (1983): A monoclonal antibody (WTI) for detecting leukemias of T cell precursors (T-ALL). *Blood*, 62:1108–1113.

192. Vogler, L. B., Crist, W. M., Bockman, D. E., Pearl, E. R., Lawton, A. R., and Cooper, M. D. (1978): Pre-B cell leukemia; a new phenotype of childhood lymphoblastic leukemia. *N. Engl. J. Med.*, 298:872–878.

193. Waldmann, T. A., Greene, W. C., Sarin, P. S., Saxinger, C., Blayney, D. W., Blattner, W. A., Goldman, C. K., Bongiovanni, K., Sharrow, S., Depper, J. M., Leonard, W., Uchiyama, T., and Gallo, R. C. (1984): Functional and phenotypic comparison of human T cell leukemia/lymphoma virus positive adult T cell leukemia with human T cell leukemia/lymphoma virus negative sezary leukemia, and their distinction using anti-Tac. *J. Clin. Invest.*, 73:1711–1718.

194. Weiss, L. M., Bindl, J. M., Picozzi, V. J., Link, M. P., and Warnke, R. A. (1986): Lymphoblastic lymphoma: An immunophenotype study of 26 cases with comparison to T cell acute lymphoblastic leukemia. *Blood*, 67:474–478.

195. Woods, G. M., Sawyer, P. J., Kirov, S. M., Lowenthal, R. M., Jupe, D. M., and Catovsky, D. (1985): Functional and phenotypic analysis of a T cell prolymphocytic leukemia. *Leuk. Res.*, 9:587–596.

196. Yamada, Y., Kamihira, S., Amagasaki, T., Kinoshita, K., Kusano, M., Chiyoda, S., Yawo, E., Ikeda, S.,

Suzuyama, J., and Ichimaru, M. (1985): Adult T cell leukemia with atypical surface phenotypes: Clinical correlation. *J. Clin. Oncol.*, 3:782–788.

197. Yamada, Y., Kamihira, S., Amagasaki, T., Kinoshita, K., Kusano, M., Ikeda, S., Toriya, K., Suzuyama, J., and Ichimaru, M. (1984): Changes of adult T cell leukemia cell surface antigens at relapse or at exacerbation phase after chemotherapy defined by use of monoclonal antibodies. *Blood*, 64:440–444.

198. Yokochi, T., Holly, R. D., and Clark, E. A. (1982): B lymphoblast antigen (BB1) expressed on Epstein-Barr virus-activated B cell blasts. B lymphoblastoid cell lines, and Burkitt's lymphomas. *J. Immunol.*, 128:823–827.

199. Yoshizaki, K., Nakagawa, T., Fukunaga, K., Kaieda, T., Maruyama, S., Kishimoto, S., Yamamura, Y., and Kishimoto, T. (1983): Characterization of human B cell growth factor from cloned T cells or mitogen-stimulated T cells. *J. Immunol.*, 130:1241–1246.

Diagnostic Immunopathology,
edited by R.B. Colvin,
A.K. Bhan, and R.T. McCluskey.
Raven Press, New York © 1988.

11 / *Lymphomas*

Nancy L. Harris

*Department of Pathology, Massachusetts General Hospital and Harvard Medical School,
Boston, Massachusetts 02114*

In the last decade, the application of monoclonal antibodies to the characterization of lymphoid cells in tissue sections has made a major contribution to the diagnosis and classification of lymphomas (19). Although the ultimate goal of a lymphoma classification based on immunophenotypic markers has not been reached, immunohistologic analysis has greatly improved diagnostic accuracy in two clinically important areas and has contributed significantly to a third. The two most important problems that can be resolved by markers are the distinction between reactive and neoplastic lymphoid infiltrates and the distinction between lymphoid and nonlymphoid neoplasms. These two differential diagnoses are among the most important problems faced by pathologists practicing diagnostic hematopathology, and the contribution of immunohistologic studies cannot be overemphasized. The third area in which immunophenotyping is clinically useful is in subclassifying lymphomas into T, B, and other cell types, and also within a given lineage. This is a more difficult and sometimes less clinically relevant area, and the role of immunophenotypic studies is still developing.

The impact of immunohistologic studies on diagnostic hematopathology is twofold. First, in an individual case, a definite diagnosis can often be made that would have been impossible, incorrect, or only presumptive, if only routine histologic sections had been available. Second, the pathologist's "eye" is improved: if routine sections are re-examined, knowing the results of the immunohistologic stains, the histologic criteria for making the diagnosis may be refined. Experience with immunohistologic stains has led, for example, to the recognition that many lymphocytic infiltrates of the orbit, lung, and gastrointestinal tract that had previously been considered to be benign "pseudolymphomas" are in fact low-grade, monoclonal B cell lymphomas. Correlating the morphologic features with the immunophenotypic studies has permitted many of these neoplasms to be recognized on routine sections, even when marker studies are unavailable. Similarly, use of the monoclonal antileukocyte antibodies has identified as lymphomas many tumors that would have been otherwise classified as undifferentiated carcinomas or sarcomas. The pathologist's index of suspicion that a poorly differentiated neoplasm may be lymphoma is increased, and the spectrum of morphologic appearances of large cell lymphoma is better understood.

The general principles of immunophenotypic studies will be presented in this chapter, followed by a review of normal B and T cell differentiation. The immunophenotypes of the currently recognized lymphomas will be briefly reviewed. A panel of the antibodies that are of greatest practical use in the diagnosis of lymphomas will be presented in detail, with a discussion of their applications and pitfalls in interpretation. The chapter will conclude with specific clinical situations in which immunohistologic studies are helpful, with suggested panels of antibodies for use with each differential diagnosis.

IMMUNOPHENOTYPIC MARKERS

Individual B and T lymphoid cells can be recognized in cell suspensions or tissue sections by the presence of surface or cytoplasmic molecules (antigens) that can be detected using antibodies labeled with either fluorescent or enzymatic (immunohistochemical) methods. Using monoclonal antibodies and acetone-fixed cryostat sections, it has been possible to characterize many types of normal and neoplastic lymphoid cells (20–27,47,48). Information derived from this type of study forms the basis for most of the conclusions presented in this review.

During each stage of differentiation, lymphoid cells undergo characteristic changes in both morphology and surface antigen expression. These features can be used to identify both normal and neoplastic lymphoid cells in tissue sections. The constellation of antigens expressed at a given time by a cell is called its immunophenotype. The nomenclature for both the morphologic stages and the surface antigens can be confusing, since different authorities use different morphologic terms, and various monoclonal antibodies with different names detect the same antigens. Three international workshops have recently developed a standardized nomenclature for many of the antigens detected by more than one monoclonal antibody (43). Selected "cluster designations (CD)" are summarized in Table 1 and will be used in this review. (See Chapter 18 for a complete list.) Commonly used morphologic synonyms are summarized in Table 2 (32–34,42,50).

Immunophenotyping with monoclonal antibodies can be done using viable cell suspensions, frozen tissue sections, or paraffin-embedded sections. In general, acetone-fixed frozen sections provide the most convenient and reliable method for the pathologist to assess the phenotype of lymphoid cells in tissues. For cells in body fluids, particularly the peripheral blood, flow cytometry with fluorescent-labeled antibodies has many advantages, which are addressed in Chapter 18. For solid tissues, however, the suspension methods have several disadvantages. First, architectural information inherent in the tissue is lost when a suspension is made. Thus, concentrations of neoplastic cells in follicles cannot be appreciated, for example, and small aggregates of tumor cells in partially involved lymph nodes may be obscured in suspension by a large number of reactive cells. Second, in the process of preparing a suspension, particularly from fibrotic specimens, fragile, large neoplastic lymphoid cells may be preferentially destroyed, leaving a predominance of reactive lymphoid cells in the suspension. Finally, viable cell suspensions must be prepared immediately, and biopsies are often performed at inconvenient times. It is often more convenient to freeze representative tissue from such specimens for later study.

For the study of lymphocyte-associated antigens, frozen sections are more useful for immunohistochemical stains that paraffin sections. The majority of antigens recognized on lymphoid cells by currently available monoclonal antibodies are masked or destroyed by formalin fixation and paraffin embedding, but are readily detected in acetone-fixed frozen sections. Two important exceptions are cytoplasmic immunoglobulin, which may be better preserved in paraffin sections than in acetone-fixed frozen sections, and the leukocyte common antigen, which is often well preserved in paraffin sections and can be extremely

TABLE 1. *Selected monoclonal antibodies of interest in the study of lymphoid neoplasia*[a]

		Antigen	
CD	Common Names	MW(Kd)	Spectrum of Reactivity
CD1	T6,OKT6,Leu6,NA1/34	45	Thymocyte/Langerhans
CD2	T11,OKT11,9.6, Leu5	50	Pan T (E Rosette receptor)
CD3	T3,OKT3,Leu4	19-29	Pan T (T receptor related)
CD4	T4,OKT4,Leu3	55	T helper (MHC class II reactive)
CD5	OKT1, Leu1	67	Pan T, rare B
CD6	T12, TU33	120	Pan T, rare B
CD7	Leu9, TU14, 3A1	41	Pan T
CD8	T8,OKT8,Leu2	32	T cytotoxic/suppressor (MHC class reactive)
CD9	J2, BA2	24	T, B, myeloid
CD10	J5, BA3, VilA1	100	Pre-B, pre-T, GC (CALLA)
CD15	Leu M1, anti X-Hapten	—	Granulocyte, monocyte, RS cells, epithelial cells
CD19	B4	95	Pan B (not plasma cell)
CD20	B1	35	Pan B (not plasma cell)
CD21	B2	145	Restricted B:PB,GC,MZ;FDC
CD22	Leu14, (To15), SHCL1	135	Pan B
CD23	Tu1, Blast 2	45	Restricted B: MZ,?GC,not PB
CD24	BA1	45,55,65	PanB; granulocyte; plasma cell
CD25	TAC	55	Activated T + B (IL2 receptor)
CD30	Ki-1	90-110	RS cells, activated T and B cells
CD45	LCA,T29/33,PD7/26	220	Leukocyte common antigen (T,B,M)
—	TdT	—	B + T precursors, cortical thymocyte
—	HLA-DR (Ia-like)	—	B (not PC), activated T(MHC IIag)

[a]Abbreviations: CALLA = common acute lymphoblastic leukemia antigen, CD = cluster designation, GC = germinal center, FDC = follicular dendritic cells, IL2 = interleukin-2, Kd = kilodaltons, MHC = major histocompatibility complex, MZ = mantle zone, PB = peripheral blood, PC = plasma cell, RS = Reed-Sternberg, TdT = terminal deoxynucleotidyl transferase. (See complete listing in Chapter 18.)

TABLE 2. *Nomenclature of lymphoid cells*

Rappaport	Lukes and Collins Working Formulation	Kiel
Well-differentiated lymphocyte	Small lymphocyte (B or T)	Lymphocyte (B or T)
Plasmacytoid lymphocyte	Plasmacytoid lymphocyte (B)	Immunocyte (B)
Poorly-differentiated lymphocyte	Small cleaved FCC[a] (B)	Centrocyte (B)
Histiocyte	Large cleaved FCC (B)	Centrocyte (B)
Histiocyte	Large noncleaved FCC (B)	Centroblast (B)
Histiocyte	Immunoblast (B or T)	Lymphoblast (B)
Undifferentiated cell	Small noncleaved FCC (B)	Lymphoblast (B)
Lymphoblast	Convoluted lymphocyte (T)	Lymphoblast, convoluted (T) Lymphoblast un-classified.

[a]FCC = Follicular center cell. This modifier is omitted in the Working Formulation terminology, as is the lineage designation (B or T).

useful in the diagnosis of poorly differentiated malignancies when frozen tissue is unavailable (54).

The study of immunohistochemical stains on frozen sections has several pitfalls that must be recognized to be avoided. First, with some antibodies, there appears to be an unavoidable level of background staining. This is most noticeable with immunoglobulins, particularly IgG, and probably reflects normal tissue concentrations of these proteins. Staining of connective tissue, necrotic areas, and intercellular material may sometimes be seen with antibodies to the leukocyte common antigen for reasons that are unclear. Background staining is less of a problem with most other lymphocyte-associated antibodies. A second problem is that the morphologic detail on acetone-fixed frozen sections is usally not good, even with hematoxylin counterstains. Difficulty may be encountered in the morphologic identification of the cells that react with a particular antibody. Thus, on a frozen section, it is often impossible to be certain whether a single positive cell is a part of the tumor in question or a reactive cell. Determinations of positivity or negativity are best made on groups or populations of cells with this technique. Finally, enumeration of cells is difficult in tissue sections; this technique is more suited to analysis of the architectural distribution of cell types than to quantitation.

Despite these limitations, frozen section immunohistochemistry remains for the present the most reliable and practical method for immunophenotyping lymphoid cells in the anatomic pathology laboratory. Several laboratories are now working on developing antibodies to formalin-resistant antigens or epitopes, so that in the near future, detection of lymphoid cell subsets in paraffin sections will likely be more reliable.

GENOTYPIC MARKERS

Although this chapter deals with immunohistologic techniques, no discussion of lymphoma diagnosis is complete without some mention of gene rearrangement. Although clinical applications of molecular genetic techniques are still in their early stages, these techniques have much to contribute to our understanding of lymphomas and therefore will be explained briefly here (18).

Differentiation of the B cell involves rearrangements of the genes involved in immunoglobulin production. The genes that encode the constant and variable regions of the immunoglobulin heavy and light chain molecules are located far apart on the chromosomes in germline cells. To produce RNA for an immunoglobulin protein, many thousands of base pairs of DNA must be deleted from the genome to bring the different portions of the immunoglobulin gene together. These rearrangements change the position of restriction sites on the DNA: points at which restriction endonucleases cleave the DNA. Thus, fragments produced by digesting B cell DNA with these enzymes will be of a different size than those produced by digesting non-B cell (germline) DNA and will migrate differently in an electrophoresis gel. When radiolabeled DNA probes (cloned segments of DNA produced by bacteria), which are complementary to specific portions of the immunoglobulin gene, are applied to such a gel, they will specifically mark the position of the immunoglobulin gene, which can be demonstrated on an autoradiograph. The exact size and therefore position on the gel (Southern blot) of each immunoglobulin gene fragment is unique to an individual B cell; thus, this technique provides not only a specific marker for B cells, but also a true marker for monoclonality (2,10,12,31).

A process of gene rearrangement analogous to that seen in the B cell system also occurs in T cell differentiation. This process involves the DNA encoding a T-cell-specific surface molecule that serves as the T cell receptor for antigen, analogous to surface immunoglobulin (SIg) on B cells. As in the B cell system, the size of restriction fragments of the DNA encoding the T cell receptor gene are specific for a single clone of T cells. Thus T cell receptor gene rearrangement is a specific marker for T cells, and also a true marker for monoclonality in T cells (1,55).

PATHWAYS OF LYMPHOCYTE DIFFERENTIATION

There are two distinct phases of development within both the T and B lymphoid cell lines: antigen-independent and antigen-dependent (Figs. 1 and 2). (See also Chapter 10.) Antigen-independent proliferation and differentiation occur in the primary lymphoid organs—bursa-equivalent (?bone marrow) and thymus—without exposure to antigen. These stages occur during fetal and neonatal development, and possibly to a lesser extent, throughout adult life. This process takes the lymphocyte from a stem cell to a mature, so-called "virgin" T or B cell, that is capable of responding to antigen but has not yet been exposed to it. On encountering an antigen that fits its surface receptor, the virgin T or B cell undergoes "blast transformation," proliferates, and differentiates into an antigen-specific effector cell. This reaction also generates antigen-specific "memory," which enables cells to produce an accelerated response on re-exposure to the same antigen. Thus, in both T and B cell systems, there are several stages of development at which proliferation occurs, as well as several resting stages (16,32,58).

B Cell Differentiation

Antigen-independent

The rearrangement of the immunoglobulin heavy chain gene is the earliest sign of B cell differentiation. The earliest recognizable B cell is one that has rearranged its immunoglobulin gene, but does not make immunoglobulin (Ig). Cells at this stage have been called B cell precursors or pre-pre-B cells (31). At the next stage of development, pre-B cells make cytoplasmic μ heavy chain, but they do not make light chain and do not express surface Ig. Both types of cells are morphologically lymphoblasts, with dispersed chromatin and visible but not prominent nucleoli. They contain the nuclear enzyme, terminal deoxynucleotidyl transferase (TdT), and express HLA-DR (Class II histocompatibility antigens, Ia) and the common acute lymphoblastic leukemia antigen (CALLA, CD10) (30,40). Some pan-B cell antigens (CD19,CD20) may be expressed at this stage (43,45,Chapter 10). Cells with these morphologic and immunologic features can be found in normal and regenerating bone marrow.

The next stage in antigen-independent B cell differentiation is that of an early B cell. The normal location of this cell is unknown. The early B cell is CALLA positive and TdT negative, and expresses a complete surface IgM molecule, with both a heavy and a light chain. Each individual B cell is committed to a single light chain, either kappa or lambda, and all of its progeny will express the same light chain.

The last stage of antigen-independent B cell differentiation is the mature (virgin) B cell, which expresses both surface IgM and IgD, lacks TdT and CALLA, and is capable of responding to antigen. These mature B cells are morphologically small lymphocytes, which

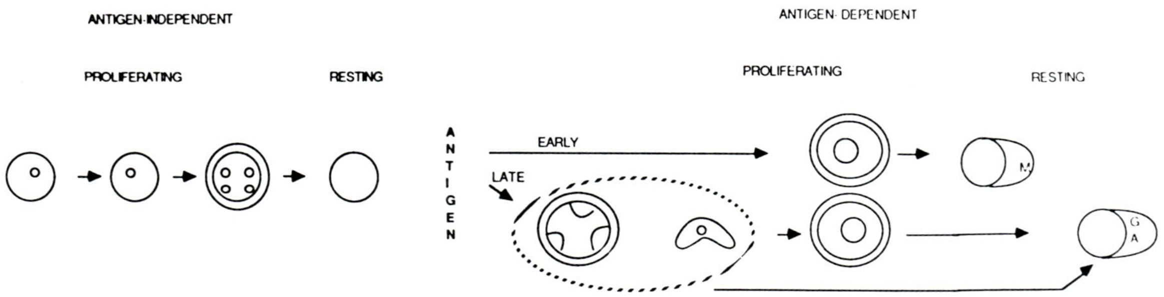

ANTIGEN-INDEPENDENT

ANTIGEN DEPENDENT

PROLIFERATING   RESTING   EARLY   LATE   ANTIGEN   PROLIFERATING   RESTING

NORMAL CELL	B-PRECURSOR	PRE B	EARLY B	MATURE B "VIRGIN"	CENTROBLAST	CENTROCYTE	B-IMMUNOBLAST	PLASMACYTOID LYMPHOCYTE	PLASMA CELL
LOCATION	BONE MARROW		?	1°FOLLICLE	GERMINAL CENTER		LYMPH NODE PARACORTEX MEDULLA	LYMPH NODE MEDULLA	BONE MARROW
Ig Gene	+	+	+	+	+	+	+	+	+
LCA	+/-	+	+	+	+	+	+	+	+
TdT	+	+	-	-	-	-	-	-	+/-
CALLA(CD10)	+	+	+/-	-	-/+	-/+	-	-	-
HLA-DR	-/+	+	+	-	+/-	-	+	+	-/+
CIg	-	+(µ)	-	-	-/+	-/+	+	+	+
SIg	-	-	+(M)	+(M+D)	+(M/G)	+(M/G)	M (early) G/A (late)	+(M)	G or A
B4 (CD19)	+	+	+	+	+	+	M (early) G/A (late)	+/-	-
B1 (CD20)	-/+	+/-	+	+	+	+	+/-	+/-	-
Leu14(CD22)	-/+	-/+	+	-/+	-/+	+/-	+/-	+/-	-
B2(CD21)	-	-	-/+	+	-/+	+/-	-	+/-	-
T1(CD5)	-	-	-	+		+/-	-	-	-

NEOPLASM	B-PRECURSOR & PRE-B ALL/LBL	BURKITT'S TUMOR	B-CLL/SL	FOLLICULAR LYMPHOMA (Both Cell Types) CENTROBLASTIC LYMPHOMA / CENTROCYTIC LYMPHOMA	B-IMMUNOBLASTIC LYMPHOMA	IMMUNO-CYTOMA	PLASMACYTOMA MYELOMA

FIG. 1. Hypothetical scheme of B cell differentiation. Location and phenotype of normal B cell stages is indicated below. Neoplasms thought to correspond to each stage are indicated at bottom. Reprinted with permission from Harris, N. L., Lymphoma 1987: An interim approach to diagnosis and classification. In: *Pathology Annual 1987*, edited by P.P. Rosen and R.E. Fechner. Appleton-Century-Crofts, East Norwalk, CT.

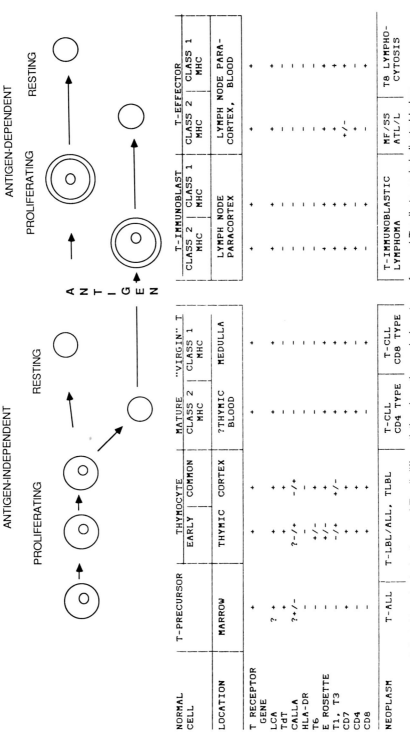

FIG. 2. Hypothetical scheme of T cell differentiation. Location and phenotype of normal T cell stages is indicated below. Neoplasms thought to correspond to each stage are listed at bottom. Reprinted with permission from Harris, N. L., Lymphoma 1987: An interim approach to diagnosis and classification. In: *Pathology Annual 1987*, edited by P.P. Rosen and R.E. Fechner. Appleton-Century-Crofts, East Norwalk, CT.

probably circulate in the blood and also reside in primary lymphoid follicles and follicle mantle zones (so-called recirculating B cells) (16). In addition to SIg, the mature B cell expresses pan-B cell antigens, HLA-DR, complement receptors and possibly the pan-T cell antigen, Leu 1 (CD5) (48). The earlier stages of B cell antigen-independent differentiation are proliferative stages, giving rise to large numbers of immunocompetent mature B cells. The mature B cell, however, is presumably in a resting stage until it encounters antigen.

Antigen-dependent

On encountering antigen, the mature B cell transforms again into a proliferating cell. Antigen-dependent B-cell proliferation and differentiation can apparently take two forms. In the primary immune response, a virgin B cell may transform directly into an immunoblast, proliferate, and differentiate into an IgM-secreting plasmacytoid lymphocyte or plasma cell, producing the IgM antibody of the primary immune response (58). The B-immunoblasts have surface IgM and acquire cytoplasmic IgM, as they mature toward plasma cells. During blast transformation, SIgD is lost, as are complement receptors (38, 46). With maturation to plasma cells, most surface antigens are lost, including pan-B cell antigens, HLA-DR, and the leukocyte common antigen, CD45 (17,21). The immunoblastic and plasma cell reaction of the early immune response occurs in the paracortex and medulla of lymph nodes (52).

In the late primary or secondary immune response, the B cell encounters antigen presented on the processes of follicular dendritic cells, and the germinal center reaction occurs (39,58). The germinal center contains two morphological types of B cells—centroblasts (large noncleaved follicle center cells) and centrocytes (cleaved follicle center cells) (Fig. 3A). The germinal center reaction gives rise to the better-fitting IgG antibody of the later primary or secondary immune response and also gives rise to B cell "memory"—the ability to respond more quickly on second exposure to antigen. The switch from IgM to IgG or A production (heavy chain class switching) occurs in individual B cells (53) and appears to involve deletion of the gene for μ (IgM) heavy chain. The cell continues to express the same light chain (kappa or lambda).

The immunophenotype of normal germinal center B cells is difficult to determine, since germinal centers are complex structures that contain in addition to B cells, T cells and follicular dendritic cells, with immunoglobulin trapped on their processes (Figs. 3B–D). While mantle-zone B cells are IgM- and IgD-positive, most germinal center cells lack IgD, and many appear to have undergone heavy chain class switching, expressing surface and/or cytoplasmic IgG or IgA (4,20,23,47,48), while others express IgM (Fig. 3B). Some germinal center B cells appear to be Ig-negative, but most express pan-B cell antigens. Most germinal centers contain a dense, apparently extracellular meshwork of immunoglobulin-containing material (Fig. 3B). This is thought to represent secreted antibody associated with dendritic cell processes. Using one monoclonal antibody (47), CALLA can be readily detected on most normal germinal center cells, while with another (25), they stain faintly or not at all. Some follicular center B cells and follicular dentritic cells have C3d complement receptors, that can be detected with monoclonal antibodies, for example, B2 (CD21) (28) (Fig. 3C). Another monoclonal antibody, anti-DRC (Dako) preferentially stains dendritic cells (48). Numerous T cells, predominantly of the helper phenotype, are also found in most germinal centers (20,41) (Fig. 3D). Rare B cells, expressing the T-associated antigen, Leu 1 (CD5), have been described in germinal centers (8).

With differentiation to the plasma cell stage, there is sequential loss of C3d receptors (B2), surface immunoglobulin, pan-B cell antigens, HLA-DR antigen, and leukocyte common antigen, and cytoplasmic IgG or IgA accumulates (21,46).

T Cell Differentiation

Antigen-independent

As in the B cell system, the earliest stages of T cell differentiation involve characteristic rearrangements of the DNA encoding the antigen receptor molecule. The earliest antigen-independent stages of T cell differentiation appear to occur in the bone marrow; later stages occur in the thymic cortex. Cortical thymocytes, particularly those in the outer cortex, have the morphologic appearance of lymphoblasts; they contain the nuclear enzyme, TdT, and have a unique constellation of surface antigens that appear to be acquired sequentially in early differentiation. These include the E-rosette receptor (CD2), CD7, the thymocyte-Langerhans cell antigen CD1 (T6), both helper- and suppressor-associated antigens CD4 and CD8, and to a variable extent, pan-T cell antigens (CD3 and CD5). Proliferation and maturation in the thymus gives rise to mature (virgin) T cells, which have the morphologic appearance of small lymphocytes. They lack TdT and CD1 and express either (but not both) CD4 or CD8, as well as pan-T antigens (5). The exact location of mature T cells is unknown, but cells with this phenotype are found in the thymic medulla.

Antigen-dependent

On encountering antigen, mature T cells transform into immunoblasts, the proliferative stage of antigen-dependent T cell differentiation. Antigen-dependent T cell reactions occur in the paracortex of lymph nodes and the periarteriolar lymphoid sheath of the spleen (16,32,58). The T immunoblasts are large cells with prominent nucleoli and basophilic cytoplasm, which may be indistinguishable from B immunoblasts. In contrast to T lymphoblasts (thymocytes), T immunoblasts are TdT and CD1 negative, strongly express pan-T cell antigens, and continue to express *either* CD4 or CD8, but not both. Resting T cells and thymocytes do not usually express HLA-DR antigens, but activated or proliferating T cells may express HLA-DR. The T immunoblastic reaction produces antigen-specific effector T cells of either CD4 or CD8 type, as well as T cell memory. Although in general, T effector cells of the CD 4 type act as helper cells and those of the CD8 type as suppressor cells *in vitro*, both types can be cytotoxic. The CD4 cells recognize HLA-DR (Class II) histocompatibility loci on target cells, whereas CD8 cells recognize HLA-ABC (Class I) antigens for cytotoxicity (36,51) (See Chapter 7). Fully differentiated T effector cells appear to be small lymphocytes, morphologically similar to other nonproliferating lymphocytes of either T or B type.

IMMUNOLOGICAL PHENOTYPES OF LYMPHOMAS

Lymphomas should be classified according to their normal counterpart in the immune system, as other tumors are classified according to their probable normal counterpart. Such a classification should predict natural history and clinical behavior. Although we do not

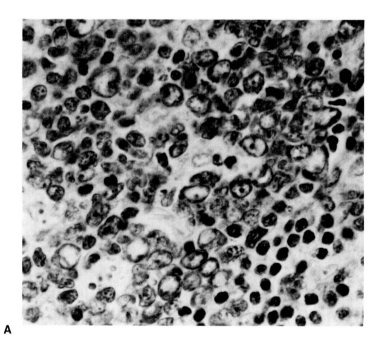

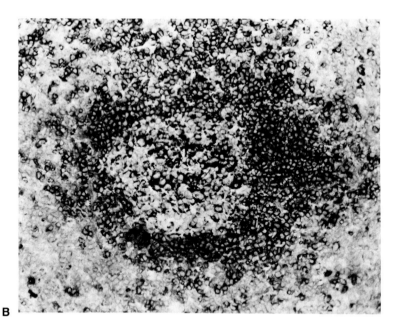

FIG. 3. Normal germinal centers. **A.** Giemsa stain showing centroblasts (large noncleaved cells) and centrocytes (cleaved cells). **B.** Immunoperoxidase stain, mu heavy chain, showing positive mantle zone lymphocytes, extracellular/cytoplasmic staining in follicle, and some negative follicle center cells. Similar staining is seen with antibodies to kappa and lambda. (*Figure continues.*)

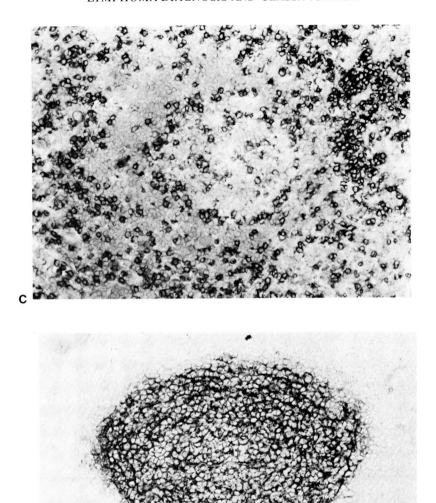

FIG. 3. (*continued*). **C**. Anti-Leu4 (CD3) showing numerous T cells within and around germinal center. **D**. Anti-B2 (CD21), showing striking dendritic pattern as well as cellular staining of lymphoid cells, particularly in the mantle (**A**. Giemsa, × 788, **B**. × 200, **C**. × 200, **D**. × 200).

have enough information about either the immune system or the lymphomas to permit this to be done in all cases, the normal counterpart of many lymphomas can be postulated with reasonable certainty. Note that the term normal counterpart does not imply the cell stage of origin. It is currently possible to determine the stage of differentiation of many lymphomas but this does not mean that neoplastic transformation necessarily occurred in a cell that had reached that stage. It may well be that neoplastic transformation occurs in a primitive cell and that the level of differentiation achieved by the tumor depends on a variety of factors, such as a specific oncogene translocation (12). Nonetheless, understanding the relationship of the lymphomas to their normal counterparts can be useful in understanding the biological behavior of these neoplasms.

Using a combination of morphologic features, immunologic studies, and clinical information, at least 17 different types of lymphoma are now recognized, in addition to Hodgkin's disease. These lymphomas differ as much from one another as they do from Hodgkin's disease and should be recognized as distinct clinicopathological entities. Although most of these entities are recognized in most classification schemes, the different classifications group and divide them in various ways (32–34,42,50). For this reason, it is most practical simply to list the lymphomas that can be recognized at present, giving synonyms where appropriate to place them in the various existing classifications (19). The morphologic and immunologic features of the major categories of lymphoproliferative disorders are summarized in Figures 1 and 2 and in Table 3.

The lymphomas are listed in order of their putative positions in the B and T cell differentiation pathway. Lymphomas and lymphoid leukemias are lumped together; the distinction between them is artificial, since lymphomas can have a leukemic phase, and diseases usually classified as leukemias may not have circulating malignant cells in all cases (See Chapter 10).

TABLE 3. *Major categories of lymphoproliferative diseases recognizable by morphology and immunologic markers*

Name	Morphologic features	Markers
B CELL NEOPLASMS		
B-Precursor lymphoblastic lymphoma/leukemia	Lymphoblasts: medium-sized cells, inconspicuous nucleoli, scant cytoplasm	TdT$^+$ CALLA$^+$ Cmu$^+$ (Ig gene rearrangement) Pan B$^+$
Burkitt's and Burkitt-like lymphomas	Medium-sized cells, multiple nucleoli, basophilic cytoplasm; "starry sky," high mitotic rate	SIgM$^+$ CALLA$^+$ Pan B$^+$
Small lymphocytic lymphoma/B-chronic lymphocytic leukemia	Small lymphocytes	SIgM$^+$ D$^+$ CD5 (CLL) Pan B$^+$
Immunocytoma (lymphoplasmacytoid lymphoma)	Plasmacytoid lymphocytes plasma cells, lymphocytes rare immunoblasts, follicular center cells	SIgM$^+$ CIg$^+$ (M-component), Pan B$^+$
Centrocytic lymphoma	Small cleaved follicular center cells	SIgM$^+$D$^+$CD5 Pan B$^+$
Germinal center lymphomas (centroblastic/centrocytic)	Mixture of centroblasts and centrocytes, usually follicular pattern	SIg$^+$ CALLA$^+$ Pan B$^+$

Large cell lymphoma (centroblastic, immuno-blastic)	Monomorphous large cells with prominent nucleoli and basophilic cytoplasm; high mitotic rate	SIg$^+$ ($^+$CIg); Pan B$^+$
Hairy cell leukemia	Small lymphocytes, "hairy" cytoplasm, low mitotic rate	SIg$^+$ (multiple heavy chains), Pan B$^+$
Plasmacytoma, myeloma	Plasma cells, plasma-blasts	CIg$^+$; PanB$^-$, Ia$^+$, LCA$^-$
T CELL NEOPLASMS		
T-lymphoblastic lymphoma/ leukemia	Lymphoblasts: medium-sized cells, ± nuclear convolu-tion, inconspicuous nucleoli	TdT$^+$ PanT$^+$ T4,T6,T8$^{+\prime}$
T-CLL	Small lymphoid cells$^\pm$ convoluted nuclei, granular cytoplasm	Pan T$^+$ T4$^+$ or 8$^+$ Ia$^+$ TdT
Large cell lymphomas	Monomorphous large cells with prominent nucleoli; may have clear cytoplasm	TdT$^-$, panT$^+$ CD4$^+$ or 8$^+$
Adult T cell lymphoma/ leukemia (endemic)	Variable proportions of atypical lymphocytes and immunoblasts	Pan T$^+$ CD4$^+$ TdT$^-$,HTLV$^+$ CD7$^+$
Nonendemic pleomorphic T cell lymphoma	Like ATL/L	Pan T$^+$ CD4$^+$ or CD8$^+$ CD7$^+$
Sezary's syndrome and mycosis fungoides	Small and large lymphoid cells with "cerebriform" nuclei	Pan T$^+$ CD4$^+$ TdT$^-$ CD7$^+$
T8 Lymphoproliferative disease	Small lymphoid cells, granular cytoplasm	Pan T$^+$, CD8$^+$
NEOPLASMS OF UNCERTAIN LINEAGE		
Hodgkin's disease	Reed-Sternberg cells Reactive cells	Mixed T&B cells RS cells; LeuM1 + Ia+LCA−
Angiocentric lymphoma	Variable proportions of atypical lymphocytes and immunoblasts, vascular invasion & necrosis	?pan T$^+$ T cell receptor gene rearranged

See text for abbreviations.

ANTIGENS USEFUL IN HEMATOPATHOLOGY

Knowing the range of expression of antigenic markers by normal and neoplastic lymph-oid cells, it is possible to predict the clinical situations in which various monoclonal anti-bodies will be useful. In practical diagnostic applications, a relatively limited panel of antibodies is needed. These markers will be presented here in approximate order of their diagnostic usefulness.

Immunoglobulin

At most stages of differentiation, B lymphocytes have immunoglobulin molecules on their surfaces (SIg). Each normal B cell produces immunoglobulin of a single light chain

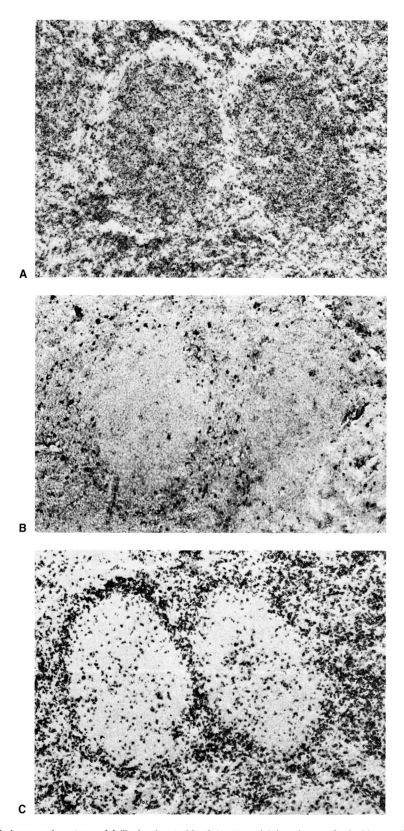

FIG. 4. Immunophenotype of follicular (centroblastic/centrocytic) lymphoma. **A**. Anti-kappa light chain, showing staining of cells in and between follicles. **B**. Anti-lambda light chain, showing only rare positive cells. **C**. Anti-Leu4 (CD3) shwoing numerous positive cells both within and between follicles. (*Figure continues.*)

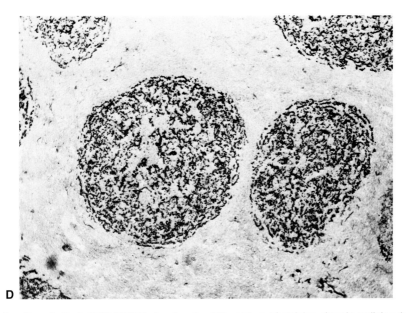

FIG. 4. (*continued*). **D**. Anti-B2 (CD21) showing dendritic pattern of staining sharply outlining the follicles (× 79).

type kappa (K) or lambda (L). Several different heavy chain classes—delta (D), gamma (G), alpha (A), or mu (M)—may be produced by a single B cell either simultaneously or at different developmental stages, but they all have the same type of light chain. With differentiation toward plasma cells, SIg is lost, and immunoglobulin accumulates in the cytoplasm and is secreted (CIg). Normally, populations of human B cells carry K or L light chains in approximately a 2 : 1 ratio. Neoplastic populations arising from a single progenitor cell (i.e., clones) should contain only a single light chain, K or L. Thus, not only can immunoglobulin be used to identify cells as B lymphocytes, but the presence of light-chain restriction (monotypic or "monoclonal" Ig) is presumptive evidence of neoplasia. The phenomenon of light chain restriction makes immunoglobulin the most useful cell marker in diagnostic hematopathology. An additional factor is that over 80% of lymphomas in the U.S. and Europe are of B cell type, so that a marker that can identify monoclonal B cell neoplasms is valuable in the majority of cases.

There are several pitfalls in interpreting sections stained with antibodies to immunoglobulin. First, since immunoglobulin is normally present in plasma, there may be a high level of "real" background staining due to immunoglobulin present in the tissues. This is particularly true for IgG, may be a problem with kappa and lambda, and is less of a problem with IgM. Experience is required to interpret such sections. Second, comparison of the slides stained for kappa and lambda is of paramount importance in interpreting immunoglobulin staining. Sections stained with each antibody must be incubated simultaneously, and antibody dilutions must be adjusted so that staining of normal cells with these antibodies is identical. Comparison of sections stained for kappa and lambda are controls for each other. Only if there is a difference between the two is it possible to be certain that the cells staining are neoplastic (Figs. 4A and B). Although not absolutely necessary, simultaneous evaluation of sections stained with antibodies to heavy chains can be helpful. If staining for one heavy chain is identical to one of the two light chains, it supports the interpretation of monotypic Ig staining. Finally, cytoplasmic immunoglobulin may not be detected as well in frozen as in paraffin sections. Apparently, acetone is a better fixative for membrane antigens than for cytoplasmic antigens; myelomas or plasmacytoid lymphomas may show very indistinct staining on frozen sections, but clear cytoplasmic staining on paraffin sections. Thus, in a neoplasm with mature plasma cells, if definite Ig staining is not seen on frozen sections, it is advisable to stain paraffin sections as well.

Pan-Leukocyte Antibodies

Several commercially available monoclonal antibodies detect a 220 Kd antigen (T200, CD45) said to be present on all hematopoietic cell lines (3). This antigen appears to be analogous to the murine leukocyte common antigen (LCA). These antibodies cannot distinguish benign from malignant lymphoid cells or lymphoid cells from myeloid or monocytic cells, but can be very useful in distinguishing lymphomas and leukemic infiltrates from nonhematologic neoplasms (3,54). This antigen is most reliably detected in frozen sections. In paraffin-embedded sections, DAKO-LCA also stains lymphoid cells. It works most reliably on B5 fixed tissues, but can also be used on formalin-fixed material. In some poorly fixed tissues, DAKO-LCA does not stain at all. Most troublesome are some large cell lymphomas (particularly B immunoblastic), as well as granulocytic sarcomas which will not be stained in paraffin sections, even when lymphocytes in the same tissue are positive. It should also be emphasized that LCA is not present on the majority of plasmacytomas and in multiple myeloma; thus, it cannot be used to distinguish anaplastic myeloma from carcinoma (21). Reed-Sternberg cells and mononuclear variants are also negative (14).

Pan B Cell Monoclonal Antibodies (CD19, 20, 22)

B1 (CD20), B4 (CD19) and Leu 14 (CD22) detect antigens expressed on normal B cells and pre-B cells, but not on plasma cells. Pan B antibodies cannot distinguish benign from malignant B cells, but may be useful in distinguishing between Ig negative B cell lymphomas and undifferentiated carcinoma or other nonlymphoid tumors. They are detected in frozen but not in paraffin sections (43,45).

From the pre-B cell stage to the pre-plasma stage, CD20 is present on B cells but is lost on differentiation to a mature plasma cell (46). CD19 appears slightly earlier than B1. The spectrum of CD22 reactivity appears to be similar but not identical to that of B1 (43,45, 46). The three antibodies differ in their staining intensity tissue sections: B4 (CD19) and B1 (CD20) frequently give poorly localized, faint staining, while that with Leu-14 (CD22) is usually strong and clear. Neoplastic lymphoid cells variably express CD20 and CD22; large cell lymphomas in particular may lack one or the other antigen.

Anti-B2 (CD21) detects an antigen present on peripheral blood, primary follicle and mantle zone lymphocytes. This antigen is variably expressed by follicular center B cells, and strongly expressed by follicular dendritic cells (FDC, also known as dendritic reticulum cells or DRC) (Fig. 4C). Recent evidence indicates that B2 is the C3d receptor and functions as a receptor for Epstein-Barr virus (EBV) (28,38). This antigen is acquired later and lost earlier in B cell differentiation than the pan-B cell antigens. It is not useful in the primary diagnosis of B cell neoplasia, but has proven to be of interest in the subclassification of these disorders. Cases of B-chronic lymphocytic leukemia (B-CLL) and small

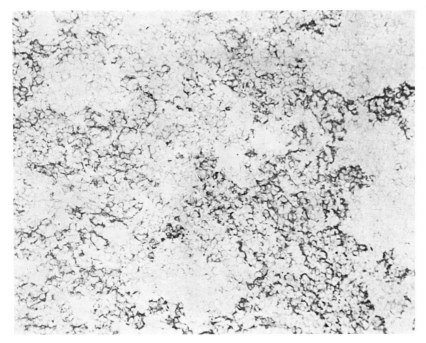

FIG. 5. Centrocytic lymphoma stained with anti-B2 (CD21), showing irregular pattern of dendritic staining, in contrast to sharply follicular pattern seen in centroblastic/centrocytic lymphoma (× 250).

lymphocytic lymphoma usually express B2, and the pattern in tissue sections is consistent with membrane staining. Centrocytic (diffuse small cleaved cell or intermediate lymphocytic) lymphomas also show membrane staining for CD21, but in addition, contain irregular aggregates of FDC, which are seen as a meshwork of processes with anti B2 (Fig. 5). These cells are also seen with anti-DRC antibody. Centroblastic/centrocytic lymphomas (follicular lymphomas) also contain FDC, but in a sharply follicular pattern (Fig. 4C). Thus, the staining of both neoplastic B cells and accessory cells with anti-B2 are characteristic for different subsets of B cell lymphomas.

With the use of pan B cell antibodies, it has become apparent that a substantial minority (10% to 20%) of both follicular and diffuse B cell lymphomas do not express Ig (13,24, 25). The B cell nature of some of these cases has been confirmed by demonstration of Ig gene rearrangement (10).

Pan-T Cell Monoclonal Antibodies

Sheep Erythrocyte Rosette Receptor (CD2)

Originally detected using suspensions of viable cells, this receptor can now be detected using monoclonal antibodies (T11a, Leu 5). This receptor is present on the majority of normal mature T cells as well as on most thymic T cells, but is absent from some early T cells. The E rosette receptor cannot be used to distinguish benign from malignant T cell populations. It can be detected in frozen sections but not in paraffin sections.

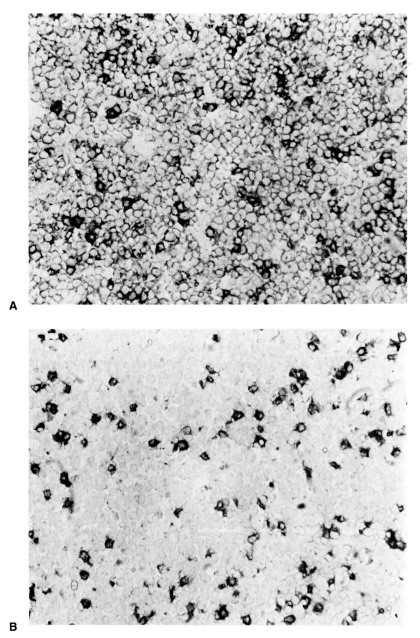

FIG. 6. Lymph node involved by B-chronic lymphocytic leukemia, IgM,D,Kappa type. **A.** Anti-Leu1 (CD5), pan-T cell antibody, showing faint staining of most cells and strong staining of a few cells. **B.** Anti-Leu4 (CD3), a T-cell specific antibody, showing only scattered strongly-stained, presumably reactive, T cells. This pattern of reactivity is characteristic of both B-CLL and centrocytic lymphoma (× 313).

CD5 (T1, Leu-1)

This antigen is present on normal peripheral blood and thymic T cells. It is also present on the cells of the majority of the cases of B cell chronic lymphocytic leukemia and centrocytic (diffuse small cleaved cell or intermediate lymphocytic) lymphomas (22,25, 48). It is unknown whether this phenomenon represents anomalous expression of antigen by neoplastic B cells or whether these neoplasms derive from small populations of normal CD5 positive B cells. Most observers favor the latter hypothesis. Rare B cells, expressing the CD5 antigen, have been detected in suspensions of lymph nodes and localized to the germinal center (8). Other writers have reported faint staining of normal primary follicle and mantle zone B cells with some anti CD5 antibodies (48). Normal peripheral blood B cells lack CD5. Since two quite distinct B cell neoplasms express this antigen, it is possible that there is more than one CD5 positive B cell subset.

In practice, staining of neoplastic B cells is usually fainter than that of benign T cells present in the tumor (Fig. 6). Comparison of sections stained with anti CD5 antibody with sections stained for a T-cell-specific antigen, such as CD3, is often necessary to confirm staining of the neoplastic B cells for CD5. The antibody is useful in detecting T cells, but perhaps more useful in subclassifying B cell lymphomas.

CD3 (OK-T3, Leu-4)

This antigen is apparently T cell specific and has not been reported to react with normal or neoplastic B cells. (Purkinje cells have been reported to stain with some anti-CD3 antibodies.) In frozen sections, Leu-4 produces good staining and is a useful T cell marker for routine screening. Like the E rosette receptor, this antigen cannot be used to distinguish benign from malignant T cell populations and cannot be demonstrated in paraffin sections. To detect Leu-1$^+$ B cell lymphomas, Leu-1 and Leu-4 must be used in parallel.

CD7 (3A1, Tu14, Leu 9)

This antigen is expressed on T cells at an early stage of development, including all thymocytes. Mature T cells also express the antigen, with the exception of a subset of CD4 cells that provide help to helper effector cells, so-called "helpers of help" (51). Other CD4 cells as well as virtually all normal peripheral blood CD8 cells express CD7. Antibodies to this antigen are useful in evaluating lymphoblastic lymphomas and some mature T cell neoplasms, which may lack other pan T cell antigens but often express CD7 (7). Mycosis fungoides cells are CD4$^+$ and CD7$^-$.

T Cell Subsets (CD4, CD8)

Like the pan T cell antigens, the T cell subset antigens are present on both benign and malignant T cell populations, and cannot reliably distinguish neoplastic from reactive T cells. The proportions of T cells reactive with CD4 or CD8 in normal blood and lymph nodes have been established in many institutions; however, the CD4/CD8 ratio may be dramatically altered in various nonneoplastic states. Thus, "subset restriction" is not a reliable indicator of monoclonality. Conversely, many T-lymphoblastic lymphomas co-express CD4 and CD8, so that lack of subset restriction does not indicate a benign lesion (56). It has been reported that many T cell lymphomas have anomalous phenotypes; that is, they lack one or another of the pan T antigens or may not express a subset antigen. In some cases, this phenomenon may be useful in distinguishing normal from neoplastic T cell populations (7).

The CD4 antigen is also present on normal monocytes and macrophages. T cell subset antigens are readily detected in frozen but not in paraffin sections. Staining for CD4 is frequently faint and diffuse; staining for CD8 is usually clearer.

The diagnosis of T cell neoplasia by immunohistological methods is difficult for several reasons: (a) none of the available monoclonal antibodies can distinguish between normal and neoplastic T cells; (b) many nonneoplastic T cells may be present in lymphomas of either T or non-T cell type; and (c) many T cell lymphomas are morphologically polymorphous. To diagnose a T cell lymphoma with confidence, T cell markers must be demonstrated on a homogeneous population of cytologically malignant cells. Given the ubiquity and wide range of morphology of reactive T cells and the morphologic heterogeneity of many putative T cell lymphomas, these conditions may be difficult to meet. The application of the Southern blot technique for detection of clonal T cell receptor gene rearrangement to the diagnosis of T cell lymphoma may help to elucidate this confusing group of neoplasms.

Terminal Deoxynucleotidyl Transferase (TdT)

TdT is a unique CNA polymerase enzyme that can add deoxynucleotides to the end of a DNA molecule without a template. Its biological function is unknown. Found chiefly in the thymus, it was initially thought to be a marker for T cell precursors, but subsequent studies have shown it to be present in bone marrow B-cell precursors as well (30). As a marker for lymphoblasts, TdT is most useful in the diagnosis of acute leukemia and lymphoblastic lymphoma. It is also present in the thymocytes of thymomas and in the blast cells of rare cases of acute myeloid leukemia. It can be detected by a biochemical method, by immuno-fluorescence on imprints or frozen sections, and by immunoperoxidase on frozen sections. Fixation is by cold methanol, rather than acetone, and sections should be placed in fixative immediately after cutting. The antibody is available only in kit form for immunofluorescence; it can be adapted for immunoperoxidase by substituting for the fluoresceine-conjugated antibody. The staining is nuclear, rather than cytoplasmic or surface, and is usually faint.

"Common ALL Antigen (CALLA)" (CD10)

Initially discovered on the cells of a case of B-precursor ALL and thought to be a true tumor antigen, CALLA has since been identified on a small fraction of normal bone marrow cells (30,40). Among the acute leukemias, it is most consistently present on "common" ALL cells; recent studies have found reactivity with some T-ALL's and T lymphoblastic lymphomas as well as many follicular and some diffuse B cell lymphomas. This marker is most useful in the subclassification of acute leukemias (40) (Chapter 10).

It is detected in frozen but not in paraffin sections. The staining is frequently faint and poorly localized. Outside of the acute leukemias, CALLA is most useful in the subclassification of follicular center cell lymphomas: centrocytic versus centroblastic/centrocytic. The former is CALLA negative and expresses CD5 (Leu 1), while the latter lacks CD5, and 80% express CALLA (25).

Lysozyme

Lysozyme is a lysosomal enzyme present in cells of the monocyte-macrophage and granulocyte series. It is not found in T or B lymphocytes and is thus useful in distinguishing myeloblasts from lymphoblasts and, theoretically, in identifying the rare large cell lymphoma of true histiocytic origin. Lysozyme is usually detected with the immunoperoxidase technique in paraffin sections. It may also be detected in frozen sections. Since normal granulocytes and macrophages contain lysozyme, and many lymphoid neoplasms contain large numbers of reactive granulocytes and macrophages, sections must be carefully evaluated to determine whether or not neoplastic cells are staining. Lysozyme has not proven to be reliable as a marker for malignant histiocytes. Most cases diagnosed morphologically and immunologically as true histiocytic neoplasms are probably neoplasms of T or B lymphoid cells (57).

CD15: Lacto-N-fucose Pentaosyl III (Leu-M1, Myl)

This granulocyte-associated antibody has been recently reported to be a marker for Reed-Sternberg (RS) cells and their variants in all types of Hodgkin's disease (HD) other than lymphocyte predominant (14). It can be detected on both frozen and paraffin sections (more reliable on B5-fixed than formalin-fixed sections). Because the morphology is better, paraffin sections are preferred. Typical Reed-Sternberg cells show both peripheral membrane staining and paranuclear (Golgi) staining. Most cases of typical mixed cellularity or nodular scleroses Hodgkin's disease have at least a few atypical cells (and often *only* a few) that show characteristic paranuclear and peripheral cytoplasmic staining with Leu-M1. The majority of cases of lymphocyte predominance Hodgkin's disease do not show staining of Reed-Sternberg cells for Leu M1. In a variety of epithelial cells, in non-neoplastic myeloid or monocytic cells, and in some cases of T cell lymphoma, Leu M1 has been shown to be present. In all of these cells, the staining is said to be diffuse, rather than having the characteristic paranuclear and peripheral staining of RS cells (14). When Hodgkin's disease cannot be definitively diagnosed histologically, the differential diagnosis often includes metastatic nonlymphoid tumor, true histiocytic lymphoma, and non-Hodgkin's lymphoma. Staining for Leu M1 would not exclude any of these diagnoses.

At present, the diagnosis of HD is important because of its characteristic clinical behavior and response to treatment. The clinical spectrum of the disease known as HD is based on cases with the characteristic *histologic* appearance of HD: scattered, characteristic, atypical cells in an inflammatory-appearing background. High-grade malignancies, characterized by solid proliferations of malignant cells that bear a superficial morphologic *or* immunohistologic resemblance to RS cells, *cannot* be assumed to have the characteristic biologic behavior of typical HD. For the present, a diagnosis of HD should continue to be made only on histologic grounds.

The utility of Leu M1 is somewhat analogous to that of tartrate-resistant acid phosphatase in the diagnosis of hairy cell leukemia. If the morphologic features are atypical or perhaps borderline, positive staining provides comforting corroboration of the diagnosis; however, its absence should not exclude the diagnosis in typical cases, and its presence is insufficient for diagnosing cases that do not meet the morphologic criteria.

Class II Antigens (HLA-DR, DQ, DP)

The HLA-D locus antigens, HLA-DR, DQ, DP or Ia (immune-associated) antigens are found on various epithelial cells as well as fibroblasts and hematopoietic cells. Among hematopoietic cells, HLA-DR antigens are found on most B lymphocytes, monocytes, and granulocytes, but are lacking on most plasma cells and T lymphocytes. Activated T cells may express HLA-DR antigens. They are present on the cells of most "null" or "common" acute lymphoid leukemias, and in conjunction with CALLA, may be used to distinguish these from T cell acute leukemias. Within the B cell system, HLA-DR may be a differentiation antigen, differentially expressed at different stages of development (17). It is not of great diagnostic utility at present.

CD30 (Ki-1)

The antibody Ki-1 was initially raised against a long-term cell line derived from a patient with Hodgkin's disease (44). It reacts with Reed-Sternberg cells and their variants in all types of Hodgkin's disease and also with rare cells in the perifollicular regions of reactive lymph nodes. Although it was initially hoped that Ki-1 might be a specific marker for Hodgkin's disease, subsequent studies showed that the antigen appeared on T or B lymphocytes that were activated *in vitro* by mitogens or viruses (49) and that it was present in some non-Hodgkin's lymphomas. Scattered Ki-1 positive cells are found in rare B-immunoblastic lymphomas and in about ¼ of T cell lymphomas; the Ki-1 positive cells are often large, binucleate Reed-Sternberg-like cells in such cases. In addition, a group of large cell lymphomas has been identified in which the majority of the cells express Ki-1. These lymphomas may be of T, B, or null phenotype, but all have a characteristic morphology: large, bizarre, anaplastic cells with single or multiple pleomorphic, hyperchromatic nuclei and abundant often basophilic cytoplasm (49). They show a cohesive growth pattern and a tendency to invade lymph node sinuses, so that they had often been misdiagnosed as non-lymphoid neoplasms—carcinoma, melanoma, or malignant histiocytosis. Large-cell anaplastic Ki-1 positive lymphomas may arise *de novo*, often in children, and often in the skin or subcutis. Lesions previously described as "regressing atypical histiocytosis" may for the most part be anaplastic T cell lymphomas that are Ki-1 positive. Ki-1 positive lymphomas with anaplastic cytologic features may also develop in patients who have been treated for Mycosis fungoides, Hodgkin's disease, and low-grade non-Hodgkin's lymphomas.

The nature of these anaplastic Ki-1 positive lymphomas remains to be elucidated. It is currently postulated that they represent neoplasms of lymphoid cells that are in an "activated" state; this view is supported by the fact that the interleukin-2 receptor (CD25) and HLA-DR are also expressed by these tumors. Their relationship to other high-grade T and B cell neoplasms and to lymphocyte-depleted Hodgkin's disease remains to be determined.

APPLICATION OF IMMUNOHISTOLOGIC MARKERS TO DIAGNOSIS (TABLES 4 & 5)

At the Massachusetts General Hospital, whenever the diagnosis of lymphoma is suspected clinically, the tissue removed surgically is sent fresh, in saline, to the frozen section laboratory. The pathologist freezes a representative slice and does a diagnostic frozen section, stained with hematoxylin-eosin. Examination of the frozen section permits: (a) determination of the adequacy of the specimen for diagnosis, and (b) a preliminary estimate of the differential diagnosis. A definite pathological diagnosis on frozen sections of lymphoid lesions is not usually rendered, but the apparent differential diagnosis is useful to guide further workup. If the frozen section shows a malignant tumor, a small piece is fixed for electron microscopy. If the frozen section shows a lymphoid infiltrate, electron microscopy is useless. In any case, the frozen tissue is saved, airtight, at − 70°C. If the diagnosis appears straightforward (e.g., hyperplasia, Hodgkin's disease, carcinoma, or follicular lymphoma) the permanent sections will be awaited, since marker studies may not be necessary for diagnosis. If the lesion appears difficult on frozen section (undifferentiated malignant tumor, extranodal lymphoid infiltrate or atypical hyperplasia) immunohistochemical stains can be requested immediately and can be ready at the same time as the permanent sections.

If the biopsy specimen is small, so that it must all be frozen, 5 to 10 additional frozen sections can be cut and stored at − 70°C. The frozen block can then be thawed and processed for permanent sections. Immunohistologic studies can be done on the pre-cut frozen sections. This compromise is particularly useful for brain biopsies and small biopsies of orbital or other extranodal lymphoid infiltrates.

When immunophenotyping is used for diagnosis, it is essential to use *panels* of antibodies, rather than a single marker for a specific tumor type. There is virtually no single marker that is absolutely diagnostic and completely reliable for any particular neoplasm.

TABLE 4. *Procedure for lymph node biopsy processing*

1. Specimen sent in saline to frozen section laboratory
2. Freeze 1 slice in cryostat and cut a diagnostic frozen section to evaluate adequacy of specimen and to get an impression of the differential diagnosis.
3. SAVE frozen tissue in an airtight container labeled with patient's name. Store at − 70° indefinitely (can remain at − 20° several days)
4. If there is no more tissue for permanent sections, cut 5-10 frozen sections and SAVE at − 20° or − 70°
5. If frozen section shows malignant tumor, fix several 1-2 mm cubes in fixative for electron microscopy; this material can be discarded if diagnosis is clear from histology or immunophenotyping.
6. Fix remaining tissue for paraffin embedding (B5 and/or formalin).
7. If the frozen section suggests non-Hodgkin's lymphoma, proceed with immunoperoxidase stains; if it strongly suggests hyperplasia, Hodgkin's disease or carcinoma, delay immunohistochemical studies until after permanent sections; in some cases markers may not be necessary for diagnosis.

TABLE 5. *Clinical application of immunophenotyping*

Differential Diagnosis	Antibody panel[a]
Reactive versus neoplastic lymphoid proliferations	Immunoglobulin heavy and light chains Pan T antibody
Lymphoma versus non-lymphoid tumor	Leukocyte common antigen Immunoglobulin heavy and light chains Pan B and pan T antibodies Cytokeratin, other antibodies as indicated by specific differential diagnosis Lysozyme (for myeloid leukemia)
Subclassification of lymphomas	Immunoglobulin heavy & light chains Pan B and pan T antibodies TdT, CALLA (CD10) T subset antibodies LCA (CD45), Leu M1 (CD15)

[a]See text for abbreviations.

The panel of antibodies to be used will depend on the differential diagnosis, based on evaluation of routine histologic sections. The staining techniques are described in Chapter 17.

Reactive Versus Neoplastic Lymphoid Proliferations

This problem arises in two different forms: (a) the distinction between extranodal inflammatory infiltrates ("pseudolymphoma") and extranodal lymphocytic lymphoma ("well-differentiated"), and (b) the distinction between reactive follicular hyperplasia and follicular lymphoma of lymph nodes. Dense infiltrates of small lymphocytes in extranodal sites present a difficult diagnostic problem, since by definition there is minimal cytologic atypia, and the architectural features used to distinguish lymphoma from hyperplasia in lymph nodes are lacking. Many of these extranodal lesions in the orbit, lung, gastrointestinal tract, and skin were formerly called pseudolymphomas, with the diagnosis of lymphoma in these sites being made only when either cytologic atypia or nodal involvement were present. With the use of immunologic studies, most have now been shown to have monotypic immunoglobulin, indicating that they are clonal B cell proliferations and thus low-grade neoplasms (11,26,37). The other problem, distinguishing between follicular hyperplasia and follicular lymphoma, occurs less often, since there are usually sufficient morphological criteria for making this diagnosis. However, follicular lymphomas with numerous large cells can mimic reactive follicles, and demonstration of monotypic immunoglobulin in the follicles can aid in the diagnosis.

In this differential diagnosis, immunoglobulin light chains are the only useful markers. Heavy chain staining is usually evaluated as well, but is not absolutely necessary. A pan-T cell antibody can be added to help localize reactive T cells within the infiltrate; however, the number and distribution of T cells do not correlate with neoplasia. Theoretically, demonstration of CD5 (Leu 1) on the B cell population would support a diagnosis of neoplasia.

This finding may be useful if present, but the majority of extranodal lymphocytic lymphomas not associated with CLL have been found to be Leu 1 negative (22). Expression of CALLA by follicular center cells is usually more prominent in lymphomatous than in reactive follicles; however it may be absent from some follicular lymphomas and present in some hyperplasias, so it is not a reliable marker for neoplasia.

An important caveat in interpreting the results of immunoglobulin staining is that the only *diagnostic* finding is that of monotypic immunoglobulin. Polyclonal B cells do *not exclude* a diagnosis of lymphoma; this result may reflect a sampling problem, a technical problem, or an immunoglobulin-negative lymphoma that contains some reactive B cells. This is particularly true when only paraffin sections are examined, but can even occur with frozen sections. In the absence of monotypic Ig, one cannot confirm the diagnosis of lymphoma, but one cannot necessarily exclude it either.

Lymphoma versus Nonlymphoid Tumor

This is an extremely common problem; lymphomas can have a wide variety of morphologic appearances and seem to have replaced syphilis as the "great imitator." The list of tumors that can be mimicked by lymphomas includes nasopharyngeal carcinoma (lymphoepithelioma), small round cell sarcomas of childhood, poorly differentiated adenocarcinoma, oat cell carcinoma, Merkel cell carcinoma, thymoma, melanoma, and even spindle cell sarcomas. The most important factor in making the correct diagnosis in these cases is a high index of suspicion—a recognition that lymphoma is in the differential diagnosis.

The most useful marker in this situation is the leukocyte common antigen (CD45, LCA), since it is expressed by the vast majority of lymphomas and can often be detected in paraffin sections. Immunoglobulin light chains and a pan-B cell antibody are useful in the initial panel, since LCA may be undetectable in lymphomas with plasmacytoid differentiation, particularly in paraffin sections, but also in frozen sections. These neoplasms often contain cytoplasmic Ig, which can be detected in paraffin sections. A pan-T cell antibody can be included to detect the occasional T large cell lymphoma. In the diagnosis of small round cell tumors of childhood, it may be necessary to include antibodies to thymic T cell antigens (CD1, CD7) and TdT, since T lymphoblastic lymphoma may lack the leukocyte common antigen as well as other markers usually found on more differentiated lymphomas.

If a nonlymphoid neoplasm is strongly suggested by the morphology on routine sections, an appropriate nonlymphoid marker can be added to the initial panel—e.g., cytokeratin, carcinoembryonic antigen, chromogranin, desmin, or S-100—depending on the type of tumor suspected. Note that vimentin is not useful in this differential diagnosis, since lymphomas variably express this intermediate filament. In addition, some lymphomas express epithelial membrane antigen so that staining with this antibody must be interpreted with caution.

Subclassification of Lymphomas

The importance of the immunologic subclassification of lymphomas is less universal than the distinction between benign and malignant lymphoid infiltrates and between lymphoid and nonlymphoid neoplasms. For the most part, the clinically relevant subclassification of lymphomas still rests primarily on morphologic features. There are certain situations, however, in which the lineage of a lymphoma may not be apparent morphologically and may be clinically significant. The most obvious example is the distinction between Hodgkin's disease and non-Hodgkin's lymphomas, which can be difficult but can be aided by immunohistologic stains. Distinction between non-Hodgkin's lymphomas of T and B cell types may also be both morphologically difficult and clinically relevant in certain cases: lymphoblastic lymphoma of T cell type versus Burkitt's tumor, chronic lymphocytic leukemia of T cell versus B cell type, and virus-associated T cell lymphoma versus diffuse lymphomas of B cell type. In other cases, such as the distinction between large cell lymphomas of B versus T cell types, there is no evidence that cell lineage is clinically relevant. Finally, there are some situations in which morphologic features are more important than phenotype. For example, the distinction between mycosis fungoides (MF) and non-MF cutaneous T cell lymphoma is impossible with marker studies and rests solely on the characteristic morphology of the former.

Even within a given lineage, immunophenotyping may be important and useful. For example, T lymphoblastic lymphomas are clinically distinct from more differentiated T cell lymphomas and can be recognized by their distinctive immunophenotype. Differences in immunophenotype between other subsets of T or B cell lymphomas are beginning to appear as panels of antibodies are applied to large series of cases. However, differences in classification schemes and antibody panels, as well as the small numbers of cases in any one study, impair the usefulness of many of these studies. For example, some studies have shown that centrocytic lymphoma, an aggressive B cell neoplasm, can be distinguished from the more indolent and morphologically similar centroblastic/centrocytic lymphoma by differences in immunophenotype (25,48). The morphologic definitions of these entities are not universally accepted, however, and different investigators have applied different antibody panels, so that it is difficult to adopt the results in diagnostic practice. Nonetheless, the use of panels of antibodies to define and refine morphological and clinical subgroups of lymphomas is an important area that will continue to be explored and should continue to produce interesting and useful information.

Hodgkin's Disease, Lymphocytic Predominance Versus B Cell Small Lymphocytic Lymphoma

Although this distinction can usually be made on morphological grounds, it may be difficult. Occasional cases of B-CLL have atypical Reed-Sternberg-like large cells in lymph nodes. Demonstration of monotypic Ig confirms the diagnosis of non-Hodgkin's lymphoma. Note that immunohistologic studies *cannot* reliably distinguish between Hodgkin's disease and T cell lymphomas, since both contain a predominance of T cells, usually of the CD 4 subset. As discussed above, Leu M1 (CD15) should be used with caution.

T- or B-precursor Lymphoblastic Lymphoma versus Burkitt's Lymphoma

The lymphoblastic lymphomas of T and B precursor type may be morphologically identical but are clinically distinct diseases (6,9,35,56). Both contain TdT, but the former expresses early or cortical thymocyte markers, while the latter expresses pan B cell antigens, CALLA and HLA-DR. Both must be distinguished from Burkitt's or Burkitt-like lymphomas, which have a different natural history and require different therapy (15). This distinction is often readily made on routine sections, but in difficult cases, demonstration of SIg and absence of TdT can be useful in confirming the diagnosis of Burkitt's lymphoma.

Virus-associated Adult T Cell Lymphoma/Leukemia (ATL/L)
versus Diffuse Lymphomas of B Cell Type

The human T lymphotrophic virus-Type I (HTLV-I) associated lymphoproliferative disorder, ATL/L, may have a variable histological picture and may be indistinguishable morphologically from diffuse small, mixed, or large cell lymphomas of B cell type. The clinical behavior of ATL/L is distinctive and can only be predicted if immunophenotyping establishes the diagnosis of T cell disease, and virologic studies are done to confirm HTLV-Infection (29). The neoplastic cells have a mature T cell phenotype, lacking TdT and expressing pan T cell antigens and the T subset antigen, CD4.

CONCLUSION

Performing and interpreting immunohistologic stains requires experience, and probably should not be attempted by laboratories that do not encounter a large number of lymphomas. In small laboratories, frozen tissue can be obtained and stored at $-20°C$ for a few days; if immunohistological studies are deemed necessary, the frozen tissue can be sent on dry ice to a reference laboratory. At present, immunophenotyping should be done in most cases of non-Hodgkin's lymphoma to provide both confirmation of the diagnosis and the prognostic information contributed by cell lineage. Lymphomas are potentially fatal, but can be curable, although the treatment is not without toxicity. It is essential that the diagnosis be correct whenever possible, and immunohistologic studies will greatly increase the frequency of correct diagnoses.

In preparing clinically important biopsy specimens for immunohistologic studies and in interpreting the results of these studies, it is important to bear in mind that excellent morphology is still crucial for the diagnosis and subclassification of hematologic neoplasia. Obtaining tissue for marker studies should not be permitted to interfere with adequate morphologic examination. Similarly, artifacts and technical problems can occasionally lead to misleading results; the immunohistologic studies must be interpreted in light of the case as a whole and should never be allowed to contradict common sense.

The contribution of immunohistologic studies to the diagnosis of lymphomas is acknowledged. Their potential contribution to subclassification has not been fully explored. More large studies are needed, combining careful morphologic subclassification, large panels of monoclonal antibodies, and clinical followup, to determine the contribution of immunophenotyping studies of the classification of this fascinating group of diseases.

ACKNOWLEDGMENTS

I am indebted to Ms. Deirdre Donoghue for her accomplished secretarial assistance, to Mr. Steven Conley and Ms. Michelle Forrestall for the photography, and to Mr. Bruce Kaynor and Ms. Kathleen Bain for the immunoperoxidase stains.

REFERENCES

1. Aisenberg, A. C., Krontiris, T. G., Mak, T. W., and Wilkes, B. M. (1985): The gene for the beta chain of the T-cell receptor is rearranged in T-cell chronic lymphocytic leukemia and allied disorders. *N. Engl. J. Med.*, 313:529–533.

2. Arnold, A., Cossman, J., Bakhshi, A., Jaffe, E. S., Waldmann, T. A., and Korsmeyer, S. J. (1983): Immunoglobulin gene rearrangements as unique clonal markers in human lymphoid neoplasms. *N. Engl. J. Med.*, 309:1594–1599.

3. Battifora, H., and Trowbridge, I. S. (1983): A monoclonal antibody useful for the differential diagnosis between malignant lymphoma and nonhematopoietic neoplasms. *Cancer*, 51:816–821.

4. Bhan, A. K., Nadler, L. M., Stashenko, P., and Schlossman, S. F. (1981): Stages of B cell differentiation in human lymphoid tissues. *J. Exp. Med.*, 154:737–749.

5. Bhan, A. K., Reinherz, E. L., Poppema, S., McCluskey, R. T., and Schlossman, S. F. (1980): Location of T cell and major histocompatibility antigens in the human thymus. *J. Exp. Med.*, 152:771–782.

6. Borowitz, M., Croker, B. D., and Metzgar, R. S. (1983): Lymphoblastic lymphoma with the phenotype of common acute lymphoblastic leukemia. *Am. J. Clin. Pathol.*, 79:387–391.

7. Borowitz, M., Reichert, T. A., Brynes, R. K., Cousar, J. B., Whitcomb, C. C., Collins, R. D., Crissman, J. D., and Byrne, G. E., Jr. (1986): The phenotypic diversity of peripheral T-cell lymphomas. *Hum. Pathol.*, 17:567–574.

8. Caligeris-Cappio, F., Cobbi, M., Bofill, M., and Janossy, G. (1982): Infrequent normal B lymphocytes express features of B chronic lymphocytic leukemia. *J. Exp. Med.*, 155:623–628.

9. Castella, A., Neuberg, R. W., Kurec, A. S., Jones, D. B., and Davey, F. R. (1982): Non-Hodgkin's lymphoma with immunologic phenotype similar to non-T non-B acute lymphocytic leukemia. *Hum. Pathol.*, 13:777–779.

10. Cleary, M. L., Trela, M. J., Weiss, L. M., Warnke, R., and Sklar, J. (1985): Most null large-cell lymphomas are B cell neoplasms. *Lab. Invest.*, 53:521–525.

11. Colby, T. V., and Carrington, C. B. (1983): Pulmonary lymphomas: Current concepts. *Hum. Pathol.*, 14:884–887.

12. Croce, C. M., and Nowell, P. C. (1985): Molecular basis of human B cell neoplasia. *Blood*, 65:1–7.

13. Doggett, R. S., Wood, G. S., Horning, S., Levy, R., Dorfman, R. F., Bindl, J., and Warnke, R. A. (1984): The immunologic characterization of 95 nodal and extranodal diffuse large cell lymphomas in 89 patients. *Am. J. Pathol.*, 115:245–252.

14. Dorfman, R. F., Gatter, K. C., Pulford, K. A. F., Mason, D. Y. (1986): An evaluation of the utility of anti-granulocyte and anti-leukocyte monoclonal antibodies in the diagnosis of Hodgkin's disease. *Am. J. Pathol.*, 123:508–519.

15. Garcia, C. F., Weiss, L. M., and Warnke, R. A. (1986): Small noncleaved cell lymphoma and immunophenotypic study of 18 cases and comparison with large cell lymphoma. *Hum. Pathol.*, 17:454–461.

16. Gutman, G. A., and Weissman, I. L. (1972): Lymphoid tissue architecture. Experimental analysis of the origin and distribution of T cells and B cells. *Immunology*, 23:465–479.

17. Halper, J. P., Fu, S. M., Wang, C. Y., Winchester, R. J., and Kunkel, H. G. (1978): Patterns of expression of IA-like antigens during the terminal stages of B cell development. *J. Immunol.*, 120:1480–1484.

18. Harris, N. L. (1985): The impact of molecular genetics on the study of lymphoid neoplasia. *Lab. Invest.*, 53:509–512.

19. Harris, N. L. (1987): Lymphoma 1987: An interim approach to diagnosis and classification. In: *Pathology Annual*, edited by P. P. Rosen and R. E. Fechner. Appleton-Century-Crofts, East Norwalk, CT.

20. Harris, N. L., and Bhan, A. K. (1983): Distribution of T cell subsets in follicular and diffuse lymphomas of B cell type. *Am. J. Pathol.*, 113:172–180.

21. Harris, N. L., and Bhan, A. K. (1985): Distribution of leukocyte common antigen in B cell neoplasia: T200 is lost in terminal B cell differentiation. *Lab. Invest.*, 52:28A. (Abstr.)

22. Harris, N. L., and Bhan, A. K. (1985): B cell neoplasms of the lymphocytic, lymphoplasmacytoid and plasma cell types: Immunohistologic analysis and clinical correlation. *Hum. Pathol.*, 16:829–837.

23. Harris, N. L., and Data, R. E. (1982): The distribution of neoplastic and normal B-lymphoid cells in nodular lymphomas: Use of an immunoperoxidase technique on frozen sections. *Hum. Pathol.*, 13:610–617.

24. Harris, N. L., Nadler, L. M., and Bhan, A. K. (1983): Immunohistologic characterization of non-Hodgkin's lymphoma with monoclonal antibodies. *Lab. Invest.*, 48:33–34A (Abstr.).

25. Harris, N. L, Nadler, L. M., and Bhan, A. K. (1984): Immunohistologic characterization of two malignant lymphomas of germinal center type (centroblastic/centrocytic and centrocytic). *Am. J. Pathol.*, 117:262–272.

26. Harris, N. L., Pilch, B. Z., Bhan, A. K., Harmon, D. C., and Goodman, M. (1984): Immunohistologic diagnosis of orbital lymphoid infiltrates. *Am. J. Surg. Pathol.*, 8:83–91.

27. Harris, N. L., Poppema, S., and Data, R. E. (1982): Demonstration of immunoglobulin in malignant lymphomas: Use of an immunoperoxidase technique on frozen sections. *Am. J. Clin. Pathol.*, 78:14–21.

28. Iida, K., Nadler, L. M., and Nussenzweig, V. (1983): Identification of the membrane receptor for the complement fragments C3d by means of a monoclonal antibody. *J. Exp. Med.*, 158:1021–1033.

29. Jaffe, E. S., Blattner, W. A., Blayney, D. W., Bunn, P. A., Jr., Cossman, J., Robert-Guroff, M., and Gallo, R. C. (1984): The pathologic spectrum of adult T-cell leukemia/lymphoma in the United States. *Am. J. Surg. Pathol.*, 8:263–275.

30. Janossy, G., Bollum, F. J., Bradstock, K. F., and Ashley, J. (1980): Cellullar phenotypes of normal and leukemic hematopoietic cells determined by selected antibody combinations. *Blood*, 56:430–441.
31. Korsmeyer, S. J., Hieter, P. A., Ravetch, J. V., Poplack, D. G., Waldman, T. A., and Leder P. (1981): Developmental hierarchy of immunoglobulin gene rearrangements in leukemic pre-B cells. *Proc. Natl. Acad. Sci. U.S.A.*, 78:7096–7100.
32. Lennert, K. (1978): *Malignant Lymphomas Other Than Hodgkin's Disease*. Springer-Verlag, New York.
33. Lennert, K. (1981): *Histopathology of Non-Hodgkin's Lymphomas: Based on the Kiel Classification*. Springer-Verlag, New York.
34. Lennert, K., Collins, R. D., and Lukes, R. J. (1983): Concordance of the Kiel and Lukes-Collins classification of non-Hodgkin's lymphomas. *Histopathology*, 7:549–559.
35. Link, M. P., Roper, M., Dorfman, R. F., Crist, W. M., Cooper, M. D., and Levy, R. (1983): Cutaneous lymphoblastic lymphoma with pre-B markers. *Blood*, 61:838–841.
36. Meuer, S. C., Schlossman, S. F., and Reinherz, E. L. (1982): Clonal analysis of human cytotoxic T lymphocytes: T4 and T8 effector T cells recognize products of different major histocompatibility regions. *Proc. Natl. Acad. Sci. U.S.A.*, 79:4395–4399.
37. Moore, I., and Wright, D. H. (1984): Primary gastric lymphoma—a tumor of mucosa—associated lymphoid tissue—A histological and immunohistochemical study of 36 cases. *Histopathology*, 8:1025–1039.
38. Nadler, L. M., Stashenko, P., Hardy, R., van Agthoven, A., Terhorst, C., and Schlossman, S. F. (1981): Characterization of a human B cell specific antigen (B2) distinct from B1. *J. Immunol.*, 126:1941–1947.
39. Nossal, G. J. V., and Ada, G. L. (1971): *Antigens, Lymphoid Cells, and the Immune Response*. Academic Press, New York.
40. Pesando, J. M., Ritz, J., Lazarus, H., Costello, S. B., Sallan, S., and Schlossman, S. F. (1979): Leukemia-associated antigens in ALL. *Blood*, 54:1240–1248.
41. Poppema, S., Bhan, A. K., Reinherz, E. L., McCluskey, R. T., Schlossman, S. F. (1981): Distribution of T cell subsets in human lymph nodes. *J. Exp. Med.*, 53:30–41.
42. Rappaport, H. (1986): Tumors of the hematopoietic system. In: *Atlas of Tumor Pathology*, Section III, Fasc. 8, A.F.I.P. Washington, D.C., 1966.
43. Reinherz, E., Haynes, B. F., Nadler, L. M., and Bernstein, I. D. (1986): *Leukocyte Typing II*. Springer-Verlag, New York.
44. Schwab, U., Stein, H., Gerdes, J., Lemke, H., Kirchner, H., Schaadt, M., Dichl, V. (1982): Production of a monoclonal antibody specific for Hodgkin and Reed-Sternberg cells of Hodgkin's disease and a subset of normal lymphoid cells. *Nature*, 299:65–67.
45. Stashenko, P., Nadler, L. M., Hardy, R., Schlossman, S. F. (1980): Characterization of a human B lymphocyte-specific antigen. *J. Immunology*, 125:1678–1685.
46. Stashenko, P., Nadler, L. M., Hardy, R., and Schlossman, S. F. (1981): Expression of cell surface markers after human B lymphocyte activation. *Proc. Natl. Acad. Sci. U.S.A.*, 78:3848–3852.
47. Stein, H., Gerdes, J., and Mason, D. Y. (1982): The normal and malignant germinal centre. *Clin. Haematol.*, 1:531–559.
48. Stein, H., and Mason, D. Y. (1985): Immunological analysis of tissue sections in diagnosis of lymphoma. In: *Recent Advances in Haematology*, edited by A. V. Hoffbrand, pp. 127–169. Churchill Livingstone, New York.
49. Stein, H., Mason, D. Y., Gerdes, N., O'Connor, N., Wainscort, J., Pallesen, G., Gatter, K., Falini, B., Delsol, G., Lemke, H., Schwarting, R., and Lennert, K. (1985): The expression of Hodgkin's Disease associated antigen Ki-1 in reactive and neoplastic lymphoid tissue: Evidence that Reed-Sternberg cells of histiocytic malignancies are derived from activated lymphoid cells. *Blood*, 66:848–858.
50. The Non-Hodgkin's Lymphoma Pathologic Classification Project. National Cancer Institute Sponsored Study of Classifications of Non-Hodgkin's Lymphomas: Summary and Description of a Working Formulation for Clinical Usage. (1982): *Cancer*, 49:2112–2135.
51. Thomas, Y., Rogozinski, L., Irigoyen, O. H., Shen, H. H., Talle, M. A., Goldstein, G., Chess, L. (1982): Functional analysis of human T cell subsets defined by monoclonal antibodies. V Suppressor cells within the activated OKT4$^+$ population belong to a distinct subset. *J. Immunol.*, 28:1386–1390.
52. Veldman, J. E., Keuning, F. J., Molenaar, I. (1978): Site of initiation of the plasma cell reaction in the rabbit lymph node. *Virchows Arch. B. Cell. Pathol.*, 8:187–202.
53. Wabl, M. R., Forni, L., Loor, F. (1978): Switch in immunoglobulin production observed in single clones of committed lymphocytes. *Science*, 199:1078–1079.
54. Warnke, R. A., Gatter, K. C., Falini, B., Hildreth, P., Woolston, R. E., Pulford, K., Cordell, J. L., Cohen, B., De Wolf-Peeters, C., Mason, D. Y. (1983): Diagnosis of human lymphoma with monoclonal antileukocyte antibodies. *N. Engl. J. Med.*, 309:1275–1281.
55. Weiss, L. M., Hu, E., Wood, G. S., Moulds, C., Cleary, M., Warnke, R., and Sklar, J. (1985): Clonal rearrangements of T cell receptor genes in mycosis fungoides and dermatopathic lymphadenopathy. *N. Engl. J. Med.*, 313:539–544.
56. Weiss, L. M., Bindl, J. M., Picozzi, V. J., Link, M. P., and Warnke, R. A. (1986): Lymphoblastic

lymphoma: An immunophenotype study of 26 cases with comparison to T cell acute lymphblastic leukemia. *Blood*, 67:474–478.

57. Weiss, L. M., Trela, M. J., Cleary, M., Turner, R. R., Warnke, R. A., and Sklar, J. (1985): Frequent immunoglobulin and T cell receptor gene rearrangement in histiocytic'' neoplasms. *Am. J. Pathol.*, 121:369–373.

58. Weissman, I. L., Warnke, R., Butcher, E. C., Rouse, R., and Levy, R. (1978): The lymphoid system. *Hum. Pathol.*, 9:25–49.

Diagnostic Immunopathology,
edited by R.B. Colvin,
A.K. Bhan, and R.T. McCluskey.
Raven Press, New York © 1988.

12 / *Endocrine Tumors*

Ronald A. DeLellis

*Department of Pathology, Tufts University School of Medicine, and the
New England Medical Center Hospital, Boston, Massachusetts 02111*

General concepts of the ontogeny, organization and functional interrelationships of the endocrine system have undergone a remarkable evolution over the past several decades (119). Originally conceived as a collection of discrete glands which maintained homeostatis by their secretion of hormones into the general circulation, it has become apparent that hormone synthesizing cells are also extensively distributed throughout a variety of nonendocrine tissues, including the brain and the heart (140). In addition to their endocrine functions, recent studies have highlighted the facts that hormones can also have neuroendocrine, neurotransmitter, paracrine and autocrine functions (46,83).

Delineation of the distributional patterns of hormone synthesizing cells and an approach to an understanding of their pathobiology were made possible by a series of key discoveries. These included the development of methods for the purification and biochemical characterization of the various hormones, the development of radioimmunoassay and other techniques for their quantitation in tissue extracts and body fluids, and the development and refinement of immunohistochemical methods for their localization at the light microscopic and ultrastructural levels (39,41,44,144). These last studies, in particular, not only have aided in the identification of new cell types but also have provided insights into their functional significance and interrelationships with other endocrine and nonendocrine cell types.

In addition to providing data on the distribution of endocrine cells in normal tissues and organs, immunohistochemical analyses have been of paramount importance in the diagnosis and classification of endocrine neoplasms and many of their precursor lesions. These techniques have also proven to be of value in establishing the primary sites of metastatic endocrine tumors of unknown origin. Moreover, immunohistochemical methods for hormones and other products of endocrine cells have played essential roles in the establishment of novel clinical and pathological concepts and in providing important prognostic data.

This chapter will present an overview of the value of immunohistochemical techniques with a particular emphasis on endocrine neoplasms. The first section will review markers of endocrine cells, including hormones and a variety of nonhormonal constituents. The second section will review endocrine tumors of specific sites with an emphasis on the use of the various markers for differential diagnosis and tumor classification.

HORMONAL AND NONHORMONAL MARKERS OF ENDOCRINE CELLS

Hormones

Immunofluorescence as well as immunoenzymatic techniques have proven to be effective for the demonstration of virtually all classes of hormones both in frozen sections and in paraffin embedded samples (Table 1). The principles of these methods are presented in Chapters 16 and 17 and in several recent publications (31,143,146).

Experimental and clinical studies have shown that the vast majority of polypeptide hormones, including the entire class of regulatory peptides, may be demonstrated by immunohistochemical techniques in Bouin's or formalin fixed paraffin embedded samples. In many instances, the use of peptide region specific antisera has permitted the localization of pre- and pre-pro-hormones in cells containing the biologically active forms of the peptides. A variety of fixatives, including formaldehyde vapor, carbodiimide and diethyl pyrocarbonate have also been used in place of formalin and these fixatives have been reported to achieve optimal fixation of small amounts of regulatory peptides such as those occurring in peptidergic nerve fibers (76,120,121).

Endocrine cells in different anatomic sites may produce identical or biosynthetically related regulatory peptide products. These observations indicate that such peptide products cannot be used as cell lineage specific markers. For example, somatostatin has a wide distribution, and has been localized to certain hypothalamic and cortical neurons, pancreatic D cells, certain gastrointestinal and bronchopulmonary endocrine cells, thymic

TABLE 1. *Hormonal and nonhormonal markers for analysis of endocrine tumors*

Hormones
Peptides and peptide releasing factors
Steroids
Amines
Iodothyronines (T_3, T_4)
Catecholamines (epinephrine, norepinephrine, dopamine)
Indolylethylamines (serotonin)

Nonhormonal markers
Enzymes
Histaminase
Tyrosine hydroxylase, dopamine beta hydroxylase, phenylethanolamine N-methyl transferase
Neuron specific enolase
Intermediate filaments
Cytokeratins, neurofilaments, vimentin, glial fibrillary acidic protein
Secretory granule matrix constituents
Chromogranins
Secretogranins
Secretory granule membrane constituents
Chromomembrin B
Synaptic vesicle constituents
Synaptophysin
Lymphoreticular antigens
S-100 protein
Thy-1, leu 7, CD11
Other antigens
E36, A2B5, CEA

endocrine cells, and a subset of thyroidal C-cells (32,127). Gastrin releasing peptide, the mammalian analogue of bombesin, is present not only in small intestine, but also occurs in certain thyroidal C-cells and in bronchopulmonary endocrine cells (74,156). Both normal and neoplastic endocrine cells are capable of expressing multiple genes encoding biosynthetically unrelated products. Growth hormone releasing hormone, for example, has been co-localized with gastrin in antral G-cells and with pancreatic polypeptide in pancreatic islets while somatostatin and calcitonin are co-localized in a subset of C-cells in the thyroid gland (17,39). Neoplasms derived from such cells would be expected to have the capacity to synthesize multiple peptides which are normally produced by the cell of origin (*eutopic* production). If the peptide products of the tumor cells differ from those of the putative cell of origin, hormone production is said to be *ectopic*. The distinction between eutopic and ectopic hormone production is somewhat artificial since microenvironmental signals may lead to apparent "ectopic" hormone production by normal endocrine cells (38,59).

Endocrine cells may produce multiple peptides derived from common biosynthetic precursors. Adrenocorticotropin (ACTH), for example, is synthesized as part of a large precursor molecule, pro-opiomelanocortin (POMC). In the anterior pituitary, POMC is processed to a 16 kd N-terminal fragment, ACTH and beta lipotropin (β-LPH). In the intermediate lobe, ACTH and β-LPH are processed to alpha MSH and beta endorphin related peptides (79). Alternative processing of the calcitonin gene results in the production both of the calcitonin gene related peptide and of calcitonin (129). In other instances, similar or identical regulatory peptides may be produced from different precursor molecules (55,89).

Immunohistochemical techniques have been effective for the demonstration of very small peptide hormones (77). Thyroid hormone releasing hormone, for example, is a tripeptide product which has been demonstrated both in formalin and acrolein fixed tissue. Many of these small peptide releasing factors have been demonstrated within the hypothalamus and in peripheral sites.

There is relatively little intracellular storage of steroids in contrast to peptide hormones. Yet steroid hormones, particularly the androgenic and estrogenic steroids, have been demonstrated in formalin fixed paraffin embedded samples of normal and neoplastic ovarian and testicular tissue (80,146). These results are somewhat surprising since tissues fixed in this fashion have been routinely dehydrated in ethanols and cleared in xylene before paraffin embedding. It is possible that fixation in formalin may have a protective effect on steroids so that they are not solubilized by treatment in organic solvents, but the exact mechanism of this effect is unknown (146). In addition to steroid hormones, receptors for steroids have been demonstrated with antibodies to receptor proteins (62). This approach has been used for the detection of estrogen and progesterone receptors in breast and uterus (123,124) (Chapter 13).

Catecholamines, and Indolylethylamines

The studies of Verhofstad and Lloyd and their co-workers have established that epinephrine and norepinephrine can be demonstrated in fresh frozen and formalin fixed paraffin embedded tissues (96,159). In the rat adrenal medulla, which shows distinct compartmentalization of catecholamines, approximately 80% of the cells contain both norepinephrine and epinephrine while 20% of the cells stain for norepinephrine alone. In the normal human adrenal, all medullary cells stain for both catecholamines. In addition, catecholamines have been demonstrated immunohistochemically in normal paraganglia and in paragangliomas. Norepinephrine has also been demonstrated in a wide variety of other normal endocrine cells including pancreatic islet and anterior pituitary cells; moreover, this amine has been detected in pituitary adenomas, medullary thyroid carcinomas, carcinoids and neuroblastomas (96).

Serotonin can be demonstrated in formalin fixed paraffin embedded tissue samples using immunohistochemical techniques (159). This amine is present in a wide variety of normal endocrine cells, including thyroid C-cells and gastrointestinal enterochromaffin cells and in many of the neoplasms which are derived from these cell types.

Catecholamine Synthesizing Enzymes and Histaminase

Immunohistochemical techniques have been of value for the demonstration of tyrosine hydroxylase (TH), dopamine beta hydroxylase (DβH) and phenylethanolamine N-methyl transferase (PNMT) (96). These enzymes distinguish cells that have the capacity to synthesize catecholamines from those which have the capacity for catecholamine uptake. Thus, normal adrenal medullary cells and pheochromocytomas are positive for DβH, but most other normal neuroendocrine cells and their corresponding neoplasms are not. Tyrosine hydroxylase activity, on the other hand, is commonly present in medullary thyroid carcinomas, although these tumors are less likely to contain DβH (96).

Histaminase (diamine oxidase) has been used as a marker for certain endocrine cells and their corresponding tumors (104). The physiologic significance of this enzyme in endocrine cells is unknown; it can degrade putrescine, the precursor of spermidine and spermine. Marked increases in histaminase levels in the serum occur in pregnancy and this enzyme has been localized immunohistochemically to decidual cells of the endometrium. Among endocrine neoplasms, histaminase is present in high concentrations in medullary thyroid carcinomas, but not in C-cell hyperplasia. Immunoreactive histaminase has also been demonstrated in small cell carcinomas of the lung and in a variety of other tumors of non-endocrine origin (104).

Neuron Specific Enolase

Neuron specific enolase (NSE, 14-3-2 protein), first isolated from beef brain by Moore in 1965, is the most acidic isoenzyme of the glycolytic enzyme, enolase (97). This enzyme has been identified by immunohistochemistry both in neurons and in neuroendocrine cells (13). Although optimal fixation is achieved by the use of picric acid paraformaldehyde, satisfactory results have been obtained with formalin fixed paraffin embedded samples. Positive staining for neuron specific enolase has been observed in a wide variety of normal neuroendocrine cells and in many of their corresponding tumors, including carcinoids, medullary thyroid carcinomas, pheochromocytomas, neuroblastomas and oat cell carcinomas. In contrast to chromogranin immunoreactivity, which typically exhibits a granular pattern of staining, neuron specific enolase is present diffusely within the cytoplasm of these cells (97).

The enolases are products of three independent gene loci which have been designated alpha, beta and gamma (97). Non-neural enolase (alpha-alpha) is present in fetal tissues, glial cells and many non-endocrine tissues except muscle while beta enolase (beta-beta) is characteristic of muscle tissues. Hybrid enolases (alpha-gamma, alpha-beta) have been identified in megakaryocytes and certain other cell types. Neuron specific enolase (gamma-

gamma) replaces non-neuronal enolase during the migration and differentiation of neurons and it has been suggested that the appearance of NSE reflects the formation of synapses and the acquisition of electrical excitability.

The specificity of neuron specific enolase as a marker for neuronal and neuroendocrine cells has been called into question recently (48,133,134,160). The presence of the gamma subunit in non-neuronal, non-neuroendocrine cells (presumably in the alpha-gamma form) has been demonstrated by Haimoto and co-workers (64). In these studies, immunoreactivity has been shown in smooth muscle, myoepithelium, renal tubular cells, lymphocytes, bronchial epithelial cells and type II alveolar epithelial cells. It is also possible that during the processes of neoplastic transformation and progression, certain cells may switch from the production of non-gamma to gamma forms of the enzyme. Accordingly, the results of immunohistochemical staining for neuron specific enolase should be interpreted with considerable caution. As stressed by Schmechel, the results obtained by immunohistochemistry should be supplemented by biochemical and immunochemical determination of the enolase isoenzymes in tissue extracts (134).

Intermediate Filaments

The major cytoskeletal proteins of mammalian cells include the actin containing microfilaments (5 to 6 nm), the tubulin containing microtubules (25 nm) and the intermediate filaments (8 to 10 nm) (25). The intermediate filaments, which include cytokeratins, glial fibrillary acidic protein, neurofilament triplet proteins, desmin and vimentin, are morphologically identical but are biochemically and immunologically distinct (8) (see Chapters 8 and 9). The distribution of the intermediate filaments has been examined in a wide variety of tumors and their corresponding normal cells (8,25,53). Immunohistochemical studies have revealed distinctive patterns of distribution in normal and neoplastic endocrine cells, and these observations will be discussed below. In addition to intermediate filaments, desmosomal proteins have also been studied to some extent in endocrine cells and tumors (111).

Chromogranins

The chromogranins (A, B, and C) constitute a widely distributed family of proteins which range in molecular weight from 76 to 120 kd. Although their functions are unknown, chromogranins are the most abundantly secreted proteins in higher organisms. Chromogranin A was first isolated from the chromaffin granules of bovine adrenal medullary cells and was later found in the human adrenal medulla. Antibodies to chromogranin A react with adrenal medullary cells and a wide variety of peptide and amine containing endocrine cells, parathyroid chief cells, cells in the nervous system and splenic cells (98,115,167). The antibodies are also reactive with a variety of neuroendocrine tumors. Multiple lower molecular weight polypeptides can be detected in immunoblots for chromogranin A with monoclonal and polyclonal antibodies (98). These smaller proteins are probably generated by the action of endogenous proteases within the chromaffin granules. Abundant evidence supports the view that chromogranin A is co-secreted with catecholamines from chromaffin cells and with other regulatory peptide products from neuroendocrine cells.

Two additional proteins have been detected in a wide variety of endocrine and neuronal cells, designated secretogranins I and II. These proteins are highly acidic because of the high content of acidic amino acids, the phosphorylation of serine, and the sulfation on tyrosine and O-linked carbohydrate (63). Chromogranin A and secretogranins I and II share a number of features, suggesting they belong to the same class of proteins. All three are acidic because of the presence of acidic amino acids and because of the post-translational modification by the addition of phosphate and sulfate groups. All three are secretory and are released upon stimulation of the target cell. Lastly, they occur in a wide variety of endocrine and neuronal cells which normally secrete peptides by a regulated pathway.

According to a recent nomenclature proposal, secretogranin I is now referred to as chromogranin B (120 kd) while secretogranin II is chromogranin C (84 kd). Antibodies to the chromogranins have revealed distinctive patterns of distribution. Both by immunoblot and immunohistochemical analyses, all three proteins have been identified in adrenal medullary cells, in the anterior pituitary and in normal and neoplastic C-cells. The parathyroid, on the other hand, contains only chromogranin A. Endocrine cells of the pancreas contain a predominance of chromogranin A with smaller amounts of the B protein. These differential patterns of chromogranin expression in normal endocrine cells suggest that similar findings may be observed with corresponding endocrine tumors.

Chromomembrins

Chromomembrin B, a chromaffin granule membrane molecule, has recently been identified as cytochrome b561. This protein transports electrons into the secretory granule matrix in order to maintain a supply of reduced ascorbic acid, which serves as an electron donor for dopamine beta hydroxylase and for amidases which modify C-terminal portions of certain neuropeptides. Antibodies to chromomembrin B may be useful for the identification of normal, hyperplastic and neoplastic neuroendocrine cells which are engaged in specific functions related to catecholamine synthesis or peptide amidation (154).

Synaptophysin

Synaptophysin is a 38 kd glycoprotein in presynaptic vesicles of neurons and adrenal medullary cells. Immunohistochemical studies with a murine monoclonal antibody (SY 38) have revealed a characteristic punctate pattern of staining in synaptic regions (58,165). Similar patterns have been observed in a wide variety of normal neuroendocrine cells and their corresponding tumors.

The studies of Wiedenmann and associates have demonstrated that synaptophysin can occur in neuroendocrine tumors of neural type which contain neurofilament antigens (165). This protein is also in neuroendocrine tumors of epithelial type, co-localized with cytokeratin proteins and desmoplakins. These findings indicate that synaptophysin is expressed independently of other neuronal differentiation markers. Consistent expression of synaptophysin has been observed in pheochromocytomas, paragangliomas, ganglioneuromas, ganglioneuroblastomas and neuroblastomas. Most, but not all carcinoids, have immunoreactive synaptophysin, as have neuroendocrine carcinomas arising in the gastrointestinal tract, bronchopulmonary system, and skin. Most neoplasms of the anterior pituitary and parathyroid glands are also synaptophysin positive. In contrast, non-neuroendocrine neoplasms, mesenchymal tumors and melanomas lack this synaptic vesicle protein (58,165).

Lymphoreticular Antigens

Normal and neoplastic neuroendocrine cells may share certain antigenic determinants in common with lymphoreticular cells. The T-lymphocyte antigen, thy-1, has been detected in certain central and peripheral neurons while macrophage antigens detectable with monoclonal antibodies OKM1, and OKM8, 9 and 10, have been detected in cell lines derived from small (oat) cell carcinomas of the lung (136).

The monoclonal antibody HNK-1 (Leu 7), which reacts with natural killer lymphocytes (Chapter 1), also reacts with myelin associated glycoprotein in the central and peripheral nervous system and with adrenal medullary chromaffin cells (90,103). In addition, this antibody stains a small proportion of cells in the anterior pituitary, pancreatic islets and the gastrointestinal tract (150). Both pheochromocytomas and small (oat) cell carcinomas of the lung may react with Leu 7 (150). While this antibody reacts with plasma membrane constituents of lymphocytes and glial cells, ultrastructural immunocytochemical studies have revealed that it reacts with a secretory granule matrix constituent of chromaffin granules. In immunoblot experiments the antibody reacts with a 75 kd constituent of chromaffin granules which differs from the myelin associated glycoprotein. The finding of lymphoreticular antigens in some neuroendocrine cells and their corresponding neoplasms suggest that these proteins may serve similar functions in these cell types. Such common functions might include certain aspects of cell to cell recognition and possible common mechanisms of release of secretory products in response to microenvironmental signals (150).

S-100 Protein

The S-100 protein is a highly acidic phenylalanine-rich protein which was first isolated from bovine brain and which has been localized in a variety of cells including Schwann cells, melanocytes, lipocytes, dendritic reticulum cells and myoepithelial cells (54,115) (Chapter 9). S-100 protein immunoreactivity is also present within thyroid follicular cells, biliary epithelium, pancreatic acinar and ductal cells and also within renal tubules (85, 158). In certain neuroendocrine tumors such as pheochromocytomas and pituitary adenomas, immunoreactivity has been found in sustentacular and folliculo-stellate cells, respectively (92,112). S-100 protein is restricted to the sustentacular cells of most carcinoids (Fig. 15), but in some it is also in the tumor cells.

Other Antigens

Acidic fractions of protein extracts of human brain have been used to generate polyclonal antisera and monoclonal antibodies that react with subsets of neuroendocrine cells. The monoclonal antibody E36, for example, reacts with the myelin sheath of peripheral nerves and the cytoplasm of astrocytes. E36 also reacts with cells in the anterior pituitary, gastrointestinal tract, pancreatic islets and adrenal medulla (131). The epitope recognized by antibody E36 is less widely distributed than chromogranin proteins, and its distribution is different from that observed with antibodies to S-100 protein and neuron specific enolase.

The monoclonal antibody A2B5 reacts with a plasma membrane component of neuroen-

TABLE 2. *Markers in endocrine pathology*

Endocrine Organ	Hormonal Markers	Nonhormonal Markers
Adenohypophysis	Growth hormone, prolactin, adrenocorticotropin, thyroid stimulating hormone, follicle stimulating hormone, luteinizing hormone, chorionic gonadotropin (alpha-chain)	Cytokeratins, chromogranins, neuron specific enolase, S-100 protein
Posterior Pituitary	Vasopressin, oxytocin, neuro-physins	Glial fibrillary acidic protein, S-100 protein
Hypothalamus	Growth hormone releasing hor-mone, gonadotropin releasing hormone, somatostatin, glucagon	Glial fibrillary acidic protein, S-100 protein, neurofilaments
Thyroid		
Follicular cells	Tri-iodothyronine, thyroxine thyroglobulin	Cytokeratins, vimentin, HLA-DR, Lactoferrin
C-cells	Calcitonin, calcitonin gene related product, somatostatin neurotensin, gastrin releasing peptide (bombesin), adreno-corticotropin, vasoactive intestinal peptide, serotonin	Keratins, neurofilaments vimentin, chromogranins, neuron specific enolase, synaptophysin, CEA
Stromal cells		Vimentin
Lymphoreticular cells		Common leukocyte antigen, immunoglobulins, T-and B-cell differentiation markers
Pancreas	Insulin, glucagon, somato-statin, pancreatic polypeptide, gastrin, vasoactive intestinal peptide, calcitonin, growth hormone releasing hormone, gastrin releasing peptide (bombesin), adrenocorticotropin enkephalins, vasopressin, para-thyroid hormone-like material, serotonin, chorionic gonadotropin	Cytokeratins, neurofilaments, chromogranins, neuron specific enolase, synap-tophysin
Gastrointestinal Tract	Gastrin, serotonin, somato-statin, cholecystokinin-pancreozymin, gastrin inhibitory peptide, vasoactive intestinal peptide motilin, gastrin releasing peptide (bombesin), pancreatic polypeptide, enkephalins, tetrin, growth hormone releasing hormone, substance P, serotonin	Cytokeratins, neurofilaments, chromogranins, neuron specific enolase, synapto-physin, CEA
Bronchopulmonary System	Serotonin gastrin releasing peptide, calcitonin, somato-statin, enkephalins, adreno-corticotropin, vasoactive intestinal peptide	Cytokeratins, neurofilaments, chromogranins, neuron specific enolase, synapto-physin
Parathyroid	Parathyroid hormone	Cytokeratins, vimentin, para-thyroid secretory protein (chromogranin)

Adrenal

Cortex	Steroids	Vimentin, cytokeratins
Medulla	Catecholamines, enkephalins, vasoactive intestinal peptide, somatostatin	Neurofilaments, chromogranins, neuron specific enolase, synaptophysin, S-100 protein
Thymus	Serotonin, somatostatin adrenocorticotropin, enkephalins	Cytokeratins, neurofilaments, neuron specific enolase, chromogranin
Skin		
(Merkel cell)	Calcitonin, enkephalins, adrenocorticotropin, pancreatic polypeptide	Cytokeratins, neurofilaments, neuron specific enolase, chromogranins

docrine cells which has been characterized as a ganglioside (49). In the nervous system, A2B5 reacts with neurons, astrocytes and oligodendrocytes. The A2B5 monoclonal antibody reacts with plasma membranes of adrenal medullary cells and pheochromocytomas; additionally, the antibody recognizes a constituent of medullary thyroid carcinoma cells but not normal C-cells.

Endocrine cells may produce a variety of oncodevelopmental antigens including carcinoembryonic antigen (7,106,125) and chorionic gonadotropin (66). These markers will be discussed in subsequent sections of this review, in relationship to specific endocrine tumor types.

TUMORS OF SPECIFIC SITES

Adenohypophysis

The cells of the anterior pituitary have been classified into acidophilic, basophilic and chromophobic types with the use of standard histological stains (78). The application of more sophisticated histochemical staining sequences revealed, however, that each cell type could be further subdivided. For example, the acidophils could be differentiated by their reactivities with orange G and erythrosin and these cells were eventually shown to contain prolactin and growth hormone, respectively with immunohistochemical methods.

The growth homone containing somatotrophs account for about 50% of the cells in the normal anterior pituitary. These cells are present predominantly in the lateral wings of the anterior lobe. Prolactin cells, also termed lactotrophs or mammotrophs, represent 15% to 25% of the cells, and are particularly numerous at the posterolateral edges of the gland. Corticotrophs account for 15% to 20% of the cells and are located in the so-called central mucoid wedge. In addition to adrenocorticotropin, these cells also contain immunoreactive beta-lipotropin and endorphins. The thyrotrophs account for approximately 5% of the anterior pituitary cells and are located in the anteromedial segments of the gland. The gonadotrophs compromise about 10% of the cells and are scattered throughout the anterior lobe with some concentration in the posterolateral region. In some gonadotrophs, follicle stimulating hormone (FSH) and luteinizing hormone (LH) can be demonstrated in the same cell while others contain only one. S-100 positive folliculo-stellate cells, which contain immunoreactive glial fibrillary acidic protein, are also present.

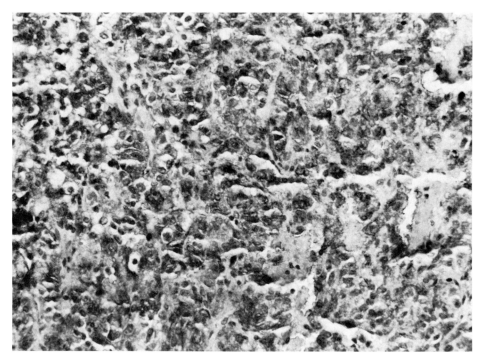

FIG. 1. Pituitary adenoma stained for chromogranin A with the monoclonal antibody LK2H10. This tumor failed to stain with antibodies directed against anterior pituitary hormones and was classified as a null cell adenoma. Chromogranin immunoreactivity is present in most of the tumor cells. Avidin biotin peroxidase complex (ABC) technique with diaminobenzidine (DAB) as the chromogen (× 400).

With the advent of immunohistochemistry, the classification of pituitary adenomas into acidophilic, basophilic and chromophobic types has been replaced by a functional classification (78). This includes: 1) densely granulated growth cell adenomas; 2) sparsely granulated growth cell adenomas; 3) densely granulated prolactinomas; 4) sparsely granulated prolactinomas; 5) mixed growth hormone-prolactin cell adenomas in which prolactin and growth hormone are present in separate cells; 6) acidophil stem cell adenomas in which growth hormone and prolactin are present in the same cells; 7) mammosomatotroph cell adenomas in which growth hormone staining is strong but prolactin is weakly stained; 8) functioning corticotroph cell adenomas; 9) silent corticotroph cell adenomas; 10) thyrotroph cell adenomas; 11) gonadotroph cell adenomas; 12) null cell adenomas in which there is no stainable hormone except in some instances of apparent alpha chain production; 13) oncocytomas in which staining for hormones is negative; 14) unclassified plurihormonal adenomas in which the hormonal content is variable.

Chromogranin A immunoreactivity has been evaluated both in normal and neoplastic anterior pituitary cells (43). With the LK2H10 monoclonal antibody, chromogranin A has been detected in TSH, FSH, LH and alpha subunit containing cells while prolactin, growth hormone and ACTH cells are unreactive. In adenomas, chromogranin immunoreactivity is restricted to those tumors storing TSH, FSH/LH or FSH/LH/TSH. Chromogranin has proven to be a particularly useful marker for null cell adenomas as well as oncocytic tumors, and in the series reported by Lloyd and co-workers, 12 of 17 null cell adenomas, including oncocytomas were chromogranin positive (Fig. 1). Neuron specific enolase occurs in anterior pituitary cells of all types and in their corresponding tumors (4). There is no apparent correlation between the degree of granularity or differentiation of the tumor and the intensity of the staining for neuron specific enolase.

Both normal and neoplastic anterior pituitary cells contain cytokeratins and the patterns of immunoreactivity are characteristic of specific cell types (67). Growth hormone producing cells exhibit a paranuclear condensation of cytokeratin filaments and this appearance is accentuated in growth hormone producing adenomas in the form of cytoplasmic fibrous bodies. Both normal and neoplastic prolactin cells show a less intense paranuclear staining pattern. Adrenocorticotropin cells, on the other hand, exhibit a more uniform and diffuse pattern of cytokeratin staining. Areas of Crooke's hyaline change are typically cytokeratin positive. FSH, LH, and TSH cells show diffuse weak staining or are completely unreactive for cytokeratins.

Hypothalamus

Hypothalamic ganglionic or gangliocytic hamartomas (choristomas) are rare lesions which usually project from the base of the brain, attached by a stalk to the tuber cinereum or mamillary bodies. These resemble hypothalamic nuclei and may show fiber connections with the hypothalamus. They also occur within the adenohypophysis, and have been termed neuronal choristomas. Asa and co-workers have reported six hypothalamic gangliocytomas associated with growth hormone production and/or acromegaly (3,5). Immunohistochemical analyses revealed that human growth hormone releasing factor (GRF) was present in the neurons of all six cases. In some, gonadotropin releasing hormone, somatostatin and glucagon were also present. The anterior pituitary adenomas associated with the gangliocytomas contained growth hormone. These data support the view that excess GRF is the primary mechanism in hypothalamic acromegaly. Analogously, precocious puberty has been found in association with hypothalamic hamartomas producing luteinizing hormone releasing hormone (LHRH).

Pineal Gland

Pineal tumors of any histological type may be associated with precocious puberty. This syndrome may result from mechanical compression that leads to activation of the hypothalamic-pituitary axis or destruction of gonadotropin inhibitory factors. Immunohistochemical studies of pituitary germinomas have demonstrated that some of these tumors secrete chorionic gonadotropin which may mediate, in part, the syndrome of precocious puberty (81).

Thyroid/Follicular Cells

The most important products of follicular cells that have been demonstrated by immunohistochemical techniques are thyroglobulin (TGB), thyroxine (T_4) and tri-iodothyronine (T_3). These constituents are demonstrable in tissues that have been fixed in formalin and embedded in paraffin or frozen and fixed by other techniques (75,168). TGB is a glycoprotein of approximately 660 kd and a sedimentation constant of 19S. Iodoproteins with higher and lower sedimentation constants have also been identified and localized immuno-

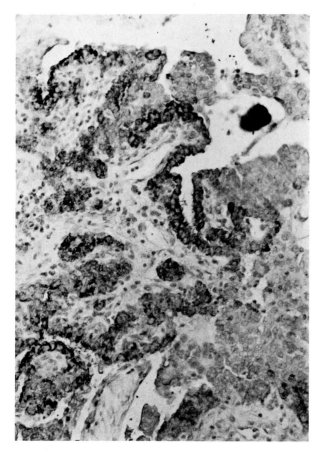

FIG. 2. Papillary carcinoma of the thyroid stained with antibodies to thyroglobulin (**A**). Thyroglobulin immunoreactivity is present diffusely throughout the cytoplasm of the tumor cells. (*Figure continues*).

A

histochemically (15,73). Normal glands show considerable variation in the staining of individual follicles for TGB. Active cuboidal to columnar cells in follicles show more intense staining than flattened and presumably atrophic cells (15,16,47). A similar variation is often seen in the staining of intraluminal colloid, and this may result from varying degrees of masking of TGB associated with different functional states. Marked variability in thyroglobulin immunoreactivity is seen in adenomatous thyroid glands while cases of Graves' disease reveal intense staining of both hyperplastic follicular cells and colloid. An intense staining is also observed in Hashimoto's disease. Autoantibodies to the thyroid in Graves' and Hashimoto's disease are described in Chapter 5.

Adenomas of follicular cells have been classified according to their ultrastructural characteristics and their patterns of TGB staining (15). In general, autonomously functioning or hyperactive adenomas show more intense TGB immunoreactivity than scintigraphically cold nodules. The macrofollicular adenomas which are lined by atrophic appearing flattened follicular cells are most often TGB negative as are pure oncocytic tumors. Clear cell adenomas show a focal dot-like pattern of TGB staining. The mitochondrion rich adenomas, which typically show numerous mitochondria within their basal regions, exhibit TGB staining in the apices of individual follicular cells. Tumors composed of so called "main"

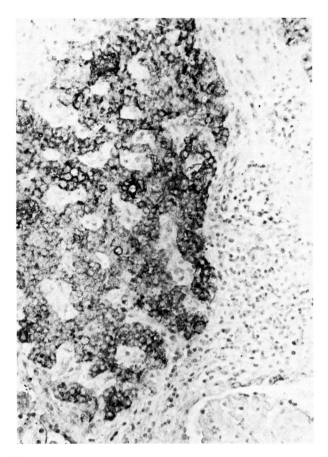

FIG. 2 (*continued*). **B.** Lymph node metastasis of follicular variant of papillary thyroid carcinoma. Staining is present diffusely throughout the cytoplasm of the tumor cells while the stroma is unreactive. ABC technique with DAB as the chromogen (× 400).

B

cells, hypertrophic cells or ergastoplasm-rich cells show diffuse TGB staining throughout their cytoplasm (15).

More than 90% of follicular and papillary carcinomas are TGB positive, including those cases presenting as metastatic lesions in lymph nodes or other sites (15,100). TGB in follicular carcinomas is often patchy in distribution and considerable variation in staining intensity has been noted in cases of papillary carcinoma (Fig. 2). Thus, while some cells show diffuse and uniform staining, others show focal apical and/or basal positivity or no staining whatsoever. In general, poorly differentiated tumors of the follicular type have shown less staining than well differentiated neoplasms. Berge-Lefranc demonstrated lower levels of TGB messenger RNA by *in situ* hybridization in less well differentiated follicular carcinomas than in better differentiated variants (12).

Undifferentiated (anaplastic) thyroid carcinomas are generally thyroglobulin negative except for small residual foci which may show papillary or follicular differentiation (15, 22,128). Most of the tumors previously classified as small cell undifferentiated carcinomas have proven to be lymphomas on the basis of their reactivity with antibodies to common leukocyte antigen, immunoglobulins or other markers of lymphoreticular cells (9,101, 151,161) (Chapter 11). TGB deposits may be seen around lymphoma cells infiltrating the

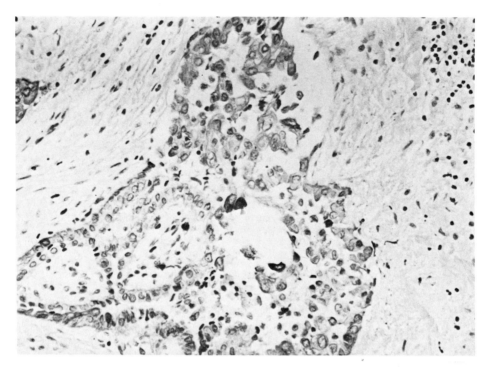

FIG. 3. Lymph node metastasis of papillary thyroid carcinoma stained with antibodies to high molecular weight cytokeratins. While most of the cells exhibit faint staining occasional cells are intensely reactive for high molecular weight cytokeratins. ABC technique with DAB as the chromogen (× 400).

thyroid; however, thyroglobulin reactivity is not seen within the cytoplasm of these cells, unless they exhibit phagocytic activity. A similar phenomenon may also be encountered in metastases to the thyroid gland. In such instances, metastatic tumors within the thyroid may surround deposits of thyroglobulin containing colloid. *In situ* hybridization for TGB messenger-RNA might be useful to discriminate synthesis of TGB by tumor cells (Chapter 19).

Carcangiu and co-workers have reported the morphologic and immunohistochemical features of 20 poorly differentiated ("insular") thyroid carcinomas (23). These contained thyroglobulin immunoreactivity which was most intense in the colloid of neoplastic follicle like structures, but was also present within the cytoplasm of tumor cells in most cases. These tumors were characteristically negative for calcitonin, but did occasionally exhibit somatostatin immunoreactivity. They suggested that this tumor type is morphologically and biologically in an intermediate position between the well differentiated papillary/follicular carcinomas and the undifferentiated/anaplastic thyroid carcinoma. They believe that it is identical to the so-called "wuchernde Strume," first described by Langhans.

Kawaoi and colleagues studied the distribution of tri-iodothyronine (T_3) and thyroxine (T_4) in a large series of thyroid adenomas and carcinomas (75). They found T_4 in 59.8% of tumors and T_3 in 78.4%. In 65 cases serially sectioned and stained for TGB, T_3 and T_4, the distribution of T_4 correlated well with TGB staining. T_3 staining did not always correlate with immunoreactivity for T_4 or thyroglobulin. Approximately two-thirds of papillary carcinomas were positive for T_3 while 95% stained for T_4. Fifty-four percent of follicular carcinomas were T_4 positive while 81% contained immunoreactive T_3. Forty percent of anaplastic carcinomas were positive for T_3, but none was positive for T_4. The significance of T_3 staining in the absence of T_4 and TGB immunoreactivity remains unknown.

In addition to thyroglobulin, T_3 and T_4, a variety of other products including lactoferrin have been demonstrated in primary thyroid neoplasms. HLA-DR antigens have also been demonstrated in the thyroid (93,157). All cases of Hashimoto's disease and most cases of Graves' disease showed HLA-DR staining both in follicular cells and in adjacent inflammatory cells. Most papillary carcinomas, including follicular variants, expressed HLA-DR in contrast to true follicular and medullary carcinomas which were negative for HLA-DR (93) (see Chapter 1 for a discussion of the significance of enhanced DR expression).

Intermediate filament analysis has proved its value in the classification and diagnosis of thyroid neoplasms (107). Antibodies to high molecular weight cytokeratins (raised to human plantar callus) reacted with some follicular cells in 1 of 12 normal thyroids, 8 of 18 thyroids with nodular hyperplasia and 12 of 12 thyroids with chronic thyroiditis. Among thyroid tumors, high molecular weight cytokeratins were identified in 100% of papillary carcinomas (12/12), 14% of follicular carcinomas (1/17), 20% of anaplastic carcinomas (2/10) and 25% of medullary carcinomas (1/14) (Fig. 3). More broadly reactive cytokeratin antibodies stained all tumor types as well as normal thyroids and cases of nodular hyperplasia and chronic thyroiditis. Follicular variants of papillary carcinoma also stained positively with antibodies to high molecular weight cytokeratins. Vimentin immunoreactivity was co-expressed with cytokeratin immunoreactivity in 4 of 4 papillary, 2 of 7 follicular, 2 of 4 medullary and 10 of 10 anaplastic carcinomas. A single case of thyroid sarcoma reported by Miettinen and co-workers was cytokeratin negative but vimentin positive (107).

Thyroid/C-cells

Parafollicular cells were first recognized in the thyroid more than 100 years ago; however, the functional significance of these cells was unknown until the 1960s when it was shown that they synthesized calcitonin. These cells also contain chromogranin proteins and neuron specific enolase in addition to other markers of neuroendocrine cells. Medullary thyroid carcinoma is derived from C-cells (39,42). These tumors may occur sporadically or as a manifestation of a genetically determined disorder with an autosomal dominant inheritance (32). The triad of medullary thyroid carcinoma, pheochromocytoma and parathyroid hyperplasia has been referred to as Sipple's syndrome or type II multiple endocrine neoplasia syndrome (MEN). Patients with medullary thyroid carcinoma have been shown to have elevated concentrations of calcitonin in the serum; moreover, administration of calcitonin secretogogues such as calcium and pentagastrin increase serum levels of the hormone (61). The latter observation has served as the basis for screening family members at high risk for the development of the inherited tumor complex. Detailed studies of such kindreds have led to the identification of C-cell hyperplasia, the precursor of medullary thyroid carcinoma (42,169).

C-cells in normal thyroid glands are concentrated at the junctions of the upper and middle thirds of the lateral lobes, as shown by immunoperoxidase techniques with antisera to synthetic human calcitonin M (29,39,42). C-cell hyperplasia is characterized by increased numbers of C-cells in these same regions. As normal C-cells, hyperplastic C-cells are exclusively intrafollicular, separated from the interstitium by the follicular basal lamina. These relationships are maintained in areas of more advanced hyperplasia where

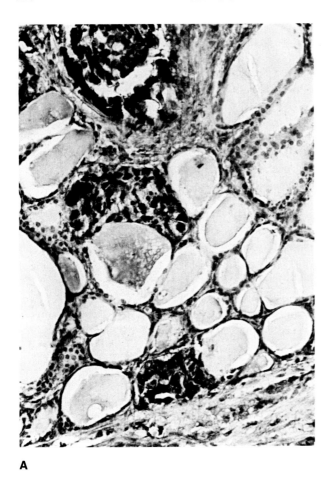

FIG. 4. Familial medullary thyroid carcinoma stained for calcitonin. Areas of C-cell hyperplasia are characterized by proliferation of C-cells within the follicular basement membranes (**A**). Foci of medullary thyroid carcinoma show evidence of stromal infiltration (*Figure continues.*)

A

C-cells often completely encircle and displace the follicular epithelium centrally. Nodular hyperplasia is characterized by the complete obliteration of the follicular space by C-cells. Medullary thyroid carcinoma is heralded by invasion of individual C-cells through defects in the follicular basal lamina (42) (Figs. 4 and 5).

C-cell hyperplasia, adjacent to medullary thyroid carcinomas or in the contralateral lobe, is a morphological marker for the familial form of this tumor (39,42). Sporadic medullary thyroid carcinomas rarely, if ever, have associated C-cell hyperplasia. The identification of C-cell hyperplasia should, therefore, alert the pathologist to the presence of the familial form of the disease and appropriate screening studies should be undertaken in other family members. Foci of nodular C-cell hyperplasia should be distinguished from a variety of other lesions in the thyroid gland including solid cell nests, foci of squamous metaplasia of follicular cells, tangential cuts of follicles and areas of palpation thyroiditis. Of these, only solid cell nests can contain immunoreactive calcitonin. Solid cell nests occur in 9.5 to 41% of thyroid glands studied at autopsy and their frequency appears to increase with the age of the population studied (6). The significance of these lesions is currently unknown since detailed endocrinology studies have not been performed in affected individuals. C-cell hyperplasia also occurs in hypercalcemia and hypergastrinemia. This type of C-cell hyperplasia has been termed "secondary," in contrast to the apparent primary C-cell hyperplasia noted in type II MEN (39,42).

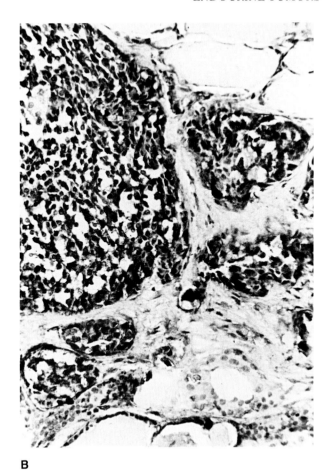

FIG. 4 (*continued*). (**B**). Peroxidase antiperoxidase (PAP) technique with DAB as the chromogen (× 400).

B

Medullary thyroid carcinomas are frequently multihormonal. These tumors may synthesize calcitonin gene-related product, somatostatin, adrenocorticotropin, β-endorphin, vasoactive intestinal peptide, serotonin and prostaglandins (34,38,51,69,139,166,170). Recently, neurotensin immunoreactivity has been identified both in human and rat medullary thyroid carcinomas (40,170) (Fig. 6). Gastrin releasing peptide (GRP) has also been demonstrated in medullary thyroid carcinoma. Kameya and co-workers have demonstrated GRP immunoreactive cells in 81% of medullary thyroid carcinomas and have also shown GRP immunoreactivity in both primary and secondary C-cell hyperplasia (74,102).

CEA has been identified in cases of medullary thyroid carcinoma and in normal C-cell cells (42). CEA and calcitonin have a similar immunohistochemical distribution in C-cell hyperplasia and medullary thyroid carcinoma grossly confined to the thyroid. In virulent disseminated tumor, on the other hand, there is an apparent inverse relationship between CEA and calcitonin content. The expression of CEA (a marker of early epithelial differentiation) in the face of loss of calcitonin (a marker for terminal differentiation) may reflect a degree of maturation block in aggressive tumors (106). One monoclonal antibody to CEA has a high specificity for medullary thyroid carcinomas (135).

Medullary thyroid carcinomas have also been studied with respect to their expression of intermediate filaments. In addition to low molecular weight cytokeratins which have been demonstrated in the majority of these tumors, medullary thyroid carcinomas may

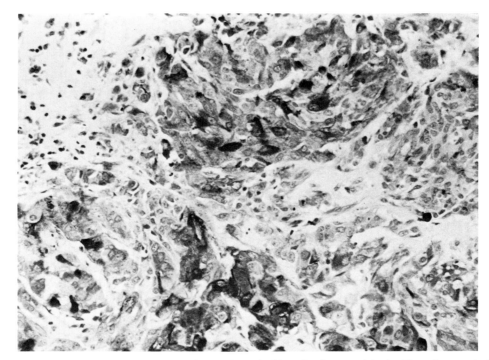

FIG. 5. Sporadic medullary thyroid carcinoma stained with antibodies to calcitonin. There is a marked degree of variation in staining intensity between individual cells of this tumor. PAP technique with DAB as the chromogen ($\times$ 400).

co-express vimentin and neurofilament proteins (107,110). Synaptophysin and desmo-plakins have also been reported (111,165).

Medullary carcinomas are typically negative for TGB except for occasional entrapped follicles or occasional isolated TGB$^+$ cells which may be dissociated follicular elements or phagocytic cells (35) (Fig. 7). In one series, thyroglobulin positive follicles or cells were identified in about two thirds of primary tumors but in no instance of metastatic tumor (35). Rarely, tumors with mixed C-cell and follicular features have been reported (91), and in several, TGB and calcitonin have been demonstrated in the same neoplastic cells. Kameda and co-workers have reported the presence of a C-cell associated TGB both in normal and neoplastic C-cells (73). The C-thyroglobulin is a 27S glycoprotein while the major fraction of TGB has a sedimentation constant of 19S. Although the precise biochemical nature of the C-thyroglobulin is unknown, some studies have indicated that it may represent a pre-cursor to calcitonin rather than being related to thyroglobulin.

Parathyroid Gland

Immunohistochemical localization of parathyroid hormone (PTH) in normal and adenomatous parathyroid tissue has proved difficult. In part, this is due to the heterogene-ity of antibodies obtained upon immunization of animals with intact PTH. While some react with the amino terminus the reactivity of other antibodies used in immunohisto-

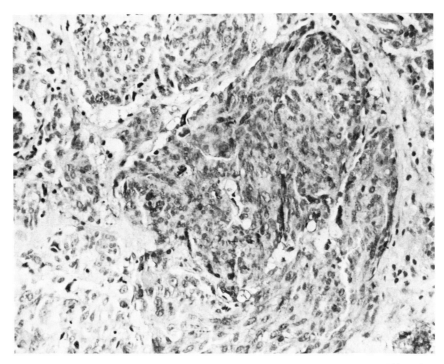

FIG. 6. Sporadic medullary thyroid carcinoma stained with antibodies to neurotensin. Although most of the tumor cells are negative, occasional cells exhibit intense immunoreactivity for neurotensin. PAP technique with DAB as the chromogen (× 400).

chemical procedures is unknown. With an antibody to bovine PTH, immunoreactivity was confined to the cytoplasm of human and bovine chief cells (52). Ultrastructurally, PTH immunoreactivity was found in the secretory granules of the chief cells. A guinea pig antibody to the biologically active aminoterminal region of bovine PTH stained functional oxyphil parathyroid adenomas (117). The antibody also stained two nonfunctional parathyroid carcinomas and an amyloid producing intrathyroid parathyroid tumor (118). Immunoreactivity for intact PTH (1-84) has been reported in four squamous cell carcinomas associated with hypercalcemia (71).

Parathyroid secretory protein (PSP) has also been localized with immunocytochemical techniques (126). The PSP is a dimer which consists of two identical subunits of 70 kd (24). A number of studies have demonstrated that PSP is secreted together with PTH, and PSP has been demonstrated by immunofluorescence in the cytoplasm of chief cells. Ultrastructurally, PSP co-localizes with PTH within the matrices of secretory granules. PSP is probably identical to chromogranin A. A positive immunoreaction in parathyroid tissue is seen after staining with the monoclonal antibody to chromogranin A (LK2H10) (98,167).

Normal, hyperplastic and neoplastic parathyroid tissues have been analyzed for intermediate filaments. The studies of Miettinen and co-workers have established that cytokeratin numbers 8 (52 kd), 18 (45 kd) and 19 (40 kd) are present in chief cells using immunoblotting and immunoperoxidase techniques (108). The chief cells of the parathyroid are, therefore, similar to other normal and neoplastic epithelial cells. High molecular weight cytokeratins on the other hand, are not expressed by parathyroid parenchymal cells. Miettinen

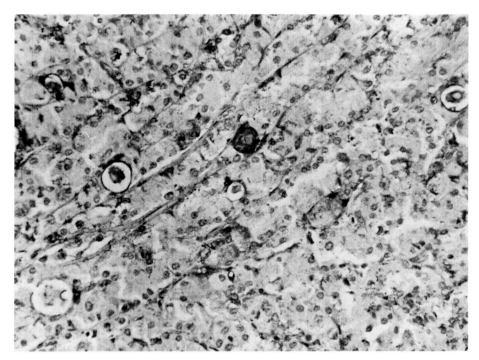

FIG. 7. Familial medullary thyroid carcinoma stained with antibodies to thyroglobulin. Occasional deposits of thyroglobulin are present within entrapped follicle like structures in this tumor. PAP technique with DAB as the chromogen (× 400).

also noted positive reactions for low molecular weight cytokeratins in water-clear and oxyphil cells; the reactivity of oxyphil cells was generally weaker than that of the chief cells. Vimentin is not expressed by the parenchymal cells but is demonstrable in stromal and vascular endothelial cells. Glial fibrillary acidic protein is not detectable in the parathyroid.

Miettinen and co-workers reported positive staining for neurofilament proteins (70 and 200 kd) in occasional cells of approximately one-third of the adenomas (108). In one, the presence of neurofilament proteins was confirmed by immunoblotting studies. Additional studies, however, will be required to resolve the question of the specificity of neurofilament proteins within parathyroid adenomas.

The oxidative enzymes of parathyroid adenomas have also been analyzed by immuno-histochemical techniques. Using an antibody to cytochrome c oxidase, Bedetti and his collaborators demonstrated an intense immunoperoxidase reaction in the cytoplasm of 10 oxyphilic parathyroid adenomas (11). Transitional type oxyphil cells stained with an intermediate intensity while the chief cells in the capsules of the adenomas stained weakly or not at all.

Lung

Argyrophilic cells, similar to those throughout the gastrointestinal tract, are present within the lungs of fetuses, newborns (145), and adults, where they have been referred to as clear cells or *Helle Zellen* (59). At the ultrastructural level, these cells contain heterogeneous secretory granules similar to those in neuroendocrine cells in other portions of the body. Subsequent studies revealed that the bronchopulmonary neuroendocrine cells could occur as solitary neuroendocrine elements or as small cellular aggregates which have been termed neuroepithelial bodies. Although the precise roles of these cells have not as yet been defined, it has been suggested that neuroepithelial bodies may serve a chemoreceptor function while isolated neuroendocrine cells may have a paracrine function. Immunohistochemical studies have demonstrated that serotonin, bombesin and calcitonin (10) are present within solitary neuroendocrine cells and neuroepithelial bodies, while leu-enkephalin is present only in solitary neuroendocrine cells (59).

Bombesin appears by about ten weeks of gestation in neuroendocrine cells and neuroepithelial bodies which increase in number with development (142). Bombesin cells are most numerous in live born infants with chronic respiratory disease. In contrast, calcitonin cells do not appear until late in the second trimester (142). Similar to bombesin, the calcitonin positive cells were most numerous in infants with chronic pulmonary disease. Serotonin containing cells were easily recognized in the lungs of first and second trimester fetuses; these were scarce in hyaline membrane disease, but were numerous in infants with chronic respiratory disease. Leu-enkephalin positive cells were found in one infant who survived 7 post-natal months of respirator care following neonatal hyaline membrane disease.

The neuroendocrine cells of the lung may undergo a series of hyperplastic changes following irritation or exposure to a variety of carcinogens (59). The studies of Gould and associates have established that mild forms of neuroendocrine cell hyperplasia retain the expression of peptides and amines normally produced by these cell types. In contrast, more severe forms of hyperplasia and dysplasia are more likely to be associated with production of ectopic products including adrenocorticotropin, vasoactive intestinal peptide and somatostatin.

Neoplasms of the bronchopulmonary neuroendocrine cells including carcinoids, atypical carcinoids and small cell (oat cell) undifferentiated carcinomas have also been studied extensively with respect to their contents of regulatory peptides and amines (19,30,59, 130,147,148,156,162,163) (Figs. 8 and 9). The most frequently encountered regulatory products include serotonin, bombesin and leu-enkephalin. Less commonly, these tumors may contain somatostatin, calcitonin, gastrin, vasoactive intestinal peptide, melanocyte stimulating hormone and adrenocorticotropin. Neuroendocrine carcinomas contain a series of similar regulatory products; however, they most commonly contain adrenocorticotropin bombesin and/or calcitonin. Said and co-workers have examined a large series of pulmonary neuroendocrine tumors with a panel of antibodies to chromogranin (Fig. 8), neuron specific enolase (Fig. 9) and bombesin (130). Neuron specific enolase was found in 100% of carcinoids and small cell carcinomas; however, this enzyme was also localized in 57% of non-neuroendocrine tumors. Bombesin was identified in 70% of carcinoids and small cell carcinomas. Chromogranin was identified in all carcinoids but in no case of small cell carcinoma. Our own studies suggest that focal chromogranin immunoreactivity is present in some small cell carcinomas, particularly after fixation in formol sublimate or Bouin's solution (Fig. 10).

Blobel and co-workers studied the desmosomal proteins and intermediate filaments in a wide spectrum of neuroendocrine neoplasms (14). Pulmonary neuroendocrine tumors contain intermediate filaments of the cytokeratin type with a predominance of cytokeratins 8, 18 and 19. Cytokeratin 19 tends to be present in small amounts in these tumors. Of the 5 neuroendocrine tumors of small cell type (oat cell), only 2 of 5 contained cytokeratins. In

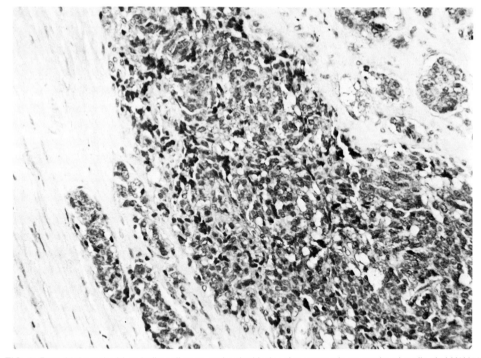

FIG. 8. Bronchial carcinoid, spindle cell type, stained with the chromogranin monoclonal antibody LK2H10. Occasional cells within this tumor exhibit intense chromogranin immunoreactivity. ABC technique with DAB as the chromogen ($\times$ 400)

contrast, all carcinoids and neuroendocrine carcinomas of intermediate type contained cytokeratins. The tumors were negative for vimentin, desmin and glial fibrillary acidic protein. The presence of neurofilament proteins in pulmonary neuroendocrine tumors has been studied by several groups with conflicting results. Lehto reported neurofilament immunoreactivity in 6 of 6 oat cell carcinomas (87), but Moll and Franke found that 8 neuroendocrine carcinomas of the oat cell and intermediate cell types were negative for neurofilaments and 4 of 7 bronchial carcinoids and 1 of 2 well-differentiated neuroendocrine carcinomas were positive (110).

In some instances, it may be impossible to distinguish metastatic oat cell carcinomas from primary cutaneous neuroendocrine (Merkel cell) tumors. Moll and Franke have reported a new cytoskeletal protein (IT) of 46 kd, (pI6.1), which may permit this distinction. The IT protein was originally found in normal human intestinal cells and in colonic carcinomas. Although the specific relationship of IT to other intermediate filaments is unknown, this protein most likely represents a cytokeratin (110). IT was present in all Merkel cell tumors, but was not found in bronchopulmonary neuroendocrine neoplasms (110).

Pancreatic Islets

With routine histochemical stains, the pancreatic islets have been divided into three cell types, designated alpha, beta, and delta (50). The beta cells, which account for 60% to

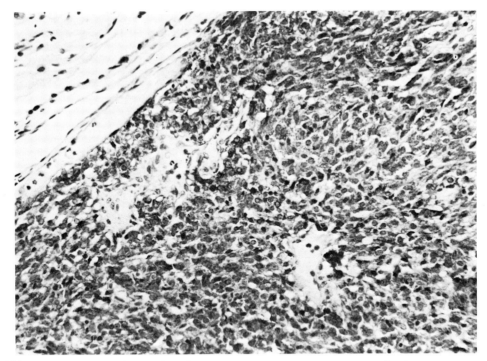

FIG. 9. Bronchial carcinoid, spindle cell type, stained with antibodies to neuron specific enolase (same case as Fig. 8). There is faint uniform reactivity for neuron specific enolase within most of the tumor cells. ABC technique with DAB as the chromogen ($\times$ 400).

80% of the cells, synthesize and store insulin. The glucagon-producing alpha cells constitute 15% to 20% of the cells and the somatostatin-producing delta cells account for 5% to 15% of the cells. Recently, a fourth cell type which produces pancreatic polypeptide (PP) has been identified (84). This cell type accounts for less than 2% of the cells and is found predominantly in the head of the gland. In many species, serotonin producing enterochromoaffin (EC) cells have also been identified within the islets; however, the existence of this cell type in humans is controversial. Endocrine cells are also present in extra-insular sites, particularly in relationship to pancreatic ducts (57).

Pancreatic endocrine tumors are biochemically heterogeneous. In addition to the eutopic hormones normally produced by islet cells, they may synthesize and secrete a variety of ectopic hormones (26,65,67), including gastrin, vasoactive intestinal peptide (VIP) (Fig. 11), adrenocorticotropin, growth hormone releasing hormone, a parathyroid hormone like substance, calcitonin, enkephalin, neurotensin, vasopressin, cholecystokinin and bombesin (41,116). Precise phenotyping of pancreatic endocrine tumors is important for several reasons. First, the predominant hormonal species stored correlates with metastatic potential. The frequency of malignancy in the various subtypes is: insulinoma (5% to 10%), PPoma (5% to 10%), glucagonoma (60%) (Fig. 12), gastrinoma (75%), VIPoma (75%), SRIFoma (75%), serotonin producing carcinoid ($>$ 75%) (65). Secondly, a small proportion of pancreatic endocrine tumors may be clinically nonfunctional. In these instances, immunohistochemistry may provide the only functional data on the biochemical composition of the

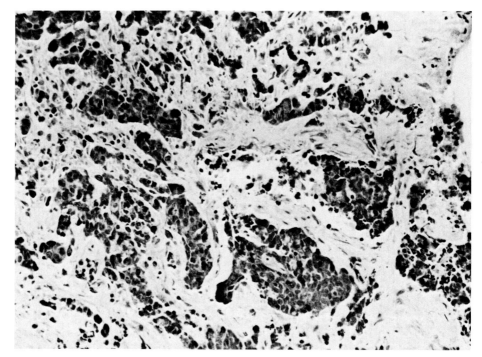

FIG. 10. Small cell undifferentiated bronchogenic carcinoma (intermediate type) stained with the monoclonal antibody to chromogranin A, LK2H10. Occasional cells within this tumor exhibit intense chromogranin immunoreactivity. ABC technique with DAB as the chromogen (× 400).

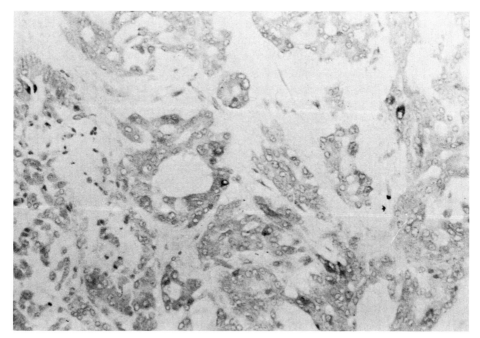

FIG. 11. Metastatic pancreatic endocrine tumor associated with the syndrome of watery diarrhea and hypokalemia, stained with antibodies to vasoactive intestinal peptide. While most of the cells are weakly reactive, occasional cells show intense staining. PAP technique with DAB as the chromogen (× 400).

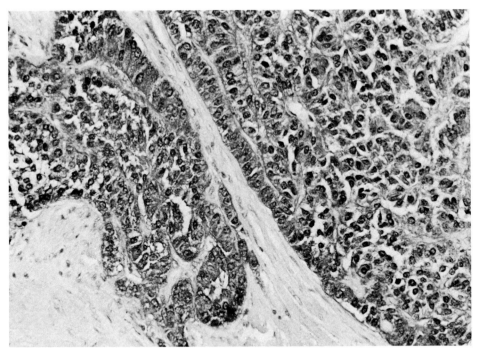

FIG. 12. Pancreatic endocrine tumor associated with the overproduction of glucagon, stained with antibodies to glucagon. Most of the cells exhibit weak to moderate glucagon immunoreactivity. PAP technique with DAB as the chromogen ($\times$ 400).

tumor. Thirdly, a significant proportion of pancreatic endocrine tumors, including those in the type I multiple endocrine neoplasia syndrome are multihormonal. Thus, the symptoms associated with overproduction of one hormone may be masked or overshadowed by the production of a second hormone. A transition from one syndrome to another may occur during the natural history of the neoplasm or during the course of chemo- and radiotherapy. Detailed analyses of pancreatic endocrine tumors have shown that somewhat more than 50% contain peptides not causing a specific clinical syndrome. Among the various peptides present in these multihormonal tumors, PP and insulin appear to be the most frequent (65,67).

In addition to the ectopic and eutopic hormones discussed above, a variety of other hormones have been identified in pancreatic endocrine tumors. The alpha chain of glycoprotein hormones has, in fact, been suggested as a marker of malignancy in functional pancreatic tumors (66). Positive staining for this marker has shown a good correlation with metastatic potential in some series.

Studies of resected pancreatic tissue in patients with type I multiple endocrine neoplasia syndrome have revealed evidence of single or multiple benign and malignant islet cell neoplasms (65). Approximately two thirds of them represent non-beta neoplasms, while the remainder have been classified as insulin producing beta cell tumors. In addition, there is often an associated hyperplasia of individual islets together with multifocal ducto-insular proliferations of endocrine cells. These foci are typically multicellular and are composed of various admixtures of insulin, glucagon, somatostatin and PP producing cells. The pancreatic tissue from infants with neonatal hypoglycemia has also been studied by immunohistochemistry. In these cases, the proportions of islet cell types are normal and are similar to those in controls.

Neuron specific enolase (13,133), chromogranin proteins (94) and synaptophysin (58) have been identified in normal and neoplastic pancreatic endocrine cells. Antibodies to neuron specific enolase stain virtually all normal and neoplastic pancreatic endocrine cell types as well as intrapancreatic nerves. Chromogranin immunoreactivity in normal islets as defined with the LK2H10 monoclonal antibody, is present predominantly in the glucagon cells while insulin cells showed considerably less reactivity. Analysis of tumors revealed that chromogranin was present in one glucagonoma, four gastrinomas and the tumors associated with multiple hormone production. Five insulinomas and one somatostatinoma were negative for chromogranins (94). Thus, both neuron specific enolase and chromogranins are expressed commonly in pancreatic endocrine tumors; however, because of the low specificity of neuron specific enolase, this marker should not be used alone for diagnosis of pancreatic endocrine tumors. Synaptophysin proteins have also been identified in pancreatic endocrine tumors of all types (58,165).

The intermediate filaments of normal pancreatic endocrine cell and their corresponding tumors are of the cytokeratin type (110). Some pancreatic endocrine tumors, however, may also express neurofilament immunoreactivity in contrast to adult and fetal pancreatic endocrine cells.

Gastrointestinal Tract

The gastrointestinal tract contains an extensive system of polypeptide hormone and amine producing cells (27). Similar to the cells of the adrenal medulla, some of the gastrointestinal endocrine cells react with potassium dichromate to form a yellow brown pigment which indicates the presence of amines. These gastrointestinal chromaffin positive cells have been referred to as enterochromaffin cells. A second population of gut endocrine cells is chromaffin negative. While the enterochromaffin cells can also be identified by their ability to reduce silver salts (argentaffinity), the non-enterochromaffin cells show variable degrees of argyrophilia. With the advent of immunohistochemistry and electron micros-

TABLE 3. *Gastrointestinal peptides and their cellular localization*

Hormone(s)	Cell Type
Gastrin, adrenocorticotropin, met-enkephalin	G
Gastrin	IG
Tetrin	TG
Somatostatin	D
Secretin	S
Cholecystokinin	I
Gastric inhibitory peptide	K
Motilin	Mo
Neurotensin	N
Enteroglucagon	L
Substance P, leu-enkephalin, serotonin	EC_1
Motilin-like peptide, leu-enkephalin, serotonin	EC_2
Serotonin, unknown product	EC_n
Unknown	ECL
Vasoactive intestinal peptide-like material	D_1
Bombesin like peptide	P
Pancreatic polypeptide	PP
PYY	PYY
Unknown	X

copy, it has been possible to classify the gut endocrine cells into at least 18 different types (Table 3) (141).

The pathophysiology of the gut endocrine cells is just beginning to be explored (27). In some cases, this goal has already been achieved and it has been possible to correlate a spectrum of proliferative abnormalities with hormone concentrations in the serum and associated clinical syndromes. Pronounced G-cell hyperplasia, for example, has been described in association with atrophic gastritis, pernicious anemia and retained excluded antrum (27). In these cases, G-cell hyperplasia probably occurs as a result of decreased hydrochloric acid bathing the gastric antrum (secondary G-cell hyperplasia). G-cell hyperplasia also occurs in association with hypercalcemia of different etiologies (28). An apparent primary G-cell hyperplasia (Fig. 13) has been found in some patients with Zollinger-Ellison syndrome unassociated with pancreatic or extra-pancreatic gastrinomas (27,88).

The understanding of normal gut hormone distribution has also profoundly influenced our knowledge of carcinoids (33) and related tumors (122,164). Carcinoids have been divided into 3 major groups on the basis of their sites of origin and their reactivities with silver stains. More recent studies have shown that there is a generally strong, although not invariable, correlation between the hormonal profiles of carcinoids and the distribution of

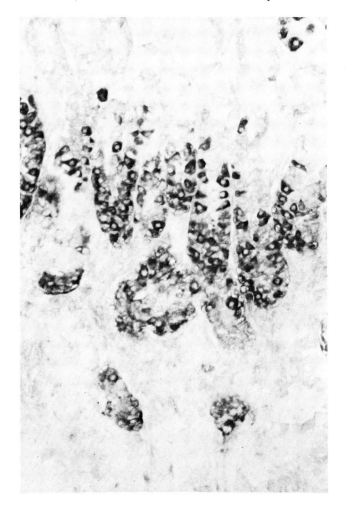

FIG. 13. Gastric antrum from a patient with primary G-cell hyperplasia, stained with antibodies to gastrin. There is a marked increase in G-cells within the gastric glands. PAP technique with DAB as the chromogen ($\times$ 400).

hormones within the normal tissues from which the tumors arise. Foregut carcinoids often contain ACTH, glucagon, somatostatin, insulin, or pancreatic polypeptide (2). Midgut carcinoids frequently contain substance P and motilin (Fig. 14) while hindgut carcinoids may contain glucagon, somatostatin, pancreatic polypeptide, substance P, enkephalin and β-endorphin (27). Gastrin releasing peptide, the mammalian analog of bombesin, has also been identified in gut carcinoids (18). S-100 positive satellite cells are observed frequently around the tumor cell clusters of carcinoids (Fig. 15).

Cytokeratins represent the major intermediate filament proteins expressed by gastrointestinal carcinoids and by corresponding normal endocrine cells present within the gastrointestinal mucosal epithelium and underlying stroma (110). Some of these tumors also contain intermediate filaments of the neurofilament type; moreover, they also exhibit reactivity for synaptophysin and desmoplakins (110,111,165). Carcinoids also apparently react with antibodies to prealbumin although the significance of this finding is unknown (21).

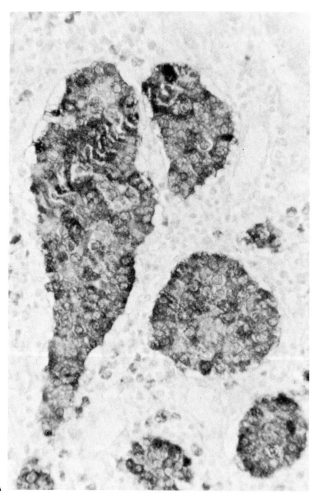

FIG. 14. Small intestinal carcinoid stained with antibodies to serotonin (**A**) and substance P (**B**). Serotonin is present uniformly within the tumor cell clusters while substance P immunoreactivity is accentuated in the peripheral cells. PAP technique with DAB as the chromogen (× 400). (*Figure continues.*)

A

Adrenal Gland

Although immunohistochemical techniques have been utilized for the localization of steroid hormones in the ovary and testis (80), there have been no published studies of steroid localization in the adrenal cortex. The intermediate filament profile of the adrenal cortex and some of its tumors, however, has been examined by Miettinen and co-workers (109). With antibodies to cytokeratin, many but not all of the normal cortical cells show a thin peripheral rim of cytoplasmic staining. There is no evidence of epidermal prekeratin in the normal cortical cells, and these cells also fail to react with antibodies to vimentin and neurofilament proteins. In cortical hyperplasia and cortical adenoma there were scattered cells which were positive for cytokeratins. In about half of the cases of cortical carcinoma, cytokeratin positive cells were identified and in 10%, occasional cells also stained positively with antibodies to epidermal prekeratin. Cortical carcinoma cells frequently revealed co-expression of vimentin and in several instances, vimentin was the only intermediate filament identified.

In contrast to the cytokeratin positivity observed in cortical cells, medullary cells are cytokeratin negative but neurofilament positive (109,132,153). With antibodies to 200 kd neurofilament proteins, positive staining was confined to axons. Antibodies reacting with

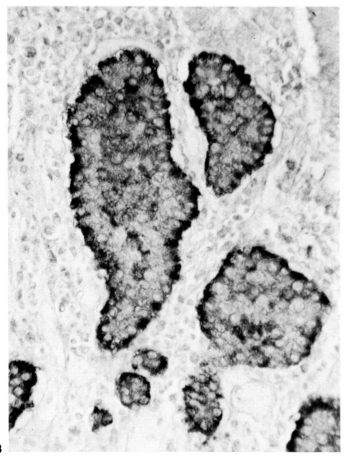

B

FIG. 14 (*continued.*)

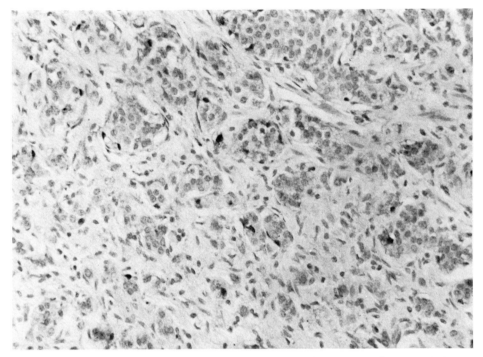

FIG. 15. Carcinoid tumor of the appendix stained with antibodies to S-100 protein. S-100 protein immunoreactivity is confined to satellite cells around the clusters of tumor cells. PAP technique with DAB as the chromogen (× 400).

68–70 and 200 kd neurofilaments on the other hand, labeled axons, ganglion cells and chromaffin cells. Pheochromocytoma cells contain neurofilament determinants reactive with antibodies to 68–70 and 200 kd proteins. Mukai and co-workers have studied a large series of human neural tumors with antibodies to neurofilament triplet proteins (113). Eight extra-adrenal paragangliomas were positively stained with antibodies to the 68 kd protein while 5 of these tumors also contained cells with reactivity for the 150 and 200 kd components. Fifteen ganglioneuromas and ganglioneuroblastomas had cells which reacted with all three neurofilament protein components. In contrast, 7 of 7 neuroblastomas contained the 68 kd component while only 3 had cells which were positive for the 150 and 200 kd neurofilament proteins.

Chromogranins, neuron specific enolase and S-100 protein have been studied in normal, hyperplastic and neoplastic adrenal medullary tissue (92,155). Generally, chromogranin immunoreactivity is more intense in normal than neoplastic adrenal medullary cells. Sustentacular cells, which are positive with antibodies to S-100 protein, are present around the nests of adrenal medullary cells. Numerous sustentacular cells have also been identified in cases of adrenal medullary hyperplasia and familial pheochromocytomas. Smaller numbers of this cell type have been noted in cases of nonfamilial (sporadic) pheochromocytoma and in extraadrenal paragangliomas (92). Variable numbers of sustentacular cells have been noted in neuroblastomas and large numbers of these cells have been found to correlate with a good prognosis (137).

Both catecholamines and catecholamine synthesizing enzymes have been demonstrated by immunofluorescent techniques in frozen sections and by immunoperoxidase techniques

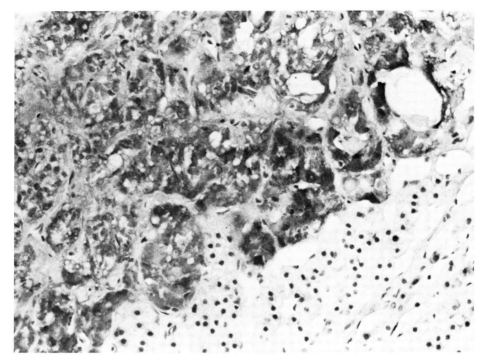

FIG. 16. Diffuse adrenal medullary hyperplasia from a patient with type II MEN stained with antibodies to leu-enkephalin. The medullary cells show strong staining for this peptide while the cortical cells are unstained. PAP technique with DAB as the chromogen ($\times$ 400).

in formalin fixed paraffin embedded samples (96). In addition to catecholamines, a variety of regulatory peptides has been identified in normal and neoplastic adrenal medullary cells (37,95). These include somatostatin, leu- and met-enkephalin (Fig. 16), adrenocorticotropin, VIP and substance P. Although VIP has been noted in some pheochromocytomas showing neuronal differentiation, this peptide may occur in pheochromocytoma cells without neuronal differentiation. In some instances, the presence of VIP in pheochromocytomas and neuroblastomas has been associated with the syndrome of watery diarrhea and hypokalemia (105,149).

Skin

Although amphibian skin is richly endowed with peptide hormones, human skin is not. Recent studies using immunohistochemical techniques, however, have demonstrated that the Merkel cells, which contain membrane bound secretory granules may be analogous to the peptide hormone producing cells of the lung, gastrointestinal tract and other sites. Much of the interest concerning the human Merkel cell has been stimulated by observations made on analysis of Merkel cell tumors (60). These small cell malignant tumors may be confused histologically with malignant lymphomas, Ewing's tumor, and metastases from bronchogenic small cell carcinomas. A variety of peptides have been identified in Merkel cell tumors: calcitonin, somatostatin, adrenocorticotropin, met-enkephalin, pancreatic polypeptide and vasoactive intestinal peptide. However, a significant proportion of these neoplasms may fail to stain with any peptide antisera (60,72,138). The tumors fail to stain with certain polyclonal antisera to CEA but up to 60% contain epithelial membrane antigen (138). These tumors may co-express neurofilament proteins with cytokeratins (68). Merkel cell tumors also contain a novel intermediate filament which has been designated IT and which may serve to distinguish them from metastatic oat cell carcinomas (110) (see above). These tumors are also commonly positive for neuron specific enolase (86) but less commonly for chromogranin proteins.

Miscellaneous Sites

Endocrine tumors may also arise from a variety of non-endocrine tissues of ectodermal, mesodermal or endodermal derivation, including the thymus, liver, cervix, prostate, kidney, and breast (20,38,45) (Chapter 13). For example, detailed immunohistochemical studies have revealed that certain gastrointestinal and pancreatic adenocarcinomas may contain subpopulations of endocrine cells which are reactive for chromogranin proteins as well as a variety of regulatory peptide products (38). Such tumors could arise from pluripotential stem cells. Alternatively, tumors with subpopulations of endocrine cells might develop as a result of plasticity of differentiated cells, microenvironmental influences or random genetic events during the course of neoplastic development and progression (38).

SUMMARY

The application of immunohistochemical techniques has had a major impact on the practice of endocrine pathology. These methods have proved effective for the localization of hormones and a wide range of non-hormonal products in normal endocrine cells and in many of their corresponding tumors. Immunohistochemical techniques have permitted the correlation of functional abnormalities with the earliest manifestations of disease at the cellular level, and have defined new clinical and pathologic entities.

ACKNOWLEDGMENTS

The author wishes to thank Drs. Yogeshwar Dayal and Paul Kwan for the use of case material, Kirsten Underwood for technical assistance, Sonia Alexander and John Gottshall for photographic assistance and Carol Ostrum for secretarial support.

REFERENCES

1. Aguirre, P., Scully, R. E., Wolfe, H. J., and DeLellis, R. A. (1984): Endometrial carcinomas with argyrophil cells. A histochemical and immunohistochemical analysis. *Hum. Pathol.*, 15:210–217.
2. Alumets, J., Falkmer, S., Grimelius, L., Hakanson, R., Ljunberg, O., Sundler, F., and Wilander, E. (1980): Immunocytochemical demonstration of enkephalin and B-endorphin in endocrine tumors of the rectum. *Acta Pathol. Microbiol. Scand. [Sect A]*, 88:103–109.
3. Asa, S. L., Bilboa, J. M., Kovacs, K., and Linfoot, J. A. (1980): Hypothalamic neuronal hamartoma associated with pituitary growth hormone cell adenoma and acromegaly. *Acta Neuropathol.*, 52:231–234.
4. Asa, S. L., Ryan, N., Kovacs, K., Singer, W., and Marangos, P. J. (1984): Immunohistochemical localization of neuron specific enolase in the human hypophysis and pituitary adenomas. *Arch. Pathol. Lab. Med.*, 108:40-43.
5. Asa, S. L., Scheithauer, B. W., Bilboa, J. M., Horvath, E., Ryan, N., Kovacs, K., Randall, R. V., Laws, E. R., Singer, W., Linfoot, J. A., Thorner, M. O., and Vale, W.(1984): A case for hypothalamic acromegaly: A clinicopathological study of six patients with hypothalamic gangliocytoma producing growth hormone releasing factor. *J. Clin. Endocrin.*, 58:796–803.

6. Autelitano, F., Santeusanio, G., diTondo, U., Costantino, A. M., Renda, F., and Autelitano, M. (1987): Immunohistochemical study of solid cell nests of the thyroid gland found from an autopsy study. *Cancer*, 59:477–483.

7. Batge, B., Bosslet, K., Sedlacek, H. H., Kern, H. F., and Kloppel, G. (1986): Monoclonal antibodies against CEA related components discriminate between pancreatic duct type carcinomas and non neoplastic duct lesions as well as nonduct type neoplasias. *Virchows Arch. (Pathol. Anat.)*, 408:361–374.

8. Battifora, H. (1985): Monoclonal antibodies in immunocytochemistry. In: *Immunocytochemistry in Tumor Diagnosis*, edited by J. Russo, pp. 31–58. Martinus Nijhoff Publishers, Boston.

9. Battifora, H., and Trowbridge, I. S. (1983): A monoclonal antibody useful for the differential diagnosis between malignant lymphoma and non-hematopoietic neoplasms. *Cancer*, 51:816–821.

10. Becker, K. L., Monaghan, K. G., and Silva, O. (1980): Immunocytochemical localization of calcitonin in Kulchitsky cells of human lung. *Arch. Pathol. Lab. Med.*, 104:196–198.

11. Bedetti, C. D., Dekker, A., and Watson, C. G. (1984): Functioning oxyphil cell adenoma of the parathyroid gland: A clinicopathologic study of 10 patients with hyperparathyroidism. *Hum. Pathol.*, 15:1121–1126.

12. Berge-Lefranc, J. L., Cartouzou, G., DeMicco, D., Fragu, P., and Lissitzky, S. (1985): Quantification of thyroglobulin of thyroglobulin messenger RNA by *in situ* hybridization in differentiated thyroid cancers. *Cancer*, 56:345–350.

13. Bishop A. E., Polak, J. M., Facer, P., Ferri, G-L., Marangos, P. J., and Pearse, A. G. E. (1982): Neuron specific enolase: A common marker for the endocrine cells and innervation of the gut and pancreas. *Gastroenterol.*, 83:902–915.

14. Blobel, G., Gould, V. E., Moll, R., Lee, I., Huszar, M., Geiger, B., and Franke, W. (1985): Co-expression of neuroendocrine markers and epithelial cytoskeletal proteins in bronchopulmonary neuroendocrine neoplasms. *Lab. Invest.*, 52:39–51.

15. Bocker, W., Dralle, H., and Dorn, G. (1981): Thyroglobulin: An immunohistochemical marker in the diagnostic pathology of thyroid disease. In: *Diagnostic Immunohistochemistry*, edited by R. A. DeLellis, pp. 37–59. Masson Publishers USA, Inc., New York.

16. Bocker, W., Dralle, H., Koch, G., DeHeer, K., and Hagemann, J. (1978): Immunohistochemical and electron microscope analysis of adenomas of the thyroid gland. I. Adenomas with specific cytological differentiation. *Virchows Arch. A Pathol. Anat. Histol.*, 380:205–220.

17. Bosman, F. T., van Assche, C., Nieuwenhuyzen-Krusaman, A. C., Jackson, S., and Lowry, P. (1984): Growth hormone releasing factor immunoreactivity in human and rat gastrointestinal tract and pancreas. *J. Histochem. Cytochem.*, 32:1139.

18. Bostwick, D. C., Roth, K. A., Barchas, J. D., and Bensch, K. (1984): Gastrin releasing peptide immunoreactivity in intestinal carcinoids. *Am. J. Clin. Pathol.*, 82:428–431.

19. Bostwick, D. C., Roth, K. A., Evans, C. J., Barchas, J. D., and Bensch, K. G. (1984): Gastrin releasing peptide, a mammalian analog of bombesin is present in human neuroendocrine lung tumors. *Am. J. Pathol.*, 117:195–200.

20. Bussolati, G., Gugliotta, P., Sapino, A., Eusebi, V., and Lloyd, R. V. (1985): Chromogranin reactive endocrine cells in argyrophilic carcinomas ("carcinoids") and normal tissue of the breast. *Am. J. Pathol.*, 120:186–192.

21. Bussolati, G., Papotti, M., and Sapino, A. (1984): Binding of antibodies against human prealbumin to intestinal and bronchial carcinoids and to pancreatic endocrine tumors. *Virchows Arch. (B)*, 45:15–20.

22. Carcangiu, M. L., Steeper, T., Zampi, G., and Rosai, J. (1985): Anaplastic thyroid cancer. A study of 70 cases. *Am. J. Clin. Pathol.*, 83:135–158.

23. Carcangiu, M. L., Zampi, G., and Rosai, J. (1984): Poorly differentiated ("insular") thyroid carcinoma. A reinterpretation of Langhans' "wuchernde struma". *Am. J. Surg. Pathol.*, 8:655–668.

24. Cohn, D. V., Elking, J. J., Frick, M., and Elde, R. (1984): Selective localization of the parathyroid secretory protein-I/adrenal medulla chromogranin family in a wide variety of endocrine cells. *Endocrinology*, 114:1963–1974.

25. Corson, J. M. (1986): Keratin protein immunohistochemistry in surgical pathology practice. *Pathol. Ann.*, 21:47–81.

26. Creutzfeldt, W. (1980): Endocrine tumors of the pancreas: Clinical chemical and morphological findings. In *The Pancreas*, International Academy of Pathology Monograph, pp. 208–230. Williams & Wilkins, Baltimore.

27. Dayal, Y. (1983): Endocrine cells of the gut and their neoplasms. In *Pathology of the Colon, Small Intestine and Anus*, edited by H. T. Norris, pp. 267–302. Churchill-Livingstone, New York.

28. Dayal, Y., and Wolfe, H. J. (1984): G-cell hyperplasia in chronic hypercalcemia: An immunocytochemical and morphometric analysis. *Am. J. Pathol.*, 116:391–397.

29. Deftos, L. J., Bone, H. G., Parthemore, J. G., and Burton, D. W. (1980): Immunohistochemical studies of medullary thyroid carcinoma and C-cell hyperplasia. *J. Clin. Endocrinol. Metab.*, 51:857–862.

30. Deftos, L. J., and Burton, D. (1980): Immunohistochemical studies of non-thyroidal calcitonin producing tumors. *J. Clin. Endocrinol. Metab.*, 50:1042–1045.

31. DeLellis, R. A. (1981): Basic techniques of immunohistochemistry. In: *Diagnostic Immunohistochemistry*, edited by R. A. DeLellis, pp. 7–16. Masson Publishers USA, Inc., New York.

32. DeLellis, R. A., Dayal, Y., Tischler, A. S., Lee, A. K., and Wolfe, H. J. (1986): Multiple endocrine neoplasia syndromes: Cellular origins and inter-relationships. *Int. Rev. Exp. Pathol.*, 28:163–190.

33. DeLellis, R. A., Dayal, Y., and Wolfe, J. H. (1984): Carcinoid tumors. Changing concepts and new perspectives. *Am. J. Surg. Pathol.*, 8:295–300.

34. DeLellis, R. A., May, L., Tashjian, A. H., Jr., and Wolfe, H. J. (1978): C-cell granule heterogeneity in man. An ultrastructural immunocytochemical study. *Lab. Invest.*, 38:263–269.

35. DeLellis, R. A., Moore, F. M., and Wolfe, H. J. (1983): Thyroglobulin immunoreactivity in human medullary thyroid carcinoma. *Lab. Invest.*, 48:20A.

36. DeLellis, R. A., Sternberger, L. A., Mann, R. B., Banks, P. M., and Nakane, P. K. (1979): Immunoperoxidase techniques in diagnostic pathology. *Am. J. Clin. Pathol.*, 71:483–488.

37. DeLellis, R. A., Tischler, A. S., Lee, A. K., Blount, M., and Wolfe, H. J. (1983): Leu enkephalin-like immunoreactivity in proliferative lesion of the human adrenal medulla and extra-adrenal paraganglia. *Am. J. Surg. Pathol.*, 7:29–37.

38. DeLellis, R. A., Tischler, A. S., and Wolfe, H. J. (1984): Multidirectional differentiation in neuroendocrine neoplasms. *J. Histochem. Cytochem.*, 32:899–904.

39. DeLellis, R. A., and Wolfe, H. J. (1981): The polypeptide hormone producing neuroendocrine cells and their tumors. An immunohistochemical analysis. *Method. Achiev. Exp. Pathol.*, 10:190–220.

40. DeLellis, R. A., and Wolfe, H. J. (1982): Neurotensin immunoreactivity in human medullary thyroid carcinoma. *J. Histochem. Cytochem.*, 30:608 (abstract).

41. DeLellis, R. A., and Wolfe, H. J. (1983): Contribution of immunohistochemistry to clinical endocrinology and endocrine pathology. *J. Histochem. Cytochem.*, 31:187–192.

42. DeLellis, R. A., and Wolfe, H. J. (1981): The pathobiology of the C-cell. *Pathol. Annual*, 16:25–40.

43. DeStephano, D. B., Lloyd, R. V., Pike, A. M., and Wilson, B. S. (1984): Pituitary adenomas. An immunohistochemical study of hormone production and chromogranin localization. *Am. J. Pathol.*, 116: 464–472.

44. DeWaele, M., DeMey, J., Renmans, W., Labeur, C., Raynaert, P., and Van Camp, B. (1986): An immunogold silver staining method for detection of cell surface antigens in light microscopy. *J. Histochem. Cytochem.*, 34:935–940.

45. diSant'Angese, P. A., Jensen, K., Churukian, C. J., and Agarwal, M. M. (1985): Human prostatic endocrine-paracrine (APUD) cells. Distributional analysis with a comparison of serotonin and neuron specific enolase immunoreactivity and silver stains. *Arch. Pathol. Lab. Med.*, 109:607–612.

46. Dockray, G. J. (1979): Evolutionary relationships of the gut hormones. *Fed. Proc.*, 38:2295–2301.

47. Dralle, H., and Bocker, W. (1977): Immunohistochemical and electron microscope analysis of adenomas of the thyroid gland. I. A comparative study of hot and cold nodules. *Virchows Arch. A. Pathol. Anat. Histol.*, 374:281–303.

48. Dranoff, G., and Bigner, D. D. (1984): A word of caution in the use of neuron-specific enolase expression in tumor diagnosis. *Arch. Pathol. Lab. Med.*, 108:535.

49. Eisenbarth, G. S., Shimizu, K., Bowring, M. S., and Wells, S. A. (1982): Expression of receptors for tetanus toxin and monoclonal antibody A2B5 by pancreatic islet cells. *Proc. Natl. Acad. Sci. U.S.A.*, 79:5066–5070.

50. Erlandsen, S. L. (1980): Types of pancreatic islet cells and their immunocytochemical identification. In: *The Pancreas*, International Academy of Pathology Monograph, pp. 140–155. Williams & Wilkins, Baltimore.

51. Falck, B., Ljungberg, O., and Rosengren, E. (1968): On the occurrence of monoamine and related substances in familial medullary thyroid carcinoma. *Acta Pathol. Microbiol. Scand.*, 74:1–10.

52. Futrell, J. M., Roth, S. I., and Su, S. P. (1979): Immunocytochemical localization of parathyroid hormone in bovine parathyroid glands and human parathyroid adenomas. *Am. J. Pathol.*, 94:615–622.

53. Gatter, K. C., Heryet, A., Alcock, C., and Mason, D. Y. (1985): Clinical importance of analyzing malignant tumors of uncertain origin with immunohistological techniques. *Lancet*, i:1302–1305.

54. Gaynor, R., Herschman, H. R., Irie, R., Jones, P., Morton, D., and Cochran, A. (1981): S-100 protein: A marker for human malignant melanoma. *Lancet*, 18:869–871.

55. Goldstein, A., Tachibana, S., Lowney, L. I., Hunkapiller, M., and Hood, L. (1979): Dynorphin (1-13), an extraordinarily potent opioid peptide. *Proc. Natl. Acad. Sci. U.S.A.*, 76:6666.

56. Gould, V. E. (1985): The co-expression of distinct classes of intermediate filaments in human neoplasms. *Arch. Pathol. Lab. Med.*, 109:984–985.

57. Gould, V. E., Chejfec, G., Shah, K., Paloyan, E., and Lawrence, A. M. (1984): Adult nesidiodysplasia. *Sem. Diag. Pathol.*, 1:43–53.

58. Gould, V. E., Lee, I., Wiedenmann, B., Moll, R., Chejfec, G., and Franke, W. W. (1986): Synaptophysin: A novel marker for neurons, certain neuroendocrine cells and their neoplasms. *Hum. Pathol.*, 17:979–983.

59. Gould, V. E., Linnoila, I., Memoli, V. A., and Warren, W. H. (1983): Neuroendocrine components of the bronchopulmonary tract: Hyperplasias, dysplasias and neoplasias. *Lab. Invest.*, 49:519–537.

60. Gould, V. E., Moll, R., Moll, I., Lee, I., and Franke, W. (1985): Neuroendocrine (Merkel) cells of the skin: Hyperplasias, dysplasias and neoplasias. *Lab. Invest.*, 52:334–353.

61. Graze, K., Tashjian, A. H., Jr., Wolfe, H. J., DeLellis, R. A., Miller, H. H., Gagel, R. F., Feldman, Z. T., Melvin, K. E. W., and Reichlin, S. (1978): Provocative tests of calcitonin secretion in the early diagnosis of medullary carcinoma and C-cell hyperplasia of the thyroid gland. *New Engl. J. Med.*, 299:980–985.

62. Greene, G. L., and Jensen, E. V. (1982): Monoclonal antibodies as probes for estrogen receptor detection and characterization. *J. Steroid Biochem.*, 16:353–359.

63. Hagn, C., Schmid, K. W., Fischer-Colbrie, R., and Winkler, H. (1986): Chromogranin, A, B, and C in human adrenal medulla and endocrine tissues. *Lab. Invest.*, 55:405–441.

64. Haimoto, H., Takahashi, Y., Koshikawa, T., Nagura, H., and Kato, K. (1985): Immunohistochemical localization of gamma enolase in normal human tissues other than nervous and neuroendocrine tissue. *Lab. Invest.*, 52:257–263.

65. Heitz, P. U. (1984): Pancreatic endocrine tumors. In: *Pancreatic Pathology*, edited by G. Kloppel and P. U. Heitz, pp. 206–232. Churchill Livingstone, Edinburgh.

66. Heitz, P. U., Kasper, M., Kloppel, G., Polak, J. M., and Vaitukaitis, J. L. (1983): Glycoprotein hormone alpha chain production by pancreatic endocrine tumors: A specific marker of malignancy. Immunocytochemical analysis of tumors in 155 patients. *Cancer*, 48:2029–2037.

67. Heitz, P. U., Kasper, M., Polak, J. M., and Kloppel, G. (1982): Pancreatic endocrine tumors. Immunocytochemical analysis of 125 tumors. *Hum. Pathol.*, 13:263–271.

68. Hoefler, H., Denk, H., and Walter, G. F. (1984): Immunohistochemical demonstration of cytokeratins in endocrine cells of the human pituitary adenomas. *Virchows Arch. [A]*, 404:359–367.

69. Hoefler, H., Kerl, H., Lackinger, E., Helleis, G., and Kenk, H. (1985): The intermediate filament cytoskeleton of cutaneous neuroendocrine carcinoma (Merkel cell tumor). *Virchows Arch. (Pathol. Anat.)*, 406:339–350.

70. Holm, R., Sobrinho-Simoes, M., Nesland, J. M., Gould, V. E., and Johannessen, J. V. (1985): Medullary carcinoma of the thyroid gland: An immunohistochemical study. *Ultrastruct. Pathol.*, 8:25–42.

71. Ilardi, C. F., and Faro, J. (1985): Localization of parathyroid hormone like substances in squamous cell carcinoma. An immunoperoxidase study with ultrastructural correlation. *Arch. Pathol. Lab. Med.*, 109:752–755.

72. Johannessen, J. V., and Gould, V. E. (1980): Neuroendocrine skin carcinoma associated with calcitonin production. A Merkel cell carcinoma? *Hum. Pathol.*, 11:586–589.

73. Kameda, Y., Harada, T., Ito, K., and Ikeda, A. (1979): Immunohistochemical study of medullary thyroid carcinoma with reference to C-thyroglobulin reaction of tumor cells. *Cancer*, 44:2071–2082.

74. Kameya, T., Bessho, T., Tsumuraya, M., Yamaguchi, K., Abe, K., Shimosato, Y., and Yanaihara, N. (1983): Production of gastrin releasing peptide by medullary carcinoma of the thyroid. *Virchows Arch. [A] Pathol. Anat. Histol.*, 401:99.

75. Kawaoi, A., Okano, T., Nemoto, N., Shina, Y., and Shikata, T. (1982): Simultaneous detection of thyroglobulin, thyroxine, and tri-iodothyronine in non-toxic thyroid tumors by the immunoperoxidase method. *Am. J. Pathol.*, 108:39–49.

76. Kendall, P. A., Polak, M., and Pearse, A. G. E. (1971): Carbodiimide fixation for immunohistochemistry. Observations on the fixation of polypeptide hormones. *Experimentia*, 27:1104–1106.

77. King, J. C., Lechan, R. M., Kugel, G., and Anthony, E. L. P. (1983): Acrolein: A fixative for immunocytochemical localization of peptides in the central nervous system. *J. Histochem. Cytochem.*, 31:62–68.

78. Kovacs, K., Horvath, E., and Ryan, N. (1981): Immunocytology of the human pituitary. In: *Diagnostic Immunohistochemistry*, edited by R. A. DeLellis, pp. 17–35. Masson Publishers USA, Inc., New York.

79. Krieger, D. T. (1984): In: *Pituitary Hyperfunction: Pathophysiology and Clinical Aspects*, edited by F. Commani and E. E. Muller, pp. 221–234. Raven Press, New York.

80. Kurman, R. J., Andrade, D., Coebelsmann, V., and Taylor, C. R. (1978): An immunohistological study of steroid localization in Sertoli-Leydig tumors of the ovary and testis. *Cancer*, 42:1772–1783.

81. Laidler, P., and Pounder, D. J. (1984): Pineal germinoma with syncytiotrophoblastic giant cells: A case with panhypopituitarism and isosexual pseudopuberty. *Human Pathol.*, 15:285–287.

82. Larsson, L. I. (1979): Pathology of the gastrin cell. *Pathol. Ann.*, 14:293–316.

83. Larsson, L.-I., Golterman, N., DeMagistris, L., Rehfield, J. F., and Schwarz, T. W. (1979): Somatostatin cell processes as pathways for paracrine secretion. *Science*, 205:1393.

84. Larsson, L. I., Schwartz, T., Lundquist, G., Chance, R. E., Sundler, F., Rehfeld, J. F., Grimelius, L., Fahrenkrug, J., Schaffalitzky De Muckadell, O., and Moon, O. (1976): Occurrence of pancreatic polypeptide in pancreatic endocrine tumors. *Am. J. Pathol.*, 85:675–684.

85. Lee, A. K., Dwarkanath, S., DeLellis, R. A., and Rosen, P. P. (1986): S-100 protein positivity in breast carcinoma. *Lab. Invest.*, 54:35A.

86. Leff, E. L., Brooks, J. S. J., and Trojanowski, J. Q. (1985): Expression of neurofilament and neuron specific enolase in small cell tumors of the skin using immunohistochemistry. *Cancer*, 56:625–631.

87. Lehto, V.-P., Stenman, S., Miettinen, M., Dahl, D., and Virtanen, I. (1983): Expression of a neural type intermediate filament as a distinguishing feature between oat cell carcinoma and other lung cancers. *Am. J. Pathol.*, 110:113–118.

88. Lewin, K., Yang, K., Ulich, T., Elashoff, J. D., and Walsh, J. (1984): Primary gastrin cell hyperplasia. Report of five cases and review of the literature. *Am. J. Surg. Pathol.*, 8:821–832.

89. Lewis, R. V., Stern, A. S., Kimura, S., Rossier, J., Stein, S., and Udenfriend, S. (1981): An about 50,000 dalton protein in adrenal medulla: A common precursor of met- and leu-enkephalin. *Science*, 208:1459–1461.

90. Lipinski, M., Braham, K., Caillaud, J. M., Carlu, C., and Tursz, T. (1983): HNK 1 antibody detects an antigen expressed on neuroectodermal cells. *J. Exp. Med.*, 158:1775–1780.

91. Ljungberg, O., Bondason, L., and Bondason, A.-C. (1984): Differentiated thyroid carcinoma intermediate type. A new tumor entity with features of follicular and parafollicular carcinoma. *Hum. Pathol.*, 15:118–228.

92. Lloyd, R. V., Blaivas, M., and Wilson, B. S. (1985): Distribution of chromogranin and S100 protein in normal and abnormal adrenal medullary tissues. *Arch. Pathol. Lab. Med.*, 109:633–635.

93. Lloyd, R. V., Johnson, T., Blaivas, M., Sisson, J. C., and Wilson, B. S. (1985): Detection of HLA-DR antigens in paraffin embedded thyroid epithelial cells with a monoclonal antibody. *Am. J. Pathol.*, 120: 106–111.

94. Lloyd, R. V., Mervak, T., Schmidt, K., Warner, T. F. C. S., and Wilson, B. S. (1984): Immunohistochemical detection of chromogranin and neuron specific enolase in pancreatic endocrine tumors. *Am. J. Surg. Pathol.*, 8:607–614.

95. Lloyd, R. V., Shapiro, B., Sisson, J. C., Kalff, V., Thompson, N. W., and Beirwaltes, W. A. (1984): An immunohistochemical study of pheochromocytomas. *Arch. Pathol. Lab. Med.*, 108:541–544.

96. Lloyd, R. V., Sisson, J. C., Shapiro, B., and Verhofstad, A. A. J. (1986): Immunohistochemical localization of epinephrine, norepinephrine, catecholamine synthesizing enzymes and chromogranin in neuroendocrine cells and tumors. *Am. J. Pathol.*, 125:45–54.

97. Lloyd, R. V., and Warner, T. F. (1984): Immunohistochemistry of neuron specific enolase. In: *Advances in Immunohistochemistry* edited by R. A. DeLellis, p. 127. Masson Publishers USA, Inc., New York.

98. Lloyd, R. V., and Wilson, B. S. (1983): Specific endocrine tissue marker defined by a monoclonal antibody. *Science*, 222:622–630.

99. Lloyd, R. V., Wilson, B. S., Kovacs, K., and Ryan, N. (1985): Immunohistochemical localization of chromogranin in human hypophyses and pituitary adenomas. *Arch. Pathol. Lab. Med.*, 109:515–517.

100. Lo Gerfo, P., LiVolsi, V., Colacchio, D., and Feind, C. (1978): Thyroglobulin production by thyroid cancers. *J. Surg. Res.*, 24:1–6.

101. Mambo, N. C., and Irwin, S. M. (1984): Anaplastic small cell neoplasms of the thyroid. An immunoperoxidase study. *Hum. Pathol.*, 15:55–60.

102. Matsubayashi, S., Yanaihara, C., Ohkubo, M., Fukata, S., Hayashi, Y., Tamai, H., Nakgawa, T., Miyanchi, A., Kuma, K., Abe, K., Suzuki, T., and Yanaihara, N. (1984): Gastrin releasing peptide immunoreactivity in medullary thyroid carcinoma. *Cancer*, 53:2472–2477.

103. McGarry, R. C., Helfand, S. L., Quarles, R. H., and Roden, J. C. (1983): Recognition of the myelin associated glycoprotein by the monoclonal antibody HNK-1. *Nature*, 306:376–378.

104. Mendelsohn, G. (1981): Histaminase localization in medullary thyroid carcinoma and small cell lung carcinoma. In: *Diagnostic Immunohistochemistry* edited by R. A. DeLellis, pp. 299–312. Masson Publishers USA, Inc., New York.

105. Mendelsohn, G., Eggleston, J. C., Olson, J. L., Said, S. I., and Baylin, S. (1979): Vasoactive intestinal peptide and its relationship to ganglion cell differentiation in neuroblastic tumors. *Lab. Invest.*, 41:144–149.

106. Mendelsohn, G., Wells, S. A., and Baylin, S. B. (1984): Relationship of tissue carcinoembryonic antigen and calcitonin to tumor virulence in medullary thyroid carcinoma. An immunohistochemical study in early, localized and virulent disseminated stages of disease. *Cancer*, 54:657–662.

107. Miettinen, M., Franssila, K., Lehto, V. P., Passivuo, R., and Virtanen, I. (1984): Expression of intermediate filament proteins in thyroid gland and thyroid tumors. *Lab. Invest.*, 50:262–270.

108. Miettinen, M., Clark, R., Lehto, B.-P., Virtanen, I., and Damjanov, I. (1985): Intermediate filament proteins in parathyroid glands and parathyroid adenomas. *Arch. Pathol. Lab. Med.*, 109:986–989.

109. Miettinen, M., Lehto, V.-P., and Virtanen, I. (1985): Immunofluorescence microscopic evaluation of the intermediate filament expression of the adrenal cortex and medulla and their tumors. *Am. J. Pathol.*, 118:-360–366.

110. Moll, R., and Franke, W. W. (1985): Cytoskeletal differences between human neuroendocrine tumors: A cytoskeletal protein of molecular weight 46,000 distinguishes cutaneous from pulmonary neuroendocrine tumors. *Differentiation*, 30:165–175.

111. Moll, R., Colvin, P., Kapprell, H.-P., and Franke, W. W. (1986): Desmosomal proteins: New markers for identification and classification of tumors. *Lab. Invest.*, 54:4–25.

112. Morris, C. S., and Hitchcock, E. (1985): Immunocytochemistry of folliculo-stellate cells in normal and neoplastic pituitary gland. *J. Clin. Pathol.*, 38:481–488.

113. Mukai, M., Torikata, C., Iri, H., Morikawa, Y., Shimizu, K., Shimoda, T., Nukina, N., Ihara, Y., and Kagayama, K. (1986): Expression of neurofilament triplet proteins in human neural tumors. An immunohistochemical study of paraganglioma, ganglioneuroma, ganglioneuroblastoma and neuroblastoma. *Am. J. Pathol.*, 122:28–35.

114. Nakajima, T., Kameya, T., Watanabe, S., Hirota, T., Shimosato, Y., and Isobe, T. (1984): S-100 protein distribution in normal and neoplastic tissues. In: *Advances in Immunohistochemistry*, edited by R. A. DeLellis, pp. 141–158. Masson Publishers USA, Inc. New York.

115. O'Connor, D. T., Burton, D., and Deftos, L. J. (1983): Chromogranin A: Immunohistology reveals its universal occurrence in normal polypeptide hormone producing endocrine gland. *Life Sci.*, 33:1657–1663.

116. Ooi, A., Kamaya, T., Tsurmuraya, M., Yamaguchi, K., Abe, K., Shimosato, Y., and Yanaihara, N. (1985): Pancreatic endocrine tumors associated with WDHA syndrome. An immunohistochemical and ultrastructural study. *Virchows Arch. (Pathol. Anat.)*, 405:311–323.

117. Ordonez, N. G., Ibanez, M. L., Mackay, B., Samaan, N. A., and Hickey, R. C. (1982): Functioning oxyphil cell adenomas of parathyroid gland: Immunoperoxidase evidence of hormonal activity in oxyphil cells. *Am. J. Clin. Pathol.*, 78:681–689.

118. Ordonez, N. G., Ibanez, M. L., Samaan, N. A., and Hickey, R. C. (1983): Immunoperoxidase study of uncommon parathyroid tumors. *Am. J. Surg. Pathol.*, 7:535–542.

119. Pearse, A. G. E. (1974): The APUD cell concept and its implications in pathology. *Pathol. Ann.*, 9:17–41.

120. Pearse, A. G. E., Polak, J. M., Adams, C., and Kendall, P. A. (1974): Diethyl pyrocarbonate, a vapor phase fixative for immunofluorescence studies on polypeptide hormones. *Histochem. J.*, 6:347–352.

121. Pearse, A. G. E., and Polak, J. M. (1975): Bifunctional reagent as vapor and liquid phase fixatives for immunohistochemistry. *Histochem. J.*, 7:179–186.

122. Perrone, T., Sibley, R. K., and Rosai, J. (1985): Duodenal gangliocytic paraganglioma. *Am. J. Surg. Pathol.*, 9:31–41.

123. Press, M. F., and Greene, G. L. (1984): An immunocytochemical method for demonstrating estrogen receptor in human uterus using monoclonal antibodies to human estrophilin. *Lab Invest.*, 50:480–488.

124. Press, M. F., Holt, J. A., Herbst, A. L., and Greene, G. L. (1985): Immunocytochemical identification of estrogen receptor in ovarian carcinomas: Localization with monoclonal estrophilin antibodies compared with biochemical assays. *Lab. Invest.*, 53:349–361.

125. Primus, F. J., Clarke, C. A., and Goldenberg, D. M. (1981): Immunohistochemical detection of carcinoembryonic antigen. In: *Diagnostic Immunohistochemistry*, edited by R. A. DeLellis, pp. 263–276. Masson Publishers USA, Inc., New York.

126. Ravazzola, M., Orci, M., Habener, J. F., and Potts, J. T. (1978): Parathyroid secretory protein: Immunocytochemical localization within cells that contain parathyroid hormone. *Lancet*, 2:371–372.

127. Reichlin, S. (1983): Somatostatin. *N. Engl. J. Med.*, 309:1495–1501; 1556–1563.

128. Rosai, J., Saxen, E. A., and Woolner, L. (1985): Undifferentiated and poorly differentiated carcinoma (thyroid). *Sem. Diag. Pathol.*, 2:123–136.

129. Rosenfeld, M. G., Amara, S. G., Birnberg, M. J., Mermod, J. J., Murdock, G. H., and Evans, R. M. (1983): Calcitonin, prolactin and growth hormone gene express as model systems for the characterization of neuroendocrine regulation. *Rec. Prog. Horm. Res.*, 39:305.

130. Said, J. W., Vinadalal, S., Nash, G., Shintaker, I. P., Heusser, R. C., Sasson, A. F., and Lloyd, R. V. (1985): Immunoreactive neuron specific enolase, bombesin and chromogranin as markers for neuroendocrine lung tumors. *Hum. Pathol.*, 16:236–240.

131. Sappino, A. P., McIhlhinney, R. A. J., Ellison, M., Monaghan, P., and Neville, A. M. (1984): A monoclonal antibody detecting neural and neuroendocrine differentiation. *J. Histochem. Cytochem.*, 32:1041–1047.

132. Sasaki, A., Ogawa, A., Nakazato, Y., and Ishida, Y. (1985): Distribution of neurofilament protein and neuron specific enolase in peripheral neuronal tumors. *Virchows Arch. (Pathol. Anat.)*, 407:33–41.

133. Schmechel, D., Marangos, P. J., and Brightman, M. (1978): Neuron specific enolase is a molecular marker for peripheral and central neuroendocrine cells. *Nature*, 17:834–836.

134. Schmechel, D. (1985): Gamma subunit of the glycolytic enzyme enolase: Non-specific or neuron specific. *Lab. Invest.*, 52:239–242.

135. Schroder, S., and Kloppel, G. (1987): Carcinoembryonic antigen and non-specific cross reacting antigen in thyroid cancer. An immunocytochemical study using polyclonal and monoclonal antibodies. *Am. J. Surg. Pathol.*, 11:100–108.

136. Seeger, R. C., Danon, Y. L., Rayner, S. A., and Hoover, F. (1982): Detection of thy-1 on human neuroblastoma, glioma, sarcoma and teratoma cells with a monoclonal antibody. *J. Immunol.*, 128:983–989.

137. Shimado, H., Aoyama, C., Chilba, T., and Newton, W. A. (1985): Prognostic subgroups for undifferentiated neuroblastoma. Immunohistochemical study with anti S-100 protein antibody. *Hum. Pathol.*, 16:471–476.

138. Sibley, R. K., and Dahl, D. (1985): Primary neuroendocrine carcinoma (Merkel cell?) of the skin. II. An immunocytochemical study of 21 cases. *Am. J. Surg. Pathol.*, 9:109–116.

139. Sikri, K. L., Varndell, I. M., Hamid, G. A., Wilson, B. S., Kameya, T., Ponder, B. A., Lloyd, R. V., Bloom, S. R., and Polak, J. M. (1985): Medullary carcinoma of the thyroid. An immunocytochemical and histochemical study of 25 cases using 8 separate markers. *Cancer*, 56:2481–2491.

140. Snyder, S. H. (1980): Brain peptides as neurotransmitters. *Science*, 209:976.

141. Solcia, E., Polak, J. M., Pearse, A. G. E., Forsmann, W. G., Larsson, L-I., Sundler, D., Lechago, J., Grimelius, L., Fujita, T., Creutzfeldt, W., Gepts, W., Falkmer, S., LeFranc, G., Heitz, P., Hage, E., Buchanan, A. M. J., Bloom, S. R., and Grossman, M. I. (1978): Lausanne 1977 Classification of gastro-entero-pancreatic endocrine cells. In: *Gut Hormones*, edited by S. R. Bloom and M. I. Grossman, pp. 40–48. Churchill Livingstone, Edinburgh.

142. Stahlman, M. T., Kasselberg, A. G., Orth, D., and Gray, M. F. (1985): Ontogeny of neuroendocrine cells in human fetal lung. II. An immunohistochemical study. *Lab. Invest.*, 52:52–60.

143. Sternberger, L. A. (1979): *Immunocytochemistry*, 2nd Ed. John Wiley & Sons, New York.

144. Tapia, F. J., Varndell, I. M., Propert, L, DeMey, J., and Polak, J. M. (1983): Double immunogold staining method for the simultaneous ultrastructural localization of regulatory peptides. *J. Histochem. Cytochem.*, 31:977–981.

145. Tateishi, R. (1973): Distribution of argyrophil cells in adult human lungs. *Arch. Pathol.*, 96:198–202.
146. Taylor, C. R. (1986): *Immunomicroscopy: A Diagnostic Tool for the Surgical Pathologist.* W. B. Saunders, Philadelphia.
147. Tischler, A. S. (1978): Small cell carcinoma of the lung: Cellular origin and relationship to other neoplasms. *Semin. Oncol.*, 5:244–252.
148. Tischler, A. S., Dichter, M. A., Biales, B., DeLellis, R. A., and Wolfe, H. J. (1976): Neural properties of cultured human endocrine tumor cells of proposed neural crest origin. *Science*, 192:902–904.
149. Tischler, A. S., Lee, A. K., Nunnemacher, G., Said, S., DeLellis, R. A., Morse, E., and Wolfe, H. J. (1981): Spontaneous neurite outgrowth and vasoactive intestinal peptide like immunoreactivity in human glomus jugulare paraganglioma cell cultures. *Cell Tissue Res.*, 219:545–555.
150. Tischler, A. S., Mobtaker, H., Mann, K., Nunnemacher, G., Jason, W. J., Dayal, Y., DeLellis, R. A., Adelman, L., and Wolfe, H. J. (1986): Antilymphocyte monoclonal antibody HNK1 (leu 7) recognizes a constituent of neuroendocrine secretory granule matrix. *J. Histochem. Cytochem.*, 34:1213–1216.
151. Tobler, A., Maurer, R., and Hedinger, C. E. (1984): Undifferentiated thyroid tumors of diffuse small cell type. Histological and immunohistochemical evidence for their lymphomatous nature. *Virchows Arch. (Pathol. Anat.)*, 404:117–126.
152. Tomita, T., Friesen, S. R., Kimmel, J. R., Doull, V., and Pollock, H. G. (1983): Pancreatic polypeptide secreting endocrine tumors. A study of three cases. *Am. J. Pathol.*, 113:134–142.
153. Trojanowski, J., and Lee, V. M. Y. (1985): Expression of neurofilament antigens by normal and neoplastic human adrenal chromaffin cells. *N. Engl. J. Med.*, 313:101–103.
154. Trotta, K., Pruss, R. M., DeLellis, R. A., Wolfe, H. J., and Tischler, A. S. (1986): Cytochrome b561 is a cell type specific marker of neuroendocrine granule membrane. *Lab. Invest.*, 54:64A.
155. Tsokos, M., Linnoila, I., Chandra, R. S., and Triche, T. J. (1984): Neuron specific enolase in the diagnosis of neuroblastoma and other small round cell tumors in children. *Hum. Pathol.*, 15:575–584.
156. Tsutsumi, Y., Osamura, R. Y., Watanabe, K., and Yanaihara, N. (1983): Immunohistochemical studies in gastrin releasing peptide and adrenocorticotrophic hormone-containing cells in the human lung. *Lab. Invest.*, 48:623–632.
157. Tuccari, G., and Barresi, G. (1985): Immunohistochemical demonstration of lactoferrin in follicular adenomas and thyroid carcinomas. *Virchows Arch. (Pathol. Anat.)*, 406:67–74.
158. Vanstapel, M.-J., Gatter, K. C., deWolf-Peeters, C., Mason, D. Y., and Desmet, V. D. (1986): New sites of human S-100 immunoreactivity detected with monoclonal antibodies. *Am. J. Clin. Pathol.*, 85:160–168.
159. Verhofstad, A. A. J., Steinbusch, H. W. M., Joosten, J. W. J., Penke, O., Varga, J., and Goldstein, M. (1983): Immunocytochemical localization of nonadrenaline, adrenaline and serotonin. In: *Immunohistochemistry, Practical Applications in Pathology and Biology*, edited by J. M. Polak and S. Van Noorden, pp. 143–168, Wright-PSG, Bristol.
160. Vinores, S. A., Bonnin, J. M., Rubinstein, L. J., and Marangos, P. J. (1984): Immunohistochemical demonstration of neuron specific enolase in neoplasms of the CNS and other tissues. *Arch. Pathol. Lab. Med.*, 108:536–540.
161. Warnke, R. A., Gatter, K. C., Falini, B., Hildreth, P., Woolston, R. E., Pulford, K., Cordell, J. L., Cohen, B., DeWolf-Peeters, C., and Mason, D. Y. (1983): Diagnosis of human lymphoma with monoclonal antileucocyte antibodies. *N. Engl. J. Med.*, 309:1275–1281.
162. Warren, W. H., Memoli, V. A., and Gould, V. E. (1984): Immunohistochemical and ultrastructural analysis of bronchopulmonary neuroendocrine neoplasm. I. Carcinoids. *Ultrastruc. Pathol.*, 6:15–28.
163. Wharton, J., Polak, J. M., Bloom, S. R., Ghatei, M. A., Solcia, E., Brown, M. R., and Pearse, A. G. E. (1978): Bombesin like immunoreactivity in the lung. *Nature*, 273:769–770.
164. Wick, M., Weatherby, R. P., and Weiland, L. H. (1987): Small cell neuroendocrine carcinoma of the colon and rectum: Clinical, histological and ultrastructural study and immunohistochemical comparison with cloacogenic carcinoma. *Hum. Pathol.*, 18:9–21.
165. Wiedenmann, B., Franke, W. W., Kuhn, C., Moll, R., and Gould, V. E. (1986): Synaptophysins: A marker protein for neuroendocrine cells and neoplasms. *Proc. Natl. Acad. Sci. U.S.A.*, 83:3500–3504.
166. Williams, E. D., Karin, S. M., and Sandler, M. (1968): Prostaglandin secretion by medullary carcinoma of the thyroid. A possible cause of the associated diarrhea. *Lancet*, 1:22–23.
167. Wilson, B. S., and Lloyd, R. V. (1984): Detection of chromogranin in neuroendocrine cells with a monoclonal antibody. *Am. J. Pathol.*, 115:458–468.
168. Wilson, M., Hitchcock, K. R., and DeLellis, R. A. (1978): Immunohistochemical localization of thyroid hormone in rat thyroid. *J. Histochem. Cytochem.*, 26:1121–1124.
169. Wolfe, H. J., Melvin, K. E. W., Cervi-Skinner, S. J., Al Saadi, A. A., Juliar, J. F., Jackson, C. E., and Tashjian, A. H., Jr. (1973): C-cell hyperplasia preceding medullary thyroid carcinoma. *N. Engl. J. Med.*, 289:437–441.
170. Zeytinoglu, F. N., Gagel, R. F., DeLellis, R. A., Wolfe, H. J., Tashjian, A. H., Jr., Hammer, R. H., and Leeman, S. E. (1983): Clonal strains of rat medullary thyroid carcinoma produce neurotensin and calcitonin. Functional and morphological observations. *Lab. Invest.*, 49:453–459.

Diagnostic Immunopathology,
edited by R.B. Colvin,
A.K. Bhan, and R.T. McCluskey.
Raven Press, New York © 1988.

13 / *Gynecological and Genitourinary Tumors*

Debra A. Bell, Robert H. Young, and Robert E. Scully

*Department of Pathology, Harvard Medical School and the James Homer Wright Pathology
Laboratories of the Massachusetts General Hospital, Boston, Massachusetts 02114*

TUMORS OF THE UTERUS

The demonstration of various antigens by immunohistochemical techniques has been used in an attempt to clarify the differential diagnosis, causation, histogenesis, malignant potential, and prognosis of uterine tumors and to identify tumor markers. A small number of the antigens detected have proved to be diagnostically or clinically useful; others have yielded information about the nature of specific tumors but have not yet been shown to be diagnostically or clinically relevant. This section will emphasize those immunohistochemical approaches that are of practical significance as well as those that have important etiologic or histogenetic implications.

Cervical Squamous Cell Carcinoma and Its Precursors

Numerous epidemiologic studies have indicated that squamous cell carcinoma of the cervix is a sexually transmissible disease, favoring an infectious agent as a cause. Immunohistochemical methods using antibodies directed against detergent-disrupted virions from pooled human plantar warts, pooled human warts from various sites, and bovine papillomavirus-type I have been employed to demonstrate the presence of human papillomavirus (HPV) structural antigens in the nuclei of cervical koilocytotic squamous cells. Positive results have been reported in 50% to 70% of cases of condyloma acuminatum or low-grade dysplasia of the cervix (Fig. 1). Specimens showing severe dysplasia or carcinoma *in situ* (CIS) are only rarely antigen-positive (86,97,167). These findings were originally interpreted as indicating that condylomas and low-grade dysplasia with koilocytosis are viral infections and not precancerous lesions. DNA hybridization studies with the use of radiolabeled probes subsequently demonstrated HPV-DNA in most dysplastic lesions either in the presence or absence of koilocytosis, implicating HPV in the development of cervical carcinoma. Recent investigations have shown that DNA hybridization can be performed on paraffin-embedded tissue sections, and the use of biotinylated rather than radiolabeled DNA-probes allows identification of specific HPV-DNA types with the use of immunoperoxidase techniques (see Chapter 19). This ability may be of clinical relevance in the future, since present data indicate that certain HPV-DNA types, such as 16 and 18, are much more

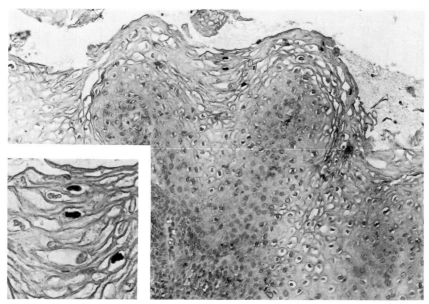

FIG. 1. Cervical condyloma. Diffuse nuclear reactivity for human papilloma virus antigen is present in a small number of koilocytotic squamous cells (× 125). *Inset,* high power view of nuclear positivity (× 640).

often associated with high grade dysplasia and invasive carcinoma than types 6 and 11, which have been identified primarily in condylomas and low-grade dysplasia.

Immunoperoxidase studies have also demonstrated the presence of a nonstructural polypeptide (VP143) of herpes simplex virus type 2 in 20% to 40% of cases of cervical dysplasia or invasive carcinoma, indicating a possible role for this virus in the development of cervical cancer (37). Studies utilizing antibodies against chlamydia antigens have failed to show a relation between this organism and cervical neoplasia (117).

Many investigations have been performed in an attempt to identify antibodies that can distinguish among normal, metaplastic, dysplastic and carcinomatous squamous cells in routine hematoxylin and eosin sections or Papanicolaou-stained cytologic smears. It has been shown that the frequency of detection of HPV structural antigens is inversely proportional to the degree of dysplasia of the epithelium. However, because HPV antigens are identified by immunohistochemical techniques in only about 50% of HPV-related lesions, because only a small number of nuclei are positive in an individual case, and because rare cases of high grade dysplasia are positive, stains for HPV are not useful in differentiating definitively between low and high grade dysplasia. They are also not helpful in identifying the HPV-DNA type (86). Early studies reported that immunohistochemical techniques using antibodies directed against carcinoembryonic antigen (CEA), epithelial membrane antigen (EMA), Ca antigen (Ca-1), involucrin, human milk fat globule 1 and 2 (HMFG 1,2), and alpha-2-macroglobulin stained normal and dysplastic squamous epithelium differently and therefore, might be of value in the diagnosis of dysplasia. Subsequent investigations, however, demonstrated that the usefulness of these techniques is limited because all of them also stain the most common lesions that mimic dysplasia, such as metaplastic and inflamed squamous epithelium and condylomas without dysplasia (18,36,81,119,142,143). Staining for chorionic gonadotropin (HCG) has been reported to be negative in normal and metaplastic cervical epithelium, but positive in only a small number of cases of cervical dysplasia or invasive carcinoma, limiting its diagnostic value (61). Antibodies against keratin and TA-4 (an antigen prepared from human cervical squamous cell carcinoma) are also not useful in this regard because both antigens have been reported to be present in most specimens of both normal and dysplastic squamous epithelium (140,173). Preliminary reports have suggested that staining for a group of monoclonal antibodies produced against human cervical cancer cells differentiated normal and neoplastic cells, but confirmatory studies have not been performed (93). Immunohistochemical studies to demonstrate laminin and type IV collagen have revealed a continuous basement membrane in relation to dysplastic epithelium and well-differentiated squamous cell carcinoma in contrast to a disrupted basement membrane adjacent to inflamed squamous epithelium and nests of anaplastic carcinoma, indicating that antibodies to these substances are not useful in differentiating non-neoplastic and neoplastic epithelium (164).

A number of studies have been performed in an attempt to correlate the presence or absence of antigens of various types with the prognosis of invasive squamous cell carcinoma. It has been shown that patients whose tumors express blood-group antigens have a better prognosis than those whose tumors do not (71% versus 37% five-year survival) (102). Several investigations have demonstrated no difference in the prognosis of patients with and without immunohistochemically detectable CEA in their tumors (104). It has also been reported that the presence or absence of CEA does not correlate with the progression of mild dysplasia (103). Although measurement of serum levels of CEA and TA-4 have not been found helpful in the early detection of cervical carcinoma, they have been shown to reflect the extent of disease in some cases and, therefore, may be useful in following patients with initially elevated serum levels.

Cervical Adenocarcinoma

Most immunohistochemical investigations of cervical adenocarcinoma have been concerned with the use of anti-CEA antibodies to distinguish well differentiated adenocarcinoma and adenoma malignum from benign glandular lesions that mimic these tumors. Microglandular hyperplasia is usually diagnosable in routinely stained sections because of its characteristic histologic features, but in some cases with atypical features differentiation from carcinoma may be difficult, and staining for CEA may be helpful. This antigen is strongly expressed in the cytoplasm of most cervical adenocarcinomas, and is absent in most cases of microglandular hyperplasia, indicating that strongly positive staining is highly suggestive of the former (160). Adenoma malignum is a predominantly very well differentiated adenocarcinoma characterized by haphazardly oriented large complex glands and small slit-like glands with sharp angulated borders, lined by mucin-filled epithelial cells that resemble closely normal cervical glandular epithelial cells. Because of the high degree of differentiation in most portions of the tumor, it is particularly difficult to diagnose in small biopsy specimens. Several investigators have suggested that it can be differentiated from benign endocervical glandular proliferations and mesonephric hyperplasia by immunohistochemical staining for CEA. Strong, diffuse cytoplasmic CEA staining has been reported to be present focally in most cases of adenoma malignum (Fig. 2) and to be absent in benign endocervical epithelium (Fig. 3), the epithelium of mesonephric remnants, and that of florid mesonephric hyperplasia and microglandular hyperplasia (16,114,160). Care must be taken in interpreting these stains, particularly in small biopsy specimens,

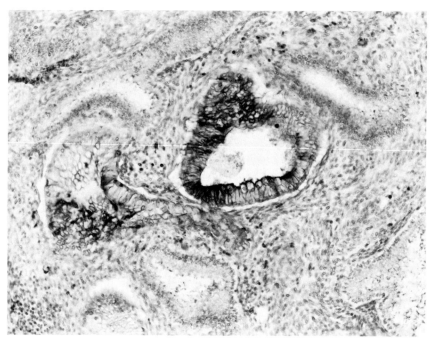

FIG. 2. Adenoma malignum, cervix. Diffuse cytoplasmic reactivity for carcinoembryonic antigen is present focally (× 125).

because reserve cell hyperplasia and immature squamous metaplasia also stain for CEA. Staining with antibodies against CEA has not proved useful in distinguishing between cervical adenocarcinoma *in situ* and invasive adenocarcinoma, since both lesions are positive in a similar proportion of cases (77). It has also been shown in a small number of cases that adenoma malignum contains cells that are immunoreactive for serotonin and gastrointestinal-pancreatic peptide-hormones; the normal endocervix rarely contains cells of this type (63).

Although the histologic differentiation of cervical and endometrial adenocarcinoma may be difficult on examination of routine sections of biopsy or curettage material, it is often possible to distinguish the two by looking for evidence of the site of origin of the tumor such as the presence of a concomitant atypical or *in situ* lesion in the cervix or endometrium, the cervical or endometrial appearance of the stroma, and the predominant site of the involvement of the tumor in the endocervical or endometrial specimen. It has been suggested that staining for CEA may also be helpful in distinguishing between the two tumors. Staining has been demonstrated in 80% to 100% of cervical adenocarcinomas in contrast to only 0% to 52% of endometrial adenocarcinomas (47,178). The staining in the former is generally strong and diffuse, whereas in the latter it is generally weak and confined to the subapical cytoplasm. It has been shown that squamous elements in endometrial adenoacanthomas and adenosquamous carcinomas stain strongly, as do areas of mucinous differentiation. Such findings indicate that although differences in CEA staining exist in large series of endometrial and cervical adenocarcinomas, staining may not be useful in an individual case because of the overlap in staining patterns.

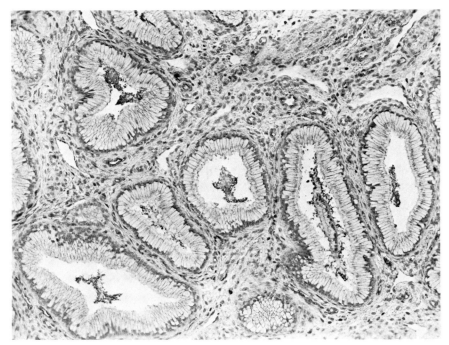

FIG. 3. Normal endocervix. The epithelium does not stain using an antibody against carcinoembryonic antigen (× 125).

Cervical Small Cell Carcinoma and Lymphoma

The majority of small cell carcinomas of the cervix contain polypeptide hormones and neuron-specific enolase, establishing their neuroendocrine differentiation (78,156). Stains for these antigens have proved useful in distinguishing among small cell carcinoma, lymphoma and granulocytic sarcoma. Lymphoma cells typically express common leukocyte antigen, and the cells of granulocytic sarcoma stain with the use of anti-lysosyme antibodies (1) (see Chapters 10 and 11). Stains for immunoglobulins have not been generally helpful in this differential diagnosis, since they have been performed in the majority of cases of cervical lymphoma on paraffin embedded sections (73). As indicated in Chapter 11 immunohistochemical studies for most lymphoid markers should be performed on frozen tissue sections to obtain optimal results. Stains with antibodies to keratin and common leukocyte antigen are of value in distinguishing between poorly differentiated large cell carcinomas and large cell lymphomas in paraffin embedded material.

Endometrial Carcinoma

A major focus of many investigators has been the use of immunohistochemical stains to differentiate severely atypical hyperplasia and well differentiated adenocarcinoma of the endometrium, but the results so far have not been encouraging. Both atypical hyperplasia and well differentiated adenocarcinoma stain with the use of antibodies to CEA, 24K protein, EMA, Ca-1, and secretory component (14,43,62,120) and retain an intact basement membrane, as shown by staining with antibodies against laminin and type IV collagen (163). A preliminary report has shown that milk fat globule membrane antigen (MAM -3) is expressed in most endometrial adenocarcinomas but is not detected in normal endometrial glands. However, stains for this antigen have not been performed on specimens of hyperplastic endometrium (172).

As in other sites, stains for intermediate filaments and common leukocyte antigen are valuable in distinguishing poorly differentiated carcinoma from sarcoma and lymphoma. It should be noted that unlike many carcinomas, pure endometrial adenocarcinomas may stain for vimentin as well as low molecular weight cytokeratins (113).

Several groups of investigators have demonstrated that 22% to 68% of histologically typical endometrial carcinomas contain argyrophil cells, and that about 11% contain serotonin, polypeptide hormones, or both, on immunohistochemical staining (4,19,79). Three types of argyrophil cells have been described, triangular or flask-shaped cells with diffuse cytoplasmic argyrophilia that resemble the enterochromaffin cells of the gut, and columnar cells with either apical or diffuse cytoplasmic argyrophilia. The argyrophilia of the latter cells is, at least in part, related to the presence of intracellular mucin or glycogen, respectively (4,79). The genesis of the enterochromaffin-like cells in endometrial carcinomas remains unclear but their presence may be due to metaplasia of the neoplastic cells to endocrine-type cells. The clinical significance of argyrophilia in endometrial carcinomas remains unclear; Sato et al. (144) have shown that patients with tumors containing argyrophil cells have hypertension or diabetes mellitus more frequently than those whose tumors lack this feature, and found that the survival of patients with grade I adenocarcinomas with argyrophil cells was worse than that of patients with similar tumors lacking argyrophilia. In contrast, another group found argyrophilia in endometrial carcinomas to be of no clinico-pathologic significance (19).

Although many endometrial adenocarcinomas are positive for estrogen receptor (estrophilin) (ER) and progesterone receptor (PR), estrogen and progesterone receptor assays are not routinely performed on these tumors in most institutions. It has been shown that the ER status can be demonstrated reliably by an immunohistochemical method with the use of an antibody raised against ER protein. The staining is localized within the nuclei of the positive cells in frozen tissue (134,138). Because this method requires only small amounts of tissue and allows precise localization of the ER-positive cells, it overcomes many of the problems associated with biochemical ER analysis of small tissue samples, such as curettage specimens, and it allows the pathologist to confirm the presence of ER in tumor cells rather than hyperplastic endometrial cells, stromal cells, or smooth muscle cells, all of which may be ER-positive.

Uterine Sarcomas

Immunohistochemical stains have proved useful in the differentiation of various types of uterine sarcoma. Perhaps the most difficult problem in this area is the distinction between sarcomas of smooth muscle and endometrial stromal type. Leiomyomas and many leiomyosarcomas are strongly positive for desmin; endometrial stromal sarcomas are strongly positive for vimentin, but may also contain scattered desmin-positive cells. Therefore, a tumor that is strongly positive for desmin is most probably of smooth muscle type (30). The diagnosis of leiomyoblastoma can be confirmed in some cases by the demonstration of desmin in the cytoplasm of the tumor cells. It has also been stated that when a tumor is strongly positive with the use of antibodies against alpha-1 antitrypsin and alpha-1 anti-chymotrypsin it is more likely to be an endometrial stromal sarcoma since leiomyosarcomas stain only focally with the use of these antibodies (110). Antibodies against smooth muscle myosin are not useful in this regard, since it may be present in both tumors and is often absent in leiomyosarcomas (110). Rhabdomyosarcomatous differentiation in malignant müllerian mixed tumors can be confirmed by the use of antimyoglobin antibodies, which are sensitive in detecting skeletal muscle differentiation, even of the small-cell category (33), and which may demonstrate skeletal muscle differentiation in a small number of cases in which it is not apparent on routinely stained sections (122).

Trophoblastic Disease

Immunohistochemical staining has a small role in the diagnosis of the two most common forms of trophoblastic disease, the hydatidiform mole and choriocarcinoma, since the diagnosis of both lesions is usually clear-cut on examination of routinely stained sections. Rare choriocarcinomas have an atypical appearance (111) and strongly positive staining of such neoplasms for HCG may support their interpretation as choriocarcinomas. It should be emphasized, however, that rare poorly differentiated carcinomas of the uterus may contain foci that resemble choriocarcinoma to varying degrees and may stain for HCG (99).

The immunohistochemical approach has been helpful in the diagnosis of the placental site trophoblastic tumor (190) and in the elucidation of its histogenesis (100). This tumor is currently considered to be composed of trophoblastic cells that are present in the normal placental site and have been designated "intermediate trophoblast" (98). Both normal intermediate trophoblast and the cells of the placental site trophoblastic tumor characteristically exhibit strongly positive staining for placental lactogen (HPL). Staining for HPL is of no help in solving the most common problem encountered in the differential diagnosis of the placental site trophoblastic tumor, namely, its distinction from an exaggerated but non-neoplastic placental site reaction. In occasional cases, however, the differential diagnosis of a placental site trophoblastic tumor and a non-trophoblastic tumor such as an endometrial carcinoma or sarcoma may be aided by staining of the neoplastic cells for HPL, which has only exceptionally been demonstrated in non-trophoblastic tumors (75). HCG is present in occasional uninucleate intermediate trophoblast cells of the placental site trophoblastic tumor but is present more often in multinucleated cells of this type that approach in appearance typical syncytiotrophoblast cells. Although staining for HPL usually predominates, staining for HCG is more striking in occasional cases, which appear to be associated with a poorer prognosis (192). Staining for HPL has also been useful in identifying intermediate trophoblast cells in decidua in curettage specimens submitted to determine whether a pregnancy is intrauterine or ectopic (12).

Unusual Uterine Tumors

The histogenesis of adenomatoid tumors of the uterus and fallopian tube has been investigated immunohistochemically. Although one group of investigators found factor VIII-related antigen staining in several cases, indicating that some of these tumors may be of vascular origin (24), subsequent studies on many cases have shown staining for cytokeratin, as seen in mesothelial cells, and negative staining for factor VIII-related antigen and

Ulex europaeus I lectin, which is also an endothelial cell marker. These findings indicate that almost all of these tumors are of mesothelial derivation (165).

GONADAL TUMORS

The great majority of gonadal tumors can be diagnosed on the basis of examination of routinely stained sections, occasionally complemented by sections stained for glycogen, mucin, argyrophil granules, and reticulum. Sometimes, evaluation of additional samples of a specimen is more helpful than the use of special stains in achieving a diagnosis. With the exception of germ cell neoplasms and occasional tumors that are metastatic or of unusual occurrence, the immunohistochemical approach to the diagnosis of gonadal tumors has been of relatively little value to date. The technique has been useful, however, in identifying antigens that can be measured in the serum and may serve as tumor markers. Immunohistochemistry has also increased our knowledge of the nature of many gonadal tumors without evident relevance to their diagnosis or management.

Germ Cell Tumors

Germinomas (testicular seminomas and ovarian dysgerminomas) are almost without exception easy to diagnose by examining hematoxylin and eosin sections, occasionally complemented by glycogen stains, which are almost always positive. In the very rare cases in which the histologic appearance is atypical, staining for intermediate filaments may be helpful. Germinomas characteristically contain vimentin but not cytokeratins, which, in contrast, are present in yolk sac tumors (endodermal sinus tumors), embryonal carcinomas, and most other carcinomas (22,115).

A diagnostic problem of clinical significance occasionally arises when the demonstration of an elevated HCG level in the serum does not correlate with a microscopical diagnosis of pure germinoma. In such a situation, the sections of the gonadal tumor should be reexamined and if the original diagnosis proves correct, the specimen should be sectioned further in search of foci of choriocarcinoma, embryonal carcinoma with syncytiotrophoblast cells, or isolated syncytiotrophoblast cells. Immunohistochemical staining for HCG or its beta subunit (Fig. 4) may help to solve the problem by accentuating the HCG-secreting cells (80). According to Mostofi et al. (121), trophoblast cells can be identified four times as frequently with the use of immunohistochemical staining as by examination of routinely stained slides. In a rare germinoma the germinoma cells themselves react positively for HCG (123).

Alpha-fetoprotein (AFP), an oncofetal antigen that is present in embryonic yolk sac and its derivatives, is also occasionally elevated in the serum in cases in which an initial diagnosis of germinoma has been made, mandating further examination of the tumor to identify foci of yolk sac differentiation. Rare yolk sac tumors with solid patterns may simulate germinomas in routinely stained specimens and can be identified with certainty only by immunohistochemical staining for AFP, which is positive in over 90% of yolk sac tumors (121). Also, small foci of yolk sac tumor lurking within germinomas and generally manifested by the formation of slit-like spaces, may be difficult to recognize without staining for this antigen.

Although typical patterns of yolk sac tumor and embryonal carcinoma are easily distinguished, these forms of germ cell neoplasia overlap in their morphological features and are

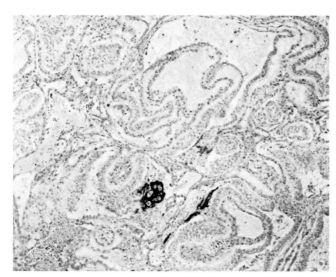

FIG. 4. Diffuse embryoma, testis. Diffuse cytoplasmic reactivity for chorionic gonadotropin is present in syncytiotrophoblast cells occurring among embryonal carcinoma cells and flattened cells within predominantly yolk sac epithelium (× 64). Reprinted by permission from de Almeida, P. C. C., and Scully, R. E. (1983): *Am. J. Surg. Pathol.* 7:633–642.

often intermixed focally or diffusely, making an appraisal of their relative proportions within a specimen difficult or impossible. In such cases, as well as within teratomas, staining for AFP has been very helpful by identifying irregular slit-like spaces, small loose networks, or thin membranes lined by AFP-positive cells (40,96,121) (Fig. 5). In teratomas, mucinous glands and cells resembling hepatocytes may stain, as well as more primitive yolk sac derivatives (38,40). Historically, the use of AFP immunostaining has enabled the pathologist to identify patterns of yolk sac neoplasia that have become recognizable subsequently as a result of examination of routine sections alone. Examples are the ovarian hepatoid yolk sac tumor (137) and a variant of yolk sac tumor that resembles endometrioid carcinoma (45); tumors with a predominance of either of those patterns may be associated with elevations of AFP in the serum.

Despite the great value of immunohistochemical staining for AFP, uncertainty remains whether all the cells that are stained, regardless of their pattern of growth, are of yolk sac nature. Sporadic reports of staining of ovarian tumors of nonendodermal type, such as serous and clear cell carcinomas (76,148) and Sertoli-Leydig cell tumors (150,168) indicate a lack of high specificity of AFP immunostaining and emphasize the need to correlate it with the appearance of the tumor in routinely stained sections.

An isoenzyme that has been studied extensively in both the serum and tissue in cases of gonadal germ cell neoplasia is *placental-like alkaline phosphatase* (PLAP). Using a polyclonal antibody prepared against this enzyme, Manivel et al. (108) reported its presence in 98% of testicular seminomas, 97% of embryonal carcinomas, 85% of yolk sac tumors, and 100% of gonadoblastomas. Its demonstration in 98% of these authors' cases of intratubular germ cell neoplasia, unclassified (carcinoma *in situ*; intratubular atypical germ cells) was a significant finding because this precancerous lesion may be overlooked in routinely stained sections. Aguirre and his associates (3) reported similar findings in testicular tumors and gonadoblastomas as well as in ovarian dysgerminomas and yolk sac tumors. These investigators obtained negative results for PLAP in seven testicular and ovarian immature teratomas and made the additional observation that three spermatocytic seminomas of the testis did not stain immunohistochemically for this enzyme.

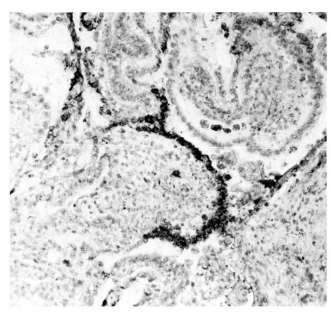

FIG. 5. Diffuse embryoma, testis. Diffuse cytoplasmic reactivity for alpha-fetoprotein in thin yolk sac epithelium (× 140). Reprinted by permission from de Almeida, P. C. C., and Scully, R. E. (1983): *Am. J. Surg. Pathol.*, 7:633–642.

Within the teratoma group of tumors, in addition to the usefulness of HCG, AFP and PLAP staining, immunohistochemical demonstration of a variety of antigens have proved helpful in identifying the various elements that may be encountered. For example, the presence of anterior pituitary tissue may be confirmed by staining of its cells with antibodies to various tropic hormones, and a dermoid cyst associated with an elevated level of ACTH and Cushing's syndrome was shown to contain a pituitary adenoma in its wall that reacted positively for ACTH (15). One of us (RES) has also demonstrated that a papillary carcinoma (in the wall of a dermoid cyst) that lacked colloid and was unassociated with recognizable thyroid tissue was a thyroid-type papillary carcinoma because of immunohistochemical staining of its cells for thyroglobulin. Prostatic tissue within teratomas can be identified by a positive reaction for prostate-specific antigen or prostate-specific acid phosphatase. Demonstration of the intermediate filaments, glial fibrillary acidic protein and neurofilament, and of neuron-specific enolase has been helpful in confirming the presence of various neuroectodermal elements within teratomas (171) and in the diagnosis of both primitive neuroectodermal tumors and ependymomas of the ovary (and broad ligament). The last two types of tumor may exist in pure or almost pure form and may be difficult to diagnose on routine staining. The immunohistochemical demonstration of thyroglobulin and thyroxin in strumal carcinoids established the presence of a thyroid component in that tumor (158), which had previously been denied. Endodermal elements within teratomas often stain positively for serotonin and a variety of peptide hormones (38).

Common Epithelial Tumors of Ovary

These tumors have been stained by antibodies raised against a wide variety of epithelial antigens, including various cytokeratins, epithelial membrane antigen and carcinoembryonic antigen, and they react as well with numerous monoclonal and polyclonal antibodies prepared against ovarian, endometrial, and other carcinomas. Some common epithelial carcinomas are positive for vimentin as well. None of the monoclonal antibodies to ovarian carcinoma tested to date has been demonstrated to be specific for this type of tumor, but some have shown limited specificity, particularly by eliciting positive reactions in mucinous and other tumors and negative reactions in serous tumors or vice versa (170). The use of several monoclonal antibodies has also proved helpful in the diagnosis and clinical management of patients with ovarian cancer. OC-125, a monoclonal antibody to a human serous carcinoma, has been employed most extensively toward these ends (84,85,92). The serum level of OC-125 has been shown to rise and fall with progression and regression of metastatic disease, and to become elevated typically several months before clinical evidence of recurrence. Initially immunostaining for OC-125 (now CA-125) was accomplished only with the use of fresh or frozen tissue, but recently a successful technique for demonstrating the antigen in paraffin-embedded tumor tissue has been described (153).

Staining for a variety of epithelial antigens, particularly cytokeratins, and for vimentin, desmin, and white cell antigens such as common leukocyte antigen may be useful in distinguishing occasional poorly differentiated carcinomas from sarcomas or lymphomas. Staining for an epithelial antigen in such cases may be very focal so that extensive sampling of the tumor may be essential to demonstrate it.

An interesting immunohistochemical finding has been the detection of cells that stain for serotonin (Fig. 6) and a variety of gastrointestinal-pancreatic peptide hormones within common epithelial tumors of the ovary, particularly mucinous tumors (149). The presence of serotonin has been demonstrated in 32% of mucinous tumors and 32% of Brenner tumors, but in much lower quantity in the latter; some endometrioid carcinomas have been shown to contain serotonin as well (5). Peptide hormones of many types have been found in 5% to 35% of mucinous tumors and less frequently in other tumors in the common epithelial category (149). In several cases mucinous cystic tumors of the ovary have been

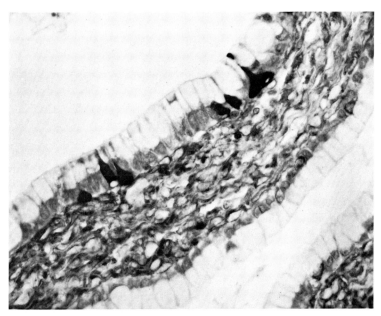

FIG. 6. Benign area of borderline mucinous tumor, ovary. Diffuse cytoplasmic reactivity for serotonin is present in flask-shaped cells distributed between columnar cells (× 640). Reprinted by permission from Aguirre, P., Scully, R. E., Dayal, Y., and DeLellis, R. A. (1984): *Am. J. Surg. Pathol.*, 8:345–356.

responsible for the development of the Zollinger-Ellison syndrome, related to oversecretion of gastrin, with the syndrome regressing after removal of the ovarian tumor; in a few cases of this type gastrin has been demonstrated immunohistochemically in isolated tumor cells within the mucinous lining epithelium (28). It is possible that subclinical secretion of serotonin and various peptide hormones might be demonstrated if their levels were measured in the circulation in cases of suspected mucinous tumors of the ovary.

Hyperamylasemia has been reported in association with serous carcinomas of the ovary, and antibodies to pancreatic amylase have been used to demonstrate this enzyme in fallopian tube epithelium and serous and endometrioid carcinomas of the ovary (174).

ER has been identified immunohistochemically in several types of common epithelial carcinoma (139). Its demonstration is of interest in view of its known presence in many of these tumors on the basis of biochemical analysis and its possible therapeutic significance.

Sex Cord-Stromal Tumors

These neoplasms, also referred to as gonadal stromal tumors, contain derivatives of the embryonic sex cords and stroma (mesenchyme) of either the female or male gonad (granulosa and Sertoli cells and theca and Leydig cells, respectively), or both in various combinations. This category of tumor includes granulosa cell tumors, thecomas and several subtypes of Sertoli-Leydig cell tumor (androblastoma; arrhenoblastoma). Rarely, a problem arises in distinguishing atypical tumors in these categories from common epithelial tumors. Earlier reports suggested that an absence of staining for cytokeratins and positive results for vimentin in granulosa cells might be helpful in the differentiation of atypical granulosa cell tumors from cytokeratin-positive common epithelial carcinomas, but we and others (25) have found that neoplastic granulosa cells stain for cytokeratins in some cases. It is possible, however, that immunohistochemical testing for a battery of epithelial cell and other markers will be successful in demonstrating consistent staining differences between neoplastic granulosa cells and common epithelial cells. The "Sertoli cell" element of Sertoli-Leydig cell tumors is commonly positive for cytokeratins as well as vimentin in contrast to the Sertoli cells of the normal adult testis, which is characteristically positive for vimentin and negative for cytokeratins (115,116). These findings have raised the question whether the so-called Sertoli cells within some tumors in the Sertoli-Leydig cell category may not be more representative of the cells lining the efferent ducts or rete of the testis rather than the Sertoli cells themselves. The demonstration of cytokeratin staining may be helpful in distinguishing a granulosa cell tumor with a theca cell component from a pure thecoma or a Sertoli-Leydig cell tumor from a tumor containing only Leydig cells or their stromal precursors.

Kurman and his associates (96) have demonstrated immunohistochemically the presence of a variety of steroid hormones, including testosterone and estradiol, in the granulosa, theca, Sertoli, Leydig, and less differentiated stromal elements of gonadal sex cord-stromal tumors. These investigators, however, have pointed out two difficulties in the interpretation of their findings. Firstly, the presence of these hormones within a cell does not distinguish among synthesis, binding and nonspecific storage. Secondly, it is possible that close chemical similarities may result in cross-reactions in immunohistochemical staining for various steroid hormones. Finally, staining of both the epithelial and stromal components of many common epithelial tumors for steroid hormones as a result of their capability to bind or synthesize these hormones (11) makes it unlikely that their immunohistochemical demonstration will prove useful in distinguishing these tumors from sex cord-stromal tumors.

Miscellaneous Tumors

A variety of unusual tumors that may be confused with the more common forms of ovarian neoplasms may be diagnosed with increased confidence by the application of immunohistochemical techniques. Such tumors include nerve sheath and smooth muscle neoplasms, both of which may resemble ovarian stromal tumors on routine staining. In one case in our experience, a pheochromocytoma, possibly metastatic, was distinguished from a steroid (lipid) cell tumor of the ovary by its staining for chromogranin (148). A rare ovarian cancer occurring in premenopausal females, a small cell carcinoma that is commonly associated with paraendocrine hypercalcemia (50), is of unknown origin and cytological nature, and stains focally for cytokeratin, epithelial membrane antigen and vimentin in most cases.

Metastatic Tumors

Metastatic carcinomas, most of which arise in the gastrointestinal tract or breast, account for approximately 5% to 10% of ovarian cancers that present clinically as adnexal masses. Metastases from the breast are almost always distinguishable from primary ovarian carcinomas because of their distinctive microscopic patterns and the presence of a known or discoverable primary tumor in the breast. Metastatic carcinomas from the gastrointestinal tract, on the other hand, often present problems in differentiation from primary mucinous adenocarcinomas of the ovary, particularly since the former may differentiate focally to form large cysts lined by well differentiated epithelium simulating that of a mucinous cystadenoma, and the glandular lining of the latter often exhibits intestinal neometaplasia, containing goblet cells, enterochromaffin cells and Paneth cells. Unfortunately, most antibodies that have been used in immunohistochemical staining of gastrointestinal carcinomas also react with mucinous carcinomas of the ovary. Thor and her associates (169), however, have recently identified a monoclonal antibody (Col-4) that recognizes an epitope of CEA that reacts strongly with colorectal carcinomas and only weakly or negatively with ovarian mucinous carcinomas.

Metastatic (as well as primary) carcinoid tumors of the ovary may simulate a variety of ovarian tumors of other types. In addition to staining for argyrophil and argentaffin cells, immunohistochemical demonstration of chromogranin, neuron-specific enolase, serotonin and a wide variety of peptide hormones may aid in the differential diagnosis. Metastatic melanomas may form cysts within the ovary and have a deceptive appearance on routine staining. Immunohistochemical demonstration of S-100 protein may be helpful in identifying their nature.

GENITOURINARY TUMORS

Prostatic Tumors

One of the areas in which immunohistochemical staining has been most useful is in the differential diagnosis of poorly differentiated tumors involving the prostate gland and ur-

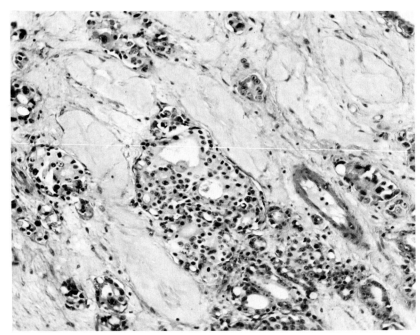

FIG. 7. Carcinoma of prostate metastatic to testis. Adenocarcinomatous glands invading among seminiferous tubules, which are hyalinized and atrophic (H&E, × 160). Reprinted by permission from Talerman, A., and Roth, L. M., editors (1986): *Pathology of the Testis and Its Adnexa*. Churchill Livingstone, New York.

inary bladder and in the establishment of the prostatic origin of metastatic tumors (Figs. 7 and 8). Although histologic differences usually enable one to distinguish prostatic and bladder carcinomas even when they are poorly differentiated, it may be impossible to do so in some cases on the basis of routine staining. The two antibodies that are useful in immunohistochemical staining to resolve this problem are those prepared against prostate-specific acid phosphatase (PSAP) (66,83,105,124–126,152,186) and prostate-specific antigen (PSA) (127,162,182,183).

A large number of publications have established the effectiveness of PSAP in confirming the prostatic nature of tumors in and around the prostate gland and at distant sites (7,13, 20,23,27,34,82,87,101,124–126,128,175,185). In one of the earliest studies (82), only one of 30 primary prostatic tumors failed to stain for PSAP and all 20 metastatic tumors of prostatic origin stained; in contrast, all 55 control tumors failed to stain. This immunocytochemical procedure can also be applied to cytological specimens (87,89). The sensitivity of PSAP staining in establishing the prostatic nature of a metastatic prostatic carcinoma is 95%, based on the combined results of three series (26,101,186). Although some investigators have found that the sensitivity of the staining was decreased in decalcified bone marrow specimens (151), this finding has not been the experience of others (101). Several groups (27,105,126) have not detected significant differences in frequency of staining for PSAP in tumors of different grades but others (21,55,152,185) have reported less intense and more variable staining of less well differentiated tumors. Staining for PSAP is maintained after prostatic carcinomas have been irradiated (107).

Despite the great utility of PSAP staining, additional staining for PSA and consideration of clinical and histologic features are essential in all cases because a variety of nonprostatic tumors, including breast carcinomas (87,89,101,185), pancreatic islet cell tumors (42,46,66,83,90), renal cell carcinomas (185), carcinoid tumors (46,66,83,159) and rare adenocarcinomas of the urinary bladder may stain for PSAP (57). In the largest study of activity of this enzyme in carcinoid tumors Sobin and his associates (159) found staining of 67% of rectal carcinoids and 15% of other gastrointestinal carcinoids. All these tumors were negative for PSA. In the study on PSAP staining of bladder tumors, five of 15 pure adenocarcinomas and three of nine tumors with mixed transitional and adenocarcinomatous patterns were positive (57). None of the tumors that stained for PSAP was also positive for PSA. The authors of this study subsequently demonstrated staining for chromogranin in some of the PSAP positive tumors, raising the question whether the PSAP staining was similar to the staining reported in some carcinoid tumors.

Although conventional histologic studies had already cast doubt on the müllerian nature of the so-called endometrioid carcinoma of the prostate gland (191), the recent demonstration of staining of the tumor cells for both PSAP and PSA (31,58,94,179) has confirmed the view that these tumors are of prostatic duct rather than müllerian origin. Staining for these antigens has also established the prostatic nature of the epithelium in the urethral polyps that have been designated prostatic-type polyps (180). Experience with immunohistochemical staining of some of the rarer forms of prostatic carcinoma with PSAP is relatively limited. Ordonez et al. (131) obtained a positive reaction in the spindle cell component of a tumor that they interpreted as a sarcomatoid prostatic carcinoma. Although Nadji and his associates have reported positive staining of small cell carcinomas of the prostate gland with PSAP (124), prostatic tumors of this type have been negative in the experience of other investigators (29,147). Several prostatic tumors that were interpreted as resembling carcinoids, at least focally (166), on histologic examination have also stained for PSAP (13,17,70,166) but others have been negative (106). Three tumors in the literature interpreted as adenoid cystic carcinomas of the prostate gland (83,95) have been stained for PSAP, all with negative results.

Although PSA has been investigated immunohistochemically less extensively than PSAP, its usefulness is also well established in the staining of both primary and metastatic prostatic carcinomas (6,87,111,127,155,161,162). PSA is more specific for prostatic epithelium than PSAP (67) and to our knowledge no staining of nonprostatic tumors has been encountered. PSA is less frequently positive in poorly differentiated than well differentiated tumors (55,67,122), and in one study (56) absent or weak staining correlated significantly with a poor prognosis. Although most prostatic tumors stain for both PSA and PSAP, the frequency of staining has differed in various studies (8,87). In the study on bone metastases referred to above (151), PSA was much more commonly positive than PSAP (86% versus 36%). Several unusual variants of prostatic carcinoma and other rare prostatic lesions have stained for PSA (9,10,71,88,109,130,188). Two cases of squamous cell carcinoma involving the prostate gland in patients with schistosomiasis were interpreted as being of prostatic origin on the basis of staining with PSA (6). One reported case of "adenoid cystic carcinoma" of the prostate gland was negative for PSA (154). Basal cell hyperplasia did not stain for PSA in one case (44).

The importance of staining for both PSA and PSAP was highlighted by the recent study of Feiner and Gonzales (60). Seven tumors they considered to be undifferentiated prostatic carcinomas were negative for PSA but six of the seven were positive for PSAP. When 108 prostatic carcinomas were stained for both antigens by Naritoku and Taylor (128) only two failed to stain for one or the other antigen.

The staining of the prostate gland and its tumors for antigens other than PSAP and PSA

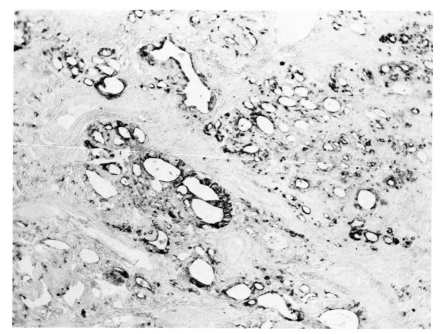

FIG. 8. Carcinoma of prostate metastatic to testis. The tumor cells stain positively for prostatic-specific antigen (× 125). Reprinted by permission from Talerman, A., Roth, L. M., editors (1986): *Pathology of the Testis and Its Adnexa*. Churchill Livingstone, New York.

has been the subject of relatively little investigation to date. In some studies prostatic columnar cells uninvolved by tumor have exhibited little (91) or no (146) staining for keratin, with most of the staining being in the basal cells (91,146), but in other studies the columnar cells have exhibited strong staining, at least focally (118). These differences are probably explicable on the basis of the presence of different keratin proteins in the columnar cells and basal cells and the use of different antibodies in these studies. Brawer et al. (32) utilized one keratin antibody that stained only the normal basal cells; it also intensely stained the cells of basal cell hyperplasia. They concluded that the study confirmed the presence of different keratin epitopes in the basal and secretory (columnar) cells, and that immunohistochemical demonstration of the presence or absence of basal cells may be useful in distinguishing benign and malignant prostatic lesions. Evaluation of the presence or absence of these cells on the basis of routine staining has also been used in this differential diagnosis. The immunohistochemical demonstration of numerous basal cells in one recently reported case of so-called sclerosing adenosis of the prostate gland supported a benign interpretation (189).

When prostatic carcinomas have been stained for cytokeratins the results have varied according to the technique and the antibody used. Molinolo et al. (118) found that these tumors stained strongly for cytokeratin independent of the degree of differentiation when the tissue had been fixed in alcohol; on the other hand, formaldehyde-fixed tissues showed only weak staining. Staining of frozen sections also gave positive results in one study (91). When paraffin-embedded material has been used, staining for keratin has usually been negative or only weakly positive (7,59,145), but occasional strongly positive staining has been reported, particularly in well differentiated tumors (41,67,132,135). The usually negative staining of paraffin embedded prostatic carcinomas contrasts with the staining of most transitional cell carcinomas and, therefore, staining for keratin with selected antibodies in addition to PSA and PSAP may be helpful in establishing whether a tumor is prostatic or urothelial in origin (7).

Prostatic carcinoma stains for epithelial membrane antigen but since transitional cell carcinoma also stains, demonstration of this antigen is not helpful in distinguishing these tumors (7,55,74,136,157). Prostatic carcinoma has also stained for CEA in a minority of cases (55,67). The small cell component of one mixed adenocarcinoma and small cell carcinoma of the prostate gland stained for neuron-specific enolase (71). In one prostatic carcinoma, which was composed of foci of moderately well differentiated adenocarcinoma and anaplastic carcinoma and was associated with Cushing's syndrome, ACTH was localized within the anaplastic tumor cells (177). A small cell carcinoma of the prostate gland that was associated with ectopic ACTH production also contained cells that were immunoreactive for ACTH (184), and similar cells were present in three of four carcinomas without hormonal manifestations in another study (39).

Recent studies have documented cells immunoreactive for a variety of peptide hormones in the prostate gland. Di Sant'Agnese and his associates (53) have identified neuron-specific enolase and serotonin in normal prostatic acini and ducts and in prostatic carcinomas that did not resemble carcinoids or small cell carcinomas. The same group has also stained the cells of normal prostatic acini and ducts for somatostatin (52), calcitonin and bombesin (51) and have identified bombesin and calcitonin-reactive cells in single cases of prostatic carcinoma (54). Fetissof and his associates (64,65) have also found cells positive for serotonin and calcitonin in normal prostatic acini and ducts, and in two prostatic carcinomas; one of the latter focally resembled a carcinoid tumor but the other was a well differentiated adenocarcinoma. The cells in both these tumors also stained for neuron-specific enolase and in one of the tumors they also stained for serotonin. These workers additionally demonstrated a few somatostatin-positive and HCG-positive cells in the normal prostate gland.

Urinary Bladder Tumors

The major area in which immunohistochemistry of the urinary bladder has been of practical importance, the distinction of its tumors from those of the prostate gland with the use of PSAP and PSA, has already been discussed. Other findings of interest have been described, but most of them have little or no practical relevance at the present time. The antigens that have been the subject of most extensive study are the blood group antigens because of the observations that ABH antigens are present in normal urothelial cells and the cells of well differentiated transitional cell carcinomas, but are often absent in the cells of more poorly differentiated tumors. It was anticipated that an absence of stainable antigens would permit the identification of grade 1 and grade 2 papillary noninvasive transitional cell carcinomas that would subsequently become invasive. This problem was initially studied with the use of red cell adherence methods but more recently by the immunoperoxidase technique applied to paraffin sections. The results have been comprehensively reviewed by Coon and Weinstein (48). In their tabulation of the literature they found that the percent of noninvasive carcinomas that subsequently invade muscle was 7 for those that were ABO-positive compared to 62% for those that were ABH-negative. Despite these results, it is premature to rely entirely on ABH testing for making a therapeutic decision in an individual case. In our opinion, other findings such as the histologic grade of the tumor and the presence or absence of dysplasia in the mucosa elsewhere in the bladder must still be considered the factors of primary therapeutic significance in patients with noninvasive tumors. It is also of note that the histologic grade correlates strongly with blood group antigen expression.

Staining of transitional cell carcinomas for keratin is relatively rarely of practical significance except, as noted above, it may help provide evidence against a diagnosis of prostatic carcinoma if appropriate antibodies to keratin are used. In the occasional bladder carcinoma that has a prominent spindle cell pattern, demonstration of keratin within the tumor cells may confirm their epithelial nature and exclude the diagnosis of a sarcoma or a pseudosarcomatous lesion. Alternatively, the absence of keratin and presence of vimentin or desmin within a spindle cell tumor supports the diagnosis of a sarcoma. Staining for keratin, vimentin, desmin and myoglobin may be helpful in identifying epithelial and mesenchymal cells in carcinosarcomas of the bladder (68,72). Immunohistochemical studies have also helped determine neuroendocrine differentiation and production of ectopic hormones in the urinary bladder tumors. In one small cell carcinoma of the bladder associated with ectopic ACTH secretion, ACTH was demonstrated immunohistochemically within the tumor cells (133). In another tumor that was interpreted as an adenocarcinoma with neuroendocrine differentiation, some of the neoplastic cells stained for chromogranin and neuron-specific enolase (2). Finally, HCG has been demonstrated in several poorly differentiated carcinomas of the bladder with focal differentiation towards choriocarcinoma (35,49,69,129,141,187).

REFERENCES

1. Abeler, V., Kjorstad, K. E., Langholm, R., and Marton, P. F. (1983): Granulocytic sarcoma (chloroma) of the uterine cervix: Report of two cases. *Int. J. Gynecol. Pathol.*, 2:88–92.
2. Abenoza, P., Manivel, C., and Sibley, R. K. (1986): Adenocarcinoma with neuroendocrine differentiation of the urinary bladder. Clinicopathologic, immunohistochemical, and ultrastructural study. *Arch. Pathol. Lab. Med.*, 110:1062–1066.
3. Aguirre, P., Scully, R. E., Dayal, Y., and DeLellis, R. A. (1986): Placental-like alkaline phosphatase in germ cell tumors of the ovary and testis. *Lab. Invest.*, 54:2A.
4. Aguirre, P., Scully, R. E., Wolfe, H. J., and DeLellis, R. A. (1984): Endometrial carcinoma with argyrophil cells: A histochemical and immunohistochemical analysis. *Hum. Pathol.*, 15:210–217.
5. Aguirre, P., Scully, R. E., Wolfe, H. J., and DeLellis, R. A. (1986): Argyrophil cells in Brenner tumors: Histochemical and immunohistochemical analysis. *Int. J. Gynecol. Pathol.*, 5:223–234.
6. Al Adnani, M. S. (1985): Schistosomiasis, metaplasia and squamous cell carcinoma of the prostate: Histogenesis of the squamous cancer cells determined by localization of specific markers. *Neoplasma*, 32:613–622.
7. Al Adnani, M. S. (1986): Origin of carcinomas causing bladder neck obstruction demonstrated by immunoperoxidase localisation of specific antigens. *Br. J. Urol.*, 58:283–286.
8. Allhoff, E. P., Proppe, K. H., Chapman, C. M., Lin, C-W., and Prout, G. P., Jr. (1983): Evaluation of prostate specific acid phosphatase and prostate specific antigen in identification of prostatic cancer. *J. Urol.*, 129:315–318.
9. Almagro, U. A. (1985): Argyrophilic prostatic carcinoma. Case report with literature review on prostatic carcinoid and "carcinoid-like" prostatic carcinoma. *Cancer*, 55:608–614.
10. Almagro, U. A., Tieu, T. M., Remeniuk, E., Kueck, B., and Strumpf, K. (1986): Argyrophilic, "carcinoid-like" prostatic carcinoma. An immunocytochemical study. *Arch. Pathol. Lab. Med.*, 110:916–919.
11. Al-Timimi, A., Buckley, C. H., and Fox, H. (1985): An immunohistochemical study of the incidence and significance of sex steroid hormone binding sites in normal and neoplastic human ovarian tissue. *Int. J. Gynecol. Pathol.*, 4:24–41.
12. Angel, E., Davis, J. R., and Nagle, R. B. (1985): Immunohistochemical demonstration of placental hormones in the diagnosis of uterine versus ectopic pregnancy. *Am. J. Clin. Pathol.*, 84:705–709.
13. Ansari, M. A., Pintozzi, R. L., Choi, Y. S., and Ladove, R. F. (1981): Diagnosis of carcinoid-like metastatic prostatic carcinoma by an immunoperoxidase method. *Am. J. Clin. Pathol.*, 76:94–98.

14. Arends, J. W., Groniowski, M. M., de Koning Gans, H. J., and Bosman, F. T. (1983): Immunohistochemical study of the distribution of secretory component and IgA in the normal and diseased uterine mucosa. *Int. J. Gynecol. Pathol.*, 2:171–181.

15. Axiotis, C. A., Lippes, H. A., Merino, M. J., de Lanerolle, N. C., Stewart, A. F., and Kinder, B. (1987): Corticotroph cell pituitary adenoma with an ovarian teratoma. A new cause of Cushing's syndrome. *Am. J. Surg. Pathol.*, 11:218–224.

16. Ayroud, Y., Gelfand, M. M., and Ferenczy, A. (1985): Florid mesonephric hyperplasia of the cervix: A report of a case with review of the literature. *Int. J. Gynecol. Pathol.*, 4:245–254.

17. Azumi, N., Shibuya, H., and Ishikura, M. (1984): Primary prostatic carcinoid tumor with intracytoplasmic prostatic acid phosphatase and prostate-specific antigen. *Am. J. Surg. Pathol.*, 8:545–550.

18. Bamford, P. N., Ormerod, M. G., Sloane, J. P., and Warburton, M. J. (1983): An immunohistochemical study of the distribution of epithelial antigens in the uterine cervix. *Obstet. Gynecol.*, 61:603–608.

19. Bannatyne, P., Russell, P., and Wills, E. J. (1983): Argyrophilia and endometrial carcinoma. *Int. J. Gynecol. Pathol.*, 2:235–254.

20. Bartziota, E. V. (1986): Fine needle aspiration cytology of prostatic adenocarcinoma metastatic to the lung confirmed by the immunoperoxidase technique. *Acta. Cytol.*, 30:497–500.

21. Bates, R. J., Chapman, C. M., Prout, G. R., Jr., and Lin, C-W. (1982): Immunohistochemical identification of prostatic acid phosphatase: Correlation of tumor grade with acid phosphatase distribution. *J. Urol.*, 127:574–580.

22. Battifora, H., Sheibani, K., Tubbs, R. R., Kopinski, M. I., and Sun, T.-T. (1984): Antikeratin antibodies in tumor diagnosis. *Cancer*, 54:843–848.

23. Baumann, M. A., Holoye, P. Y., and Choi, H. (1984): Adenocarcinoma of the prostate presenting as brain metastasis. *Cancer*, 54:1723–1725.

24. Bell, D. A., and Flotte, T. J. (1982): Factor VIII related antigen in adenomatoid tumors. Implications for histogenesis. *Cancer*, 50:932–938.

25. Benjamin, E., Bobrow, L., and Law, S. (1986): Intermediate filament distribution in adult and developing ovaries and their expression in ovarian sex cord stromal tumours. *J. Pathol.*, 149:247A.

26. Bentz, M. S., Cohen, C., Demers, L. M., and Budgeon, L. R. (1982): Immunohistochemical demonstration of prostatic origin of metastases. *Urology*, 14:584–586.

27. Bentz, M. A., Cohen, C., Demers, L. M., and Budgeon, L. R. (1982): Immunohistochemical acid phosphatase level and tumor grade in prostatic carcinoma. *Arch. Pathol. Lab. Med.*, 106:476–480.

28. Bhagavan, B. S., Slavin, R. E., Goldberg, J., and Rao, R. N. (1986): Ectopic gastrinoma and Zollinger-Ellison syndrome. *Hum. Pathol.*, 17:584–592.

29. Bleichner, J. C., Chun, B., and Klappenbach, R. S. (1986): Pure small-cell carcinoma of the prostate with fatal liver metastasis. *Arch. Pathol. Lab. Med.*, 110:1041–1044.

30. Bonazzi del Poggetto, C., Virtanen, I., Lehto, V-P., Wahlstrom, T., and Saksela, E. (1983): Expression of intermediate filaments in ovarian and uterine tumors. *Int. J. Gynecol. Pathol.*, 1:359–366.

31. Bostwick, D. G., Kindrachuk, R. W., and Rouse, R. V. (1985): Prostatic adenocarcinoma with endometrioid features. Clinical, pathologic, and ultrastructural findings. *Am. J. Surg. Pathol.*, 9:595–609.

32. Brawer, M. K., Peehl, D. M., Stamey, T. A., and Bostwick, D. G. (1985): Keratin immunoreactivity in the benign and neoplastic human prostate. *Cancer Res.*, 45:3663–3667.

33. Brooks, J. J. (1982): Immunohistochemistry of soft tissue tumors. Myoglobin as a tumor marker for rhabdomyosarcoma. *Cancer*, 50:1757–1763.

34. Burns, J. (1977): Prostatic acid phosphatase in tissue sections revealed by the unlabelled antibody peroxidase-antiperoxidase method. *Biomedicine*, 27:7–10.

35. Burry, A. F., Munn, S. R., Arnold, E. P., and McRae, C. U. (1986): Trophoblastic metaplasia in urothelial carcinoma of the bladder. *Br. J. Urol.*, 58:143–146.

36. Bychkov, V., Rothman, M., and Bardawil, W. A. (1983): Immunocytochemical localization of carcinoembryonic antigen (CEA), alpha-fetoprotein (AFP), and human chorionic gonadotropin (HCG) in cervical neoplasia. *Am. J. Clin. Pathol.*, 79:414–420.

37. Cabral, G. A., Fry, D., Marciano-Cabral, F., Lumpkin, C., Mercer, L., and Goplerud, D. (1983): A herpes virus antigen in human premalignant and malignant cervical biopsies and explants. *Am. J. Obstet. Gynecol.*, 145:79–86.

38. Calame, J., Bosman, F. T., Schaberg, A., and Louwerens, J. W. K. (1984): Immunocytochemical localization of neuroendocrine hormones and oncofetal antigens in ovarian teratomas. *Int. J. Gynecol. Pathol.*, 3:92–100.

39. Capella, C., Usellini, L., Buffa, R., Frigerio, B., and Solcia, E. (1981): The endocrine component of prostatic carcinomas, mixed adenocarcinoma-carcinoid tumours and non-tumour prostate. Histochemical and ultrastructural identification of the endocrine cells. *Histopathology*, 5:175–192.

40. Cardoso de Almeida, P. C., and Scully, R. E. (1983): Diffuse embryoma of the testis, a distinctive form of mixed germ cell tumor. *Am. J. Surg. Pathol.*, 7:755–771.

41. Chastonay, P., Hurlimann, J., and Gardiol, D. (1986): Biological tissue markers in benign and malignant disease of the human prostate. *Virchows Arch. A.*, 410:221–229.

42. Choe, B-K., Pontes, E. J., Rose, N. R., and Henderson, M. D. (1978): Expression of human prostatic acid phosphatase in a pancreatic islet cell carcinoma. *Invest. Urol.*, 15:312–318.

43. Ciocca, D. R., Puy, L. A., Edwards, D. P., Adams, D. J., and McGuire, W. L. (1985): The presence of an estrogen-regulated protein detected by monoclonal antibody in abnormal human endometrium. *J. Clin. Endocrinol. Metab.*, 60:137–143.

44. Cleary, K. R., Choi, H. Y., and Ayala, A. G. (1983): Basal cell hyperplasia of the prostate. *Am. J. Clin. Pathol.*, 80:850–854.

45. Clement, P. B., Young, R. H., and Scully, R. E. (1987): Endometrioid-like variant of ovarian yolk sac tumor. A clinicopathologic analysis of eight cases. *Am. J. Surg. Pathol.*, 11:767–778.

46. Cohen, C., Bentz, M. S., and Budgeon, L. R. (1983): Prostatic acid phosphatase in carcinoid and islet cell tumors. *Arch. Pathol. Lab. Med.*, 107:277.

47. Cohen, C., Shulman, G., and Budgeon, L. R. (1982): Endocervical and endometrial adenocarcinoma. An immunoperoxidase and histochemical study. *Am. J. Surg. Pathol.*, 6:151–157.

48. Coon, J. S., and Weinstein, R. S. (1986): Blood group-related antigens as markers of malignant potential and heterogeneity in human carcinomas. *Hum. Pathol.*, 17:1089–1106.

49. Dennis, P. M., and Turner, A. G. (1984): Primary choriocarcinoma of the bladder evolving from a transitional cell carcinoma. *J. Clin. Pathol.*, 37:503–505.

50. Dickersin, G. R., Kline, I. W., and Scully, R. E. (1982): Small cell carcinoma of the ovary with hypercalcemia. *Cancer*, 49:188–197.

51. di Sant'Agnese, P. A. (1986): Calcitonin-like immunoreactive and bombesin-like immunoreactive endocrine-paracrine cells of the human prostate. *Arch. Pathol. Lab. Med.*, 110:412–415.

52. di Sant'Agnese, P. A., and de Mesy Jensen, K. L. (1984): Somatostatin and/or somatostatin-like immunoreactive endocrine-paracrine cells in the human prostate gland. *Arch. Pathol. Lab. Med.*, 108:693–696.

53. di Sant'Agnese, P. A., de Mesy Jensen, K. L., Churukian, C. J., and Agarwal, M. M. (1985): Human prostatic endocrine-paracrine (APUD) cells. Distributional analysis with a comparison of serotonin and neuron-specific enolase immunoreactivity and silver stains. *Arch. Pathol. Lab. Med.*, 109:607–612.

54. di Sant'Agnese, P. A., de Mesy Jensen, K. L., and O'Toole, K. (1986): Neuroendocrine differentiation in prostatic carcinoma. *Lab. Invest.*, 54:16A.

55. Ellis, D. W., Leffers, S., Davies, J. S., and Ng, A. B. P. (1984): Multiple immunoperoxidase markers in benign hyperplasia and adenocarcinoma of the prostate. *Am. J. Clin. Pathol.*, 81:279–284.

56. Epstein, J. I., and Eggleston, J. C. (1984): Immunohistochemical localization of prostate-specific acid phosphatase and prostate-specific antigen in Stage A_2 adenocarcinoma of the prostate: Prognostic implications. *Hum. Pathol.*, 15:853–859.

57. Epstein, J. I., Kuhajda, F. P., and Liberman, P. H. (1986): Prostate-specific acid phosphatase immunoreactivity in adenocarcinomas of the urinary bladder. *Hum. Pathol.*, 17:939–942.

58. Epstein, J. I., and Woodruff, J. M. (1986): Adenocarcinoma of the prostate with endometrioid features. A light microscopic and immunohistochemical study of ten cases. *Cancer*, 57:111–119.

59. Espinoza, C. G., and Azar, H. A. (1982): Immunohistochemical localization of keratin-type proteins in epithelial neoplasms. Correlation with electron microscopic findings. *Am. J. Clin. Pathol.*, 78:500–507.

60. Feiner, H. D., and Gonzalez, R. (1986): Carcinoma of the prostate with atypical immunohistological features. Clinical and histologic correlates. *Am. J. Surg. Pathol.*, 10:765–770.

61. Fenoglio, C. M., Crum, C. P., Hayata, T., and Richart, R. M. (1982): The expression of human chorionic gonadotropin in the female genital tract. Localization by the immunoperoxidase technique. *Diag. Gynecol. Obstet.*, 4:97–103.

62. Fenoglio, C. M., Crum, C. P., Pascal, R. R., and Richart, R. M. (1981): Carcinoembryonic antigen in gynecologic patients. II. Immunohistological expression. *Diag. Gynecol. Obstet.*, 3:291–299.

63. Fetissof, F., Berger, G., Dubois, M. P., Philippe, A., Lansac, J., and Jobard, P. (1985): Female genital tract and Peutz-Jeghers syndrome: An immunohistochemical study. *Int. J. Gynecol. Pathol.*, 4:219–229.

64. Fetissof, F., Bertrand, G., Guilloteau, D., Dubois, M. P., Lanson, Y., and Arbeille, B. (1986): Calcitonin immunoreactive cells in prostate gland and cloacal derived tissues. *Virchows Arch. Pathol. Anat.*, 409:523-533.

65. Fetissof, F., Bruandet, P., Arbeille, B., Penot, J., Marboeuf, Y., Le Roux, J., Guilloteau, D., and Beaulieu, J-L. (1986): Calcitonin-secreting carcinomas of the prostate. An immunohistochemical and ultrastructural analysis. *Am. J. Surg. Pathol.*, 10:702–710.

66. Fishleder, A., Tubbs, R. R., and Levin, H. S. (1980): An immunoperoxidase technique to aid in the differential diagnosis of prostatic carcinoma. *Clev. Clin. Q.*, 48:331–335.

67. Friedmann, W., Steffens, J., Lobeck, H., Blumcke, S., Nagel, R. (1985): Immunohistochemical demonstration of tumor-associated antigens in prostatic carcinomas of various histological differentiations. *Eur. Urol.*, 11:52–56.

68. Fromowitz, F. B., Bard, R. H., and Koss, L. G. (1984): The epithelial origin of a malignant mesodermal mixed tumor of the bladder: Report of a case with long-term survival. *J. Urol.*, 132:978–981.

69. Gallagher, L., Lind, R., and Oyasu, R. (1984): Primary choriocarcinoma of the urinary bladder in association with undifferentiated carcinoma. *Hum. Pathol.*, 15:793–795.

70. Ghali, V. S., and Garcia, R. L. (1984): Prostatic adenocarcinoma with carcinoidal features producing adrenocorticotropic syndrome. Immunohistochemical study and review of the literature. *Cancer*, 54:1043–1048.

71. Ghandur-Mnaymneh, L., Satterfield, S., and Block, N. L. (1986): Small cell carcinoma of the prostate gland with inappropriate antidiuretic hormone secretion: Morphological, immunohistochemical and clinical expressions. *J. Urol.*, 135:1263–1266.

72. Grossman, H. B., Sonda, L. P., Lloyd, R. V., and Gikas, P. W. (1984): Carcinosarcoma of bladder. Evaluation by electron microscopy and immunohistochemistry. *Urology*, 24:387–389.

73. Harris, N. L., and Scully, R. E. (1984): Malignant lymphoma and granulocytic sarcoma of the uterus and vagina. A clinicopathologic analysis of 27 cases. *Cancer*, 53:2530–2545.

74. Heyderman, E., Brown, B. M. E., and Richardson, T. C. (1984): Epithelial markers in prostatic, bladder, and colorectal cancer: An immunoperoxidase study of epithelial membrane antigen, carcinoembryonic antigen, and prostatic acid phosphatase. *J. Clin. Pathol.*, 37:1363–1369.

75. Heyderman, E., Chapman, D. V., Richardson, T. C., Calvert, I., and Rosen, S. W. (1983): Immunoperoxidase localization of placental proteins in non-trophoblastic extra-gonadal tumors; correlation with serum levels. *J. Pathol.*, 140:148–149.

76. Higuchi, Y., Kouno, T., Teshima, H., Akizuki, S., Kikuta, M., Ohyumi, M., and Yamamoto, S. (1984): Serous papillary cystadenocarcinoma associated with α-fetoprotein production. *Arch. Pathol. Lab. Med.*, 108:710–712.

77. Hurlimann, J., and Gloor, E. (1984): Adenocarcinoma *in situ* and invasive adenocarcinoma of the uterine cervix. An immunohistologic study with antibodies specific for several epithelial markers. *Cancer*, 54:103–109.

78. Inoue, M., Ueda, G., Nakajima, T. (1985): Immunohistochemical demonstration of neuron-specific enolase in gynecologic malignant tumors. *Cancer*, 55:1686–1690.

79. Inoue, M., Ueda, G., Yamasaki, M., Tanaka, Y., Hiramatsu, K. (1984): Immunohistochemical demonstration of peptide hormones in endometrial carcinomas. *Cancer*, 54:2127–2131.

80. Jacobsen, G. K., and Jacobsen, M. (1983): Alpha-fetoprotein (AFP) and human chorionic gonadotropin (HCG) in testicular germ cell tumours. A prospective immunohistochemical study. *Acta Pathol. Microbiol. Immunol. Scand. [Sect. A.]*, 91:165–176.

81. Jha, R. S., Wickenden, C., Anderson, M. C., and Coleman, D. V. (1984): Monoclonal antibodies for the histopathological diagnosis of cervical neoplasia. *Br. J. Obstet. Gynaecol.*, 91:483–488.

82. Jöbsis, A. C., De Vries, G. P., Anholt, R. R. H., and Sanders, G. T. B. (1978): Demonstration of the prostatic origin of metastases. An immunohistochemical method for formalin-fixed embedded tissue. *Cancer*, 41:1788–1793.

83. Jöbsis, A. C., De Vries, G. P., Meijer, A. E. F. H., and Ploem, J. S. (1981): The immunohistochemical detection of prostatic acid phosphatase: Its possibilities and limitations in tumour histochemistry. *Histochem. J.*, 13:961–973.

84. Kabawat, S. E., Bast, R. C., Jr., Bhan, A. K., Welch, W. R., Knapp, R. C., and Colvin, R. B. (1983): Tissue distribution of a coelomic-epithelium-related antigen recognized by the monoclonal antibody OC125. *Int. J. Gynecol. Pathol.*, 2:275–285.

85. Kabawat, S. E., Bast, R. C., Welch, W. R., Knapp, R. C., and Colvin, R. B. (1983): Immunopathologic characterization of a monoclonal antibody that recognizes common surface antigens of human ovarian tumors of serous, endometrioid, and clear cell types. *Am. J. Clin. Pathol.*, 79:98–104.

86. Kadish, A. S., Burk, R. D., Kress, Y., Calderin, S., and Romney, S. L. (1986): Human papillomaviruses of different types in precancerous lesions of the uterine cervix: Histologic, immunocytochemical and ultrastructural studies. *Hum. Pathol.*, 17:384–392.

87. Katz, R. L., Raval, P., Brooks, T. E., and Ordonez, N. G. (1985): Role of immunocytochemistry in diagnosis of prostatic neoplasia by fine needle aspiration biopsy. *Diagn. Cytopathol.*, 1:28–32.

88. Kendall, A. R., Stein, B. S., Shea, F. J., Petersen, R. O., and Senay, B. (1986): Cystic pelvic mass. *J. Urol.*, 135:550–553.

89. Keshgegian, A. A., and Kline, T. S. (1984): Immunoperoxidase demonstration of prostate acid phosphatase in aspiration biopsy cytology (ABC). *Am. J. Clin. Pathol.*, 82:586–589.

90. Kimura, N., and Sasano, N. (1986): Prostate-specific acid phosphatase in carcinoid tumors. *Virchows Arch. A.*, 410:247–251.

91. Kitajima, K., and Tokés, Z. A. (1986): Immunohistochemical localization of keratin in human prostate. *The Prostate*, 9:183–190.

92. Knauf, S., Anderson, D. J., Knapp, R. C., and Bast, R. C., Jr. (1985): A study of the NB/70K and CA 125 monoclonal antibody radioimmunoassays for measuring serum antigen levels in ovarian cancer patients. *Am. J. Obstet. Gynecol.*, 152:911–913.

93. Koprowska, I., Zipfel, S., Ross, A. H., and Herlyn, M. (1986): Development of monoclonal antibodies that recognize antigens associated with human cervical carcinoma. *Acta. Cytol.*, 30:207–213.

94. Kuhajda, F. P., Gipson, T., and Mendelsohn, G. (1984): Papillary adenocarcinomas of the prostate. An immunohistochemical study. *Cancer*, 54:1328–1332.

95. Kuhajda, F. P., and Mann, R. B. (1984): Adenoid cystic carcinoma of the prostate. A case report with immunoperoxidase staining for prostate-specific acid phosphatase and prostate-specific antigen. *Am. J. Clin. Pathol.*, 81:257–260.

96. Kurman, R. J., Ganjei, P., and Nadji, M. (1984): Contributions of immunocytochemistry to the diagnosis and study of ovarian neoplasms. *Int. J. Gynecol. Pathol.*, 3:3–26.

97. Kurman, R. J., Jenson, A. B., and Lancaster, W. D. (1983): Papillomavirus infection of the cervix. II. Relationship to intraepithelial neoplasia based on the presence of specific viral structural proteins. *Am. J. Surg. Pathol.*, 7:39–51.

98. Kurman, R. J., Main, C. S., Chen, H-C. (1984): Intermediate trophoblast: A distinctive form of trophoblast with specific morphological, biochemical and functional features. *Placenta*, 5:349–370.

99. Kurman, R. J., and Norris, H. J. (1982): Chapter 13 in *Pathology of the Female Genital Tract*, 2nd Ed., edited by A. Blaustein, p. 336. Springer Verlag, New York.

100. Kurman, R. J., Young, R. H., Norris, H. J., Main, C. S., Lawrence, W. D., and Scully, R. E. (1984): Immunocytochemical localization of placental lactogen and chorionic gonadotropin in the normal placenta and trophoblastic tumors, with emphasis on intermediate trophoblast and the placental site trophoblastic tumor. *Int. J. Gynecol. Pathol.*, 3:101–121.

101. Li, C. Y., Lam, W. K., and Yam, L. T. (1980): Immunohistochemical diagnosis of prostatic cancer with metastasis. *Cancer*, 46:706–712.

102. Lindgren, A., Stendahl, U., Brodin, T., Lundblad, A., Sallstrom, J., and Busch, C. (1986): Blood group antigen expression and prognosis in squamous cell carcinoma of the uterine cervix. *Anticancer Res.*, 6:-255–258.

103. Lindgren, J., Vesterinen, E., Purola, E., and Wahlstrom, T. (1986): Prognostic significance of tissue carcinoembryonic antigen in mild dysplasia of the uterine cervix. *Tumour Biol.*, 6:465–470.

104. Lindgren, J., Wahlstrom, T., and Seppala, M. (1979): Tissue CEA in premalignant epithelial lesions and epidermoid carcinoma of the uterine cervix: Prognostic significance. *Int. J. Cancer*, 23:448–453.

105. Lippert, M. C., Bensimon, H., and Javadpour, N. (1982): Immunoperoxidase staining of acid phosphatase in human prostatic tissue. *J. Urol.*, 128:1114–1116.

106. Mahadevia, P. S., Ramaswamy, A., Greenwald, E. S., Wollner, D. I., and Markham, D. (1983): Hypercalcemia in prostatic carcinoma. Report of eight cases. *Arch. Intern. Med.*, 143:1339–1342.

107. Mahan, D. E., Bruce, A. W., Manley, P. N., and Franchi, L. (1980): Immunohistochemical evaluation of prostatic carcinoma before and after radiotherapy. *J. Urol.*, 124:488–491.

108. Manivel, J. C., Jessurun, J., Wick, M. R., and Dehner, L. P. (1987): Placental alkaline phosphatase immunoreactivity in testicular germ-cell neoplasms. *Am. J. Surg. Pathol.*, 11:21–29.

109. Manivel, J. C., Shenoy, B. V., Wick, M. R., and Dehner, L. P. (1986): Cystosarcoma phyllodes of the prostate. *Arch. Pathol. Lab. Med.*, 110:534–538.

110. Marshall, R. J., and Braye, S. G. (1985): Alpha-1-antitrypsin, alpha-1-antichymotrypsin, actin, and myosin in uterine sarcomas. *Int. J. Gynecol. Pathol.*, 4:346–354.

111. Matsumoto, I., Furusato, M., Inomata, I., Wada, T., and Aizawa, S. (1986): Prostatic cancer presenting as metastatic adenocarcinoma of sphenoid sinus. *Acta Pathol. Jpn.*, 36:1753–1756.

112. Mazur, M. T., Lurain, J. R., and Brewer, J. I. (1982): Fatal gestational choriocarcinoma. Clinicopathologic study of patients treated at a trophoblastic disease center. *Cancer*, 50:1833–1846.

113. McNutt, M. A., Bolen, J. W., Gown, A. M., Hammar, S. P., and Vogel, A. M. (1985): Coexpression of intermediate filaments in human epithelial neoplasms. *Ultrastr. Pathol.*, 9:31–43.

114. Michael, H., Grawe, L., and Kraus, F. T. (1984): Minimal deviation endocervical adenocarcinoma: Clinical and histologic features, immunohistochemical staining for carcinoembryonic antigen, and differentiation from confusing benign lesions. *Int. J. Gynecol. Pathol.*, 3:261–276.

115. Miettinen, M., Virtanen, I., and Talerman, A. (1985): Intermediate filament proteins in human testis and testicular germ-cell tumors. *Am. J. Pathol.*, 120:402–410.

116. Miettinen, M., Wahlstrom, T., Virtanen, I., Talerman, A., and Astengo-Osuna, C. (1985): Cellular differentiation in ovarian sex-cord-stromal and germ-cell tumors studied with antibodies to intermediate-filament proteins. *Am. J. Surg. Pathol.*, 9:640–651.

117. Mitao, M., Reumann, W., Winkler, B., Richart, R. M., Fujiwara, A., and Crum, C. P. (1984): Chlamydial cervicitis and cervical intraepithelial neoplasia: An immunohistochemical analysis. *Gynecol. Oncol.*, 19:90–97.

118. Molinolo, A. A., Meiss, R. P., Leo, P., and Sens, A. I. (1985): Demonstration of cytokeratins by immunoperoxidase staining in prostatic tissue. *J. Urol.*, 134:1037–1040.

119. Morris, H. B., Gatter, K. C., Pulford, K., Haynes, P., Charnock, M., Taylor-Papadimitriou, J., Lane, E. B., and Mason, D. Y. (1983): Cervical wart virus infection, intraepithelial neoplasia and carcinoma; an immunohistological study using a panel of monoclonal antibodies. *Br. J. Obstet. Gynaecol.*, 90:1069–1081.

120. Morse, A. R., Curran, G. J. (1985): Distribution of epithelial membrane antigen in normal and abnormal endometrial tissue. *Br. J. Obstet. Gynaecol.*, 92:1286–1290.

121. Mostofi, F. K., Sesterhenn, I. A., and David, C. J., Jr. (1985): Immunopathology of testicular tumors. In: *Immunocytochemistry in Tumor Diagnosis*, edited by J. Russo, pp. 321–336. Martinus Nijhoff Publishing, Boston.

122. Mukai, K., Varela-Duran, J., and Nochomovitz, L. E. (1980): The rhabdomyoblast in mixed müllerian tumors of the uterus and ovary. An immunohistochemical study of myoglobin in 25 cases. *Am. J. Clin. Pathol.*, 74:101–104.

123. Mullin, T. J., and Lankerani, M. R. (1986): Ovarian dysgerminoma: Immunocytochemical localization of human chorionic gonadotropin in the germinoma cell cytoplasm. *Obstet. Gynecol.*, 68:80S–83S.

124. Nadji, M., and Morales, A. R. (1982): Prostatic acid phosphatase measurement: Its role in detection and management of prostatic cancer. In: *Annals of the New York Academy of Sciences*, Vol. 390, edited by L. M. Shaw, N. A. Romas, and H. Cohen, pp. 133–141. New York Academy of Sciences, New York.

125. Nadji, M., Tabei, S. Z., Castro, A., Morales, A. R. (1979): Immunohistological demonstration of prostatic origin of malignant neoplasms. *Lancet*, 1:671–672.

126. Nadji, M., Tabei, S. Z., Castro, A., Chu, T. M., and Morales, A. R. (1980): Prostatic origin of tumors. An immunohistochemical study. *Am. J. Clin. Pathol.*, 73:735–739.

127. Nadji, M., Tabei, S. Z., Castro, A., Murphy, G. P., Wang, M. C., and Morales, A. R. (1981): Prostatic-specific antigen: An immunohistochemical marker for prostatic neoplasms. *Cancer*, 48:1229–1232.

128. Naritoku, W. Y., and Taylor, C. R. (1983): Immunohistologic diagnosis of 2 cases of metastatic prostate cancer to breast. *J. Urol.*, 130:365–367.

129. Obe, J. A., Rosen, N., and Koss, L. G. (1983): Primary choriocarcinoma of the urinary bladder. Report of a case with probable epithelial origin. *Cancer*, 52:1405–1409.

130. Odom, D. G., Donatucci, C. F., and Deshon, G. E. (1986): Mucinous adenocarcinoma of the prostate. *Hum. Pathol.*, 17:863–865.

131. Ordonez, N. G., Ayala, A. G., von Eschenbach, A. C., Mackay, B., and Hanssen, G. (1982): Immuno-peroxidase localization of prostatic acid phosphatase in prostatic carcinoma with sarcomatoid changes. *Urology*, 14:210–214.

132. Osborn, M., and Weber, K. (1983): Biology of disease. Tumor diagnosis by intermediate filament typing: A novel tool for surgical pathology. *Lab. Invest.*, 48:372–394.

133. Partanen, S., and Asikainen, U. (1985): Oat cell carcinoma of the urinary bladder with ectopic adrenocor-ticotropic hormone production. *Hum. Pathol.*, 16:313–315.

134. Pertschuk, L. P., Beddoe, A. M., Gorelic, L. S., and Shain, S. A. (1986): Immunocytochemical assay of estrogen receptors in endometrial carcinoma with monoclonal antibodies. Comparison with biochemical assay. *Cancer*, 57:1000–1004.

135. Pinkus, G. S., Etheridge, C. L., and O'Connor, E. M. (1986): Are keratin proteins a better tumor marker than epithelial membrane antigen? A comparative immunohistochemical study of various paraffin-embedded neoplasms using monoclonal and polyclonal antibodies. *Am. J. Clin. Pathol.*, 85:269–277.

136. Pinkus, G. S., and Kurtin, P. J. (1985): Epithelial membrane antigen—A diagnostic discriminant in surgical pathology: Immunohistochemical profile in epithelial, mesenchymal, and hematopoietic neoplasms using paraffin sections and monoclonal antibodies. *Hum. Pathol.*, 16:929–940.

137. Prat, J., Bhan, A. K., Dickersin, G. R., Robboy, S. J., and Scully, R. E. (1982): Hepatoid yolk sac tumor of the ovary (endodermal sinus tumor with hepatoid differentiation). *Cancer*, 50:2344–2368.

138. Press, M. F., and Greene, G. L. (1984): An immunocytochemical method for demonstrating estrogen receptor in human uterus using monoclonal antibodies to human estrophilin. *Lab. Invest.*, 50:480–486.

139. Press, M. F., Holt, J. A., Herbst, A. L., and Greene, G. L. (1985): Immunocytochemical identification of estrogen receptor in ovarian carcinomas. *Lab. Invest.*, 53:349–361.

140. Puts, J. J. G., Moesker, O., Kenemans, P., Vooijs, G. P., and Ramaekers, F. C. S. (1985): Expression of cytokeratins in early neoplastic epithelial lesions of the uterine cervix. *Int. J. Gynecol. Pathol.*, 4:300–313.

141. Rodenburg, C. J., Nieuwenhuyzen Kruseman, A. C., de Maaker, H. A., Fleuren, G. J., and van Oosterom, A. T. (1985): Immunohistochemical localization and chromatographic characterization of human chorionic gonadotropin in a bladder carcinoma. *Arch. Pathol. Lab. Med.*, 109:1046–1048.

142. Saksela, O., Wahlstrom, T., Meyer, B., and Vaheri, A. (1984): Presence of alpha-2-macroglobulin in normal but not in malignant cervical epithelium. *Cancer Res.*, 44:2942–2946.

143. Sassoon, A. F., Said, J. W., Nash, G., Shintaku, I. P., and Banks-Schlegel, S. (1985): Involucrin in intraepithelial and invasive squamous cell carcinomas of the cervix: An immunohistochemical study. *Hum. Pathol.*, 16:467–470.

144. Sato, Y., Ozaki, M., Ueda, G., and Tanizawa, O. (1986): Clinical significance of argyrophilia in endo-metrial carcinomas. *Gynecol. Oncol.*, 25:53–60.

145. Schlegel, R., Banks-Schlegel, S., McLeod, J. A., and Pinkus, G. S. (1980): Immunoperoxidase localization of keratin in human neoplasms. *Am. J. Pathol.*, 101:41–50.

146. Schlegel, R., Banks-Schlegel, S., and Pinkus, G. S. (1980): Immunohistochemical localization of keratin in normal human tissues. *Lab. Invest.*, 42:91–96.

147. Schron, D. S., Gipson, T., and Mendelsohn, G. (1984): The histogenesis of small cell carcinoma of the prostate. An immunohistochemical study. *Cancer*, 53:2478–2480.

148. Scully, R. E. (1985): Immunohistochemistry of ovarian tumors. In: *Immunocytochemistry in Tumor Diagnosis*, edited by J. Russo and I. Russo, pp. 293–320. Martinus Nijhoff Publishing, Boston.

149. Scully, R. E., Aguirre, P., and DeLellis, R. A. (1984): Argyrophilia, serotonin, and peptide hormones in the female genital tract and its tumors. *Int. J. Gynecol. Pathol.*, 3:51–70.

150. Sekiya, S., Inaba, N., Iwasawa, H., Kobayashi, O., Takamizawa, H., Matsuzaki, O., and Nagao, K. (1985): AFP-producing Sertoli-Leydig cell tumor of the ovary. *Arch. Gynecol.*, 236:187–196.

151. Shah, N. T., Tuttle, S. E., Strobel, S. L., and Gandhi, L. (1985): Prostatic carcinoma metastatic to bone: Sensitivity and specificity of prostate-specific antigen and prostatic acid phosphatase in decalcified material. *J. Surg. Oncol.*, 29:265–268.

152. Shevchuk, M. M., Romas, N. A., Ng, P. Y., Tannenbaum, M., and Olsson, C. A. (1983): Acid phosphatase localization in prostatic carcinoma. A comparison of monoclonal antibody to heteroantisera. *Cancer,* 52:1642–1646.

153. Shishi, J., Ghazizadeh, M., Oguro, T., Aihara, K., and Araki, T. (1986): Immunohistochemical localization of CA 125 antigen in formalin-fixed paraffin sections of ovarian tumors with the use of Pronase. *Am. J. Clin. Pathol.,* 85:595–598.

154. Shong-San, C., and Walters, M. N. (1984): Adenoid cystic carcinoma of prostate. Report of a case. *Pathology,* 16:337–338.

155. Siegel, A. L., Tomaszewski, J. E., Wein, A. J., and Hanno, P. M. (1986): Invasive carcinoma of prostate presenting as rectal carcinoma. *Urology,* 27:162–164.

156. Silva, E. G., Kott, M. M., Ordonez, N. G. (1984): Endocrine carcinoma intermediate cell type of the uterine cervix. *Cancer,* 54:1705–1713.

157. Sloane, J. P., and Ormerod, M. G. (1981): Distribution of epithelial membrane antigen in normal and neoplastic tissues and its value in diagnostic tumor pathology. *Cancer,* 47:1787–1795.

158. Snyder, R. R., and Tavassoli, F. A. (1986): Ovarian strumal carcinoid: Immunohistochemical, ultrastructural, and clinicopathologic observations. *Int. J. Gynecol. Pathol.,* 5:187–201.

159. Sobin, L. H., Hjermstad, B. M., Sesterhenn, I. A., and Helwig, E. B. (1986): Prostatic acid phosphatase activity in carcinoid tumors. *Cancer,* 58:136–138.

160. Speers, W. C., Picaso, L. G., and Silverberg, S. G. (1983): Immunohistochemical localization of carcinoembryonic antigen in microglandular hyperplasia and adenocarcinoma of the endocervix. *Am. J. Clin. Pathol.,* 79:105–107.

161. Stein, B. S., and Shea, F. J. (1983): Metastatic carcinoma of the prostate presenting radiographically as lymphoma. *J. Urol.,* 130:362–364.

162. Stein, B. S., Petersen, R. O., Vangore, S., and Kendall, A. R. (1982): Immunoperoxidase localization of prostate-specific antigen. *Am. J. Surg. Pathol.,* 6:553–557.

163. Stenback, F., Risteli, J., Risteli, L., and Wasenius, V-M. (1985): Basement membrane laminin and Type IV collagen in endometrial adenocarcinoma: Relation to differentiation and treatment. *Oncology,* 42:370–376.

164. Stenback, F., Wasenius, V-M., Risteli, J., and Risteli, L. (1985): Basement membranes in progressing intraepithelial cervical neoplasia. An ultrastructural and immunohistochemical study with antibodies against human type IV collagen and laminin. *Gynecol. Obstet. Invest.,* 20:158–166.

165. Stephenson, T. J., and Mills, P. M. (1986): Adenomatoid tumours: An immunohistochemical and ultrastructural appraisal of their histogenesis. *J. Pathol.,* 148:327–335.

166. Stratton, M., Evans, D. J., and Lampert, I. A. (1986): Prostatic adenocarcinoma evolving into carcinoid: Selective effect of hormonal treatment? *J. Clin. Pathol.,* 39:750–756.

167. Syrjanen, K. J. (1983): Human papillomavirus lesions in association with cervical dysplasias and neoplasias. *Obstet. Gynecol.,* 62:617–624.

168. Tetu, B., Ordonez, N. G., and Silva, E. G. (1986): Sertoli-Leydig cell tumor of the ovary with α-fetoprotein production. *Arch. Pathol. Lab. Med.,* 110:65–68.

169. Thor, A., Muraro, R., Gorstein, F., Ohuchi, N., Viglione, M., Szpak, C. A., Johnston, W. W., and Schlom, J. (1987): An adjunct to the diagnostic distinction between adenocarcinomas of the ovary and the colon utilizing a monoclonal antibody (COL-4) with restricted CEA reactivity. *Cancer Res ,* 47:505–512.

170. Thor, A., Ohuchi, N., Szpak, C. A., Johnston, W. W., and Schlom, J. (1987): Monoclonal antibodies and immunopathology: Applications to human carcinomas. In: *Tumor Associated Antigens and Other Related Markers,* edited by B. Ghosh and L. Ghosh, pp. 238–268. McGraw Hill, New York.

171. Trojanowski, J. Q., and Hickey, W. F. (1984): Human teratomas express differentiated neural antigens. An immunohistochemical study with anti-neurofilament, anti-glial filament, and anti-myelin basic protein monoclonal antibodies. *Am. J. Pathol.,* 115:383–389.

172. Tsubura, A., Morii, S., Hilkens, J., and Hilgers, J. (1985): Expression of MAM-3 and MAM-6 antigens in endometrial and endocervical adenocarcinomas. *Virchows Arch. [Pathol. Anat.],* 407:59–67.

173. Ueda, G., Inoue, Y., Yamasaki, M., Inoue, M., Tanaka, Y., Hiramatsu, K., Saito, J., Nishino, T., and Abe, Y. (1984): Immunohistochemical demonstration of tumor antigen TA-4 in gynecologic tumors. *Int. J. Gynecol. Pathol.,* 3:291–298.

174. Ueda, G., Yamasaki, M., Inoue, M., Tanaka, Y., Abe, Y., and Ogawa, M. (1985): Immunohistochemical study of amylase in common epithelial tumors of the ovary. *Int. J. Gynecol. Pathol.,* 4:240–244.

175. Venable, D. D., Hastings, D., and Misra, R. P. (1983): Unusual metastatic patterns of prostate adenocarcinoma. *J. Urol.,* 130:980–985.

176. Vernon, S. E., and Williams, W. D. (1983): Pretreatment and post-treatment evaluation of prostatic adenocarcinoma for prostatic specific acid phosphatase and prostate specific antigen by immunohistochemistry. *J. Urol.,* 130:95–98.

177. Vuitch, M. F., and Mendelsohn, G. (1981): Relationship of ectopic ACTH production to tumor differentiation: A morphologic and immunohistochemical study of prostatic carcinoma with Cushing's syndrome. *Cancer,* 47:296–299.

178. Wahlstrom, T., Korhonen, M., Lindgren, J., and Seppala, M. (1979): Distinction between endocervical and

endometrial adenocarcinoma with immunoperoxidase staining of carcinoembryonic antigen in routine histological tissue specimens. *Lancet*, 2:1159–1160.

179. Walker, A. N., Mills, S. E., Fechner, R. E., and Perry, J. M. (1982): "Endometrial" adenocarcinoma of the prostatic urethra arising in a villous polyp. A light microscopic and immunoperoxidase study. *Arch. Pathol. Lab. Med.*, 106:624–627.

180. Walker, A. N., Fechner, R. E., Mills, S. E., and Perry, J. M. (1983): Epithelial polyps of the prostatic urethra. A light-microscopic and immunohistochemical study. *Am. J. Surg. Pathol.*, 7:351–356.

181. Walther, M. M., Nassar, V., Harruff, R. C., Mann, B. B., Jr., Finnerty, D. P., and Hewen-Lowe, K. O. (1985): Endometrial carcinoma of the prostatic utricle: A tumor of prostatic origin. *J. Urol.*, 134:769–773.

182. Wang, M. C., Papsidero, L. D., Kuriyama, M., Valenzuela, L. A., Murphy, G. P., and Chu, T. M. (1981): Prostate antigen: A new potential marker for prostatic cancer. *The Prostate*, 2:89–96.

183. Wang, M. C., Valenzuela, L. A., Murphy, G. P., and Chu, T. M. (1979): Purification of a human prostate specific antigen. *J. Urol.*, 17:159–163.

184. Wenk, R. E., Bhagavan, B. S., Levy, R., Miller, D., and Weisburger, W. (1977): Ectopic ACTH, prostatic oat cell carcinoma, and marked hypernatremia. *Cancer*, 40:773–778.

185. Yam, L. T., Janckila, A. J., Lam, W. K. W., and Li, C. Y. (1981): Immunohistochemistry of prostatic acid phosphatase. *The Prostate*, 2:97–107.

186. Yam, L. T., Winkler, C. F., Janckila, A. J., Li, C. Y., and Lam, K. W. (1983): Prostatic cancer presenting as metastatic adenocarcinoma of undetermined origin. Immunodiagnosis by prostatic acid phosphatase. *Cancer*, 51:283–287.

187. Yamase, H. T., Wurzel, R. S., Nieh, P. T., and Gondos, B. (1985): Immunohistochemical demonstration of human chorionic gonadotropin in tumors of the urinary bladder. *Ann. Clin. Lab. Sci.*, 15:414–417.

188. Yokota, T., Yamashita, Y., Okuzono, Y., Takahashi, M., Fujihara, S., Akizuki, S., Ishihara, T., Uchino, F., and Iwata, T. (1984): Malignant cytosarcoma phyllodes of prostate. *Acta Pathol. Jpn.*, 34:663–668.

189. Young, R. H., and Clement, P. B. (1987): Sclerosing adenosis of the prostate. *Arch. Pathol. Lab. Med.*, 111:363-366.

190. Young, R. H., and Scully, R. E. (1984): Placental site trophoblastic tumor. Current status. *Clin. Obstet. Gynecol.*, 27:248–258.

191. Zaloudek, C., Williams, J. W., and Kempson, R. L. (1976): "Endometrial" adenocarcinoma of the prostate. A distinctive tumor of probable prostatic duct origin. *Cancer*, 37:2255-2262.

192. Zhang, J., and Kraus, F. T. (1986): Placental site trophoblastic tumor (PSTT): Immunocytochemical correlations. *Lab. Invest.*, 54:73A.

Diagnostic Immunopathology,
edited by R.B. Colvin,
A.K. Bhan, and R.T. McCluskey.
Raven Press, New York © 1988.

14 / *Soft Tissue Tumors*

Mark R. Wick and Paul E. Swanson

Division of Surgical Pathology, Department of Laboratory Medicine and Pathology,
University of Minnesota School of Medicine, Minneapolis, Minnesota 55455

The microscopic diagnosis of soft tissue tumors is a forbidding topic for many pathologists. Such neoplasms are capable of assuming a wide array of overlapping histologic appearances, making attention to accompanying clinical details and other supplementary information invaluable in their identification. Several major reference works have been devoted especially to this topic (39,56,118), but these have focused mainly upon conventional light microscopic findings in neoplasms of the soft tissues. Relatively little can be found on the ultrastructural or immunohistochemical attributes of these lesions, in textual form. This chapter will discuss the latter subject with respect to both benign and malignant soft tissue tumors. It is not intended to be exhaustive, either in overall scope, or in relation to coverage of the tumor entities which are included. Rather, a working approach to the immunohistochemical delineation of diagnostically-troublesome soft tissue neoplasms will be provided, and related to their conventional microscopic features. Tumors that are confined to the skin and superficial subcutis are not addressed. Because paraffin-embedded tissues currently comprise the basic substrate of surgical pathology, immunologic markers that are suitably preserved in such specimens (Chapter 8) will be emphasized.

BENIGN TUMORS OF THE SOFT TISSUES

The soft tissues often express their potential for neoplastic transformation in malignant form, and the spectrum of sarcomas is therefore greater than that of benign lesions. Of the latter, those which are most often diagnostic problems are discussed in the following sections.

Fibromatoses/Proliferative Fibroblastic Lesions

Several forms of (myo-) fibromatosis are recognized. These include congenital myofibromatoses, and variants which occur predominantly in adults, and differ only in their locations—abdominal, penile, palmar, and plantar. Other rare forms include hyaline gingival and digital fibromatosis (39,125).

All lesions in these categories are characterized by a moderately cellular proliferation of cytologically-bland oval or spindle cells, embedded in a variably collagenous stroma. Sup-

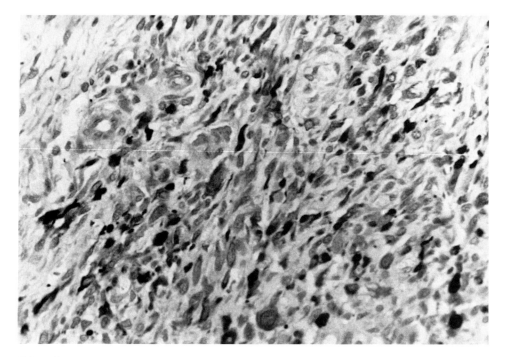

FIG. 1. Cytoplasmic reactivity for desmin, in spindle cells of abdominal fibromatosis ("desmoid tumor").

porting stromal vessels are invested with a prominent muscular coat, allowing them to maintain an open configuration despite the density of surrounding collagen.

These lesions may be confused with hemangiopericytoma, leiomyoma, low-grade fibrosarcoma, and Schwann cell tumors (39). The first three possibilities in this differential diagnostic list can usually be excluded by attention to conventional clinicopathologic details; indeed, this process is that by which a discrimination *must* be made, since their immunohistologic similarities to fibromatoses are many. Hemangiopericytoma, leiomyoma, fibrosarcoma, and fibromatoses all share reactivity for vimentin, the intermediate filament protein (IFP) of mesenchymal cells (95,103). In addition, though one publication has asserted that desmin (the muscular IFP) is absent in myofibroblasts (109) (the actual proliferating cell type in most fibromatoses), we do not agree with this conclusion. Using a highly specific antibody to desmin, our laboratory has observed reactivity in 8/11 fibromatosis cases of various types (Fig. 1). This protein is potentially common to hemangiopericytomas and leiomyomas as well (see below), as is actin, another muscle-related protein (84).

A distinction between fibromatoses and Schwann cell lesions can be made with antibody to S100 protein. The latter determinant has been found in virtually all cases of neurofibroma studied to date (117), whereas it is consistently lacking in myofibroblastic and fibroblastic proliferations.

Reactive (non-neoplastic) fibroblastic proliferations also may present themselves as tumefactive masses. Nodular fasciitis, proliferative fasciitis, and keloids are included in this category. Their immunohistochemical characteristics are as described above, in reference to fibromatoses.

Neurofibromas and Neurilemmomas

The two benign Schwannian tumors of soft tissue are the neurofibroma and the neuri-lemmoma. From an immunohistochemical standpoint, they are equivalent phenotypically (117). However, each evokes different alternatives in differential diagnosis; neurofibromas are commonly confused with myxomas, "neuratizing" nevi, or organizing scar tissue, while neurilemmomas may resemble leiomyomas (39).

Peripheral nerve sheath neoplasms display S100 protein (65,117), and also show reactiv-ity for Leu 7 (a myelin-associated glycoproteinaceous antigen) in approximately 50% of cases (100). Nevi and leiomyomas may exhibit these antigens as well, but they are absent in myxomas and scars. Neurofibromas fail to react with HMB-45, a monoclonal antibody to a melanocytic determinant (53), while nevi are positive. In addition, we have observed myelin basic protein (MBP) in benign peripheral nerve sheath tumors, at variance with the findings of Clark et al. (23); MBP is not seen in nevi (99). Neurilemmomas and neurofi-bromas share vimentin-positivity with leiomyomas, but smooth muscle tumors consistently display desmin and actin, both of which are not found in neurilemmomas. Conversely, peripheral nerve sheath tumors occasionally manifest reactivity for glial fibrillary acidic protein (51); leiomyomas do not do so.

Leiomyomas

Many of the immunohistologic features of leiomyomas have just been described above. In addition, antigenic markers that are specific for such tumors, among all histologically-similar lesions, include smooth-muscle myosin (35) and Z-band protein (85). Documenta-tion of such determinants is desirable in cases with unusual histologic patterns, such as myxoid or hyalinized leiomyomas. The latter may be confused with myxomas and nerve sheath tumors, or proliferative fibrous lesions, respectively.

Myxomas

The microscopic attributes of myxomas overlap with those of myxoid peripheral nerve sheath tumors. The dissimilar clinical settings of these possibilities notwithstanding, it is sometimes desirable to confirm their histogenesis by immunohistochemical means. Myxo-mas exhibit actin and desmin, but lack S100 protein (60); the converse of this profile obtains in cases of peripheral nerve sheath tumor.

Proliferative Tenosynovitis

"Proliferative tenosynovitis" exhibits a spectrum of histologic appearances, and may occur in superficial or deep soft tissues. We have seen several cases which presented as mass lesions, in the buttocks and other unusual locations; nevertheless, the typical clinical setting for this proliferation is as a nodular growth on the distal extremities ("giant cell tumor of tendon sheath") (39). The "fibrohistiocytic" character of most cases of prolifera-tive tenosynovitis is apparent on conventional microscopy. However, some examples are composed of monotonous collections of small and round, or large and polygonal cells, leading to confusion with such malignant neoplasms as neuroepithelioma, extraskeletal

Ewing's sarcoma, rhabdomyosarcoma, and epithelioid sarcoma. Since peripheral tenosyn-ovitis may be mitotically-active, it is in the latter cases that immunostaining procedures are particularly rewarding.

In contrast to most of the other possibilities just cited (the exception being epithelioid sarcoma) (17), peripheral tenosynovitis exhibits reactivity for alpha-1-antitrypsin (AAT) and alpha-1-antichymotrypsin (AACT)—two enzymatic markers typifying fibrohistiocytic proliferations (108). It shares vimentin-positivity with all differential diagnostic alternatives except neuroepithelioma (52), but lacks desmin- and cytokeratin-reactivity, as expected in rhabdomyosarcoma (95) and epithelioid sarcoma (17), respectively.

Capillary Hemangioma/Hemangioendothelioma

Benign vascular lesions having a dense cellularity and relatively little overt vasogenesis may prove diagnostically troublesome. Again, the differential diagnosis of such tumors primarily concerns malignant neoplasms as alternatives; both capillary (juvenile) heman-gioma and hemangioendothelioma can be confused with epithelioid sarcoma or hemangio-pericytoma, in selected cases. Assessment of *Ulex europaeus* I lectin (UEL) binding is valuable in this context, inasmuch as this agglutinin labels endothelial proliferations with a high level of sensitivity (75). However, concomitant immunostains for cytokeratin and epithelial membrane antigen must be negative in order to equate UEL-reactivity with a vascular histogenesis. This is so because of the potential binding of the lectin in question to normal epithelial cells (94) and those of epithelioid sarcomas (130).

Hemangiopericytomas do not display UEL-affinity in their extravascular proliferating cell population, and likewise lack epithelial determinants (103); all three neoplasms under consideration in this section are potentially reactive for vimentin (103). Although factor VIII-related antigen is a specific endothelial marker (83), our experience and that of others (15) has shown a disappointing lack of its presence in densely-cellular benign vascular tumors.

Rhabdomyomas

Rhabdomyomas are most commonly seen in the soft tissues of the head and neck. They may assume the "adult" or "fetal" forms, microscopically; the former shows abundant eosinophilic cytoplasm within tumor cells (39), whereas the latter type exhibits small, rather undifferentiated cells mixed with others having the appearance of fetal muscle (29). We have studied three examples of each type of rhabdomyoma immunohistochemically; all six lesions displayed unequivocal reactivity for vimentin, desmin, actin, and myoglobin. These results are useful in distinguishing fetal rhabdomyoma from fibromatoses, which lack myoglobin. However, immunohistochemistry is of no assistance in separating benign from malignant tumors of striated muscle; this goal must be accomplished on morphologic grounds alone.

Granular Cell Tumors

Benign granular cell tumors may arise at virtually any anatomic site. Furthermore, they may show a compact, cohesive cellular growth pattern, or alternately exhibit irregular permeation of surrounding connective tissue. The principal differential diagnostic considerations in such cases are rhabdomyoma, fibroxanthoma, and epithelioid neurofibroma (39). Granular cell tumors are reactive for S100 protein (116) and carcinoembryonic antigen (CEA) (113), but lack myoglobin and desmin, unlike rhabdomyoma. Fibroxanthoma displays immunopositivity for vimentin, AAT, and AACT, but not for CEA, desmin, myoglobin, or S100 protein. The immunophenotype of epithelioid neurofibroma is essentially identical to that of granular cell tumor, and in view of the fact that these two lesions are both thought to be of peripheral nerve sheath origin (89), a distinction between the two may be artificial.

MALIGNANT TUMORS OF SOFT TISSUE

Sarcomas of the somatic soft tissues may be divided into four generic groups, based on their light microscopic growth patterns. These include small round-cell tumors, spindle-cell neoplasms, epithelioid polygonal cell tumors, and pleomorphic lesions. The constituents of each category are considered in the following sections.

Small Round-cell Neoplasms (Table 1)

The small round-cell tumors of soft tissue are embryonal rhabdomyosarcoma, extraskeletal Ewing's sarcoma, peripheral neuroepithelioma, mesenchymal chondrosarcoma, extralymphoreticular lymphoma and leukemia, and "polyhistioma."

Embryonal Rhabdomyosarcoma

Embryonal tumors are the most common variants of rhabdomyosarcoma, and are the most difficult to identify diagnostically. These lesions favor pediatric patients, and have a

TABLE 1. *Immunoreactivity of small round-cell neoplasms of soft tissue*

Tumor	Determinants							
	DES	VIM	NSE	Leu 7	S100	LCA	CK	EMA
Embryonal rhabdomyosarcoma	+	+	+/−	+/−	0	0	0	0
Extraskeletal Ewing's sarcoma	0	+	+/−	+/−	0	0	0	0
Peripheral neuroectodermal tumor	0	0	+	+	0	0	0	0
Mesenchymal chondrosarcoma	0	+	+/−	+/−	+[a]	0	0	0
Lymphoma/leukemia	0	+/−	0	0	0	+	0	0
"Polyhistioma"	+/−	+/−	+/−	+/−	0	0	+/−	+/−

[a]S100 protein is seen only in chondroid islands of mesenchymal chondrosarcoma
+/− = Variable reactivity.
DES = Desmin. VIM = Vimentin. NSE = Neuron-specific enolase.
S100 = S100 protein. LCA = Leukocyte common antigen (CD45).
CK = Cytokeratin. EMA = Epithelial membrane antigen.

tendency to occur in the head and neck region or on the trunk (39). These features, as well as a less-uniform histologic appearance than those of Ewing's sarcoma, neuroepithelioma, and hematopoietic tumors, often provide helpful differential diagnostic clues. "Strap" cells, large eosinophilic myoblasts, and myxoid stroma may be seen focally in embryonal rhabdomyosarcoma (ERMS), but not in its microscopic mimics. Nevertheless, a significant number of ERMS cases show only densely-packed, lymphocyte-like tumor cells, which defy definitive interpretation on hematoxylin and eosin stains (34).

It is in this more limited subset of neoplasms that immunohistochemical analysis proves to be most helpful. Stains for intermediate filament proteins (3,4,31,49,77,97,99), "fast" myosin (30), myoglobin (13,25), and selected other proteins (42) are most relevant to the identification of ERMS. Among these, desmin and vimentin are most consistently detectable in paraffin-embedded specimens (3,4,41,76,81,95) (Fig. 2). Myoglobin-reactivity has been reported in 33% to 100% of embryonal rhabdomyosarcomas (13,25,41,110); however, if one analyzes the details of such accounts, they show that only the large, differentiating cells of these neoplasms are positive for this determinant. Our experience in 21 cases has paralleled this observation. On the other hand, desmin is consistently demonstrable in ERMS, even in those lesions that are of the primitive, "solid" type (34.41). Scupham et al. have assessed the comparative reactivity of ERMS for actin, alpha-actinin, tropomyosin, myoglobin, and myosin (110). Of these determinants, myosin was most often present; however, its prevalence was still short of that of desmin, as reflected by the results

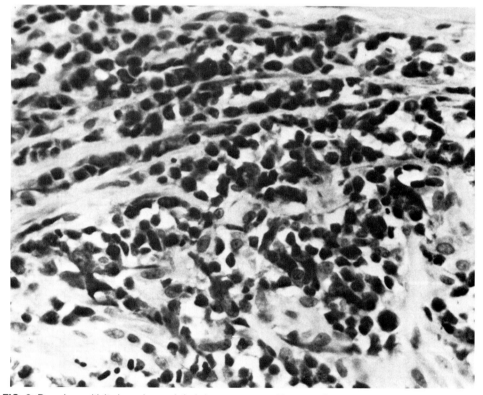

FIG. 2. Desmin-positivity in embryonal rhabdomyosarcoma. Tumor cells contain dark, globular, cytoplasmic foci of reactivity.

of several other studies. Our own experience has shown that immunostains for desmin are 100% sensitive in ERMS, and that other small round-cell neoplasms of soft tissue uniformly lack this protein. An oft-cited drawback of desmin immunostains is that they cannot distinguish between neoplasms of striated and smooth muscle. However, because a small-cell variant of leiomyosarcoma has not been reported to date, this problem appears to be factitious in the context under discussion.

Additional markers of striated muscle differentiation include Z-band protein (85), creatine kinase isozyme MM (126), and titin (96). Currently, insufficient data are available on these discriminants to make meaningful statements on their relative sensitivities for ERMS in paraffin sections. A perplexing observation in regard to this neoplasm is that it also may exhibit reactivity for neuron-specific enolase (NSE), a determinant usually associated with primitive neurogenous tumors (122) (see below).

Extraskeletal Ewing's Sarcoma/Peripheral Neuroectodermal Tumor

Considerable attention is currently being given to the validity of the premise that extraskeletal Ewing's sarcoma (EES) is a reproducible, verifiable tumor entity, distinct from peripheral primitive neuroectodermal tumors of soft tissue ("peripheral neuroepitheliomas" and "Askin's tumors") (16,59,64,70,73). A controversy has arisen over this point, with some authors contending that the two tumors are identical, and others asserting that they are indeed distinguishable from one another. Traditionally, EES has been defined as a neoplasm with ultrastructural and immunohistochemical features similar to those of classic Ewing's sarcoma of bone; i.e., one showing cytoplasmic glycogen pools, intercellular junctional complexes, and immunonegativity for all determinants except vimentin (78,90). (Fig. 3). However, recent studies have purported to demonstrate reactivity for neuron-specific enolase and Leu 7 in EES (66), as well as in osseous Ewing's sarcoma (16). These antigens usually have been seen in neuroendocrine and neuroectodermal neoplasms, including neuroblastoma and neuroepithelioma (28,122) (Fig. 4). Still other theories contending that Ewing's tumors are endothelial, lymphoreticular, or fibrohistocytic in nature have been convincingly disproven, in that none of these lesions exhibit positivity for factor VIII-related antigen, affinity for *Ulex europaeus*, or reactivity for leukocyte common antigen (LCA), AAT, or AACT (68,78,90). Muscle-related proteins are likewise absent in EES (34).

A new "neuroendocrine" marker, synaptophysin (SP), has been demonstrated in virtually all neuroectodermal tumors (50). We have observed its presence in three of nine cases with ultrastructural findings that were "classic" for Ewing's sarcoma, providing additional support for the view that it is related to the former lesions.

Moreover, using more conventional antibody reagents, our own experience mirrors that of the literature; two of ten skeletal and extraskeletal Ewing's sarcomas analyzed in our laboratory have displayed NSE and Leu 7. All of these neoplasms had the electron microscopic appearance of "classic" Ewing's tumor of bone. Preliminary clinicopathologic data show no differences in the behaviors of NSE/Leu 7-positive and -negative neoplasms of this type. Nevertheless, purists may prefer to employ these observations to define "true" EES (lacking NSE and Leu 7), and a related form of peripheral neuroepithelial tumor (expressing one or the other of the specified determinants). Before making such an equation, mention should be made of the fact that *most* peripheral neuroectodermal neoplasms exhibit characteristic ultrastructural features, differing from those of Ewing's tumor (91).

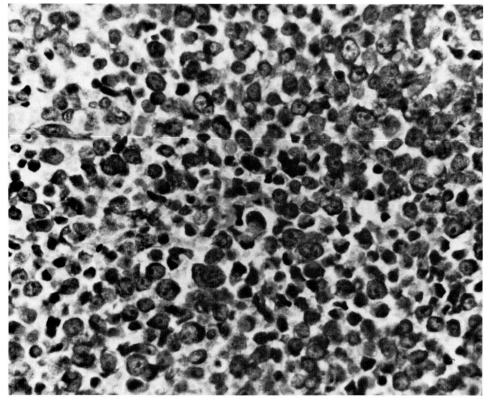

FIG. 3. Vimentin in Ewing's sarcoma of soft tissue.

In addition, the former neoplasms lack vimentin-reactivity (52), while Ewing's sarcoma regularly displays this intermediate filament (78). Certainly, this is an area of soft tissue pathology which will require additional study for resolution of the above-cited dilemma.

Mesenchymal Chondrosarcoma

Mesenchymal chondrosarcoma (MESCS) is a particularly aggressive cartilaginous neoplasm that is seen most often in young adults, and commonly occurs in extraskeletal locations (10). It is typified by a small-cell constituency like that of Ewing's tumor, with the exception that "islands" of primitive cartilage are interspersed throughout the former lesion.

Relatively few studies have addressed the immunophenotypic characteristics of MESCS (82,88). However, it differs from conventional chondrosarcoma in that it lacks uniform reactivity for S100 protein; rather, this determinant is seen only in areas of overt chondroid differentiation (82). Our own experience with this neoplasm has shown a rather surprising similarity to peripheral neuroepithelioma. All of five examples of soft-tissue MESCS studied showed diffuse immunoreactivity for NSE, and four also displayed Leu 7 (Fig. 5). Desmin, actin, myoglobin, and LCA were universally absent. Since ERMS may exhibit chondroid areas, and also may show Leu 7-positivity, these observations and others out-

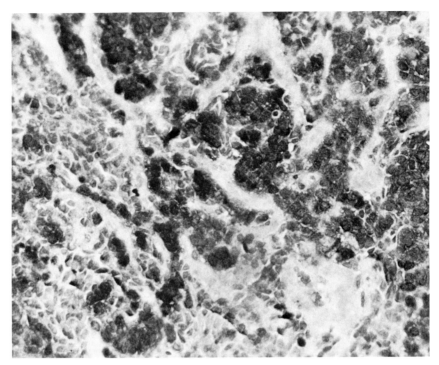

FIG. 4. Reactivity for neuron-specific enolase, in primitive peripheral neuroectodermal tumor ("peripheral neuroepithelioma").

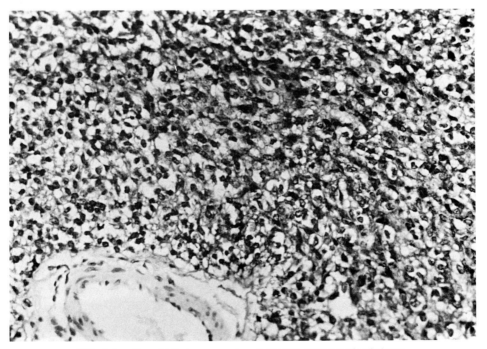

FIG. 5. Leu 7-positivity in mesenchymal chondrosarcoma of soft tissue.

lined above imply that the distinction between embryonal neural and musculoskeletal tumors may not be as clear-cut as was thought formerly. Again, additional analyses will be required to assess this possibility in greater depth.

Leukemia and Malignant Lymphoma in the Soft Tissues

Hematopoietic neoplasms only rarely present with a soft tissue mass, and this event is particularly uncommon in pediatric patients, in whom small round-cell tumors are most prevalent. Nevertheless, the immunohistologic diagnosis of such lesions is straightforward, using antibodies to leukocyte common antigen (CD45). This determinant is present on the membranes of virtually all hematopoietic cells, and is preserved in part in paraffin sections (68). Some antibody reagents to LCA are reactive only with frozen sections (e.g., T29/33 [6]), whereas others yield adequate labeling of both fresh and formalin-fixed material (68) (Chapter 11).

The specificity of LCA is such that reactivity for this discriminant may be equated with a diagnosis of a hematopoietic proliferation, with absolute certainty. Some cases of lymphoma or leukemia may also demonstrate positivity for vimentin, but NSE, muscle-related proteins, and Leu 7 are universally lacking. Once a round-cell neoplasm has been identified as hematopoietic, additional stains for lymphoid markers should be performed on frozen tissue sections (see Chapters 11 and 17). Markers such as LN-2 (40), UCHL-1 (92), and Leu M1 (112) may be employed to assess the B-cell, T-cell, or myeloid nature of the process, even if only paraffin sections are available for analysis.

"Polyhistioma"

Jacobsen proposed that occasional small-cell tumors of soft tissue could pursue several lines of differentiation, simultaneously; the name "polyhistioma" was chosen to describe such lesions (63). Although retrospective assessment has shown that most "polyhistiomas" in Jacobsen's series were actually mesenchymal chondrosarcomas (10), we believe that the former tumors do indeed exist. This opinion is based on our analysis of three neoplasms of the soft tissue in children, which had the light microscopic features of primitive neuroectodermal tumors. Each of these proliferations demonstrated immunoreactivity for vimentin, desmin, NSE, Leu 7, neurofilament protein, cytokeratin, and epithelial membrane antigen, in dissimilar cell populations. Moreover, careful clinical analysis showed the tumors to be primary in all cases. Whether one prefers to label such lesions as "primitive neuroectodermal tumors with divergent differentiation" or as polyhistiomas, their immunophenotypic characteristics clearly differ from those of other small-cell tumors. All three cases manifested aggressive clinical behaviors and proved fatal.

With these observations in mind, it would seem prudent to study all small-cell pediatric neoplasms of the soft tissue for the above-cited markers. The total number of cases showing epithelial differentiation is likely to be miniscule, but only by such means will additional data on these enigmatic tumors be gathered.

Spindle-cell Tumors (Table 2)

The malignant spindle-cell neoplasms of the deep soft tissues are fibrosarcoma, leiomyosarcoma, malignant schwannoma, monophasic synovial sarcoma, and angiosarcoma.

TABLE 2. *Immunoreactivity of spindle-cell neoplasms*

Tumor	Determinants								
	F8	UL	DES	VIM	CK	EMA	S100	MBP	Leu 7
Fibrosarcoma	0	0	0	+	0	0	0	0	0
Leiomyosarcoma/ hemangiopericytoma	0	0	+	+	0	0	0[a]	+/−	+/−
Malignant schwannoma	0	0	+/−[b]	+	0	0	+/−[b]	+/−[b]	+/−[b]
Synovial sarcoma	0	+/−	0	+	+	+	0	0	+/−
Spindle-cell Angiosarcoma	+/−	+	0	+	0	0	0	0	0

[a]Occasional leiomyosarcomas may show S100-positivity.
[b]Roughly 10% malignant schwannomas are desmin-reactive, 65% are S100-reactive; 35% are myelin basic protein-reactive; 50% are Leu 7-reactive.
F8 = Factor VIII-related antigen. UL = *Ulex europaeus* lectin binding.
DES = Desmin. VIM = Vimentin. CK = Cytokeratin.
EMA = Epithelial membrane antigen. S100 = S100 protein.
MBP = Myelin basic protein. +/− = Variable reactivity.

Immunohistochemical reagents that may be used effectively in their identification include antibodies to vimentin, desmin, actin, S100 protein, myelin basic protein, Leu 7, cytokeratin, epithelial membrane antigen, and *Ulex europaeus* lectin.

Fibrosarcoma

Until 20 years ago, fibrosarcoma was thought to be the most common soft tissue malignancy (62). With the advent of more sophisticated pathologic techniques, it is now known that this tumor is probably one of the *rarest* sarcomas (39). It most often occurs in middle adulthood, but also may be seen in infancy as a congenital lesion; in the latter setting, fibrosarcoma displays histologic features that overlap with those of the fibromatoses (20).

Because most reports on the immunohistology of fibrosarcoma have not provided other pathologic details to support such a diagnosis (77,95), some uncertainty has existed as to the immunophenotype of this tumor. We have studied four examples that were verified by electron microscopy. All of them displayed vimentin-immunoreactivity, to the exclusion of other determinants. Accordingly, we are skeptical of reports purporting to show positivity for actin and desmin in fibrosarcoma (77).

Leiomyosarcoma/Hemangiopericytoma

Sarcomas displaying smooth muscle differentiation are most commonly found in the retroperitoneum, in adults of middle age or older. They rarely occur in the deep soft tissues of the extremities, but may be seen in more superficial sites, particularly in the dermis and subcutis. Related lesions with pericytic features are more diffusely distributed anatomically.

In our experience, the great majority of leiomyosarcomas exhibit reactivity for desmin, in a diffuse cytoplasmic pattern (Fig. 6); actin is also commonly expressed (Table 2).

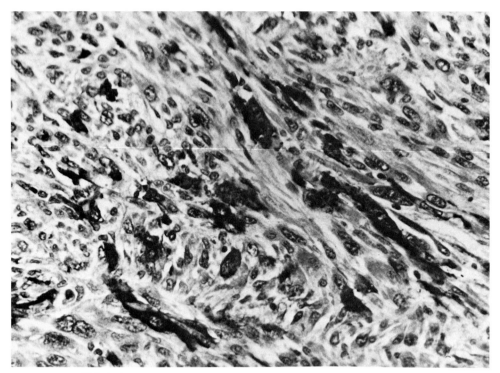

FIG. 6. Desmin-immunoreactivity in leiomyosarcoma of retroperitoneum.

Several other investigators have noted similar findings (31,49,77,95), but Hashimoto et al. obtained positive immunostaining for desmin in only nine of 19 leiomyosarcomas (58). Interestingly, four of their cases also displayed AACT, in areas that were pleomorphic microscopically. The latter point suggests that the series just cited may have been skewed in favor of poorly-differentiated or "dedifferentiated" neoplasms.

Hemangiopericytoma less commonly manifests reactivity for muscle-related proteins, despite its close relationship to leiomyosarcoma. Vimentin is most commonly observed in this tumor, without other accompanying determinants (103).

Donner et al. reported positivity for smooth-muscle myosin in only 30% of leiomyosarcomas (35), and Pertschuk (101) failed to label any of these tumors with an antibody to human smooth muscle. On the other hand, promising results obtained with another muscle-specific reagent, anti-Z-band protein, were reported by Mukai and colleagues; 90% of leiomyosarcomas reacted with this probe (85). However, it is not commercially available at present.

Malignant Schwannoma

Malignant schwannoma ("neurofibrosarcoma;" "neurogenic sarcoma;" "malignant peripheral nerve sheath tumor") is now recognized as a relatively frequent form of soft tissue sarcoma (39). It may occur in patients with and without von Recklinghausen's neurofibromatosis (VRN), and also has the potential for divergent rhabdomyoblastic, chondro-osseous, and epithelial differentiation (38). Examples of this lesion that are unassociated with clinical stigmata of VRN commonly resemble fibrosarcoma microscopically. Some may arise in major nerve trunks, providing a significant biologic clue to their identification; however, this is true of only a minority.

Perhaps because of its facility for histopathologic mimicry of other sarcomas, a goodly number of publications have addressed the immunohistochemical features of malignant schwannoma (26,32,72,120,128,132). The determinant that is most often associated with the latter neoplasm is S100 protein, inasmuch as normal Schwann cells regularly display its expression (128). However, a careful review of the literature on this topic shows that only 50% to 65% of malignant schwannomas are S100-reactive (26,32,72,128). Such has also been our experience, but we have found that inclusion of concomitant immunostains for Leu 7 and myelin basic protein allows one to label a somewhat greater percentage of these tumors (132) (Fig. 7).

Nevertheless, these results are not definitive in the identification of malignant schwannoma. Leiomyosarcoma also has the potential for S100-, Leu 7-, and MBP-expression (120), and monophasic synovial sarcoma may exhibit the second of these three determinants as well (1). Moreover, 12% of malignant schwannoma cases demonstrate focal desmin-positivity (120,132). All three neoplasms are reactive for vimentin.

These observations emphasize the value of an antibody *panel* approach to immunohistologic diagnosis, but in addition, they demonstrate its failings. Synovial sarcoma may be separated from fibrosarcoma-like malignant schwannoma by reactivity for cytokeratin (1,47,108), and negativity for MBP and S100 (120), but even under optimal circumstances leiomyosarcoma cannot be excluded as a possibility in selected cases of neurogenic tumors. Therefore, this is one setting in which electron microscopy is diagnostically superior to immunohistochemistry.

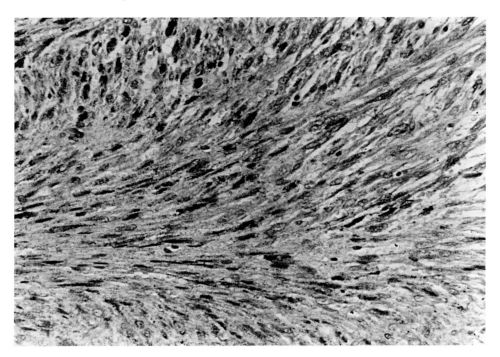

FIG. 7. Cytoplasmic reactivity for myelin basic protein, in tumor cells of spindle-cell malignant schwannoma.

Monophasic Synovial Sarcoma

Among all spindle-cell soft tissue neoplasms, the monophasic variant of synovial sarcoma (MSS) is unique in its immunohistologic characteristics. This is the only such lesion which demonstrates epithelial markers (i.e., cytokeratin and epithelial membrane antigen) (1,47,108,120) (Fig. 8). They are not present diffusely in any given tumor, but are observed in virtually all cases. Vimentin-reactivity is also typical of MSS (80).

Fisher (47) and our group (1) have shown that, in contradistinction to the situation described above for MS, ultrastructural studies are inferior to immunohistochemical analyses for the diagnosis of MSS. Monophasic synovial sarcoma also can exhibit reactivity for actin and AACT (1); however, these markers are vastly inferior in specificity to that of epithelial determinants.

Controversy has arisen over the propriety of the term "synovial" sarcoma. Miettinnen and Virtanen (80), Salisbury and Isaacson (108), and Abenoza et al. (1) demonstrated that this sarcoma does not mirror the immunohistologic qualities of proliferative synovial tissue, or of benign tumors commonly accepted as synovial in origin. In light of these observations, we would agree that synovial sarcoma is probably misnamed (80), but it is unlikely that a new designation would successfully supplant this time-honored appellation.

Spindle-cell Angiosarcoma

Angiosarcomas most commonly occur in the skin, breast, bone, and various internal organs, but also may arise in the deep somatic soft tissues in rare instances. A distinctive

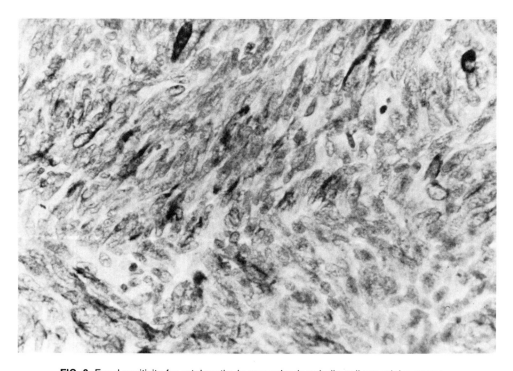

FIG. 8. Focal positivity for cytokeratin, in monophasic spindle-cell synovial sarcoma.

form of this neoplasm is typified by a poorly-differentiated spindle-cell growth pattern, showing only rudimentary formation of vascular lumina (5). Hence, it may be confused with other spindle-cell sarcomas.

Ulex europaeus I lectin labels the great majority of spindle-cell angiosarcomas (SCA) (Fig. 9), but less than 30% demonstrate factor VIII-related antigen-reactivity. As expected, all are vimentin-positive.

These observations are useful in combination with the results of other immunostains. SCA do not display cytokeratin or epithelial membrane antigen (EMA) (5), thus distinguishing them from MSS, which may also manifest vimentin- and UEL-reactivity (80). In addition, angiosarcomas fail to demonstrate positivity for S100 protein, MBP, Leu 7, and desmin.

SCA should not be confused with Kaposi's sarcoma or spindle-cell hemangioendothelioma, because of significant histopathologic and clinical differences between these lesions. The characteristic features of each have been well-documented (12,127), and will not be recounted here.

Polygonal-cell Tumors (Table 3)

A number of soft tissue sarcomas are composed of large, epithelioid, polygonal cells, yielding an appearance like that of carcinomas. These lesions include epithelioid sarcoma, epithelioid monophasic synovial sarcoma, clear-cell sarcoma, alveolar soft part sarcoma, epithelioid leiomyosarcoma, epithelioid angiosarcoma, "histiocytic" malignant fibrous histiocytoma, epithelioid malignant schwannoma, and malignant granular cell tumors.

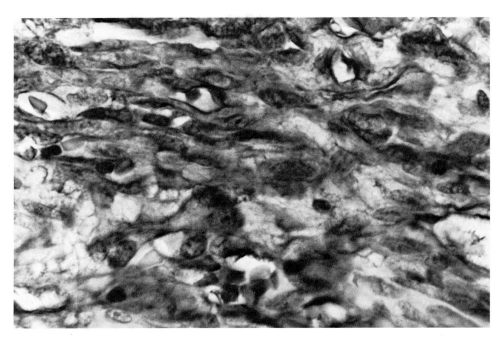

FIG. 9. Binding of *Ulex europaeus* I lectin, by tumor cells of spindle-cell angiosarcoma.

TABLE 3. *Immunoreactivity of epithelioid neoplasms of soft tissue*

Tumor	Determinants									
	CK	EMA	CEA	VIM	DES	F8	UEL	S100	MBP	Leu 7
Epithelioid sarcoma	+	+	+/−	+	0	0	+/−	+/−	0	+/−
Epithelioid synovial sarcoma	+	+	+/−	0	0	0	+/−	0	0	+/−
Epithelioid angiosarcoma	0	0	0	+	0	+	+	0	0	0
Clear-cell sarcoma[a]	0	0	0	+	0	0	0	+	0	+/−
Epithelioid malignant schwannoma[b]	0	0	0	+	0	0	0	+	+/−	+/−
Epithelioid leiomyosarcoma	0	0	0	+	+/−	0	0	0	0	0
Alveolar soft part sarcoma	0	0	0	+	+/−	0	0	0	0	0
"Histiocytic" MFH	0	0	0	+	0	0	0	0	0	0

[a]Clear-cell sarcoma is reactive with antibody HMB-45 (see text).
[b]Rare examples of epithelioid malignant schwannoma may display EMA-reactivity; this tumor is non-reactive with antibody HMB-45.
+/− = Variable reactivity.
CK = Cytokeratin. EMA = Epithelial membrane antigen.
CEA = Carcinoembryonic antigen. VIM = Vimentin. DES = Desmin.
F8 = Factor VIII-related antigen. UEL = *Ulex europaeus* lectin binding.
S100 = S100 protein. MBP = Myelin basic protein.

Epithelioid Sarcoma

Epithelioid sarcoma (ES) has a characteristic growth pattern, simulating necrobiotic granuloma or metastatic carcinoma (17,18). It most commonly arises on the extremities in young individuals, and demonstrates an indolent but potentially fatal clinical course.

ES shares many immunohistologic similarities with MSS, in that both are reactive for cytokeratin and EMA (17,18,71) (Fig. 10). In addition, ES and MSS may display positivity for carcinoembryonic antigen (CEA) in a minority of cases (17). S100 protein has been reported in ES, but not in MSS (17,120). The latter determinant is always accompanied by cytokeratin or EMA, providing a means for distinguishing ES from other S100-positive polygonal-cell neoplasms (see below).

Immunohistochemical studies do not allow for the separation of ES from metastatic carcinomas of soft tissue; such a distinction instead must be made on clinical grounds alone. However, they do supply the pathologist with a means for differentiating between epithelioid sarcomas and isolated necrobiotic granulomas. A granuloma would be expected to manifest reactivity for LCA, while ES does not; conversely, the former of these lesions is cytokeratin- and EMA-negative (131). Vimentin-positivity has been documented in both.

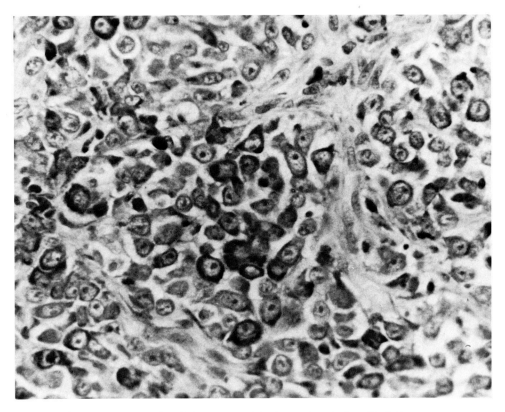

FIG. 10. Intense cytoplasmic immunoreactivity for cytokeratin, in epithelioid sarcoma.

Epithelioid Monophasic Synovial Sarcoma

As just outlined, the homologies between synovial sarcoma and ES are many. The first of these two neoplasms also may assume a "pure" epithelioid growth pattern, heightening this confusion (44). However, epithelioid synovial sarcoma is typically seen in deep soft tissues, in contrast to the more superficial location of ES. In addition, the former exhibits the formation of true glandular lumina, at least focally.

Immunohistochemical reports have not been focused specifically on monophasic epithelioid synovial sarcoma. However, we have analyzed two examples of this neoplasm; our results show striking similarities to the immunophenotype of epithelioid sarcoma, including reactivity for cytokeratin, EMA, and CEA. Neither lesion demonstrated vimentin- or S100-positivity.

Epithelioid Hemangioendothelioma (Low-Grade Angiosarcoma)

In 1982, Weiss and Enzinger first reported the pathologic features of a peculiar, endothelial, polygonal-cell tumor of soft tissues, with a microscopic resemblance to ES and metastatic carcinoma (126). This was given the designation of "epithelioid hemangioendothelioma;" subsequent studies have shown that histologically-similar tumors also occur in

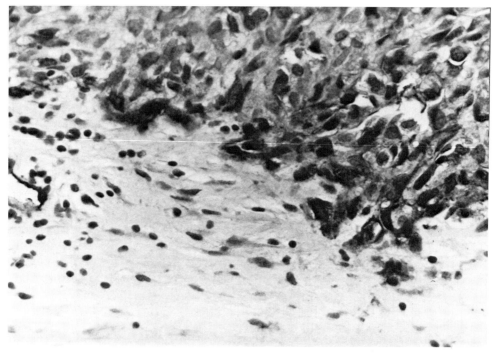

FIG. 11. Factor VIII-related antigen-reactivity in epithelioid hemangioendothelioma (borderline epithelioid angiosarcoma).

such visceral organs as the liver (27) and lung (11). Such neoplasms are of "borderline" malignancy, and may metastasize.

The majority of epithelioid hemangioendotheliomas (EH) display binding of UEL, with or without reactivity for blood group isoantigens A, B, and H and factor VIII-related antigen (FVIIIRAG) (126,130) (Fig. 11). They are negative for cytokeratin, EMA, and S100 protein.

The latter observations assume particular importance in this context, since ES is capable of expressing blood group isoantigens and binding UEL. Hence, UEL and blood group isoantigens are useful as endothelial determinants only in the concurrent absence of epithelial markers. Reactivity for FVIIIRAG is, however, diagnostically specific for EH among all polygonal-cell soft tissue tumors.

Clear-cell Sarcoma

Recent reassessment has made it appear likely that a distinctive tumor of the tendons and aponeuroses, originally called "clear-cell" sarcoma, is actually the primary soft-tissue counterpart of cutaneous malignant melanoma (21). This neoplasm is typified by the compartmentalized growth of polygonal cells with prominent nucleoli and optically-lucent cytoplasm; melanin pigment may or may not be observed.

The immunohistochemical attributes of clear-cell sarcoma (CCS) strengthen its relationship to malignant melanoma. These include reactivity for vimentin and S100 protein (Fig. 12), and the absence of cytokeratin and EMA (21,87). Moreover, two examples studied in

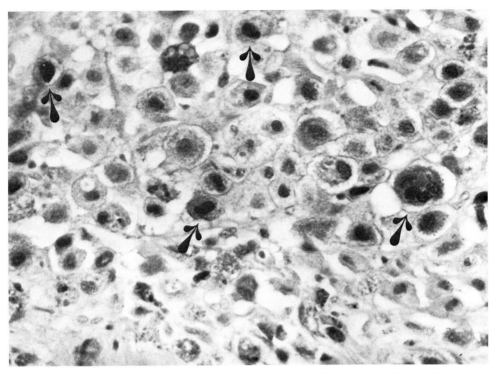

FIG. 12. S100 protein-positivity in clear cell sarcoma of Achilles tendon. Arrows indicate nuclear staining of the tumor cells.

our laboratory failed to demonstrate CEA, FVIIIRAG, binding of UEL, or expression of BGI. In accord with the observations of Wilson et al. (133), and Gown and colleagues (53), in reports on cutaneous melanomas, we have also observed the HLA-DR antigen and reactivity with HMB-45 in these cases of CCS.

Epithelioid Malignant Schwannoma and Malignant Granular Cell Tumor

The above-cited sketch of the clinical features of spindle-cell malignant schwannoma also applies to its polygonal-cell counterpart (33,132). However, epithelioid and spindle-cell malignant schwannoma have dissimilar differential diagnoses, with the former resembling the other neoplasms considered in this section. Malignant granular cell tumors differ from polygonal-cell malignant schwannoma in their composition by cells with strikingly granular cytoplasm; however, both are probably closely-related lesions and will be discussed together.

Epithelioid malignant schwannoma exhibits S100 protein in 70% of cases, with or without MBP, Leu 7, and HLA-DR (132). It lacks cytokeratin, but rare examples are capable of focal EMA-expression (132). Carcinoembryonic antigen is consistently absent, as are FVIIIRAG, UEL, blood group isoantigens, and the HMB-45 antigen. Malignant granular cell tumors manifest a similar immunophenotype, except for the potential expression of CEA (113).

Epithelioid Leiomyosarcoma

The existence of a polygonal-cell variant of leiomyosarcoma ("leiomyoblastoma") in the soft tissues has not received much attention, presumably because of its rarity (39). Correspondingly, data on its immunocytochemical characteristics are anecdotal. As in the stomach and uterus, soft tissue leiomyoblastoma (LMBL) usually is composed of sheets and clusters of epithelioid cells, with vacuolated or granular cytoplasm. Mitotic figures are variable in number, but may be altogether absent. Despite this feature, Enzinger and Weiss have cautioned that all tumors of this type should be considered malignant and capable of metastasizing (39).

We have studied five cases of LMBL, four of which were retroperitoneal and seeded the peritoneum extensively, and one of which was located within the deltoid muscle and recurred repeatedly. All were reactive for vimentin, four showed actin-positivity, and three contained desmin as well. None displayed S100, cytokeratin, EMA, FVIIIRAG, blood group isoantigens, UEL binding, or CEA.

Alveolar Soft Part Sarcoma

Ever since its initial description (19), alveolar soft part sarcoma (ASPS) has been the object of debate and controversy, over its lineage of cellular differentiation. One theory proposed that this neoplasm was endocrine in nature and related to paraganglioma (123), while another favored a myogenous histogenesis (46).

Recent immunohistochemical studies by Mukai and colleagues give further support to the latter view (86), which also seems most likely on the basis of the usual intramuscular location of ASPS. These investigators demonstrated reactivity for actin, Z-band protein, or desmin in the majority of alveolar soft part sarcomas. Three cases analyzed in our laboratory were vimentin-positive, and one manifested reactivity for desmin as well (Fig. 13). None have expressed neuron-specific enolase, Leu 7, or chromogranin (another neuroendocrine-specific marker), in contrast to the usual characteristics of paragangliomas. Similarly, we have not observed cytokeratin, EMA, FVIIIRAG, blood group isoantigens, CEA, S100, or UEL binding in ASPS.

"Histiocytic" Malignant Fibrous Histiocytoma

Occasional examples of malignant fibrous histiocytoma (MFH) of the soft tissues are wholly comprised by uniform, polygonal cells, with a sheetlike growth pattern. These have been designated as representative of a "histiocytic" variant of this neoplasm (39).

The very existence of "fibrohistiocytic" neoplasms is currently being challenged, on immunohistochemical grounds (134). Several authors have proposed the theory that MFH is actually a form of fibrosarcoma, based on a lack of antigenic expression like that of histiocytic proliferations. This argument will be discussed in greater detail subsequently. In general, MFH displays reactivity for AAT, AACT, and ferritin (37,67), while fibrosarcoma does not. With specific reference to the differential diagnostic context being considered here, histiocytic MFH also lacks the expression of cytokeratin, EMA, desmin, actin, FVIIIRAG, blood group isoantigens, CEA, S100, MBP, Leu 7, and the HMB-45 antigen. However, we have observed HLA-DR in the majority of such tumors analyzed in our laboratory.

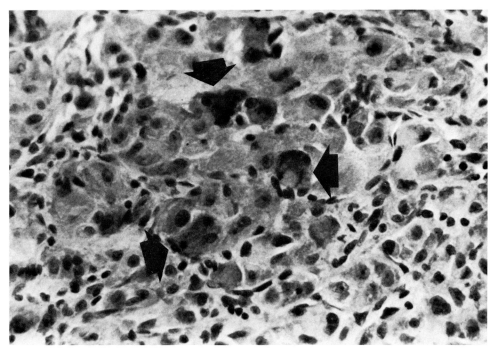

FIG. 13. Focal reactivity for desmin (arrows) in alveolar soft part sarcoma of thigh.

Admittedly, the immunohistochemical diagnosis of histiocytic MFH is one of exclusion, since other soft tissue sarcomas also share the capacity for AAT-, AACT-, and ferritin-expression (17,67). The latter include ES, monophasic epithelioid synovial sarcoma, clear-cell sarcoma, and epithelioid MS. Nonetheless, these tumors display reactants that are not seen in MFH, as described in the foregoing discussion.

Pleomorphic Tumors of Soft Tissue (Table 4)

Those soft tissue sarcomas that may display a pleomorphic microscopic appearance include MFH, pleomorphic rhabdomyosarcoma, pleomorphic and dedifferentiated liposarcoma, dedifferentiated leiomyosarcoma, and malignant schwannoma.

Pleomorphic Malignant Fibrous Histiocytoma

Malignant fibrous histiocytoma is currently accepted as the most common form of soft tissue sarcoma in adults (39). Despite its relative frequency, the exact nature of this neoplasm is in doubt, as referenced in the preceding section. Ozzello et al. were the first to postulate that MFH was related to tissue histiocytes, based on its characteristics in tissue culture (98). Subsequently, shared reactivity for AAT, AACT, ferritin, and binding of peanut agglutinin was demonstrated between MFH and histiocytic proliferations (37,67, 104). These points notwithstanding, Wood et al. (134) and Roholl and colleagues (105) have documented dissimilarities between the two lesions in immunohistologic analyses of

TABLE 4. *Immunoreactivity of pleomorphic neoplasms*

Tumor	Determinants						
	DES	VIM	MB	S100	MBP	Leu 7	ACT
Malignant fibrous histiocytoma[a]	0	+	0	0	0	0	+
Pleomorphic rhabdomyosarcoma	+	+	+	0	0	0	+/−
Pleomorphic and dedifferentiated liposarcoma[b]	0	+	0	+	0	0	+/−
Dedifferentiated leiomyosarcoma[c]	+/−	+	0	0	+/−	+/−	+/−
Malignant schwannoma[d]	0	+	0	+/−	+/−	+/−	+/−

[a]Occasional MFH cases are focally desmin-positive.
[b]Lipoblastic cells in pleomorphic liposarcoma are reactive for S100 protein.
[c]Reactivity for desmin, MBP and Leu 7 refer only to well-differentiated areas of dedifferentiated leiomyosarcoma.
[d]Approximately 65% of malignant schwannomas are S100-reactive; approximately 35% are reactive for myelin basic protein.
DES = Desmin. VIM = Vimentin. MB = Myoglobin.
S100 = S100 protein. MBP = Myelin basic protein.
ACT = Alpha-1-antichymotrypsin. +/− = Variable reactivity.

frozen sections, using antibodies to macrophage-related antigens. The former of these groups of investigators also questioned the specificity of other markers used to identify MFH, including AAT, AACT, lysozyme, ferritin, "nonspecific esterase," and complement receptors. Both studies contended that MFH should be regarded as a primitive mesenchymal neoplasm, more closely related to fibrosarcoma than to any other soft tissue tumor. Additional confusion has been introduced by the findings of Strauchen and Dimitriu-Bona (119), who purportedly *did* observe macrophage-related determinants in MFH.

From a practical point of view, this issue is irrelevant to the immunohistochemical diagnosis of "fibrohistiocytic" sarcomas. As already stated, they exhibit AAT, AACT, and ferritin, in conjunction with vimentin (Fig. 14). It is likely that an MFH-like histologic appearance and the antigenic reflection of this pattern are "final common denominators" for several primary soft tissue sarcomas (14). However, determinants that are associated with these other malignant tumors are absent in MFH. These include myoglobin, S100 protein, myelin basic protein, and Leu 7 (13,120). Focal desmin-reactivity has been reported in this neoplasm (95), as has similar positivity for actin (84). These observations are thought to correlate with the "myofibroblastic" differentiation seen in some cells of MFH by electron microscopy (22). Wood et al. failed to detect HLA-DR in their series (134), but we have observed this determinant in the majority of malignant fibrous histiocytomas. Strauchen and Dimitriu-Bona (119) and Roholl et al. (105) have reported similar results.

Pleomorphic Rhabdomyosarcoma

Among the various forms of rhabdomyosarcoma, the pleomorphic type is the most uncommon. However, it is also the easiest to diagnose immunohistologically, because of a

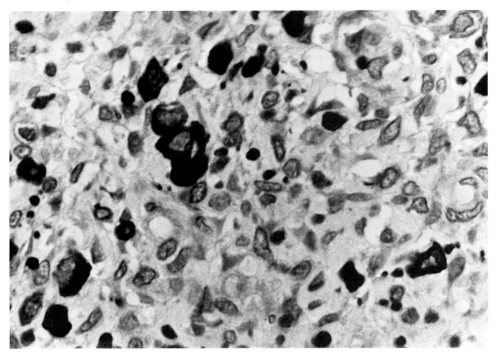

FIG. 14. Positivity for alpha-1-antichymotrypsin, in pleomorphic malignant fibrous histiocytoma.

uniform expression of myoglobin (13). This finding is associated with the comparatively high level of striated muscle differentiation seen in pleomorphic rhabdomyosarcoma, reflected by the presence of "strap" cells on conventional microscopy. It is well-known that myoglobin appears relatively late in the ontogeny of rhabdomyoblasts, in comparison with desmin, actin, and myosin (96). Correspondingly, the latter proteins are also vividly displayed by this tumor (3,85,96). Although we have mentioned the occasional positivity for desmin and actin that may be observed in MFH, the magnitude and scope of expression of these antigens by pleomorphic rhabdomyosarcoma dwarfs those seen in the former neoplasm. Conversely, AAT, AACT, and ferritin may be seen focally in this form of striated muscle sarcoma. S100 protein and neural determinants such as MBP and Leu 7 are uniformly lacking in differentiated rhabdomyosarcomas, as is the HLA-DR antigen.

Pleomorphic and "Dedifferentiated" Liposarcomas

Pleomorphic liposarcoma is defined as a neoplasm with an overall microscopic resemblance to MFH, except for the regular interspersion of signet ring-cell or multivacuolated lipoblasts in the former lesion. "Dedifferentiated" liposarcoma presents a similar histologic appearance, but differs from the pleomorphic variant in that it is found in apposition to well-differentiated liposarcoma (43), or represents a recurrence-related change in the latter tumor (114).

Hence, it should not be surprising that pleomorphic and dedifferentiated liposarcomas manifest the potential expression of most of the determinants seen in MFH (e.g., AAT, AACT, and ferritin). However, these adipose tissue tumors also exhibit S100 protein-immunoreactivity in their lipoblastic constituents (24,57), unlike pure fibrohistiocytic neoplasms. Although S100 is best-known as a neural determinant, mature adipocytes and their precursors also are capable of its synthesis (128). Myelin basic protein, Leu 7, desmin, and myoglobin are absent in poorly-differentiated liposarcomas.

"Dedifferentiated" Leiomyosarcoma

In a foregoing section on spindle-cell leiomyosarcoma, mention was made of the observations of Hashimoto et al., with respect to three examples of this tumor in their series (58). These lesions were analogous to the just-cited "dedifferentiated" liposarcoma, in that microscopic fields of typical leiomyosarcoma blended with others having the appearance of MFH. Correspondingly, the former component was diffusely desmin-reactive but lacked AAT and AACT, whereas the reverse of these findings obtained in the pleomorphic constituent. Again, such observations support the contention that MFH may be a "final common pathway" for soft tissue sarcomas undergoing biological transition. Further antigenic expression was not evaluated in this study, and we have not had the opportunity to assess any examples of "dedifferentiated" leiomyosarcoma in our laboratory. Thus, comment cannot be made upon the potential presence of S100, myoglobin, MBP, or Leu 7 in this tumor.

Pleomorphic Malignant Schwannoma

In addition to its spindle-cell and epithelioid forms, malignant schwannoma may assume a pleomorphic appearance (61). This eventuality does not seem to represent another example of dedifferentiation, at least in the same sense as that conveyed up to this point. Such a statement is based on the fact that pleomorphic MS retains the ability to express S100 proteins, MBP, and Leu 7 even in the poorly-differentiated cells of this tumor; nonetheless, positivity for AACT, AAT, and ferritin also may be present. Myoglobin and desmin are uniformly absent.

Immunohistologic Findings in Other Primary Neoplasms of the Soft Tissue

Some primary tumors of the soft tissue do not fit neatly into one of the categories presented thus far. Chordoma, extra-osseous myxoid chondrosarcoma ("chordoid" sarcoma), extraskeletal osteosarcoma, aggressive angiomyxoma, and some liposarcoma variants are included in this group.

Chordoma/Extra-osseous Myxoid Chondrosarcoma

Typical chordoma and "chordoid" sarcoma share several histologic features. Both are composed of plump, vacuolated epithelioid cells in clusters and linear arrays, embedded in a loose myxo-chondroid matrix and growing in a lobular configuration. Mitotic figures are rare, and necrosis is usually absent (39). These two tumors also share the capacity to undergo "dedifferentiation" (9,48), yielding a component which resembles MFH, as described above. Finally, although accepted dogma states that chordoma is confined to the axial portion of the body, because of a proposed origin from the notochord, recent studies indicate that identical neoplasms may arise in the peripheral soft tissues as well (102). This heightens their similarity to chordoid sarcomas.

Several reports have demonstrated that, despite these clinicopathologic homologies, there are immunophenotypic differences between chordoma and chordoid sarcoma. The first of these tumors exhibits cytokeratin, with or without vimentin, whereas the extra-skeletal myxoid chondrosarcoma displays only vimentin (2,74,107). Also, chordoma is reactive for EMA and other milk-fat globule proteins (74,107), but chordoid sarcoma is not. Both commonly demonstrate synthesis of S100 protein (74), and we also have seen Leu 7 in the majority of chordomas and chordoid sarcomas.

We have studied one case each of dedifferentiated chordoma and dedifferentiated chordoid sarcoma. As expected, the pleomorphic components of each neoplasm exhibited an immunophenotype like that of MFH (i.e., AAT-, AACT-, and ferritin-positive). However, rare cells in these high-grade areas retained S100-reactivity, unlike the phenotype in de novo MFH. Others have reported similar findings (9,48).

Extraskeletal Osteosarcoma

Osteosarcoma rarely arises entirely in the soft tissues, without a connection to subjacent bones. The histologic variants of this tumor in osseous sites are well-known, and include fibroblastic, osteoblastic, chondroblastic, and pleomorphic forms (39). The common feature to all subtypes is, of course, the production of verifiable osteoid matrix.

In keeping with the aforementioned microscopic diversity, the immunohistologic features of extraskeletal osteosarcoma are varied. In our experience, the cells in the fibro-blastic form of this tumor manifests only vimentin-reactivity, without the presence of any other epithelial or mesenchymal determinants. The osteoblastic variant demonstrates posi-

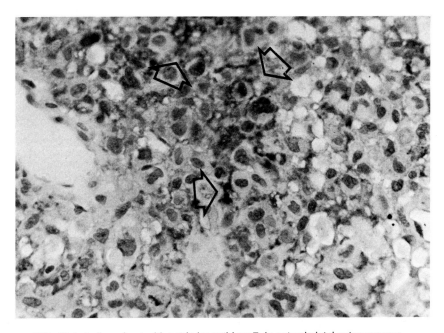

FIG. 15. Labeling of osteoid matrix by anti-Leu 7, in extraskeletal osteosarcoma.

tivity for alkaline phosphatase as well. Chondroblastic osteosarcomas of the soft tissue are reactive for S100 protein in areas of cartilaginous differentiation (88), but not in osteogenic foci; again, vimentin and alkaline phosphatase are diffusely present. Finally, pleomorphic extraskeletal osteosarcoma shows an immunophenotype like that of MFH, with or without focal alkaline phosphatase-reactivity as well.

The immunohistochemical "common thread" in extraskeletal osteosarcoma variants is a reactivity of the osteoid matrix with anti-Leu 7 (Fig. 15). It has been established that this reagent recognizes glycoproteinaceous determinants (100), one of which is presumably present in osteoid. In a comparative study of other sarcomas with osteoid-*like* matrices (synovial sarcoma, fibrosarcoma, MFH), the latter have failed to label with anti-Leu 7 in every instance. We would emphasize at this point that this statement refers *only* to the matrix, and not to tumor cells themselves, although chondroblastic extraskeletal osteosarcoma does indeed manifest cellular Leu 7-positivity as well.

Aggressive Angiomyxoma

A peculiar neoplasm of the female pelvis has been described recently by Steeper and Rosai (115). This lesion features a composition by loosely-arranged, bland, stellate cells, embedded in a myxoid matrix which is punctuated by numerous venule- and capillary-sized blood vessels. It is considered to be a low-grade malignancy by virtue of its frequent recurrence, although metastasis has not been observed to date.

Begin and colleagues studied five examples of aggressive angiomyxoma immunocytochemically, with antibodies to actin, S100 protein, and FVIIIRAG (8). Reactivity in the stellate cells was observed for actin only. We have analyzed an additional eight cases; our series showed positivity for vimentin, desmin, and actin while FVIIIRAG, S100 protein, MBP, and Leu 7 were lacking. These data are useful in confirming the "myofibroblastic" nature for this tumor that was proposed by Begin et al. on ultrastructural grounds (8), and in excluding Schwannian, endothelial, and lipoblastic tumors in differential diagnosis. The specified immunophenotype of aggressive angiomyxoma is virtually identical to that of intramuscular myxoma (60), but these lesions can be separated from one another on conventional clinicopathologic grounds alone.

Liposarcoma Variants

Liposarcoma is easily-recognized by most pathologists in its well-differentiated form. Nevertheless, myxoid and round-cell variants of this neoplasm may be the sources of consternation in differential diagnosis with other histologically-similar tumors. Pleomorphic and dedifferentiated liposarcomas have already been considered in an earlier section.

Myxoid liposarcoma expresses the array of antigens just enumerated in connection with aggressive angiomyxoma. In addition, however, this lesion is also focally S100-reactive, in the signet ring-cell- or multivacuolated lipoblasts which define its categorization (57). Myelin basic protein and Leu 7 are not detectable, allowing for a distinction from myxoid peripheral nerve sheath tumors, in conjunction with the morphologic features of the S100-positive constituents in each (120).

Round-cell liposarcoma is itself a heterogeneous neoplasm, which may resemble either chordoid sarcoma or cellular Schwannian sarcomas (39). S100- and vimentin-reactivity is common to all three tumors, but the "branching" form of round cell liposarcoma differs from its histologic mimic, chordoid sarcoma, in that Leu 7 is absent in the former and present in the latter. Malignant schwannomas that are similar microscopically to round cell liposarcoma also display Leu 7 and MBP (120,132), but again, both of these antigens are lacking in lipoblastic neoplasms.

METASTASES OF NONSARCOMATOUS NEOPLASMS

Just as immunohistochemistry is incapable of separating benign from malignant tumors, it also is not infallible in distinguishing between primary and secondary neoplasms of the soft tissue. Nonetheless, the latter topic is less laden with fatalism, since immunopheno-typing *can* identify metastatic sarcomatoid carcinomas that mimic primary mesenchymal malignancies. Renal cell carcinoma is particularly important in this respect, due to its well-known abilities to simulate virtually any other neoplasm. Hence, it is our practice to include antibodies to cytokeratin and EMA in all immunohistochemical analyses of puta-tive soft tissue sarcomas. This provision is of no assistance in cases where epithelioid or synovial sarcomas are diagnostic possibilities, due to their shared reactivity for epithelial markers. Nevertheless, we have encountered several examples of metastatic pulmonary or renal carcinomas in the soft tissue, in which the primary tumor was occult and single secondary deposits were originally regarded as sarcomas.

Similar comments apply to metastases of malignant melanoma, but these may be more difficult to recognize. This problem stems from the nonepithelial nature of melanomas, and their shared expression of vimentin with most sarcomas, in the absence of cytokeratin and EMA (79). An important clue to the possibility that one may be dealing with metastatic melanoma and not sarcoma is the presence of S100 protein, based on the morphologic features of the lesion in question. Other melanoma-related determinants such as the HMB-45 antigen promise to supply additional means for the recognition of this tumor (53), but additional work is needed on this point.

SUMMARY AND PROSPECTS

This discussion has been an attempt to provide the surgical pathologist with an outline of the determinants of greatest differential diagnostic interest, in dealing with soft tissue sar-comas. It is not an all-inclusive review, and represents an admittedly biased approach based on our personal experience with this area of diagnostic pathology.

One important stipulation in regard to immunohistochemical studies is that they are *not* a substitute for skilled interpretation of conventionally-stained microscopic specimens. In other words, a poor morphologist is also likely to be a poor immunohistochemist! In addition, not all of the immunohistochemical reagents discussed in connection with each tumor entity are *necessary* to reach a final diagnosis. In keeping with the latter statement, we have provided abbreviated flow-charts for this purpose (Figs. 16 to 19), documenting the "essentials" of the immunohistochemical diagnosis of sarcomas.

Finally, it may be stated with relative certainty that this area of immunohistology is in its infancy. We expect that the near future will supply information on an expanded array of increasingly more specific determinants in soft tissue tumors. These may include collagen types (93,106), collagenase (69), adrenergic receptor proteins (129), lipoprotein lipase (45), synemin (54), prostacyclin (124), morphogenetic bone protein (7), onconeural anti-gen (111), and others (36,55). It is anticipated that such discriminants, in combination with

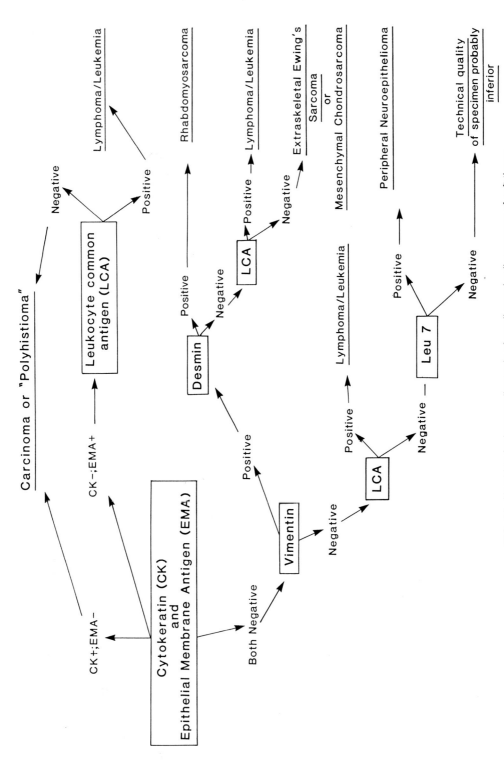

FIG. 16. Algorithm for immunodiagnosis of small round-cell sarcomas of soft tissue.

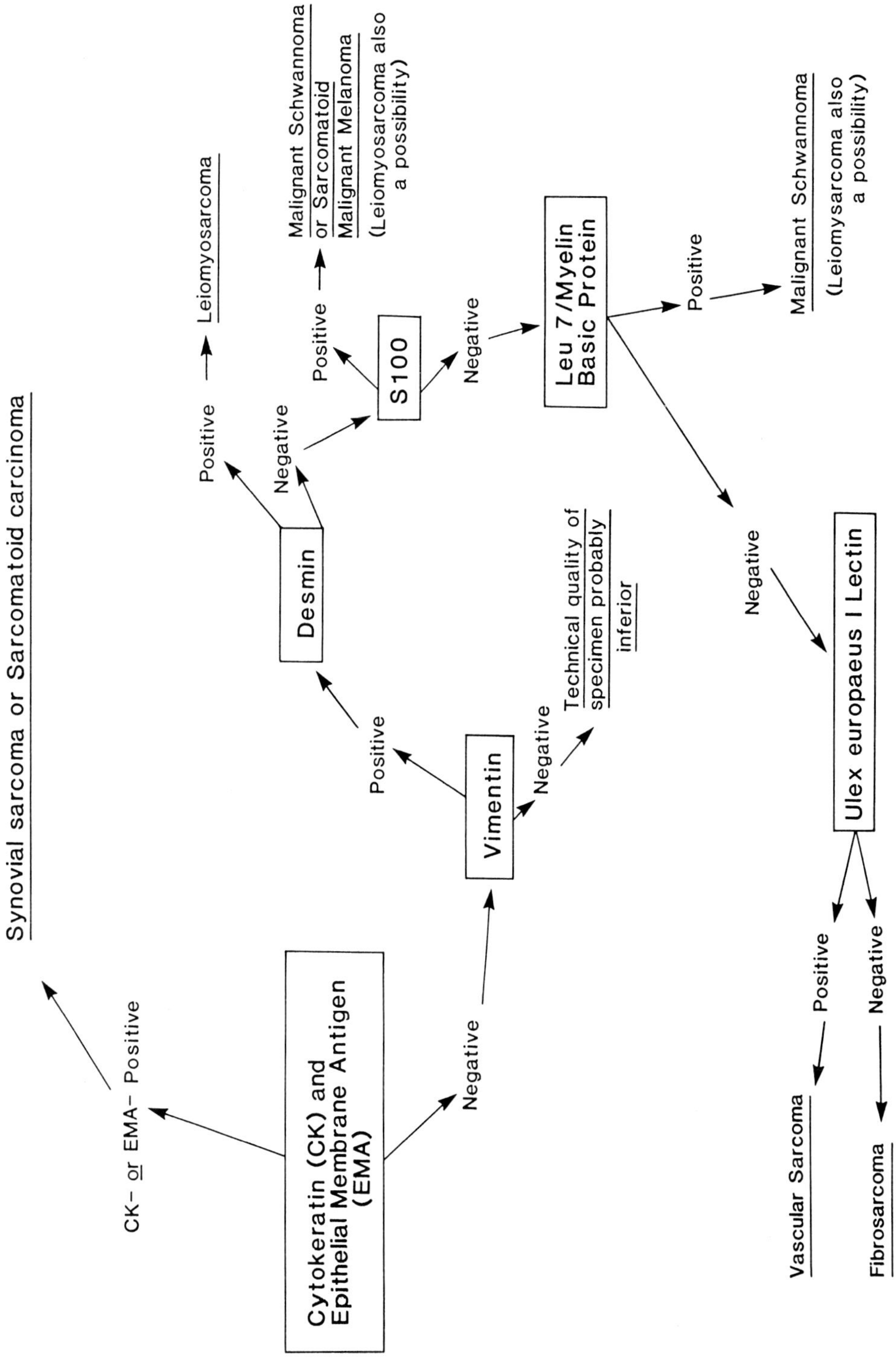

FIG. 17. Algorithm for immunodiagnosis of spindle-cell sarcomas of soft tissue.

393

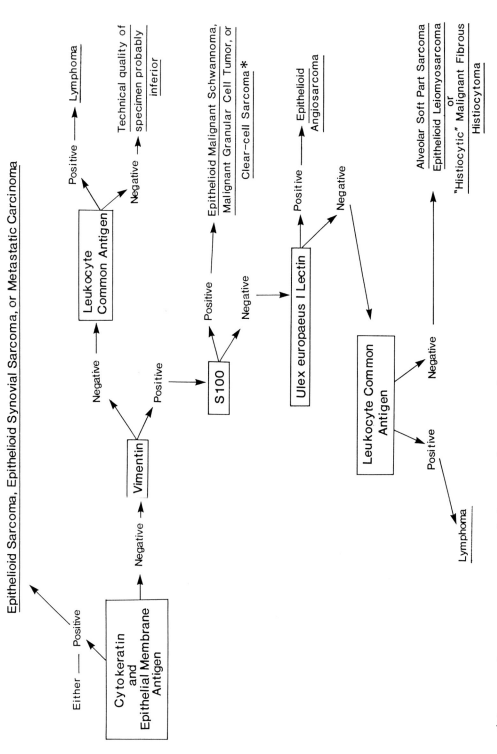

FIG. 18. Algorithm for immunodiagnosis of epithelioid polygonal-cell sarcomas of soft tissue.

*See text for additional discriminatory immunostains in these groups

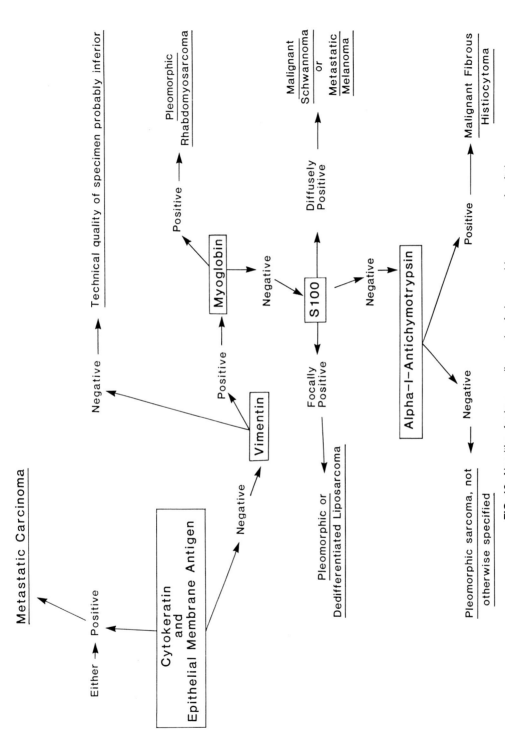

FIG. 19. Algorithm for immunodiagnosis of pleomorphic sarcomas of soft tissue.

395

continuing advances in immunostaining technique, will remove much of the "art" (and uncertainty) from the immunohistochemical diagnosis of soft tissue neoplasms, and make this field a more practical reality for all pathologists.

ACKNOWLEDGMENTS

Dr. Wick is the recipient of a Career Development Award in Oncology from the American Cancer Society.

REFERENCES

1. Abenoza, P., Manivel, J. C., Swanson, P. E., and Wick, M. R. (1986): Synovial sarcoma: An ultrastructural study, and an immunocytochemical analysis using a combined PAP-ABC procedure. *Hum. Pathol.*, 17: 1107–1115.
2. Abenoza, P., and Sibley, R. K. (1986): Chordoma: An immunohistologic study. *Hum. Pathol.*, 17:744– 747.
3. Altmannsberger, M., Osborn, M., Treuner, J., Holschr, A., Weber, K., and Schauer, A. (1982): Diagnosis of human childhood rhabdomyosarcoma by antibodies to desmin, the structural protein of muscle specific intermediate filaments. *Virchows Arch. Cell. Pathol.*, 39:203–215.
4. Altmannsberger, M., Weber, K., Droste, R., and Osborn, M. (1985): Desmin is a specific marker for rhabdomyosarcomas of human and rat origin. *Am. J. Pathol.*, 118:85–95.
5. Auclair, P. L., Langloss, J. M., Weiss, S. W., and Corio, R. L. (1986): Sarcomas and sarcomatoid neoplasms of the major salivary gland regions. A clinicopathologic and immunohistochemical study of 67 cases and review of the literature. *Cancer*, 58:1305–1315.
6. Battifora, H., and Trowbridge, I. S. (1983): A monoclonal antibody useful for the differential diagnosis between malignant lymphoma and nonhematopoietic neoplasms. *Cancer*, 51:816–821.
7. Bauer, F., and Urist, M. (1981): Human osteosarcoma-derived soluble bone morphogenetic protein. *Clin. Orthop.*, 154:291–295.
8. Begin, L. R., Clement, P. B., Kirk, M. E., Jothy, S., McCaughey, W. T. E., Ferenczy, A. (1985): Aggressive angiomyxoma of pelvic soft parts: A clinicopathologic study of nine cases. *Hum. Pathol.*, 16:621–628.
9. Belza, M. G., and Urich, H. (1986): Chordoma and malignant fibrous histiocytoma: Evidence for transformation. *Cancer*, 58:1082–1087.
10. Bertoni, F., Picci, P., Bacchini, P., Capanna, R., Innas, V., Bacci, G., and Campanacci, M. (1983): Mesenchymal chondrosarcomas of bone and soft tissues. *Cancer*, 52:533–541.
11. Bhagavan, B. S., Dorfman, H. D., Murthy, M. S. N., and Eggleston, J. C. (1982): Intravascular bronchioloalveolar tumor (IVBAT): A low-grade sclerosing epithelioid angiosarcoma of lung. *Am. J. Sur. Pathol.*, 6:41–52.
12. Blumenfield, W., Egbert, B. M., and Sagebiel, R. W. (1985): Differential diagnosis of Kaposi's sarcoma. *Arch. Pathol. Lab. Med.*, 109:123–127.
13. Brooks, J. J. (1982): Immunohistochemistry of soft tissue tumors. Myoglobin as a tumor marker for rhabdomyosarcoma. *Cancer*, 50:1757–1763.
14. Brooks, J. J. (1986): The significance of double phenotypic patterns and markers in human sarcomas. A new model of mesenchymal differentiation. *Am. J. Pathol.*, 125:113–123.
15. Burgdorf, W. H. C., Mukai, K., and Rosai, J. (1981): Immunohistochemical identification of factor VIII-related antigen in endothelial cells of cutaneous lesions of alleged vascular nature. *Am. J. Clin. Pathol.*, 75:167–171.
16. Cavazzana, A., Ross, R., Miser, J. S., and Triche, T. J. (1986): Experimental evidence for a neural origin of Ewing's sarcoma (abstract). *Lab. Invest.*, 54:10A.
17. Chase, D. R., and Enzinger, F. M. (1985): Epithelioid sarcoma. Diagnosis, prognostic indicators, and treatment. *Am. J. Surg. Pathol.*, 9:241–263.
18. Chase, D. R., Enzinger, F. M., Weiss, S. W., and Langloss, J. M. (1984): Keratin in epithelioid sarcoma: An immunohistochemical study. *Am. J. Surg. Pathol.*, 8:435–441.
19. Christopherson, W. M., Foote, F. W., and Stewart, F. W. (1952): Alveolar soft part sarcomas. Structurally characteristic tumors of uncertain histogenesis. *Cancer*, 5:100–111.
20. Chung, E. B., and Enzinger, F. M. (1976): Infantile fibrosarcoma. *Cancer*, 38:729–739.
21. Chung, E. B., and Enzinger, F. M. (1983): Malignant melanoma of soft parts. A reassessment of clear-cell sarcoma. *Am. J. Surg. Pathol.*, 7:405–423.
22. Churg, A. M., and Kahn, L. B. (1977): Myofibroblasts and related cells in malignant fibrous and fibrohistiocytic tumors. *Hum. Pathol.*, 8:205–218.

23. Clark, H. B., Minesky, J. J., Agrawal, D., and Agrawal, H. C. (1985): Myelin basic protein and P2 protein are not immunohistochemical markers for Schwann cell neoplasms: A comparative study using antisera to S100, P2, and myelin basic proteins. *Am. J. Pathol.*, 121:96–101.

24. Cocchia, D., Lauriola, L., Stolfi, V. M., Tallini, G., and Michetti, F. (1983): S100 antigen labels neoplastic cells in liposarcoma and cartilaginous tumors. *Virchows Arch. Pathol. Anat.*, 402:139–145.

25. Corson, J. M., and Pinkus, G. S. (1981): Intracellular myoglobin—a specific marker for skeletal muscle differentiation in soft tissue sarcoma. An immunoperoxidase study. *Am. J. Pathol.*, 103:384–389.

26. Daimaru, Y., Hashimoto, H., and Enjoji, M. (1985): Malignant peripheral nerve sheath tumors (malignant schwannomas): An immunohistochemical study of 29 cases. *Am. J. Surg. Pathol.*, 9:434–444.

27. Dean, P. J., Haggitt, R. C., and O'Hara, C. J. (1985): Malignant epithelioid hemangioendothelioma of the liver in young women. Relationship to contraceptive use. *Am. J. Surg. Pathol.*, 9:695–704.

28. Dehner, L. P. (1986): Peripheral and central primitive neuroectodermal tumors: A nosologic concept seeking a consensus. *Arch. Pathol. Lab. Med.*, 110:997–1005.

29. Dehner, L. P., Enzinger, F. M., and Font, R. L. (1972): Fetal rhabdomyoma. An analysis of nine cases. *Cancer*, 30:160–166.

30. DeJong, A. S. H., Van Vark, M., Albus-Lutter, C. E., Van Raamsdonk, W., and Voute, P. A. (1984): Myosin and myoglobin as tumor markers in the diagnosis of rhabdomyosarcoma: A comparative study. *Am. J. Surg. Pathol.*, 8:521–528.

31. Denk, H., Krepler, R., Artlieb, U., Gabbiani, G., Rungger-Brandle, E., Leoncini, P., and Franke, W. W. (1983): Proteins of intermediate filaments: An immunohistochemical and biochemical approach to the classification of soft tissue tumors. *Am. J. Pathol.*, 110:193–208.

32. Dewit, L., Albus-Lutter, C. E., DeJong, A. S. H., and Voute, P. A. (1986): Malignant schwannoma with a rhabdomyoblastic component, a so-called Triton tumor: A clinicopathologic study. *Cancer*, 58:1350–1356.

33. DiCarlo, E. F., Woodruff, J. M., Bansal, M., and Erlandson, R. A. (1986): The purely epithelioid malignant peripheral nerve sheath tumor. *Am. J. Surg. Pathol.*, 10:478–490.

34. Dickman, P. S., and Triche, T. J. (1986): Extraosseous Ewing's sarcoma versus primitive rhabdomyosarcoma: Diagnostic criteria and clinical correlation. *Hum. Pathol.*, 17:881–893.

35. Donner, L., DeLanerolle, P., and Costa, J. (1983): Immunoreactivity of paraffin-embedded normal tissues and mesenchymal tumors for smooth muscle myosin. *Am. J. Clin. Pathol.*, 80:677–681.

36. Donner, L., Triche, T. J., Israel, M. A., Seeger, R. C., and Reynolds, C. P. (1985): A panel of monoclonal antibodies which discriminate neuroblastoma from Ewing's sarcoma, rhabdomyosarcoma, neuroepithelioma, and hematopoietic malignancies. *Prog. Clin. Biol. Res.*, 175:347–366.

37. DuBoulay, C. E. H. (1982): Demonstration of alpha-1-antitrypsin and alpha-1-antichymotrypsin in the fibrous histiocytomas using the immunoperoxidase technique. *Am. J. Surg. Pathol.*, 6:559–564.

38. Ducatman, B. S., and Scheithauer, B. W. (1984): Malignant peripheral nerve sheath tumors with divergent differentiation. *Cancer*, 54:1049–1057.

39. Enzinger, F. M., and Weiss, S. W. (1983): *Soft Tissue Tumors.* C.V. Mosby, St. Louis, Missouri.

40. Epstein, A. L., Marder, R. J., Winter, J., and Fox, R. I. (1984): Two new monoclonal antibodies (LN-1, LN-2) reactive in B5-fixed, paraffin-embedded tissues with follicular center and mantle zone human B lymphocytes and derived tumors. *J. Immunol.*, 133:1028–1036.

41. Eusebi, V., Ceccarelli, C., Gorza, L., Schiaffino, S., and Bussolati, G. (1986): Immunocytochemistry of rhabdomyosarcoma: The use of four different markers. *Am. J. Surg. Pathol.*, 10:293–299.

42. Eusebi, V., Rilke, F., Ceccarelli, C., Fedeli, F., Schiaffino, S., and Bussolati, G. (1986): Fetal heavy chain skeletal myosin: An oncofetal antigen expressed by rhabdomyosarcoma. *Am. J. Surg. Pathol.*, 10:680–686.

43. Evans, H. L. (1979): Liposarcoma. A study of 55 cases with a reassessment of its classification. *Am. J. Surg. Pathol.*, 3:507–523.

44. Farris, K. B., and Reed, R. J. (1982): Monophasic, glandular, synovial sarcomas and carcinomas of the soft tissues. *Arch. Pathol. Lab. Med.*, 106:129–132.

45. Fielding, C., and Havel, R. (1977): Lipoprotein lipase. *Arch. Pathol. Lab. Med.*, 101:225–229.

46. Fischer, E. R., and Reidbord, H. (1971): Electron microscopic evidence suggesting the myogenous derivation of the so-called alveolar soft part sarcoma. *Cancer*, 27:150–159.

47. Fisher, C. (1986): Synovial sarcoma: Ultrastructural and immunohistochemical features of epithelial differentiation in monophasic and biphasic tumors. *Hum. Pathol.*, 17:996–1088.

48. Fukuda, T., Ishikawa, H., Ohnishi, Y., Tachikawa, S., Onizuka, S., and Sakashita, I. (1986): Extraskeletal myxoid chondrosarcoma arising from the retroperitoneum. *Am. J. Clin. Pathol.*, 85:514–519.

49. Gabbiani, G., Kapanci, Y., Barrazone, P., and Franke, W. W. (1981): Immunochemical identification of intermediate-sized filaments in human neoplastic cells. A diagnostic aid for the surgical pathologist. *Am. J. Pathol.*, 104:206–216.

50. Gould, V. E., Lee, I., Wiedenmann, B., Moll, R., Chejfec, G., and Franke, W. W. (1986): Synaptophysin: A novel marker for neurons, certain neuroendocrine cells, and their neoplasms. *Hum. Pathol.*, 17:979–983.

51. Gould, V. E., Moll, R., Moll, I., Lee, I., Schwechheimer, K., Franke, W. W. (1986): The intermediate filament complement of the spectrum of nerve sheath neoplasms. *Lab. Invest.*, 55:463–474.

52. Gown, A. M., and Vogel, A. M. (1985): Monoclonal antibodies to intermediate filament proteins. III. Analysis of tumors. *Am. J. Clin. Pathol.*, 84:413–424.

53. Gown, A. M., Vogel, A. M., Hoak, D., and McNutt, M. (1986): Monoclonal antibodies specific for melanocytic tumors distinguish subpopulations of melanocytes. *Am. J. Pathol.*, 123:195–203.

54. Granger, B. L., and Lazarides, E. (1980): Synemin: A new high molecular weight protein associated with desmin and vimentin filaments in muscle. *Cell*, 22:727–738.

55. Gross, N., Beck, B., Carrel, S., and Munoz, M. (1986): Highly selective recognition of human neuro-blastoma cells by mouse monoclonal antibody to a cytoplasmic antigen. *Cancer Res.*, 46:2988–2994.

56. Hajdu, S. I. (1979): *Pathology of Soft Tissue Tumors*. Lea & Febiger, Philadelphia.

57. Hashimoto, H., Daimaru, Y., and Enjoji, M. (1984): S100 protein distribution in liposarcoma. An immuno-peroxidase study with special reference to the distinction of liposarcoma from myxoid malignant fibrous histiocytoma. *Virchows Arch. Pathol. Anat.*, 405:1–10.

58. Hashimoto, H., Daimaru, Y., Tsuneyoshi, M., and Enjoji, M. (1986): Leiomyosarcoma of the external soft tissues: A clinicopathologic, immunohistochemical, and electron microscopic study. *Cancer*, 57:2077–2088.

59. Hashimoto, H., Enjoji, M., Nakajima, T., Kiryu, H., and Daimaru, Y. (1983): Malignant neuroepithelioma (peripheral neuroblastoma). A clinicopathologic study of 15 cases. *Am. J. Surg. Pathol.*, 7:309–318.

60. Hashimoto, H., Tsuneyoshi, M., Daimaru, Y., Enjoji, M., and Shinohara, N. (1986): Intramuscular myxoma: A clinicopathologic, immunohistochemical, and electron microscopic study. *Cancer*, 58:740–747.

61. Herrera, G. A., Reimann, B. E. F., and Salinas, J. A. (1982): Malignant schwannomas presenting as malignant fibrous histiocytomas. *Ultrastruct. Pathol.*, 3:253–261.

62. Ivins, J. C., Dockerty, M. B., and Ghormley, R. K. (1950): Fibrosarcoma of the soft tissues of the extremities: A review of 78 cases. *Surgery*, 28:495–508.

63. Jacobsen, S. A. (1977): Polyhistioma: A malignant tumor of bone and extraskeletal tissues. *Cancer*, 40:2116–2130.

64. Jaffe, R., Santamaria, M., Yunis, E. J., Hrinia-Tannery, N., Agostini, R. M., Medina, J., and Goodman, M. (1984): Neuroectodermal tumor of bone. *Am. J. Surg. Pathol.*, 8:885–898.

65. Kahn, H. J., Marks, A., Thom, H., and Baumal, R. (1983): Role of antibody to S100 protein in diagnostic pathology. *Am. J. Surg. Pathol.*, 7:341–347.

66. Kawaguchi, K., and Koike, M. (1986): Neuron-specific enolase and Leu 7 immunoreactive small round cell neoplasm. The relationship to Ewing's sarcoma in bone and soft tissue. *Am. J. Clin. Pathol.*, 86:79–83.

67. Kindblom, L-G., Jacobsen, G. K., and Jacobsen, M. (1982): Immunohistochemical investigations of tumors of supposed fibroblastic-histiocytic origin. *Hum. Pathol.*, 13:834–840.

68. Kurtin, P. J., and Pinkus, G. S. (1985): Leukocyte common antigen—a diagnostic discriminant between hematopoietic and nonhematopoietic neoplasms in paraffin sections using monoclonal antibodies. Correlation with immunologic studies and ultrastructural localization. *Hum. Pathol.*, 16:353–365.

69. Labrosse, K. R., and Liener, I. E. (1978): Collagenolytic activities in methyl-cholanthrene-induced fi-brosarcomas in mice. *Mol. Cell. Biochem.*, 181–189.

70. Linnoila, R. I., Tsokos, M., Triche, T. J., Marangos, P. J., and Chandra, R. S. (1986): Evidence for neural origin and PAS-positive variants of the malignant small cell tumor of thoracopulmonary region ("Askin tumor"). *Am. J. Surg. Pathol.*, 10:124–133.

71. Manivel, J. C., Wick, M. R., Sibley, R. K., and Dehner, L. P. (1987): Epithelioid sarcoma: An immuno-histochemical study. *Am. J. Clin. Pathol.*, 81:319–326.

72. Matsunou, H., Shimoda, T., Kakimoto, S., Yamashita, H., Ishikawa, E., and Mukai, M. (1985): Histopa-thologic and immunohistochemical study of malignant tumors of peripheral nerve sheath (malignant schwannoma). *Cancer*, 56:2269–2279.

73. Mierau, G. W. (1985): Extraskeletal Ewing's sarcoma (peripheral neuroepithelioma). *Ultrastruct. Pathol.*, 9:91–98.

74. Miettinen, M. (1984): Chordoma: Antibodies to epithelial membrane antigen and carcinoembryonic antigen in differential diagnosis. *Arch. Pathol. Lab. Med.*, 108:891–892.

75. Miettinen, M., Holthofer, H., Lehto, V.-P., Miettinen, A., Virtanen, I. (1983): *Ulex europaeus* I lectin as a marker for tumors derived from endothelial cells. *Am. J. Clin. Pathol.*, 79:32–36.

76. Miettinen, M., Lehto, V.-P., Badley, R. A., and Virtanen, I. (1982): Alveolar rhabdomyosarcoma: Demonstration of the muscle type of intermediate filament protein, desmin, as a diagnostic aid. *Am. J. Pathol.*, 10:246–251.

77. Miettinen, M., Lehto, V.-P., Badley, R. A., and Virtanen, I. (1982): Expression of intermediate filaments in soft tissue sarcomas. *Int. J. Cancer*, 30:541–546.

78. Miettinen, M., Lehto, V.-P., and Virtanen, I. (1982): Histogenesis of Ewing's sarcoma. An evaluation of intermediate filaments and endothelial cell markers. *Virchows Arch. Cell. Pathol.*, 41:277–284.

79. Miettinen, M., Lehto, V.-P., and Virtanen, I. (1983): Presence of fibroblastic-type intermediate filaments (vimentin) and absence of neurofilaments in pigmented nevi and malignant melanomas. *J. Cutan. Pathol.*, 10:188–192.

80. Miettinen, M., and Virtanen, I. (1984): Synovial sarcoma—a misnomer. *Am. J. Pathol.*, 117:18–25.

81. Molenaar, W. M., Oosterhuis, J. W., Oosterhuis, A. M., and Ramaekers, F. C. S. (1985): Mesenchymal and muscle-specific intermediate filaments (vimentin and desmin) in relation to differentiation in childhood rhabdomyosarcomas. *Hum. Pathol.*, 16:838–843.

82. Monda, L., and Wick, M. R. (1985): S100 protein immunostaining in the differential diagnosis of chondroblastoma. *Hum. Pathol.*, 16:287–293.

83. Mukai, K., and Rosai, J. (1984): Factor VIII-related antigen: An endothelial marker. In: *Diagnostic Immunohistochemistry*, edited by R. A. DeLellis, pp. 253–261. Masson Publishing USA, Inc., New York.

84. Mukai, K., Schollmeyer, J. V., and Rosai, J. (1981): Immunohistochemical localization of actin. Applications in surgical pathology. *Am. J. Surg. Pathol.*, 5:91–97.

85. Mukai, M., Iri, H., Torikata, C., Kageyama, K., Morikawa, Y., and Shimizu, K. (1984): Immunoperoxidase demonstration of a new muscle protein (Z-protein) in myogenic tumors as a diagnostic aid. *Am. J. Pathol.*, 114:164–170.

86. Mukai, M., Torikata, C., Iri, H., Mikata, A., Hanuoka, H., Kato, K., and Kageyama, K. (1986): Histogenesis of alveolar soft part sarcoma. An immunohistochemical and biochemical study. *Am. J. Surg. Pathol.*, 10:212–218.

87. Mukai, M., Torikata, C., Iri, H., Mikata, A., Kawai, T., Hanaoka, H., Yakumaru, K., and Kageyama, K. (1984): Histogenesis of clear-cell sarcoma of tendons and aponeuroses. An electron microscopic, biochemical, enzyme-histochemical, and immunohistochemical study. *Am. J. Pathol.*, 114:264–272.

88. Nakamura, Y., Becker, L. E., and Marks, A. (1983): S100 protein in tumors of cartilage and bone. An immunohistochemical study. *Cancer*, 52:1820–1824.

89. Nakazato, Y., Ishizebi, J., Takahishi, K., and Yamaguchi, H. (1982): Immunohistochemical localization of S100 protein in granular cell myoblastoma. *Cancer*, 49:1624–1628.

90. Navas-Palacios, J. J., Aparicio-Duque, R., and Valdes, M. D. (1984): On the histogenesis of Ewing's sarcoma. An ultrastructural, immunohistochemical, and cytochemical study. *Cancer*, 53:1882–1901.

91. Nesland, J. M., Sobrinho-Simoes, M. A., Holm, R., and Johannessen, J. V. (1985): Primitive neuroectodermal tumor (peripheral neuroblastoma). *Ultrastruct. Pathol.*, 9:59–64.

92. Norton, A. J., Ramsay, A. D., Smith, S. H., Beverley, P. C. L., and Isaacson, P. G. (1986): Monoclonal antibody (UCHL1) that recognises normal and neoplastic T cells in routinely fixed tissues. *J. Clin. Pathol.*, 39:399–405.

93. Ogawa, K., Oguchi, M., Yamabe, H., Nakashima, Y., and Hamashima, Y. (1986): Distribution of collagen type IV in soft tissue tumors: An immunohistochemical study. *Cancer*, 58:269–277.

94. Ordonez, N. G., and Batsakis, J. G. (1984): Comparison of *Ulex europaeus* I lectin with factor VIII-related antigen in vascular lesions. *Arch. Pathol. Lab. Med.*, 108:129–132.

95. Osborn, M., Altmannsberger, M., Debus, E., and Weber, K. (1985): Differentiation of the major human tumor groups using conventional and monoclonal antibodies specific for individual intermediate filament proteins. *Ann. N.Y. Acad. Sci.*, 455:649–668.

96. Osborn, M., Hill, C., Altmannsberger, M., and Weber, K. (1986): Monoclonal antibodies to titin in conjunction with antibodies to desmin separate rhabdomyosarcomas from other tumor types. *Lab. Invest.*, 55:101–108.

97. Osborn, M., and Weber, K. (1983): Tumor diagnosis by intermediate filament typing. A novel tool for surgical pathology. *Lab. Invest.*, 48:372–394.

98. Ozzello, L., Stout, A. P., and Murray, M. R. (1963): Cultural characteristics of malignant fibrous histiocytomas and fibrous xanthomas. *Cancer*, 16:331–334.

99. Penneys, N. S., Mogollon, R., Kowalcyzk, A., Nadji, M., and Adachi, K. (1984): A survey of cutaneous neural lesions for the presence of myelin basic protein. An immunohistochemical study. *Arch. Dermatol.*, 120:210–213.

100. Perentes, E., and Rubinstein, L. J. (1985): Immunohistochemical recognition of human nerve sheath tumors by anti-Leu 7 (HNK-1) monoclonal antibody. *Acta Neuropathol. (Berl)*, 68:319–324.

101. Pertschuk, L. P. (1975): Immunofluorescence of soft-tissue tumors with anti-smooth muscle and anti-skeletal-muscle antibodies. *Am. J. Clin. Pathol.*, 63:332–342.

102. Povysil, C., and Matejovsky, Z. (1985): A comparative ultrastructural study of chondrosarcoma, chordoid sarcoma, chordoma, and chordoma periphericum. *Pathol. Res. Pract.*, 179:546–559.

103. Roholl, P. J. M., De Jong, A. S. H., and Ramaekers, F. C. S. (1985): Application of markers in the diagnosis of soft tissue tumours. *Histopathol.*, 9:1019–1035.

104. Roholl, P. J. M., Kleyne, J., Pijpers, H. W., and Van Unnik, J. A. M. (1985): Comparative immunohistochemical investigation of markers for malignant histiocytes. *Hum. Pathol.*, 16:763–771.

105. Roholl, P. J. M., Kleyne, J., and Van Unnik, J. A. M. (1985): Characterization of tumor cells in malignant fibrous histiocytoma and other soft tissue tumors in comparison with malignant histiocytes. II. Immunoperoxidase study on cryostat sections. *Am. J. Pathol.*, 121:269–274.

106. Sakai, L. Y., Engvall, E., Hollister, D. W., and Burgeson, R. E. (1982): Production and characterization of a monoclonal antibody to human type IV collagen. *Am. J. Pathol.*, 108:310–318.

107. Salisbury, J. R., and Isaacson, P. G. (1985): Demonstration of cytokeratins and an epithelial membrane antigen in chordomas and human fetal notochord. *Am. J. Surg. Pathol.*, 9:791–797.

108. Salisbury, J. R., and Isaacson, P. G. (1985): Synovial sarcoma: An immunohistochemical study. *J. Pathol.*, 147:49–57.

109. Schurch, W., Seemayer, T. A., Lagace, R., and Gabbiani, G. (1984): The intermediate filament cytoskeleton of myofibroblasts: An immunofluorescence and ultrastructural study. *Virchows Arch. Pathol. Anat.*, 403:323–336.

110. Scupham, R., Gilbert, E. F., Wilde, J., and Wiedrich, T. A. (1986): Immunohistochemical studies of rhabdomyosarcoma. *Arch. Pathol. Lab. Med.*, 110:818–821.
111. Seeger, R. C., Zeltzer, P. M., and Rayner, S. A. (1979): Onco-neural antigen: A new neural differentiation antigen expressed by neuroblastoma, oat cell carcinoma, Wilms' tumor, and sarcoma cells. *J. Immunol.*, 122:1548–1555.
112. Sheibani, K., Battifora, H., Burke, J. S., and Rappaport, H. (1986): Leu M1 antigen in human neoplasms. An immunohistologic study of 400 cases. *Am. J. Surg. Pathol.*, 10:227–236.
113. Shousha, S., and Lyssiotis, T. (1979): Granular cell myoblastoma is positive staining for carcinoembryonic antigen. *J. Clin. Pathol.*, 32:219–226.
114. Snover, D. C., Sumner, H. W., and Dehner, L. P. (1982): Variability of histologic pattern in recurrent soft tissue sarcomas originally diagnosed as liposarcoma. *Cancer*, 49:1005–1015.
115. Steeper, T. A., Rosai, J. (1983): Aggressive angiomyxoma of the female pelvis and perineum. Report of nine cases of a distinctive type of gynecologic soft tissue neoplasm. *Am. J. Surg. Pathol.*, 7:463–475.
116. Stefansson, K., and Wollmann, R. L. (1982): S100 protein in granular cell tumors (granular cell myoblastomas). *Cancer*, 49:1834–1838.
117. Stefansson, K., Wollmann, R. L., and Jenkovic, M. (1982): S100 protein in soft tissue tumors derived from Schwann cells and melanocytes. *Am. J. Pathol.*, 106:261–268.
118. Stout, A. P., and Lattes, R. (1967): Tumors of the soft tissue. In: *Atlas of Tumor Pathology*, Second Series, Fascicle 1, Armed Forces Institute of Pathology, Washington, D.C.
119. Strauchen, J. A., and Dimitriu-Bona, A. (1986): Malignant fibrous histiocytoma: Expression of monocyte/macrophage differentiation antigens detected with monoclonal antibodies. *Am. J. Pathol.*, 124:303–309.
120. Swanson, P. E., Manivel, J. C., and Wick, M. R. (1987): Immunoreactivity for Leu 7 in neurofibrosarcoma and other spindle-cell sarcomas of soft tissue. *Am. J. Pathol.*, 126:546–560.
121. Tsokos, M., Howard, R., and Costa, J. (1983): Immunohistochemical study of alveolar and embryonal rhabdomyosarcoma. *Lab. Invest.*, 48:148–155.
122. Tsokos, M., Linnoila, R. I., Chandra, R. S., and Triche, T. J. (1984): Neuron-specific enolase in the diagnosis of neuroblastoma and other small round cell tumors in children. *Hum. Pathol.*, 15:575–584.
123. Unni, K. K., and Soule, E. H. (1975): Alveolar soft part sarcoma: An electron microscopic study. *Mayo Clin. Proc.*, 50:591–598.
124. Vane, J. R., and Moncada, S. (1980): Prostacyclin. In: *Blood Cells and Vessel Walls: Functional Interactions*, pp. 79–97. (Ciba Foundation Symposium 71). Excerpta Medica, New York.
125. Weiss, S. W. (1986): Proliferative fibroblastic lesions: From hyperplasia to neoplasia. *Am. J. Surg. Pathol.*, 10 [Suppl. 1]:14–25.
126. Weiss, S. W., and Enzinger, F. M. (1982): Epithelioid hemangioendothelioma: A vascular tumor often mistaken for a carcinoma. *Cancer*, 50:970–981.
127. Weiss, S. W., and Enzinger, F. M. (1986): Spindle-cell hemangioendothelioma: A low-grade angiosarcoma resembling a cavernous hemangioma and Kaposi's sarcoma. *Am. J. Surg. Pathol.*, 10:521–530.
128. Weiss, S. W., Langloss, J. M., and Enzinger, F. M. (1983): Value of S100 protein in the diagnosis of soft tissue tumors with particular reference to benign and malignant Schwann cell tumors. *Lab. Invest.*, 49:299–308.
129. Whitsett, J. A., Burdsall, J., Workman, L., Hollinger, B., and Neely, J. (1983): Beta-adrenergic receptors in pediatric tumors: Uncoupled B-1-adrenergic receptor in Ewing's sarcoma. *JNCI*, 71:779–786.
130. Wick, M. R., and Manivel, J. C. (1987): Epithelioid sarcoma and epithelioid hemangioendothelioma: An immunohistochemical and lectin-histochemical comparison. *Virchows Arch. Pathol. Anat.*, 410:309–316.
131. Wick, M. R., and Manivel, J. C. (1986): Epithelioid sarcoma and isolated necrobiotic granuloma: An immunohistochemical comparison. *J. Cutan. Pathol.*, 13:253–260.
132. Wick, M. R., Swanson, P. E., Scheithauer, B. W., and Manivel, J. C. (1987): Malignant peripheral nerve sheath tumor: An immunohistochemical study of 62 cases. *Am. J. Clin. Pathol.*, 87:425–433.
133. Wilson, B. S., Herzig, M. A., and Lloyd, R. V. (1984): Immunoperoxidase staining for Ia-like antigens in paraffin-embedded tissues from human melanoma and lung carcinoma. *Am. J. Pathol.*, 115:102–116.
134. Wood, G. S., Beckstead, J. H., Turner, R. R., Hendrickson, M. R., Kempson, R. L., and Warnke, R. A. (1986): Malignant fibrous histiocytoma tumor cells resemble fibroblasts. *Am. J. Surg. Pathol.*, 10:323–335.

Diagnostic Immunopathology,
edited by R.B. Colvin,
A.K. Bhan, and R.T. McCluskey.
Raven Press, New York © 1988.

15 / *Tumor Stroma*[1]

Harold F. Dvorak

*Departments of Pathology, Beth Israel Hospital and Harvard Medical School, and the
Charles A. Dana Research Institute, Beth Israel Hospital, Boston, Massachusetts 02215*

Solid tumors are composed of two distinct but interdependent compartments: the malignant cells themselves and the stroma that they induce and in which they are dispersed (65,78). In carcinomas, tumors of epithelial cell origin, a basal lamina often separates clumps of tumor cells from stroma. However, the basal lamina may be incomplete, especially at points of tumor invasion. In other types of tumors, such as sarcomas and lymphomas, malignant cells abut directly on and may intermingle with stromal elements (55,65).

Tumor stroma interposes connective tissue between malignant cells and normal host tissues. On the one hand, this connective tissue stroma is essential for tumor growth. Stroma provides the vascular supply that tumors require for obtaining nutrients, gas exchange, and waste disposal. All solid tumors, regardless of their type or cellular origin, require stroma if they are to grow beyond a minimal size of 1 to 2 mm (33). On the other hand, stroma may also limit the influx of inflammatory cells, or, alternatively, could limit tumor expansion (17,24). Stroma, therefore, at once provides both a lifeline for the tumor and imposes a barrier that inhibits and may regulate interchange of fluids, gases and cells with the host.

Over the past decade considerable interest has been focused on one aspect of tumor stroma, angiogenesis. The major types of collagen deposited in tumor stroma have been identified, and a beginning has been made at investigation of tumor associated glycosaminoglycans (GAG). It has also been established that two plasma proteins, fibrinogen and fibronectin, are regular components of tumor stroma, particularly the provisional tumor stroma that is subsequently transformed into mature connective tissue. In this chapter I will review selected aspects of our current understanding of tumor stroma, the pathogenesis of its generation, and its biologic significance. While no specific diagnostic applications are possible at this time, a number of studies suggest that the correlations with tumor behavior might be found in the future.

---

[1]Portions of this chapter were adapted from a review article by the author entitled *Tumors: Wounds that do not heal*, that appeared in the New England Journal of Medicine, 315:1650–1659, 1986.

COMPOSITION OF TUMOR STROMA

Tumor stroma consists of interstitial connective tissue and in the case of epithelial tumors, basal lamina. Basal lamina is organized as a structural lattice of type IV collagen and laminin and also includes GAG; limited amounts of water and plasma-derived proteins, such as fibronectin may also be found in basal lamina. Components of basal lamina aside from plasma protein and water are thought to be products of tumor cell themselves.

The great bulk of tumor stroma is composed of interstitial connective tissue. This connective tissue is formed from elements that are derived both from the circulating blood and from the adjacent connective tissues. Plasma components include water, plasma proteins, and various types and numbers of inflammatory cells. Almost any element found in the various normal connective tissues of the body may be represented in tumor interstitial stroma, even including, for example, bone and cartilage. Generally speaking, the major components of interstitial tumor stroma can be categorized as follows: structural proteins; interstitial fluid; GAG, both sulfated and nonsulfated; new blood vessels; interstitial collagens (types I, III, and, to a lesser extent, type V); fibrin; fibronectin; and cells of two general types, fixed tissue cells such as fibroblasts that reside in normal connective tissue and inflammatory cells that are derived from the blood.

The composition of tumor stroma is not static. Studies of transplantable tumors have revealed the important insight that tumor stroma undergoes a characteristic series of changes with time (Table 1) (17,18,22,24); as we shall see, these changes closely resemble the progression of events associated with normal wound healing (13,54).

Although the same basic building blocks comprise all tumor stroma, pathologists have long recognized that tumors differ markedly from each other in stromal content. Sometimes these differences are primarily *quantitative*. At one extreme, for example, are desmoplastic tumors, such as many carcinomas of the breast, stomach, and pancreas, in which up to

TABLE 1. *Major stromal components at successive intervals after tumor transplantation*

Components	Provisional Stroma	Mature Stroma	
		Early	Late
Structural proteins	Abundant fibrin–fibronectin gel	↓ Fibrin	↓ ↓ Fibrin
		↑ Fibronectin in at least some tumors	↑ Fibronectin in at least some tumors
		↑ Interstitial Collagens[a]	↑ ↑ Interstitial Collagens[a]
Interstitial fluid	Abundant	Abundant	Often Less
Glycosaminoglycans	0	Hyaluronic acid + Sulfated GAG	Hyaluronic acid + Sulfated GAG
New blood vessels	0	Many	Fewer
Connective tissue cells (fibroblasts)	0	Many	Fewer
Inflammatory cells	Variable	Variable	Variable

[a]Type I > type III > type V; elastin and other structural components of mature connective tissue may also appear in tumors.

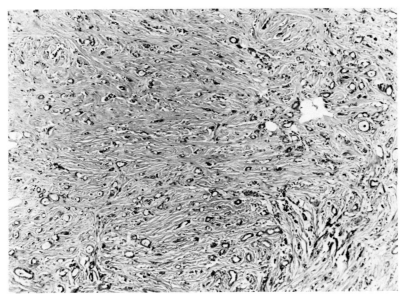

FIG. 1. Typical scirrhous ductal carcinoma of the breast illustrating tumor cells dispersed in an extensive fibrous connective tissue stroma. H&E ($\times$ 160).

90% of the total tumor mass consists of stroma (Fig. 1). At the other extreme are tumors such as medullary carcinomas of the breast in which only minimal stroma is deposited.

In other cases, the differences in stromal content between different tumors are largely *qualitative*. For example, fibroadenomas of the breast may have a stroma composed of loosely arranged, cellular and vascular connective tissue or, alternatively, the stroma may consist of dense, scirrhous collagen. Some tumors induce an extensive lymphocytic infiltrate; others may induce none. Even within a single tumor there may be significant variations in stromal composition from one area to another.

FIBRIN: A MISSING LINK IN TUMOR STROMA GENERATION

The association between malignancy and abnormal hemostasis dates back at least to Trousseau in the middle of the last century (reviewed in 11), but the presence of fibrin in tumors was not firmly established until quite recently. O'Meara first proposed that fibrin was deposited in tumors in the 1950s (60) but his light microscopic evidence was unpersuasive. Others subsequently found that if radiolabeled fibrinogen or antibodies to fibrinogen were given intravenously to tumor-bearing animals or patients, these tracers concentrated selectively in tumors (10,73). Fibrinogen-related proteins were also demonstrated in tumors by immunofluorescence staining of tissue sections (45). However, interest in these data was tempered by several concerns. It was felt that tumor-associated fibrin might simply be the result of clotting that occurred at sites of tumor necrosis or during surgical removal or transplantation of tumors, rather than being evidence that fibrin deposition represented an intrinsic property of malignancy. As will be discussed later, tumors contain procoagulants that rapidly generate fibrin clots after exposure to plasma. Another criticism of these earlier studies concerned the specificity of the antibodies used to detect fibrin.

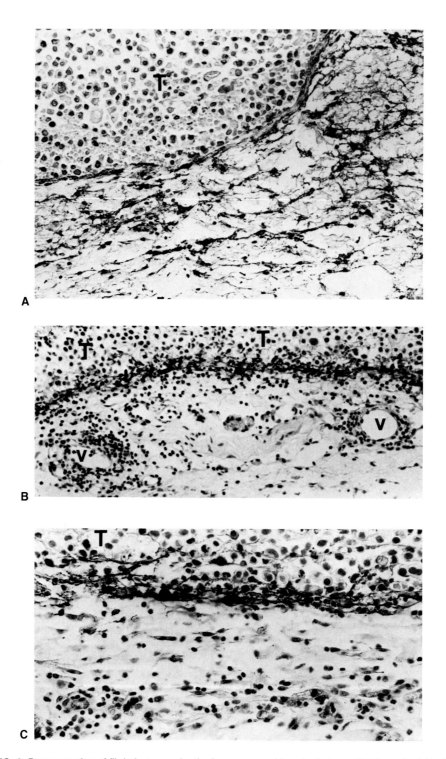

FIG. 2. Demonstration of fibrin in tumors by the immunoperoxidase technique. (**A**) Transplantable line 10 bile duct carcinoma (T, upper left) growing in subcutaneous space of a syngeneic strain two guinea pig. Note abundant enveloping fibrin-rich stroma. Fibrin is delineated by a monoclonal antibody specific for fibrin kindly provided by Dr. Gary Matsueda. Counterstained with methyl green, (× 170). (**B and C**) Mouse ovarian tumor (T) growing in the subcutaneous space of C3H female mice. Fibrin, demonstrated here with a heteroantiserum to fibrinogen, is deposited as a thin meshwork layer separating tumor above from stroma below. Note that lymphocytes and other mononuclear cells form cuffs around venules (v) and extend up to the fibrin meshwork but do not actually penetrate it to come into contact with tumor cells. **B**: (× 210); **C**: (× 330).

Nearly all heteroantisera to fibrinogen have also been found to contain antibodies to fibronectin, a protein that was first recognized in the plasma in the 1940s, but that is now itself known to be a regular component of tumor stroma. Thus, the fibrin thought to have been observed in tumors could have instead represented crossreacting fibronectin.

Recent experiments have now dispelled these objections. Fibrin can be demonstrated in both autochthonous and transplanted solid tumors with heteroantisera or with monoclonal antibodies of proven specificity, even when elaborate precautions have been taken to avoid artifacts such as surgically associated or postmortem coagulation (20) (Fig. 2). Therefore, there can be little doubt that fibrin itself is a regular constituent of solid tumor stroma.

Distribution of Fibrin in Solid Tumors

The anatomic distribution of fibrin in tumors varies somewhat depending on the tumor type (15,24,25,42). In carcinomas, fibrin is deposited between tumor cells or tumor cell clumps and is often particularly abundant peripherally, at the tumor-host interface. Fibrin deposits are less prominent in older, more central portions of tumor stroma which consist largely of sclerotic collagen. Fibrin may be deposited in zones of tumor necrosis.

Recent evidence indicates that fibrin is also selectively deposited in the basal lamina zones of certain carcinomas (4). However, this acquired staining tends to be lost with malignant progression, and particularly at sites of tumor invasion. Thus, loss of acquired fibrin staining, like the loss of basal lamina staining for type IV collagen and laminin, affords a potentially useful marker for tumor invasion.

In lymphomas, and apparently also in sarcomas, fibrin may be observed between individual malignant tumor cells as well as between adjacent, morphologically reactive lymphoid cells.

Biochemical Nature of Fibrin in Tumors

Fibrinogen is a 340 kd hexamer composed of three pairs of nonidentical polypeptide chains (alpha, beta, and gamma); these are bound together covalently in a dimeric structure by disulfide bonds (59). When thrombin clots fibrinogen, it cleaves, in sequence, fibrinopeptides A and B from the A-alpha and B-beta chains, respectively, thereby generating soluble fibrin monomers. These join together spontaneously to form fibrin polymers that are at first linked together non-covalently. Only with the further action of clotting factor XIIIa (32), a transglutaminase that is itself activated by thrombin, does fibrin become covalently cross-linked via its gamma and alpha chains to yield the urea-insoluble molecule most commonly referred to as "fibrin". If present, plasma fibronectin is also incorporated into the fibrin clot by the action of factor XIIIa (58).

Heteroantibodies prepared against fibrinogen react not only with fibrinogen but also with fibrin and with a variety of fibrinogen and fibrin degradation products (18), and generally cannot distinguish among them. Thus, reactivity with such antibodies in immunohistochemical preparations may give little information as to the nature of the fibrinogen or fibrin present in tumors. Recently, however, monoclonal antibodies have become available that react with the amino terminus of beta chains from which fibrinopeptide B has been cleaved. These antibodies react with fibrin but do not distinguish among its several types; however, they do not recognize fibrinogen.

In order to define the biochemical nature of the fibrin deposited in tumors it has been necessary to apply biochemical methods (4a, 4b, 20). Urea insolubility, electrophoresis, and Western blotting methods have now been applied to the study of five transplantable solids tumors in guinea pigs and mice; in all instances the bulk of tumor fibrin was found to be crosslinked. This finding raises an important parallel with healing wounds in which deposition of crosslinked fibrin is also a central early event. Other parallels also exist (13). It will therefore be useful at this point to present an overview of wound healing and to compare it with tumor stroma generation.

OVERVIEW OF WOUND HEALING AND OF TUMOR STROMA GENERATION

Local tissue injury typically results in leakage of plasma or in frank hemorrhage from damaged blood vessels (6,13,46,54). These fluids clot rapidly upon contact with tissue procoagulants that are present in most normal tissues; tissue factor is the most prominent of these (1). The initial clot is a gel composed of fibrin, fibronectin, and platelets that entraps soluble plasma proteins, water and blood cells. Platelets are important in wound healing because they contribute clotting factors (50), provide a surface for prothrombinase assembly (77), and also provide mitogens and chemoattractants for connective-tissue cells (11,71).

The clot that forms at the site of wounding serves as a provisional stroma into which inflammatory cells, particularly monocyte-derived macrophages, migrate; invading macrophages are thought to ingest debris and degrade the gel locally (5,6,18). New blood capillaries and fibroblasts follow close behind. Fibroblasts synthesize and deposit many of the same matrix components that were earlier described as components of tumor stroma (Table 1); namely, fibronectin, interstitial collagens, and GAG. The result is a cellular, edematous, and highly vascular tissue that retains for a limited time remnants of the original fibrin-fibronectin gel matrix. This tissue is called "granulation tissue"—an old clinical term that refers to the granular appearance of the young connective tissue that fills open wounds (6,46,65). Granulation tissue then matures with deposition of more interstitial collagen. Subsequently this tissue is remodeled as blood vessels are resorbed and fibroblasts disappear (18,65), leaving behind a relatively avascular and acellular scar.

The events taking place in solid tumors closely resemble those just described in healing wounds. The initial tumor stroma consists largely of fibrin-fibronectin gel that entraps extravasated plasma proteins and water (Table 1); however, in contrast to wounds, platelets are generally absent. Over time, this provisional stroma is transformed progressively into mature connective tissue by a succession of events that, at least descriptively, closely resemble those of normal wound healing. Blood-derived monocytes enter the area and differentiate into macrophages. Fibroblasts and blood vessels from adjacent connective tissue replicate. Macrophages, blood vessels, and fibroblasts all migrate into the fibrin-fibronectin gel, gradually replacing the fibrin-fibronectin matrix with an immature connective tissue that mimics the granulation tissue of healing wounds. With the passage of time, this connective tissue undergoes further maturation; more collagen is deposited and both vascularity and cellularity decrease. The result is dense, fibrous connective tissue, similar to the scar tissue of healed wounds.

There are, however, differences between wound healing and tumor stroma generation that deserve mention. First, as already noted, platelets are found in healing wounds but not outside of blood vessels in solid tumors. Platelets participate in the hemostatic phase of wound healing and may also be important at later stages because they produce, among other products, platelet-derived growth factor, a potent mitogen and chemoattractant for fibroblasts (11,71). It is noteworthy that tumor cells perform certain of the functions ascribed to platelets in healing wounds. Among these are the expression of procoagulant activity and the secretion of transforming growth factors that function as mitogens and chemoattractants (74).

Second, fibrin and, to an even greater extent, fibronectin, persist in tumor stroma, whereas both proteins appear only transiently in wounds that heal normally (18,52,75). This difference is attributable at least in part to differences in vascular permeability. In wounds, normal vascular permeability is restored within a few days of injury. By contrast, persistent increased vascular permeability to plasma proteins is a hallmark of tumor blood vessels (20). Thus, at the same time that provisional stroma is being transformed to mature connective tissue in more central portions of growing tumors, new provisional tumor is continuously being laid down at the tumor periphery as fibrinogen and other plasma proteins extravasate from leaky blood vessels (13,20). In a sense, therefore, tumors are wounds that do not heal!

THE GENERATION OF PROVISIONAL TUMOR STROMA

Tumor fibrin generally results from the extravasation and extravascular clotting of plasma fibrinogen (17,25). Only tumors of hepatocellular origin have been found to synthesize fibrinogen. For fibrin to deposit in solid tumors, or for that matter at any site outside blood vessels, the microvasculature's normally low permeability to plasma proteins must increase significantly so that fibrinogen and other plasma clotting proteins can escape. In addition, a mechanism must exist for clotting extravasated fibrin. A third regulatory step, that of fibrin degradation, may also be anticipated because tumor cells are rich in plasminogen activators, enzymes that initiate the fibrinolytic cascade (64). The pathogenesis of tumor-associated fibrin deposition thus requires an understanding of how local microvascular permeability is increased and how extravascular coagulation and fibrinolysis interrelate and are regulated. Recent work has established that tumor cells have an important role in each of these three important regulatory steps (Fig. 3).

Heightened Permeability of the Tumor Microvasculature to Plasma Proteins

The tumor microvasculature exhibits strikingly increased permeability to plasma proteins (13,17,20,22,24,25,62). Radiolabeled fibrinogen, for example, enters a number of experimental tumors about five times more rapidly than it enters control tissues (20). A number of hypotheses have been put forth to explain the general state of hyperpermeability of tumor vessels, only to be rejected (24,25), but recently a satisfactory general explanation has been proposed (13,22,24,25,69).

Tumor cells of guinea pig, mouse, rat, hamster, and human origin all secrete the peptide vascular permeability factor (VPF), which causes normal blood vessels to become leaky to plasma proteins (69,70). Concentrations of VPF are particularly high in tumor ascites, suggesting that this peptide has an important role in malignant fluid accumulation in body cavities as well as in solid tumors. VPF has now been purified more than 10,000-fold from animal and human tumor sources and has a molecular weight of 36,000 to 42,000. It is active at picogram levels, and on a molar basis is more than 1000 times as active as histamine in enhancing microvascular permeability.

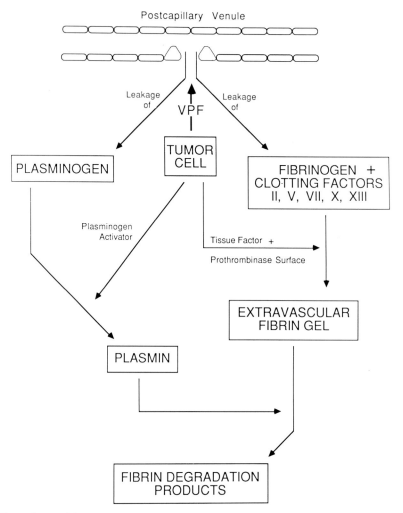

FIG. 3. Tumor-host cell interactions that regulate fibrinogen influx, extravascular coagulation, fibrin deposition and fibrin turnover in solid tumors. VPF denotes vascular permeability factor. Reprinted from ref. 13, with permission.

Like histamine, VPF induces reversible contractile separation of endothelial cells in venules without injuring these cells, and does not of itself provoke inflammatory-cell accumulation. Studies of its mechanism of action are incomplete; however, VPF does not act through basophils or mast cells or by way of other classic inducers of increased vascular permeability such as histamine, kinins, or products of arachidonic acid metabolism (24, 25). At present, a specific rabbit antibody is the only known inhibitor of VPF (69).

Coagulation and Fibrinolysis of Extravasated Plasma Fibrinogen

Once fibrinogen leaves the plasma and enters tissues, it is clotted, transglutaminated to crosslinked fibrin, and degraded proteolytically (22,61,64). These processes occur rapidly

(20); most fibrinogen that extravasates from leaky blood vessels is clotted and crosslinked within a matter of minutes. Also, catabolism of extravasated fibrinogen occurs rapidly and at more that 90% of the rate of fibrinogen influx (20). Such rapid kinetics would not necessarily have been anticipated from morphologic studies, which depict net fibrin accumulation at a single moment of time, and which provide no information as to the relative rates of fibrinogen influx, clotting, and fibrinolysis. However, immunohistochemical assessments of tumor fibrin content agree closely with independent measurements of net tumor fibrin accumulation made by tracer methods (17,18,20).

Tumor cell procoagulants are undoubtedly important in the clotting of extravasated fibrinogen (12,14,22–25,27,28,40,63,81). The procoagulant that has been most carefully documented in tumor cells is tissue factor, a phospholipoprotein that initiates the extrinsic pathway of the coagulation cascade (1). Tissue factor acts as a cofactor that increases the activity of clotting factor VIIa by several orders of magnitude, thus greatly enhancing the catalysis of clotting factor X to Xa. Living tumor cells as well as tumor cell homogenates express substantial tissue factor activity (12,23,27,28). In addition, many tumor cells release tissue factor into ascites fluid and into tissue culture medium in the form of nanometer-sized membrane vesicles; these vesicles are shed from the tumor plasma membrane (23).

Not all of the procoagulant activity expressed by tumor cells or by shed tumor vesicles can be attributed to tissue factor, however. A variety of tumor cells are also active later in the coagulation cascade, at the level of prothrombinase generation (81). Prothrombinase cleaves prothrombin to thrombin, forming an enzyme complex when clotting factors Va, Xa, and prothrombin assemble on an appropriate surface in the presence of calcium ions (59). Critical to this association is a phospholipid surface that binds factor Va with high affinity. Tumor cells and their shed vesicles provide such a surface, bind factor Va avidly ($K_d = 4 \times 10^{-10}M$) and promote efficient prothrombinase assembly (81). This step is important, because activation of the coagulation pathway at earlier steps, for example, by tissue factor, would be unproductive in the absence of a functional prothrombinase capable of completing the cascade, generating thrombin from prothrombin and, thence, fibrin from fibrinogen. Several other coagulation-initiating activities have been ascribed to tumor cells (40,63), but their role *in vivo* remains to be established.

Although tumor procoagulants have attracted much interest, the capacity to effect coagulation in tissues is not a unique property of malignant cells. In several normal tissues, an increase in microvascular permeability sufficient to cause extravasation of plasma proteins leads inevitably to the same rapid extravascular deposition of crosslinked fibrin that occurs in tumors (26). In these tissues, prominent nidi of fibrin form on the surfaces of otherwise normal appearing tissue fibrocytes and histiocytes. This result is not surprising when one recalls that the fundamental purpose of the clotting system is to minimize blood loss after injury. Thus, one would expect that normal peripheral tissues would contain procoagulants capable of clotting extravasated blood or plasma after injury. I conclude that tumor-associated procoagulants are not newly acquired functions of malignant cells, as has been widely believed; rather, they appear to be activities that are shared by a variety of cells in normal tissues and that are retained after malignant transformation.

The extent of microvascular permeability, rather than the availability of tissue procoagulants, is the rate-limiting step that governs coagulation in both normal tissues and tumors (26). However, fibrinolysis is of critical importance in determining the extent of net tumor fibrin accumulation. Fibrinogen influx and initial clotting have been found to be similar in experimental tumors that express significantly different amounts of fibrin (20); in these tumors, the large differences in observed fibrin content are primarily attributable to differences in rates of plasminogen activator release and consequent fibrinolysis (13).

TRANSFORMATION OF PROVISIONAL FIBRIN-FIBRONECTIN MATRIX INTO MATURE TUMOR STROMA

The fibrin-fibronectin gel that initially invests solid tumors is transformed over time into a vascular and collagenous matrix (Fig. 4). This metamorphosis involves the ordered replication, differentiation and migration of several types of blood cells and connective tissue cells. To a large extent, the factors regulating this series of events are poorly understood but recent progress has occurred on several fronts. For example, it has been found that cell replication may be controlled by tumor-secreted growth factors that serve as chemoattractants, as mitogens or, in some instances, as inhibitors of fibroblast and endothelial cell division (44,67,74).

Cell Migratory Events

The first step in the transformation of provisional fibrin matrix into mature stroma is the inward migration of macrophages, fibroblasts, and endothelial cells. Cellular migration in

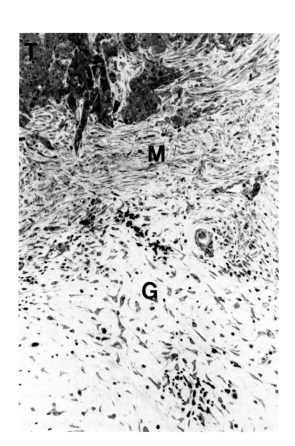

FIG. 4. Generation of mature stroma in the scirrhous line 1 bile duct carcinoma growing in a syngeneic strain two guinea pig host. The provisional matrix has been largely replaced by edematous, vascular granulation tissue (G) that continues to stain strongly for both fibrin and fibronectin by immunohistochemical methods (not shown). Granulation tissue, in turn, is being replaced by mature fibrous connective tissue stroma (M) in zones adjacent to tumor cells (T). The figure is a 1 μm Epon section (Giemsa stain). Reprinted from ref. 13, with permission. (× 210).

fibrin gels is only now beginning to be studied and solid data are presently available only for macrophages (5).

Depending upon fibrin and thrombin concentrations and on the extent of fibrin cross-linking, fibrin matrices can either enhance or inhibit macrophage migration. When prepared at sub-plasma concentrations of fibrinogen (e.g., 1 mg/ml), crosslinked fibrin gels afford a preferred substrate for macrophage migration; however, macrophages find higher fibrin concentrations (e.g., $\geq$ 5 mg/ml), to be virtually impenetrable. Additional variables such as thrombin concentration and the extent of factor XIII crosslinking also serve to determine final gel structure and therefore the suitability of matrix for inflammatory cell migration. Crosslinking of fibrin alpha chains is particularly inhibitory to macrophage migration (5).

Macrophages are unable to penetrate cellulose nitrate filters having a pore size below 5 μm, but they nonetheless migrate readily in fibrin gels having a mean pore size below 3 μm. Apparently, macrophages migrate through the much smaller pores of fibrin gels by: (1) pushing apart the relatively elastic fibrin fibrils, thereby transiently increasing effective gel pore diameter, and/or (2) lysing the gel by secreting proteases such as plasminogen activator. Of course, neither of these strategies is available to macrophages migrating through cellulose filters whose relatively rigid fibers are insusceptible to digestion by macrophage proteases. However, only small amounts of lysis, amounting to < 4% of the total fibrin gel, accompanied maximal macrophage migration (5); therefore, if fibrinolysis has a role in facilitating macrophage migration through fibrin gels, it must be highly selective and localized. Macrophage migration in fibrin gels of appropriate composition was unaffected by fibronectin contamination. However, macrophage surface receptors for fibrinogen (7,39,72) could have played a role in that their presence would favor a positive selective interaction between the cell surface and the fibrin matrix. The capacity of fibroblasts, vascular endothelium, and other stromal cells to migrate in fibrin gels is only now being investigated. Of interest, fibroblasts also express surface receptors for fibrinogen (8).

Angiogenesis

It has been known for some time that fibrin gels implanted in the subcutaneous space of experimental animals induce local angiogenesis (17). This work has been difficult to extend for want of a suitable methodology that affords the necessary reproducibility and quantitation. Recently, however, a new assay system has been developed (19) that satisfies these and additional criteria.

Cylindrical plexiglass chambers, enclosed except for a dozen small pores opening on one face, were filled with contents to be tested for their ability to induce angiogenesis (19). Chambers were implanted in the subcutaneous space of guinea pigs and were removed at appropriate intervals thereafter for varying periods, generally 4 to 6 days. Angiogenesis was scored by morphometry.

Chambers filled with homologous crosslinked fibrin gels, or with clotted plasma, regularly induced angiogenesis. New blood vessels entered the chambers through the pores that had been bored in one surface; vessels then extended radially from each pore into the fibrin gel, both laterally and vertically. The kinetics of angiogenesis were similar to those of new blood vessel formation in solid tumors and in wound healing; the intensity of angiogenesis was significantly enhanced when zymogen-activated serum, platelet derived growth factor, or the chemoattractant f-met-leu-phe were included in the fibrin gel. Angiogenesis involved the gradual replacement of fibrin gel with new blood vessels and associated collagen. Turnover of fibrin in chambers corresponded to the replacement of fibrin gel by vessel ingrowth.

In contrast to fibrin, gels prepared from type I collagen or agarose over a range of concentrations failed to initiate new blood vessel formation, whether or not supplemented with serum or ZAS. However, collagen did not inhibit the angiogenic response when it was included in chambers along with fibrin. Angiogenesis was strongly inhibited by hyaluronic acid (HA) at the high concentrations found in umbilical cord (30) but not at the much lower concentrations reported in tumors (41). HA binds to fibrinogen and may be expected to alter fibrin gel structure (53,58); it has also been reported to inhibit angiogenesis in another assay (30).

It is not yet clear how these new data relate to earlier studies of angiogenesis. A large number of angiogenesis factors has now been described (37). Some of these are cell mitogens, whereas the mechanism of action of others is unknown. Because fibrin is regularly found in tumors that acquire a vascular supply, it may be that certain of the angiogenesis factors act by inducing fibrin deposition; in that sense, VPF and tumor procoagulants may be considered to represent "angiogenesis factors." In any event, the chamber experiments here cited demonstrate conclusively that new vessel growth requires a suitable extravascular matrix and that fibrin provides such a matrix.

Collagen Synthesis

Ingress of macrophages, fibroblasts, and capillaries transforms the fibrin-fibronectin provisional matrix deposited about tumors into a highly cellular, highly vascular tissue resembling granulation tissue (17,18) (Fig. 4). Collagen is often deposited initially in intimate association with preexisting fibrin (42). Subsequently, the granulation-like tissue about tumors acquires more collagen, loses its cellularity and vascularity, and comes to resemble scar tissue. This sequence of events closely resembles the transformation of fibrin-fibronectin gel to mature collagenous stroma that occurs in wound healing.

Recently, the structural proteins deposited in tumor and wound stroma have been analyzed immunohistochemically and biochemically (Table 1) (2,6,18,36,55,56). Fibrin staining is at first substantial in both, but declines more rapidly and completely in healing wounds than in tumors. Staining for fibronectin also increases initially in both wounds and tumors but then declines precipitously in the former, while persisting in the latter. Deposits of types I and III collagen progessively increase in both processes. Thus, mature tumor stroma, like that of healed wounds, is composed largely of interstitial collagens.

Identification of the cell or cells responsible for synthesizing the individual components of the tumor stroma has not been finally resolved. Majority opinion has long held that the collagen and other structural proteins that compose tumor stroma are products of benign fibroblasts that are induced to participate in the development of desmoplastic tumors (18, 29,36,65,78). On the other hand, almost all nucleated mammalian cells can synthesize one or more types of collagen (reviewed in 36). Generally, malignant cells retain the ability to synthesize the collagen type or types associated with their cell of origin, though often in reduced amounts. Therefore, some have argued that tumor cells themselves synthesize desmoplastic stroma (reviewed in 18).

This controversy entered a new phase when it was realized that collagens of type I and III, and (more recently) type V (2), composed the bulk of tumor stroma interstitium, whereas type IV collagen was confined to basal laminae such as those that envelop blood vessels and epithelial tumor cells (2,18,55,56). A number of benign and malignant epithelial cells synthesize type IV collagen, and, in at least some instances, these same tumor cells were found *not* to make types I, III, and V collagen (18,36). Conversely, fibroblasts taken from several sources synthesize collagen types I and III and, to a lesser extent, type V, but not collagen type IV. I am persuaded, therefore, that benign fibroblasts of host origin are generally responsible for synthesizing the several types of collagen that compose the desmoplastic stroma of carcinomas, whereas epithelial tumor cells synthesize primarily the type IV collagen deposited in their basement membranes. However, there may be exceptions to this rule. At least some benign and malignant epithelial cells do synthesize interstitial collagens in tissue culture (2,34). To discover whether they also do so *in vivo* will require the use of newer methods, such as *in situ* hybridization, that allow identification of the cellular sources of individual collagen types. Interstitial collagens would of course, be the expected product of tumors derived from connective-tissue cells such as sarcomas.

Synthesis of Glycosaminoglycans and Proteoglycans

Glycosaminoglycans (GAG) are regular components of mature tumor stroma, just as they are of the stroma of normal connective tissue (41,47–49,51,57,76). They are complex carbohydrates that fall into two major categories: 1. nonsulfated GAG, primarily hyaluronic acid (HA) and 2. sulfated GAG, including heparin sulfate, chondroitin sulfate (CS), keratin sulfate and dermatan sulfate. In both benign and malignant tissues the sulfated GAG are normally linked covalently to protein cores, forming proteoglycans; HA is thought not to be so bound (57), though it may be joined to other sulfated GAG by "link proteins" (47). HA is the largest of the GAG with a MW varying from 10^5 to several million. It is a polyanion that occupies an enormous hydrodynamic volume in solution (about 1,000 times that of its dry volume) because of the mutual repulsion that exists between the negatively charged carboxyl groups of its glucuronate moieties. Thus, HA is thought to play an important role in tissue hydration (9).

HA is present in significant amounts in the stroma of a number of animal and human tumors (51). This finding is of particular interest because of the correlation that exists between HA and differentiation. Very high concentrations of HA have also been found in embryogenesis, in tissue remodeling, and in wound healing, states in which mesenchymal cells migrate and proliferate actively (76). Conversely, cessation of mesenchymal cell migration and the onset of cell differentiation are accompanied by an abrupt termination of HA synthesis, the expression of increased hyaluronidase activity, and elevated synthesis of sulfated GAG. These findings led Toole and associates (51,76) to the view that HA, because of its capacity to restrict the movement of tissue water and cause tissue swelling, provided a favorable matrix for cell migration and proliferation. It follows that these same conditions would favor tumor cell invasiveness. Indeed, HA was found to be present in much higher concentrations in an experimental tumor (V-2 carcinoma) when it was grown in rabbits under conditions where it was highly invasive than when the same tumor was grown in nude mice where it was not invasive (reviewed in 51).

HA is actively synthesized by some but not all transformed cells and tumor cell lines in culture (51). Often, transformed mesenchymal cells synthesize less HA than their non-transformed counterparts. Also, a number of tumors that contain high concentrations of HA when grown *in vivo* synthesize little or no HA when grown in tissue culture. It has been postulated that interactions between tumor and host-derived connective tissue cells could explain this apparent discrepancy; i.e., that tumor cells might induce fibroblasts to synthesize increased amounts of HA. Indeed, in a careful study Knudson et al. (51) have found that a variety of tumor cells stimulate fibroblasts to produce increased amounts of HA but only under culture conditions that allow direct contacts between tumor cells and fibroblasts; i.e., tumor culture medium could not duplicate the stimulatory effect of living tumor cells. On the other hand, Iozzo (48,49) has recently reported that, in another tumor system, tumor culture supernatants can stimulate fibroblast HA production.

Sulfated GAG may also be found in tumors at elevated concentrations, presumably in the form of proteoglycan complexes (47,48). Studies of human colonic carcinoma revealed both quantitative and qualitative changes in sulfated GAG composition (49). Total sulfated GAG were increased approximately 3-fold, but nearly all of this increment was attributable to an increase in CS which increased 12-fold above levels found in normal colonic tissue. Only a minor component of normal colonic tissue, CS accounted for some 60% of total sulfated GAG in colonic carcinomas. This increased CS was found primarily in the intercellular matrix of the connective tissue stroma; autoradiography revealed that connective tissue cells, not the tumor cells themselves, were the primary site of CS synthesis. There were also qualitative changes in the CS produced; electron microscopy of ruthenium red-stained sections revealed proteoglycan granules that were several times more numerous but about 23% smaller in size than in normal tissue. That is, in tumors there was a larger number of smaller granules and these were packed more closely together than in normal colon. As with HA production, tumor cells have been found to stimulate fibroblasts to produce increased amounts of CS. Iozzo (47,48) has reported that tumor-secreted factors are capable of effecting this stimulation. Whether or not this stimulation is tumor-specific must await purification of a tumor product.

In summary, available data indicate the presence of both sulfated and nonsulfated GAG in mature tumor stroma. The HA deposited in maturing stroma would appear to assume at least one of the functions exerted by the fibrin gel in primordial tumor stroma; namely, that of a water-trapping gel. Existing evidence suggests that although proteoglycan metabolism is regularly deranged in tumors, there may be no single proteoglycan alteration that is shared by all tumors. Rather, since proteoglycans are tissue specific (47), it may be more fruitful to compare the proteoglycan profile of different tumors with that of its tissue of origin, rather than with that of other tumors.

SIGNIFICANCE OF TUMOR STROMA FOR
HOST IMMUNOLOGICAL DEFENSE MECHANISMS

As intimated earlier, tumor stroma may have a role in regulating host immunological defense mechanisms against tumors. Immunologists generally assume that tumors possess specific antigens, that these antigens elicit an immunological response, and that the resulting immunological response affords the host some degree of protection against tumors (79,82). A further assumption is also generally implied; namely, that the immunologic response actually generated in animals or patients with progressively growing tumors is quantitatively or qualitatively defective, and for this reason the host is unable to rid itself of tumor. It is to this last point that tumor immunologists have devoted considerable attention. To circumvent the presumed immunologic deficiency of tumor-bearing hosts, immunologists have attempted either to stimulate the endogenous immune response [e.g., with BCG (3) or, more recently, with agents such as Interleukin-2 (66)] or to provide an exogenous supplement of specific cytotoxic antibodies, activated T cells, etc. The underlying premise is that a better or more powerful immune response will rid the host of tumor.

There is little doubt that specific antibodies and/or inflammatory cells effectively kill tumor cells *in vitro*. An immune response may also be highly effective at destroying certain experimental solid tumors *in vivo* [e.g., line 1 carcinoma in the guinea pig (17)]; however, with many other tumors, both the host's endogenous immune response and immunotherapy prove ineffective. One major, and heretofore largely neglected, explanaton for the failure of the immune response to rid the host of solid tumors *in vivo* is the tumor stroma and its barrier function (17). In patients or animals, the cells that comprise solid tumors are enmeshed in stroma and do not grow in suspension or as monolayers as do the same tumor cells when they are cultured *in vitro*. In order to make contact with tumor cells *in vivo*, therefore, antibodies or inflammatory cells must first penetrate a "cocoon" of provisional or mature stroma. That such penetration may not be a trivial undertaking is suggested by histological studies of growing autochthonous and transplantable human and animal tumors (13,16,17,24,25,80). In the case of many, perhaps most carcinomas, such lymphocytes as are called forth to tumor sites remain confined to the tumor periphery, and only a minority actually penetrates stroma and makes contact with tumor cells (Fig. 2A,B). In some instances, of course, lymphocytes do penetrate tumor stroma and do make direct contact with tumor cells. Such penetration is particularly common in tumors where stromal connective tissue is poorly developed (e.g., seminomas, medullary carcinomas of the breast).

It may be useful to examine the factors that regulate the passage of antibodies and inflammatory cells out of blood vessels and into solid tumors. Clearly, two barriers must be penetrated: the vessel wall and the tumor stroma. With regard to the former, entry of antibodies into the tumor interstitium should be facilitated by the generally leaky state of tumor vessels. After leaving vessels, antibody movement is subject to the physical laws that govern macromolecular diffusion and convection in fibrin, HA, or other gels (9,41).

Entry of inflammatory cells into tumors is a more complex issue. Generalized leakiness of the tumor microvasculature to plasma proteins would not be expected of itself to affect the exodus of inflammatory cells from the blood. Inflammatory cells do not usually leave blood vessels because of increased permeability; rather, they first adhere selectively to the endothelium, migrate to interendothelial junctions, and then penetrate these junctions as well as the underlying basal lamina. None of these steps is well understood in molecular terms. However, it is known that the inflammatory cell-endothelial cell contacts that initiate diapedesis are highly specific in at least two respects: (1) All such attachments take place on a specialized endothelium, that of post-capillary venules. Regardless of type, inflammatory cells exit the blood only from venules. (2) The inflammatory cell-endothelial cell interaction is subject to highly specific and selective regulation. That is, in any given type of inflammatory reaction, leukocytes of certain classes, but not of others, attach to endothelium and emigrate; e.g., lymphocytes and monocytes, but not the much more numerous granulocytes, selectively populate human delayed hypersensitivity reactions.

Inflammatory cells that have overcome the first or blood vascular barrier must then penetrate either provisional or mature connective tissue stroma before they can make contact with tumor cells. Only very recently have initial attempts been made to analyze the capacity of such cells to migrate in a simplified connective tissue matrix, fibrin gels of defined composition. As was described in an earlier section, crosslinked fibrin gels, prepared at fibrinogen concentrations below plasma levels, provide a matrix that facilitates macrophage migration (5). However, as fibrin concentrations were increased above plasma levels, the resulting gels formed a progressively impermeant barrier to macrophage migration. Above about 5 mg/ml, macrophages could not enter fibrin gels at all. Since fibrin concentrations in some tumors have been measured in excess of 7 mg/ml (20), it follows that the fibrin stromal matrix may indeed present a biologically significant barrier to macrophage penetration. Fibrin, therefore, may contribute to the paucity of macrophages and perhaps of lymphocytes and other inflammatory cells found in some tumors.

A somewhat gloomy conclusion follows from this discussion, namely, that an enveloping fibrin or other connective tissue cocoon may thwart the immune response from rejecting tumors. High titers of cytotoxic antibodies and large numbers of circulating cytotoxic inflammatory cells may not necessarily lead to the control of tumor growth. In addition to providing specific cells and antibodies in the circulation, tumor immunologists will also have to devise a means of delivering these effectors in such a way that they are able to make intimate contact with tumor cells. Certainly in the case of desmoplastic tumors, the stromal cocoon may present a formidable barrier to both antibodies and cells and, as a consequence, to effective immunotherapy.

Vascular factors may also be important. At least one reason for the concentration of inflammatory cells at the tumor periphery may be the availability there, and not in more central portions of tumor, of suitably differentiated venules that can support cell attachment and therefore allow lymphocyte emigration. Intratumor blood vessels are generally poorly differentiated, and their endothelial cells may lack the receptors with which leukocytes need to interact if they are to emigrate from vessels.

SUMMARY AND CONCLUSION

Tumor stroma generation shares many important properties with normal wound healing. Both processes begin with the spillage of plasma proteins, among them fibrinogen, fibronectin, and plasminogen. In both processes, extravasated fibrinogen is clotted and crosslinked to itself and to fibronectin, inserting into the tissues an insoluble, water-holding gel. In both, this extravascular fibrin-fibronectin clot serves as a provisional stroma, providing a matrix for the immigration of macrophages, fibroblasts, and new capillaries. In both, the fibrin-fibronectin gel is degraded and transformed into granulation tissue and eventually into dense, relatively acellular collagenous connective tissue.

The recognized differences between tumor stroma generation and wound healing are minor and can be attributed primarily to the distinct mechanisms that initiate each. In most wounds, extravascular fibrin gel is laid down for only a limited interval after injury. In contrast, tumors constitutively secrete a vascular permeability factor that renders local blood vessels permeable to plasma proteins for protracted periods of time. A second obvious difference, the participation of platelets in wounds but not in tumors, may be less important because tumor cells themselves are able to perform several critical functions of platelets, i.e., the capacity to express procoagulants and to secrete chemotactic and mitogenic factors that regulate both inflammatory and connective-tissue cells.

Very likely the presence of stroma also has profound consequences for tumor immunology. Stroma is a barrier that separates tumor cells from host defense mechanisms, whether humoral or cellular. In order to destroy solid tumors, antibodies or effector cells must first penetrate stroma; depending on the extent and nature of stroma deposited in an individual tumor, this may be a greater or lesser problem. Tumor immunologists have been slow to consider the possibility that tumor stroma might provide a serious obstacle to effective immunotherapy. This is particularly surprising given the rather disappointing results obtained to date with monoclonal antibodies and with other forms of immunotherapy.

By taking into account the stroma that supplies and, to a variable extent, isolates solid tumors, tumor immunologists will at the very least have a more realistic view of the problems they face in directing antibodies or sensitized cells to tumors and will be in a better position to overcome these problems. However, tumor immunologists should not regard stroma in an entirely negative light. Tumor stroma may itself offer an attractive target for immunotherapy! If tumors are to grow beyond a minimal size of 1 to 2 mm, they must develop stroma (33). Therefore, any therapy that destroys stroma or thwarts its generation would be expected to have profound consequences for tumor growth and survival. Indeed, precedents for such an approach already exist. For example, the microvasculature is recognized as the primary target of the immune response in the first set rejection of skin and heart allografts in several species (21,35). It is also a major target in at least several examples of cell-mediated tumor rejection in guinea pigs and mice (17,25,38).

ACKNOWLEDGMENTS

This work was supported by US Public Health Service Research Grants CA-28471 and CA-40624, and under terms of a contract from the National Foundation for Cancer Research.

REFERENCES

1. Bach, R., Nemerson, Y., and Konigsberg, W. (1981): Purification and characterization of bovine tissue factor. *J. Biol. Chem.*, 256:8324–8331.
2. Barsky, S., Rao, C., Grotendorst, G., and Liotta, L. (1982): Increased content of type V collagen in desmoplasia of human breast carcinoma. *Am. J. Pathol.*, 108:276–283.
3. Bast, R. C., Jr., Zbar, B., Borsos, T., and Rapp, H. J. (1974): BCG and cancer. *N. Engl. J. Med.*, 290:1458–1469.
4. Brown, L. F., Chester, J. F., Malt, R. A., and Dvorak, H. F. (1987): Fibrin deposition in autochthonous Syrian hamster pancreatic adenocarcinomas induced by the chemical carcinogen N-nitro-bis(2 oxopropyl)amine. *J. Natl. Cancer Inst.*, 78:979–986.
4a. Brown, L. F., Asch, B., Harvey, V. S., Buchinski, B., and Dvorak, H. F. (1988): Fibrinogen influx and accumulation of cross-linked fibrin in mouse carcinomas. *Cancer Res.*, 48:1920–1925.
4b. Brown, L. F., VanDeWater, L., Harvey, V. S., and Dvorak, H. F. (1988): Fibrinogen influx and accumulation of cross-linked fibrin in healing wounds and in tumor stroma. *Am. J. Pathol.*, 130:455–465.
5. Ciano, P., Colvin, R., Dvorak, A. M., McDonagh, J., and Dvorak, H. F. (1986): Macrophage migration in fibrin gel matrices. *Lab. Invest.*, 54:62–70.
6. Clark, R. A. F., and Colvin, R. B. (1985): Wound repair. In: *Plasma Fibronectin: Structure and Function*, edited by J. McDonagh, pp. 197–262. Marcel Dekker, Inc., New York.
7. Colvin, R., and Dvorak, H. F. (1975): Fibrinogen/fibrin on the surface of macrophages: Detection, distribution, binding requirements and possible role in macrophage adherence phenomena. *J. Exp. Med.*, 142:1377–1390.
8. Colvin, R., Gardner, P., Roblin, R., Verderber, E., Lanigan, J., and Mosesson, M. (1979): Cell surface fibrinogen-fibrin receptors on cultured human fibroblasts. *Lab. Invest.*, 41:464–473.
9. Comper, W. D., and Laurent, T. C. (1978): Physiological function of connective tissue polysaccharides. *Physiological Rev.*, 58:255–315.
10. Day, E., Planisek, J., and Pressman, D. (1959): Localization *in vivo* of radioiodinated anti-rat fibrin antibodies and radioiodinated rat fibrinogen in the Murphy rat lymphosarcoma and in other transplantable rat tumors. *J. Natl. Cancer Inst.*, 22:413–426.
11. Deuel, T., and Huang, J. (1984): Platelet-derived growth factor. Structure, function, and roles in normal and transformed cells. *J. Clin. Invest.*, 74:669–676.
12. Donati, M. (1984): Hemostatic abnormalities in tumor-bearing animals. In: *Hemostatic Mechanisms and Metastases*, edited by K. V. Honn, and B. F. Sloane, pp. 62–71. Martinus Nijhoff, Boston.

13. Dvorak, H. F. (1986): Tumors: Wounds that do not heal. *N. Engl. J. Med.*, 315:1650–1659.

14. Dvorak, H. F. (1987): Abnormalities of hemostasis in malignancy. In: *Hemostasis and Thrombosis*, 2nd Edition, edited by R. W. Colman, J. Hirsh, V. J. Marder, and E. W. Salzman, pp. 1143–1157. J.B. Lippincott, Philadelphia.

15. Dvorak, H. F., Dickersin, G., Dvorak, A. M., Manseau, E., and Pyne, K. (1981): Human breast carcinoma: Fibrin deposits and desmoplasia. Inflammatory cell type and distribution. Microvasculature and infarction. *J. Natl. Cancer Inst.*, 67:335–345.

16. Dvorak, H. F., and Dvorak, A. M. (1982): Immunohistological characterization of inflammatory cells that infiltrate tumors. In: *Tumor Immunity in Prognosis*, edited by S. Haskill, pp. 279–307. Marcel Dekker, New York.

17. Dvorak, H. F., Dvorak, A. M., Manseau, E., Wiberg, L., and Churchill, W. (1979): Fibrin gel investment associated with line 1 and line 10 solid tumor growth, angiogenesis, and fibroplasia in guinea pigs. Role of cellular immunity, myofibroblasts, microvascular damage, and infarction in line 1 tumor regression. *J. Natl. Cancer Inst.*, 62:1459–1472.

18. Dvorak, H. F., Form, D., Manseau, E., and Smith, B. (1984): Pathogenesis of desmoplasia. Immunofluorescence identification and localization of some structural proteins of line 1 and line 10 guinea pig tumors and of healing wounds. *J. Natl. Cancer Inst.*, 73:1195–1205.

19. Dvorak, H. F., Harvey, V. S., Estrella, P., Brown, L. F., McDonagh, J., and Dvorak, A. M. (1987): Fibrin containing gels induce angiogenesis: A new assay with implications for tumor stroma generation and wound healing. *Lab. Invest.*, 57:673–686.

20. Dvorak, H. F., Harvey, V. S., and McDonagh, J. (1984): Quantitation of fibrinogen influx, deposition and turnover in line 1 and line 10 guinea pig carcinomas. *Cancer Res.*, 44:3348–3354.

21. Dvorak, H. F., Mihm, M. C., Jr., Dvorak, A. M., Barnes, B. A., and Galli, S. J. (1980): The microvasculature is the critical target of the immune response in vascularized skin allograft rejection. *J. Invest. Dermatol.*, 74:280–284.

22. Dvorak, H. F., Orenstein, N. S., Carvalho, A. C., Churchill, W. H., Dvorak, A. M., Galli, S. J., Feder, J., Bitzer, A. M., Rypysc, J., and Giovinco, P. (1979): Induction of a fibrin-gel investment: An early event in line 10 hepatocarcinoma growth mediated by tumor secreted products. *J. Immunol.*, 122:166–174.

23. Dvorak, H. F., Quay, S., Orenstein, N. S., Dvorak, A. M., Hahn, P., and Bitzer, A. M. (1981): Tumor shedding and coagulation. *Science*, 212:923–924.

24. Dvorak, H. F., Senger, D. R., and Dvorak, A. M. (1983): Fibrin as a component of the tumor stroma: Origins and biological significance. *Cancer Metastasis Rev.*, 2:41–73.

25. Dvorak, H. F., Senger, D. R., and Dvorak, A. M. (1984): Fibrin formation: Implications for tumor growth and metastasis. In: *Hemostatic Mechanisms and Metastasis*, edited by K. V. Honn and B. S. Sloane, pp. 96–114. Martinus Nijhoff, Boston.

26. Dvorak, H. F., Senger, D. R., Harvey, V. S., and McDonagh, J. (1985): Regulation of extravascular coagulation by microvascular permeability. *Science*, 227:1059–1061.

27. Dvorak, H. F., VanDeWater, L., Bitzer, A. M., Dvorak, A. M., Anderson, D., Harvey, V. S., Bach, R., Davis, G. L., DeWolf, W., and Carvalho, A. C. A. (1983): Procoagulant activity associated with plasma vesicles shed by cultured tumor cells. *Cancer Res.*, 43:4334–4342.

28. Edwards, R., and Rickles, F. (1984): Hemostatic alterations in cancer patients. In: *Hemostatic Mechanisms and Metastases*, edited by K. V. Honn and B. F. Sloane, pp. 342–354. Martinus Nijhoff, Boston.

29. El-Torky, M., Giltman, L., and Mustafa, D. (1985): Collagens in scar carcinomas of the lung. *Am. J. Pathol.*, 121:322–326.

30. Feinberg, R. N., and Beebe, D. C. (1983): Hyaluronate in vasculogenesis. *Science*, 220:1177–1179.

31. Fett, J. W., Strydom, D. J., Lobb, R. R., Alderman, E. M., Bethune, J. L., Riordan, J. F., and Vallee, B. L. (1985): Isolation and characterization of angiogenin, an angiogenic protein from human carcinoma cells. *Biochemistry*, 24:5480–5486.

32. Folk, J., and Finlayson, H. (1977): The epsilon (gamma-glutamyl) lysine cross-link and the catalytic role of transglutaminases. *Adv. Protein Chem.*, 31:1–133.

33. Folkman, J. (1985): Tumor angiogenesis. *Adv. Cancer Res.*, 43:175–203.

34. Folkman, J. (1986): How is blood vessel growth regulated in normal and neoplastic tissue? *Cancer Res.*, 46:467–473.

35. Forbes, R. D. C., Guttmann, R. D., Gomersall, M., and Hibberd, J. (1983): A controlled serial ultrastructural tracer study of first-set cardiac allograft rejection in the rat. *Am. J. Pathol.*, 111:184–196.

36. Form, D., VanDeWater, L., Dvorak, H. F., and Smith, B. (1984): Pathogenesis of tumor desmoplasia. Collagens synthesized by line 1 and line 10 guinea pig carcinoma cells and by syngeneic fibroblasts *in vitro*. *J. Natl. Cancer Inst.*, 73:1207–1214.

37. Furcht, L. (1986): Critical factors controlling angiogenesis: Cell products, cell matrix, and growth factors. *Lab. Invest.*, 55:505–509.

38. Galli, S. J., Bast, R. C., Jr., Bast, B. S., Isomura, T., Zbar, B., Rapp, H. J., and Dvorak, H. F. (1982): Bystander suppression of tumor growth: Evidence that specific targets and bystanders are damaged by injury to a common microvasculature. *J. Immunol.*, 129:1790–1799.

39. Gonda, S., and Shainoff, J. (1982): Adsorptive endocytosis of fibrin monomer by macrophages: Evidence of a receptor for the amino terminus of the fibrin alpha chain. *Proc. Natl. Acad. Sci. (U.S.A.)*, 79:4565–4569.

40. Gordon, S. (1984): Evidence for a tumor proteinase in blood coagulation. In: *Hemostatic Mechanisms and Metastases*, edited by K. V. Honn and B. F. Sloane, pp. 72–82. Martinus Nijhoff, Boston.

41. Gullino, P. M. (1975): Extracellular compartments of solid tumors. In: *Cancer. A Comprehensive Treatise*, edited by F. F. Becker, pp. 327–354. Plenum Press, New York.

42. Harris, N., Dvorak, A. M., Smith, J., and Dvorak, H. F. (1982): Fibrin deposits in Hodgkin's disease. *Am. J. Pathol.*, 108:119–129.

43. Heimark, R., Twardzik, D. R., and Schwartz, S. M. (1986): Inhibition of endothelial regeneration by type-beta transforming growth factor from platelets. *Science*, 233:1078–1080.

44. Heldin, C, and Westermark, B. (1984): Growth factors: Mechanism of action and relation to oncogenes. *Cell*, 37:9–20.

45. Hiramoto, R., Bernecky, J., and Jurandowski, J. (1960): Fibrin in human tumors. *Cancer Res.*, 20:592–593.

46. Hunt, T. K. (1980): *Wound Healing and Wound Infection*. Appleton-Century-Crofts, New York.

47. Iozzo, R. V. (1984): Proteoglycans and neoplastic-mesenchymal cell interactions. *Hum. Pathol.*, 15:2–10.

48. Iozzo, R. V. (1985): Biology of disease. Proteoglycans: Structure, function, and role in neoplasia. *Lab. Invest.*, 53:373–396.

49. Iozzo, R. V., Bolender, R. P., and Wight, T. N. (1982): Proteoglycan changes in the intercellular matrix of human colon carcinoma. *Lab. Invest.*, 47:124–138.

50. Karpatkin, S., and Holmsen, H. (1983): Biochemistry and function of platelets. In: *Hematology*, 3rd Edition, edited by W. J. Williams, E. Beutler, A. J. Erslev, and M. A. Lichtman, pp. 1136–1149. McGraw Hill, New York.

51. Knudson, W., Biswas, C., and Toole, B. P. (1984): Interactions between human tumor cells and fibroblasts stimulate hyaluronate synthesis. *Proc. Natl. Acad. Sci. (U.S.A.)*, 81:6767–6771.

52. Labat-Robert, J., Birembaut, P., Robert, L., and Adnet, J. (1981): Modification of fibronectin distribution pattern in solid human tumors. *Diag. Histopathol.*, 4:299–306.

53. LeBoeuf, R. D., Raja, R. H., Fuller, G. M., and Weigel, P. H. (1986): Human fibrinogen specifically binds hyaluronic acid. *J. Biol. Chem.*, 261:12586–12592.

54. Leibovich, S. J., and Ross, R. (1975): The role of the macrophage in wound repair: A study with hydrocortisone and antimacrophage serum. *Am. J. Pathol.*, 78:71–92.

55. Liotta, L. (1984): Tumor invasion and metastases: Role of the basement membrane. *Am. J. Pathol.*, 117:339–348.

56. Liotta, L., Rao, C., and Barsky, S. (1983): Tumor invasion and the extracellular matrix. *Lab. Invest.*, 49:636–649.

57. Mason, R. M., d'Arville, C., Kimura, J. H., and Hascall, V. C. (1982): Absence of covalently linked core protein from newly synthesized hyaluronate. *Biochem. J.*, 207:445–457.

58. McDonagh, J. (1985): *Plasma Fibronectin: Structure and Function*. Marcel Dekker, New York.

59. Mosesson, M., and Doolittle, F. (1983): Molecular biology of fibrinogen and fibrin. *Ann. N.Y. Acad. Sci.*, 408:1–672.

60. O'Meara, R., and Jackson, R. (1958): Cytological observations on carcinomas. *Br. J. Med. Sci.*, 6:327–328.

61. Orenstein, N., Bucynski, A., and Dvorak, H. F. (1983): Cryptic and active plasminogen activators secreted by line 10 tumor cells in culture. *Cancer Res.*, 43:1783–1789.

62. Peterson, H-I. (1979): *Tumor Blood Circulation: Angiogenesis, Vascular Morphology and Blood Flow of Experimental and Human Tumors*. CRC Press, Boca Raton, Florida.

63. Pineo, G., Brain, M., Gallus, A. S., Hirsch, J., Hatton, M., and Regoeczi, E. (1974): Tumors, mucus production, and hypercoagulability. *Ann. N.Y. Acad. Sci.*, 230:262–270.

64. Reich, E. (1975): Plasminogen activator: Secretion by neoplastic cells and macrophages. In: *Proteases and Biological Control*, edited by E. Reich, D. B. Rifkin, and E. Shaw, pp. 333–341. Cold Spring Harbor, New York.

65. Robbins, S., Cotran, R., and Kumar, V. (1984): *Pathologic Basis of Disease*. W.B. Saunders Co., Philadelphia.

66. Rosenberg, S. A., Spiess, P., and Lafreniere, R. (1986): A new approach to the adoptive immunotherapy of cancer with tumor-infiltrating lymphocytes. *Science*, 233:1318–1321.

67. Saloman, D., Liotta, L., and Kidwell, W. (1981): Differential response to growth factor by rat mammary epithelium plated on different collagen substrata in serum-free medium. *Proc. Natl. Acad. Sci. (U.S.A.)*, 78:382–386.

68. Schreiber, A. B., Winkler, M. E., and Derynck, R. (1985): Transforming growth factor alpha: A more potent angiogenic mediator than epidermal growth factor. *Science*, 232:1250–1253.

69. Senger, D. R., Galli, S. J., Dvorak, A. M., Perruzzi, C., Harvey, V. S., and Dvorak, H. F. (1983): Tumor cells secrete a vascular permeability factor that promotes accumulation of ascites fluid. *Science*, 219:983–985.

70. Senger, D. R., Perruzzi, C. A., Feder, J., and Dvorak, H. F. (1986): A highly conserved vascular permeability factor secreted by a variety of human and rodent tumor cell lines. *Cancer Res.*, 46:5629–5632.

71. Seppa, H., Grotendorst, G., Seppa, S., Schiffmann, E., and Martin, G. (1982): Platelet-derived growth factor is chemotactic for fibroblasts. *J. Cell Biol.*, 92:584–588.

72. Sherman, L. (1983): Binding of soluble fibrin to macrophages. *Ann. N.Y. Acad. Sci.*, 408:611–620.

73. Spar, I., Bale, W., Marrak, D., Dewy, W., McCardle, R., and Harper, P. (1967): ^{131}I-labeled antibodies to human fibrinogen: Diagnostic studies and therapeutic trials. *Cancer*, 20:865–870.

74. Sporn, M., and Roberts, A. (1985): Autocrine growth factors and cancer. *Nature*, 313:745–747.

75. Szendroi, M., Lapis, K., Zalatnai, A., Robert, L., and Labat-Robert, J. (1984): Appearance of fibronectin in putative preneoplastic lesions and in hepatocellular carcinoma during chemical hepatocarcinogenesis in rats and in human hepatomas. *J. Exper. Pathol.*, 1:189–199.

76. Toole, B. P. (1981): Glycosaminoglycans in morphogenesis. In: *Cell Biology of Extracellular Matrix*, edited by E. D. Hay, pp. 259–293. Plenum Press, New York.

77. Tracy, P., Nesheim, M., and Mann, K. (1981): Coordinate binding of Factor Va and Factor Xa to the unstimulated platelet. *J. Biol. Chem.*, 256:743–751.

78. Tremblay, G. (1979): Stromal aspects of breast carcinoma. *Exp. Mol. Pathol.*, 31:248–260.

79. Uhr, J. W. (1984): Immunotoxins: Harnessing nature's poisons. *J. Immunol.*, 133:i–x.

80. Vaage, J., and Pepin, K. (1985): Morphological observations during developing concomitant immunity against a C3H/He mammary tumor. *Cancer Res.*, 45:659–666.

81. VanDeWater, L., Tracy, P., Aronson, D., Mann, K., and Dvorak, H. F. (1985): Tumor cell generation of thrombin via functional prothrombinase assembly. *Cancer Res.*, 45:5521–5525.

82. Waters, H., editor (1978): *The Handbook of Cancer Immunology*, Vols. 1–5. Garland STPM Press, New York.

Diagnostic Immunopathology,
edited by R.B. Colvin,
A.K. Bhan, and R.T. McCluskey.
Raven Press, New York © 1988.

16 / *Immunofluorescence*

A. Bernard Collins

*Immunopathology Unit, Department of Pathology, Massachusetts General Hospital,
and, Harvard Medical School, Boston, Massachusetts 02114*

Immunofluorescence is a well established immunohistochemical technique used for the detection of a wide variety of antigens in tissues or on cells in suspension (5,23). Coons developed immunofluorescence in the 1940s, with the blue fluorescing compound, β-anthracene coupled to rabbit antisera and was able to localize pneumococcal antigens in formalin fixed tissue (13). To differentiate from the blue tissue autofluorescence he switched to fluorescein isocyanate, which produces green fluorescence. In the 1950s, the more stable isothiocyanate derivatives of fluorescein and rhodamine were synthesized and became commercially available, and immunofluorescence techniques became widely used. The value of immunofluorescence in diagnostic studies was apparent soon after its introduction, and has become routine in the diagnosis of immunologically mediated diseases of the kidney (11,22,33,34) (Chapter 3) and skin (1,4,7,14) (Chapter 4) the demonstration of circulating antibodies, such as autoantibodies or antibodies (3,6,24,26) (Chapter 5). Optimal immunofluorescence results require attention to tissue preparation and sectioning.

FLUORESCENCE MICROSCOPE

Fluorescence microscopy depends upon the principle that certain molecules, such as fluorescein, have electrons that are readily excited to unstable higher energy states by "absorbing" photons of light of certain energies (25,37). When these electrons return to a more stable energy state, they release the stored energy as light, but at a lower energy level and a longer wave length, which is emitted as fluorescent light. An excitation filter is chosen to provide incident photons of optical energy at the correct wave length, and the barrier filter is chosen to block out most of the photons of excitation energy and allow only those with the lower energies of the "fluorescent" or emitted photons to pass through. Fluorescein is maximally excited at about 490 nm and has a peak emission at around 510 to 517 nm. FITC interference and excitation filters developed in recent years take advantage of the strong absorption of fluorescein at 490 nm; they are combined with a barrier filter which blocks energy with a wave length of less than 500 nm. This combination of filters results in an apple-green color with fluorescein labeled antibodies. Rhodamine is maximally excited at 550 nm its peak emission at 580 nm and appears cherry red with the appropriate corresponding excitation and interference filters (18,37).

Tissues stained with fluorescein conjugates can be examined with light microscopes equipped with appropriate excitation and barrier filters to visualize the green color of fluorescein or the red color of rhodamine and phycoerythrin. The optics are fully described in (37). Epi-illumination employs a vertical illuminator and dichroic mirrors developed by Ploem (49). The excitation energy is focused directly on the specimen and the emitted fluorescent light is transmitted directly to the eye through the dichroic mirror. The dichroic mirror acts both as the excitation and barrier filter, since it allows the passage of excitation in one direction and the emission energy in the other. One limitation of epi-illumination is that the light at lower magnification is considerably less than with a dark field condenser. However, there are several advantages of epi-illumination over transmitted illumination using a dark field condenser: no oil is needed; the intensity of illumination is constant, once the objective is focused so that the brightness of staining in different specimens can be more reliably compared; viewing can be combined with standard phase microscopy, which is important for cell suspension studies and for defining morphologic detail in tissue sections: and examination in double staining studies is easier due to interchangeable FITC and TRITC filter systems.

Most fluorescence microscopes are illuminated by a high pressure mercury or xenon lamp. Halogen lamps are also available as a cheaper source of illumination, but the amount of light available is less than with the mercury lamp. The brightness of fluorescence is due to the efficiency of the fluorochrome in converting incident light to fluorescent light, the concentration of the fluorochrome in specimen and the intensity of the light source.

METHODS

Tissue Preparation and Processing

Tissue for immunofluorescence studies should be obtained fresh and kept moist until rapidly frozen. If freezing can be performed within 20 min, the tissue can be kept on a saline moistened piece of gauze or filter paper in a closed vial or small petri dish. Specimens transported long distances can be placed in Michel's transport fixative (36,39) which can be obtained commercially (Zeus Scientific, Inc., Raritan, NJ) or prepared according to the method given in Beutner (4). The solution contains an anti-autolytic agent, N-ethyl-maleimide to preserve tissue bound immunoglobulins. Since it also contains $(NH4)_2SO_4$ the specimen must be washed at least three times in the wash buffer provided by the supplier or phosphate buffered saline before freezing. Otherwise, ammonium sulfate crystals may form, resulting in poor morphology.

Tissue for immunofluorescence studies can be obtained by percutaneous needle biopsy, open wedge biopsy or excision. Percutaneous needle biopsies, which usually range in length from 0.5 to 1.0 cm, can be divided in such a manner as to insure that adequate tissue is available for histologic, immunofluorescence, and electron microscopy studies (28). An example of how a renal biopsy approximately 1.0 cm in length can be divided is illustrated in (Fig. 1).

Skin biopsies (usually 4 mm punch biopsies) can also be divided for histologic and immunofluorescence studies, but usually a second biopsy specimen is obtained if electron microscopic studies are indicated. Tissue obtained at autopsy may be suitable for certain immunofluorescence studies, but frequently the results are difficult to interpret because of high background staining, which probably results from autolysis and nonspecific trapping of serum proteins.

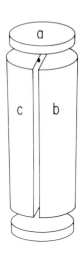
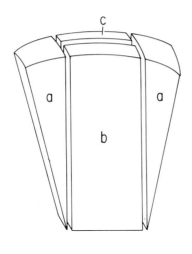

FIG. 1. Schematic illustration of the division of a closed needle and an open surgical renal biopsies for (**A**) Electron microscopy. (**B**) Direct immunofluorescence and (**C**) Light microscopic studies.

Freezing

Many of the difficulties in immunofluorescence are related to suboptimal freezing or subsequent storage. Slower freezing favors the formation of larger ice crystals, which is the cause of structural disruption. The standard method in our laboratory is to freeze the specimen in a cryostat. Properly oriented tissue is immersed in a small amount of O.C.T. compound, a water soluble resin (Miles Laboratories, Inc., Naperville, IL), on a precooled metal chuck in the cryostat and sprayed gently with MCB Tissue Freeze (Matheson, Coleman and Bell Manufacturing Chemists, Norwood, OH). Comparable results are obtained if a metal heat sink is used. Tissue frozen in this manner is ready for sectioning in less than three minutes.

In order to preserve the greatest activity of certain enzymes, such as ATPase in muscle, the tissue must be frozen even more rapidly, in isopentane and liquid nitrogen. This combination reduces the bubbling and irregular cooling caused by the low thermal conductivity of liquid nitrogen alone. The isopentane is precooled by placing it into a beaker, which is immersed in liquid nitrogen. The isopentane should be removed when opaque droplets appear in the bottom of the beaker, which indicates that it is near its own freezing point ($-160°C$). Tissue is placed on filter paper or placed properly oriented onto a layer of frozen O.C.T. contained in metal mold or a "boat" made with aluminum foil and then covered with more O.C.T. compound. The tissue contained in the "boat" is immersed with tongs in the precooled isopentane for approximately 10 sec; if it remains too long the tissue may crack.

Another method of freezing is in CO_2 and alcohol (25). Small blocks of dry ice are added to 100% alcohol contained in a wide-mouth thermos until the temperature reaches approximately $-70°C$. Small pieces of tissue are snap-frozen by placing them on the inner wall of a glass boiling tube and immersing the tube into the slurry so that the tissue is below the level of the mixture. Care should be taken to avoid entrance of alcohol into the tube, since it will act as a fixative and prevent proper freezing.

Fixation

Most diagnostic studies using direct and indirect immunofluorescence techniques are performed on unfixed tissue sections, because many antigens of interest are destroyed by fixation. For certain diffusible antigens, however fixation is necessary (e.g., plasma cell Ig, surface antigens) (18,37). Fixation of cryostat sections, cytospin preparations or touch imprints can be achieved with 100% acetone, paraformaldehyde-lysine-periodate fixative (38), 95% to 100% ethanol, methanol, 1 : 1 mixture of 95% ethanol and anhydrous ether, or 2% to 3% paraformaldehyde. In addition, alcoholic fixation and paraffin embedding may be carried out following the method of Sainte-Marie (47). Optimal fixation conditions must be determined empirically for the particular antigen under study.

Storage

The specimens should be stored frozen at $-70°C$ in a small plastic bag with as little air as possible. It is important to avoid touching the frozen block, since heat from the hands will melt the O.C.T. compound. At $-70°C$ it is possible to store blocks for long periods, often for years, and still obtain adequate results. Tissue can be stored at $-20°C$, but at this temperature satisfactory preservation usually does not exceed several months. Major reasons for deterioration during storage are ice crystal formation and desiccation.

Cryostat Sections

Tissue sections cut at a thickness of 2 to 4 microns provide generally satisfactory resolution by fluorescence microscopy. The sections should be cut from frozen blocks equilibrated in a cryostat at $-25°C$ to $-20°C$. I recommend the use of alcohol washed, Histostik coated (Accurate Scientific, Inc., Westbury, NY), single-end frosted glass slides, which facilitate labeling and decrease the chance that tissue will accidently be wiped off the wrong side. When the slide at room temperature is brought near the knife surface the tissue attaches because of the temperature difference. The tissue thaws quickly unless the section is extremely large. Slides can then be air dried and stained forthwith, or they can be frozen by placing them in a slide box, which is then covered with aluminum foil or plastic wrap and stored at $-20°C$ until they are to be stained. Storing slides overnight is convenient and allows effective organization of a technician's time. Frozen tissue for auto-antibody assay is processed similarly (Chapter 5).

Immunofluorescence

There are two basic methods of immunofluorescence: direct and indirect (Fig. 2). The direct method, is a one step procedure in which a fluorochrome label is covalently conjugated directly to the primary antibody reactive with the antigen of interest. The indirect method requires two incubations, first with primary unlabeled antisera or antibody and then with a fluorochrome labeled antibody specific for the primary antibody. The fluorochromes used commonly are fluorescein isothiocyanate (FITC) tetramethylrhodamine isothiocyanate (TRITC), or phycoerythrin (PE).

PE is a fluorochrome of high quantum yield (19). These highly fluorescent proteins are

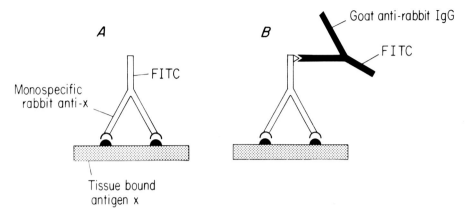

FIG. 2. (A) Direct and **(B)** indirect immunofluorescence staining techniques.

found in the light gathering organelles of certain algae and are highly hydrophilic. When coupled to macromolecules, such as biotin or antibody, they form stable biocomplexes that are useful as fluorescent probes (31,40). Since the incident energy required for excitation of phycoerythrin is the same as that of FITC they are particularly useful in two color analysis in histocytochemistry and cell suspension studies (Chapter 18).

Direct Immunofluorescence

Cryostat sections (2–4 μm) must be dry before staining or they will detach and wash away. If they are to be stained on the day of preparation they can be air dried with warm air from a hair dryer, (medium setting for 30 min) but adherence is improved by placing the air dried tissue sections in a slide box that is wrapped in aluminum foil and stored overnight at $-20°C$. The next morning the slides are removed from the freezer and air dried at room temperature for 20 to 30 min before staining. It is useful to mark around the location of small tissue sections with a diamond pencil, since it can be difficult to find the tissue after sections are coverslipped.

1. Prior to staining, it is necessary to remove unbound serum proteins, which can contribute significantly to background staining. The slides are loaded into a staining rack of a Tissue-Tek II slide staining unit, which is placed on a clinical rotator adjusted to give gentle stirring. The sections are washed for 5 minutes in 0.01 M sodium phosphate-buffered saline 0.15 M NaCl, pH 7.3 (PBS).

2. After the washing, one slide at a time is removed and blotted around the specimen to remove excess PBS. One drop (25–50 μl) of appropriately diluted fluorescein conjugate is applied to the tissue section while it is still moist. Methods for determining appropriate dilutions will be discussed in the fluorescent reagents section. The drop of conjugate should be applied immediately adjacent to the tissue section, rather than directly over the section, since this will often detach the tissue from the slide. The section should be completely covered; this is best accomplished by gently tipping the slide to one side and then the other after the drop of conjugate is pipetted. Renal and skin biopsies are routinely stained in our Immunopathology Laboratory with IgG fractions of fluoresce-

inated monospecific antisera to IgG, IgA, IgM, C3, Clq, fibrin/ogen, albumin, kappa, and lambda. Slides are incubated in a moist, level chamber for 30 min at room temperature. A single chamber large enough to accommodate the slides or several 22 mm petri dishes containing a moistened piece of filter paper can be used. It is imperative that tissue remain moistened after being hydrated.

3. After incubation, the slides are tipped to one side to allow the excess conjugate to run off.
4. The slides are washed as in Step (1) in PBS 4 times for 8 to 10 min to remove unbound fluorochrome-labeled conjugate.
5. Excess PBS is blotted from around the specimen and the moistened tissue is cover-slipped. Mounting media are described below.

Indirect Immunofluorescence

An important advantage of the indirect method is its increased sensitivity (generally $10-15 \times$), which results from amplification (18,37). An additional advantage is that it obviates the need for conjugation of the primary antibody and is thus the method of choice for the detection of antibodies in serum. The procedure is the same as in the direct method, except that the primary antibody used in step 2 is unlabeled and a step is added, in which 50 μl of FITC-labeled antibodies specific for the IgG of the primary antiserum is applied to the tissue section and incubated as with the primary unlabeled antiserum.

The standard indirect immunofluorescence technique is used routinely in our laboratory for the detection of the following circulating autoantibodies to the glomerular and tubular basement membranes (32,51), skin basement membrane and epidermal antigens (3,16, 26,27) (see Chapters 3 and 4). Similar techniques are used for ANA and other autoantibodies (Chapter 5). Complement fixation is a modification of the indirect technique performed according to (45) and used to demonstrate circulating anti-BMZ antibodies associated with herpes gestationis (8). Complement binding to the basement membrane is necessary in order to detect the presence of these low titer antibodies (29).

Mounting Medium

The simplest and most commonly used mounting preparation for immunofluorescence slides is the one described by Coons (13), 9 parts glycerol and 1 part PBS. It requires that the coverslip be immobilized, which can be accomplished by ringing the perimeter of the coverslip with nail polish or permount used for permanent mounting of histology sections.

In our experience the best mounting medium for preparations that can be stored for long periods of time is a mixture of polyvinyl alcohol-glycerol-PBS (46). This sets into a semi-solid gel and does not require immobilization of the coverslip. Polyvinyl alcohol is a water soluble resin (Monsanto, St. Louis). Available as "Gelvatol, grade 20-30," previously referred to as Elvanol (E.I. du Pont de Nemours and Company, Wilmington, DL) by Goldman (18). To prepare the medium, 20 g of Gelvatol are added to 80 ml of cold PBS, contained in 250 ml Erlenmeyer flask with a magnetic stir bar. The polyvinyl alcohol should be added while gently stirring the liquid, otherwise it will clump and be difficult to dissolve. The mixture is then heated to 70°C in a water bath until it dissolves, which usually occurs in approximately 30 to 45 min. When it is cool, 40 ml of glycerol is added. It is important to make sure the glycerol is mixed completely, because of differences in the two densities. For most purposes the pH of mounting medium should be neutral. However, the pH of mounting media can be manipulated to achieve more intense fluorescence, or to emphasize one color over another, which is particularly helpful when performing double staining. The green fluorescence of fluorescein is quenched at lower pH, that accents the visualization of the red fluorescence of rhodamine; at high alkaline pHs both fluorochromes fluoresce yellow. If slides are mounted in Gelvatol and stored at 4°C or frozen the fluorescence is preserved for at least four to eight weeks, and even longer if the staining is very intense.

Rapid fading of fluorescence after excitation is one of the most serious disadvantages of immunofluorescence techniques which limits the reexamination of slides for further interpretation, unless the initial intensity of staining is very high. Photography can be used to document results, but for careful evaluation, examination under the microscope is necessary. One means of insuring that unfaded tissue is available is to place mutiple sections on the same slide or stain sections in duplicate.

Fading is probably related to a combination of factors, including photochemical reactions, fluorochrome oxidation and the physical-chemical properties of the FITC-conjugate. Additions to the mounting medium can retard fading. Platt and Michael reported in 1983 that the addition of a reducing agent, p-phenylenediamine, to glycerol-PBS (9 : 1) prolonged fluorescence without affecting antibody binding (44). Subsequently Valnes and Brandtzaeg (50) recommended the use of Gelvatol mounting media either with p-phenylenediamine (0.2–2 g/L) or n-propyl gallate (6 g/L) for the preservation of fluorescence. The reducing agents must be added to the mounting medium just prior to coverslipping to avoid quenching, and the preparation must be examined within 2 days. If the p-phenylenediamine was added to Gelvatol and stored at 4°C before mounting it decreased the initial intensity noticeably and an even more significant reduction was seen after 8 days. If p-phenylenediamine was added to the Gelvatol ahead of time and stored at 4°C it turned brown, due to oxidation and could not be used because of significant quenching of the initial fluorescence intensity. The suggested mechanism by which these reducing agents retard fading of FITC-fluorescent preparations is suppression of photodecomposition in the excited state of the fluorochrome. Rhodamine emission does not appear to be quenched, which is an important consideration in double labeling studies.

Use of Monoclonal Antibodies with Indirect Immunofluorescence

Monoclonal antibodies have been successfully used as primary antibodies in the indirect immunofluorescence technique and have been employed to detect a variety of antigens including immunoglobulin subclasses (12), viral (11) and bacterial antigens (17). Advantages of monoclonal antibodies include the potential availability of unlimited quantities of antibody, high titer and specificity (30,35). The homogeneity of monoclonal antibody preparations makes it possible to compare reactivities between laboratories. Furthermore, monoclonal antibodies can be prepared against a range of immunogens that cannot be used successfully for the production of polyclonal antisera since many antigens cannot be prepared or purified in sufficient quantities for immunization, absorption and quality control studies. However, there are several theoretical and practical disadvantages associated with the use of monoclonal antibodies in immunochemical techniques. Paradoxically, one of the most important problems is related to the specificity of these antibodies. Conventional antisera present a mixture of antibodies with a range of affinities for several antigenic determinants on a particular molecule. On the other hand, the single antigenic determinant recognized by a monoclonal antibody can and is often denatured or destroyed by fixation, which is a frequent problem in formalin fixed tissue but not usually in frozen material. Further discussion concerning the use of monoclonal antibodies in immunohistochemistry techniques is contained in Chapter 17.

Double Staining Techniques

The codistribution of two antigens in tissue can be visualized by the use of two color fluorescence, using either double direct or indirect immunofluorescence techniques employing FITC and PE (or TRITC) labeled antisera (18,31,37,40,43). The direct method of double staining has a somewhat limited application primarily due to its low sensitivity, which is critical if either of the antigens under study is present in low concentration. It is, however, possible to amplify the reaction by using unlabeled primary antibodies and different fluorochrome-labeled secondary antibodies. The primary and secondary antibodies must be derived from different species. Biotin-Avidin-FITC conjugates can be used also (2,9,21,52) (Chapter 17). Appropriate controls are necessary to rule out cross-reactivities, and usually require that secondary labeled antibodies be cross species absorbed.

RECORDING RESULTS AND PHOTOGRAPHY

Slides should be examined preferably on the day of staining, and a detailed record of the results kept on work sheets. It is wise to run positive and negative controls with each biopsy, until one gains confidence in the specificity of staining with a given conjugated antibody. Unexpected results should be confirmed before reporting.

Photography is the only permanent record one has of the immunofluorescence findings. Black and white Tri-X (ASA 400), and high speed Ektachrome (ASA 200, 400, 800, or 1,000) for color slides are recommended. Rapid processing and "pushing" to higher ASA is available for Ektachrome film. Exposure time is determined empirically. Automatic exposure meters are generally not particularly helpful, unless they have spot metering. Average exposure times vary from 5 to 10 sec for fast (ASA 400) black and white film, and from 30 to 60 sec for (ASA 400) color film. A log book in which exposure times are recorded is useful in determining correct exposure times. Unless the fluorescence is extremely bright, it is difficult to overexpose.

PROBLEMS AND PITFALLS

Fluorescent Reagents

High background often results from antibodies that are too heavily conjugated with fluorescein (F/P molar ratio > 4); these molecules adhere nonspecifically to tissue because of their negative charge. High background staining may also be the result of partial drying of tissue sections after the staining procedure has begun. The best reagents for tissue staining are IgG fractions (of FITC- or TRITC-labeled) antisera recovered by DEAE cellulose chromatography from the sera of animals that have been immunized with highly purified immunogens (10). The reagents should contain 2 to 4 molecules of FITC per molecule of antibody protein. More highly labeled antibodies, with F/P ratios greater than 4, which can be eluted with higher ionic strength buffers, may be suitable for detecting cell surface antigens in suspension studies.

The polyclonal and monoclonal fluoresceinated IgG available from a number of commercial companies are generally satisfactory for diagnostic purposes. If conjugation is necessary, the dialysis method of Goldman (18) is recommended, since this results in low F/P ratios. Most commercial conjugates are supplied in a lyophilized form and require reconstitution with distilled water, or in diluent supplied by the manufacturer. Data from the supplier should include immunoelectrophoresis results, total protein concentration, antibody concentration and the fluorescein/protein ratio.

The undiluted stock should be divided into volumes of (0.10–0.50 ml) and stored frozen ($-20°C$) until ready to be diluted. Monoclonal antibodies are particularly sensitive to freeze-thaw denaturation and should be stored at 4°C or in aliquots at $-70°C$. Optimal dilutions of the conjugates are determined empirically using known positive and negative control. The range of working dilutions for direct immunofluorescence is usually 1 : 4– 1 : 32 or (about 40–300 μg/ml antibody protein); these diluted conjugates should be stored at 4°C with merthiolate (1 : 10,000) or sodium azide (0.02%) and not refrozen, since freezing and thawing can be detrimental to antibody activity, particularly at dilute concentrations. The range of working dilutions for indirect immunofluorescence is usually greater than with direct immunofluorescence because of an amplification effect. The correct dilution should be determined by chessboard titrations as described in Beutner (4). Conjugates should be centrifuged before using (8,000 $\times$ g for 15 min), to remove aggregates that may form as a result of storage.

Antibody Specificity

Specificity and high degree of reactivity are the two most important prerequisites of FITC-labeled antisera or antibodies used in immunofluorescence studies. Presently many commercial suppliers produce monospecific fluorochrome-labeled reagents that require no further purification or modification. However, confirmation of specificity and sensitivity is the responsibility of the user.

One method for determining the specificity of FITC-labeled reagents is by the consistency of reactivity with known positive and negative tissue controls. For example, a biopsy specimen of membranous glomerulonephritis, which has previously been shown to contain only IgG, but not IgA is very helpful in defining the specificity of a FITC-labeled anti-human IgG. Specificity can sometimes be established by blocking or absorption studies (37). To block staining, the tissue is incubated with unlabeled specific antibody prior to being incubated with the specific fluorescent antibody. Although this sometimes results in diminished fluorescence, complete prevention of staining is rarely seen. In the second approach the tissue is incubated with specific fluorescent antibody after it has been absorbed with antigen coupled to an insoluble matrix, such as cyanogen bromide activated sepharose beads (15).

Polyclonal antibody preparations usually contain unwanted specific antibodies, largely because preparations used for immunization are not usually pure; very small amounts of unwanted highly immunogenic proteins stimulate antibody production. Furthermore, even when antibodies are directed against a purified macromolecular protein, some of the reactivities may be undesirable. For example, if intact human IgG is used to immunize an animal the resultant anteserum will generally detect all classes of immunoglobulins because they share light chains. Such reactivity can be removed by absorbing the antibody with a preparation of light chains, as is done in the preparation of commercially available heavy chain specific antisera (15,37). Cross species antigenic similarity of immunoglobulin can result in problems in indirect immunofluorescence studies; for instance, goat anti-rabbit IgG may cross-react with human IgG. If, for example, one is attempting to detect human IgG in immune deposits using antibodies of rabbit and goat origin as the primary and secondary antibodies respectively, it is essential that the goat anti-rabbit IgG be absorbed with human IgG until no cross-reactivity remains (15,37). It is wise to include a control slide with deposits of IgG, which is incubated with normal rabbit serum (diluted to the same extent as the antiserum) followed by FITC labeled goat anti-rabbit antibodies IgG. Positive staining indicates that the goat antibodies have not been properly absorbed.

Frequently sera obtained from immunized animals (or even hybridoma ascites) contain antibodies to environmental antigens, or tissue antigens, in particular antinuclear and anti-smooth muscle antibodies. Many unwanted antibodies can be screened for by testing pre-immune sera in parallel studies with the FITC conjugate in question. Pre-immune sera is sometimes available from the supplier of the anti-serum. Alternatively, normal serum from the species immunized can be used. Culture supernatants of hybridomas can be checked to validate the origin of the reactivity in ascites.

Commercial suppliers of antibodies usually provide a profile of the specificity and sensitivity of the antisera. These often include the results of Ouchterlony or immunoelectrophoresis analysis (41,48). It should be noted that these techniques are not sufficiently sensitive to detect minor contaminating antibodies. The most satisfactory means of determining antibody reactivity and specificity is through the appropriate use of positive and negative tissue controls. Positive controls for immunoglobulins include touch preparations or frozen tissue sections of tonsil or small intestine. Another useful approach is to compare new and old lots of antisera with respect to their ability to detect a known antigen. Rigorous proof of antibody specificity, although often required in research applications, is usually not necessry in diagnostic studies, particularly if one has evidence of specificity of a particular reagent either by immunodiffusion or electrophoresis, and reactivity and lack of reactivity with positive and negative tissue controls respectively.

Unwanted antibodies can often be removed by incubation of the antiserum with appropriate insoluble preparations, such as tissue homogenates or washed red blood cells (37). It is important to use insoluble antigens, since soluble complexes cannot be removed effectively by centrifugation and may bind to the tissue and interfere. One of the best ways of insolubilizing proteins is to conjugate them to cyanogen bromide activated Sepharose beads (Pharmacia, Uppsala, Sweden) (15).

Evaluation of Staining Results

Tissue

The fluorescence staining should be described according to location, extent, pattern, and intensity. In the glomerulus, examples of location are mesangial or capillary wall and in the skin basement membrane zone or intraepidermal (Chapters 3 and 4). The extent of the staining should be described; this is usually expressed by the terms focal or diffuse in the case of the kidney. It may be necessary to counterstain the section with Evans blue 0.01% or stain adjacent sections with toluidine blue in order to determine the exact location of immunofluorescence staining, since morphology can be difficult to visualize. In addition to location and extent of staining, the pattern must be described. A granular pattern (see Fig. 3) is suggestive of immune complex deposition and a linear pattern (see Fig. 4) is characteristic of autoantibodies bound to basement membranes, as in anti-GBM disease or bullous pemphigoid. Intensity is assessed in a subjective manner usually on a graded scale of 0−4 +. There is often a need to compare relative intensities of staining between positive and background staining in control slides, particularly when screening for autoantibodies. Many factors affect intensity, principally antibody characteristics (dilution, avidity, F/P ratio), thickness of the section, the light path and filter system of the fluorescence microscope.

Autofluorescence, due to fluorescence found intrinsically in the tissue, is recognized usually by its color, which is generally yellow or orange with the usual FITC-filter system (blue with UV filters) and is easily distinguishable from the apple green color of fluorescein. Pigments, such as lipofuscin, are frequently responsible for autofluorescence, particularly in brain and cardiac tissue, where they usually appear as orange granules. Elastic fibers, particularly the elastic lamina of vessels, exhibit autofluorescence and can be misinterpreted as specific staining by inexperienced observers. Examination of an unstained section can be helpful in judging autofluorescence.

As already noted nonspecific fluorescence due to a nonimmunologic reaction of fluorescein conjugated antibody with the tissue is most often due to the use of FITC-labeled antibodies that are too heavily conjugated with fluorescein. Several methods can be used to remove highly charged negative molecules. The simplest involves absorption of the conjugate with tissue powder, prepared by acetone treatment and drying (37). Alternatively,

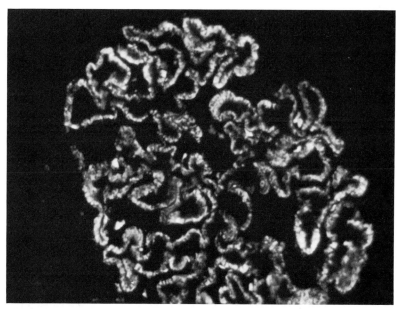

FIG. 3. Direct immunofluorescence of a frozen section of a human kidney biopsy from a patient with membranous glomerulonephritis stained with FITC-goat anti-human IgG showing granular deposits of IgG along the glomerular basement membrane (× 800).

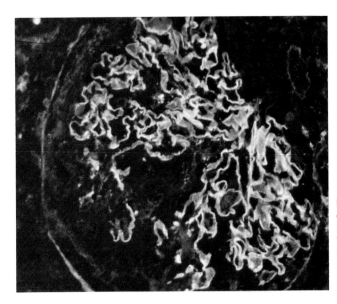

FIG. 4. Direct immunofluorescence of a frozen section of a human kidney biopsy from a patient with anti-GBM disease stained with FITC-goat anti-human IgG showing linear staining along the glomerular basement membrane (× 710).

highly conjugated molecules can be removed by anion exchange chromatography (DEAE 52) (18). Further fractionation is usually not necessary, since commercially prepared conjugates are available from a variety of sources that have been chromatographed in order to obtain fractions with F/P ratios of 2 to 4. Highly charged molecules usually precipitate in conjugates upon storage at 4°C, so that if background staining is only a marginal problem, it may disappear in time. Other methods that can be used to prevent nonspecific fluorescence include the addition of a negatively charged molecule, such as bovine serum albumin, which competes with the conjugate for binding sites in the tissue, or prestaining the tissue with a negative dye, such as Evans blue 0.01%. Usually these procedures are not necessary for diagnostic studies. Nonspecific fluorescence can also result from free fluorochrome, which can be removed by dialysis against PBS or by gel filtration using Sephadex (G-25) (18).

Another mechanism by which antibodies can bind nonspecifically to tissues or to cells in suspensions is by reaction of Fc receptors on the surface of cells or of anti IgG antibodies in immune complex deposits with the Fc portion of IgG antibody molecules, especially aggregated IgG. Aggregates can be removed by ultracentrifugation (100,000 g for 45 min). Binding by Fc receptor activity can be excluded by the use of F(ab')$_2$ or Fab fragments, both of which are available commercially for a variety of antibodies. Alternatively, these fragments can be prepared by either pepsin or papain digestion according to the method of (42). F(ab')$_2$ or Fab fragments are only occasionally required for tissue immunofluorescence studies.

Cell Suspensions

Direct or indirect immunofluorescence performed on tissue sections is usually not satisfactory for the demonstration of cell surface antigens but, such antigens can often be demonstrated in cell suspensions by fluorescence microscopy or flow cytometry (Chapter

18). The relative advantages are discussed in Chapters 10 and 18. To determine percentages of stained cells in suspensions one must be able to count negative cells, which is almost impossible to do without the aid of phase microscopy.

Dead cells take up conjugates and appear diffusely positive. Nonspecific binding of antibodies by means of Fc receptors found on B cells, K cells, NK cells and monocytes frequently accounts for nonspecific staining. This can be avoided by using $F(ab')_2$ or Fab conjugates. However, the use of these conjugates does not permit distinction between membrane Ig on B cells and endogenous IgG (which may be in the form of complexes) bound to Fc receptors. These two possibilities are distinguished by removing the IgG by trypsinization or capping, and incubating the cells in IgG free media to determine if the Ig regenerates. Mobility (patching, capping) ingestion, and shedding of conjugates can occur in living cell preparations and can be prevented by using Fab fragments, incubation at 4°C or addition of sodium azide.

REFERENCES

1. Ahmed, A. R., and Provost, T. T. (1979): Incidence of a positive lupus band test using sun-exposed and un-sun-exposed skin. *Arch. Dermatol.*, 115:228–229.
2. Berman, J. W., Basch, R. S. (1980): Amplification of the biotin-avidin immunofluorescence technique. *J. Immunol. Method*, 36:335–338.
3. Beutner, E. H., and Jordan, R. E. (1964): Demonstration of skin antibodies in sera of pemphigus vulgaris patients by indirect immunofluorescent staining. *Proc. Soc. Exp. Biol. Med.*, 117:505–510.
4. Beutner, E. H., Nisengard, R. J., and Kumar, V. (1979): Defined immunofluorescence: Basic concepts and their application to clinical immunodermatology. In: *Immunopathology in the Skin*, edited by E. H. Beutner, T. P. Chorzelski, and S. F. Bean, pp. 29–75. John Wiley & Sons, New York.
5. Beutner, E. H., Nisengard, R. J., and Albini, B., editors (1983): *Defined Immunofluorescence and Related Cytochemical Methods*. The New York Academy of Sciences, New York.
6. Briggs, W. A., Johnson, J. P., Teichman, S., Yeager, H. C., and Wilson, C. B. (1979): Antiglomerular basement membrane antibody-mediated glomerulonephritis and Goodpasture's Syndrome. *Medicine*, 58:348–353.
7. Burnham, T. K., Neblett, T. R., and Fine, G. (1963): The application of fluorescent antibody technique to the investigation of lupus erythematosus and various dermatoses. *J. Invest. Dermatol.*, 41:541–556.
8. Carruthers, J. A., Black, M. M., and Ramnarain, N. (1977): Immunopathological studies in herpes gestationis. *Br. J. Dermatol.*, 96:35–43.
9. Chaiet, L., and Wolf, F. S. (1964): The properties of streptavidin, a biotin binding protein produced by Streptomyces. *Arch. Biochem. Biophys.*, 106:1–5.
10. Chase, M. W. (1968): Production of antiserum. In: *Methods in Immunology and Immunochemistry*, Vol. 1, edited by C. A. Williams, and M. W. Chase, pp. 81–118. Academic Press, New York.
11. Collins, A. B., Bhan, A. K., Dienstag, J. L., Colvin, R. B., Haupert, G. T., Jr., Mushahwar, I. K., and McCluskey, R. T. (1983): Hepatitis B. Immune complex glomerulonephritis: Simultaneous glomerular deposition of Hepatitis B surface and e antigens. *Clin. Immunol. and Immunopathol.*, 26:137–153.
12. Conley, M. E., Cooper, M. D., and Michael, A. F. (1980): Selective deposition of immunoglobulin A_1 in immunoglobulin A nephropathy, anaphylactoid purpura and systemic lupus erythematosus. *J. Clin. Invest.*, 66:1432–1436.
13. Coons, A. H., Creech, H. J., Jones, R. N., and Berliner, E. (1942): The demonstration of pneumococcal antigen in tissues by the use of fluorescent antibody. *J. Immunol.*, 45:159–170.
14. Dahl, M. V. (1983): Usefulness of direct immunofluorescence in patients with lupus erythematosus. *Arch. Dermatol.*, 119:1010–1017.
15. Fuchs, S., and Sela, M. (1986): Immunoadsorbents. In: *Handbook of Experimental Immunology*, Vol. 1, edited by D. M. Weir, pp. 16.1–16.5. Blackwell Scientific Publications, Oxford.
16. Gammon, W. R., Briggaman, R. A., and Inman, A. O. (1984): Differentiating anti-lamina lucida and anti-sublamina densa anti-BMZ antibodies by indirect immunofluorescence on 1.0 M sodium chloride separated skin. *J. Invest. Dermatol.*, 82:139–144.
17. Gillis, T. P., and Buchanan, T. M. (1982): Production and partial characterization of monoclonal antibodies to *Mycobacterium leprae*. *Infect. Immun.*, 37:172–180.
18. Goldman, M. (1968): *Fluorescent Antibody Methods*. Academic Press, New York.
19. Grabowsky, J., and Gantt, E. (1978): Photophysical properties of phycobiliproteins from phycobilisomes: Fluorescence lifetimes, quantum yields, and polarization spectra. *Photochem. Photobiol.*, 28:39–45.

20. Harrist, T. J., and Mihm, M. C. (1979): Cutaneous immunopathology. The diagnostic use of direct and indirect immunofluorescence techniques in dermatologic disease. *Hum. Pathol.*, 10:625–653.

21. Heggeness, M. H., and Ash, J. F. (1977): Use of the avidin-biotin complex for the localization of actin and myosin with fluorescence microscopy. *J. Cell. Biol.*, 73:783–788.

22. Heptinstall, R. H., editor (1974): *Pathology of the Kidney*. Little, Brown, Boston.

23. Hijmans, W., and Schaeffer, M., editors (1975): *Fifth International Conference on Immunofluorescence and Relating Staining Techniques*. New York Academy of Science, New York.

24. Jablonska, S., Chorzelski, T. P., and Beutner, E. H. (1979): Indication for skin and serum immuno-fluorescence in dermatology. In: *Immunopathology of the Skin*, edited by E. H. Beutner, T. P. Chorzelski, and S. F. Bean, pp. 3–28. John Wiley & Sons, New York.

25. Johnson, G. D, and Holborow, E. J. (1986): Preparation and use of fluorochrome conjugates. In: *Handbook of Experimental Immunology*, Vol. 1, edited by D. M. Weir, pp. 28.1–28.15. Blackwell Scientific Publications, Oxford.

26. Jordan, R. E., Beutner, E. H., and Witebsky, E. (1967): Basement membrane zone antibodies in bullous pemphigoid. *JAMA*, 200:751–756.

27. Judd, K. P., and Lever, W. F. (1976): Correlation of antibodies in skin and serum with disease activity. *Arch. Dermatol.*, 115:428–432.

28. Karnovsky, M. J. (1965): A formaldehyde-glutaraldehyde fixation of high osmolality for use in electron microscopy. *J. Cell Biol.*, 27:137 (Abstr.).

29. Katz, S. I., Hertz, K. C., Yoaita, H. (1976): Herpes gestationis: Immunopathology and characterization of the HG factor. *J. Clin. Invest.*, 57:1434–1441.

30. Kohler, G., and Milstein, C. (1975): Continuous cultures of fused cells secreting antibody of predefined specificity. *Nature*, 256:495–497.

31. Kronick, M. N., and Grossman, P. (1983): Immunoassay techniques with fluorescent phycobiliprotein conju-gates. *Clin. Chem.*, 29:1582–1586.

32. Lerner, R. A., Glassock, R. J., and Dixon, F. J. (1967): The role of antiglomerular basement membrane antibody in pathogenesis of human glomerulonephritis. *J. Exp. Med.*, 117:989–1004.

33. McCluskey, R. T., and Bhan, A. K. (1981): Immune complexes and renal diseases. In: *Clinics in Immunol-ogy and Allergy*, edited by A. S. Fauci, pp. 397–414. W.B. Saunders, London.

34. McCluskey, R. T., and Collins, A. B. (1983): The value of immunofluorescence in the study of renal disease. In: *Defined Immunofluorescence and Related Cytochemical Methods*, edited by E. H. Beutner, R. J. Nisengard, and B. Albini, pp. 302–308. The New York Academy of Sciences, New York.

35. McMichael, A. J., and Fabre, J. W., editors (1982): *Monoclonal Antibodies in Clinical Medicine*. Academic Press, New York.

36. Michel, B., Milner, Y., and David, K. (1972): Preservation of tissue-fixed immunoglobulins in skin biop-sies of patients with lupus erythematosus and bullous diseases—preliminary report. *J. Invest. Dermatol.*, 59:449–452.

37. Nairn, R. C., editor (1976): *Fluorescent Protein Tracing*. Churchill Livingstone, Edinburgh.

38. McLean, I. W., and Nakane, P. K. (1974): Periodate-lysine-paraformaldehyde fixative. A new fixative for immunoelectron microscopy. *J. Histochem. Cytochem.*, 22:1077–1083.

39. Nisengar, R. J., Blaszczyk, M., Chorzelski, T., and Beutner, E. (1978): Immunofluorescence of biopsy specimens: Comparison of methods of transportation. *Arch. Dermatol.*, 114:1329–1332.

40. Oi, V. T., Glazer, A. N., and Stryer, L. (1982): Fluorescent phycobiliprotein conjugates for analyses of cells and molecules. *J. Cell Biol.*, 93:981–986.

41. Ouchterlony, O., and Nilsson, L. A. (1986): Immunodiffusion and immunoelectrophoresis. In: *Handbook of Experimental Immunology*, edited by D. M. Weir, Vol. 1, pp. 32.1–32.15. Blackwell Scientific Publica-tions, Oxford.

42. Parham, P. (1986): Preparation and purification of active fragments from mouse monoclonal antibodies. In: *Handbook of Experimental Immunology*, edited by D. M. Weir, Vol. 1, pp. 14.1–14.23. Blackwell Scien-tific Publications, Oxford.

43. Pizzolo, G., and Chilosi, M. (1984): Double immunostaining of lymph node sections by monoclonal anti-bodies using phycoerythrin labeling and haptenated reagents. *Am. J. Clin. Pathol.*, 82:44–47.

44. Platt, J. L., and Michael, A. F. (1983): Retardation of fading and enhancement of intensity of immuno-fluorescence by p-phenylenediamine. 31:840–842.

45. Provost, T. T., Yaoita, H., and Katz, S. I. (1979): Herpes gestationis. In: *Immunopathology of the Skin*, edited by E. H. Beutner, T. P. Chorzelski, and S. F. Bean, pp. 273–282. John Wiley & Sons, New York.

46. Rodriquez, J. E., and Deinhardt, F. (1960): Preparation of a semi-permanent mounting medium for fluores-cent antibody studies. *Virology*, 12:316–371.

47. Sainte-Marie, G. (1962): A paraffin embedding technique for studies employing immunofluorescence. *J. Histochem. Cytochem.*, 10:250–256.

48. Stites, D. P. (1982): Clinical laboratory methods for detection of antigens and antibodies. In: *Basic and Clinical Immunology*, edited by D. P. Stites, J. D. Stobo, H. H. Fudenberg, and J. V. Wells, pp. 325–365. Lange, Los Altos, CA.

49. Ploem, J. S. (1967): The use of vertical illuminator with interchangeable dichroic mirrors for fluorescent microscopy with incident light. *Z. Wiss. Mikr.*, 68:129–142.

50. Valnes, K., and Brandtzaeg, P. (1985): Retardation of immunofluorescence during microscopy. *J. Histochem. Cytochem.*, 33:755–761.

51. Wilson, C. B. (1979): Immunopathology of antibasement membrane antibodies. In: *Mechanisms of Immunopathology*, edited by S. Cohen, D. A. Ward, and R. T. McCluskey, pp. 181–201. John Wiley & Sons, New York.

52. Woods, G. S., and Warnke, R. (1981): Suppression of endogenous avidin-binding activity in tissue and its relevance to biotin-avidin detection system. *J. Histochem. Cytochem.*, 29:1196–1204.

Diagnostic Immunopathology,
edited by R.B. Colvin,
A.K. Bhan, and R.T. McCluskey.
Raven Press, New York © 1988.

17 / *Immunoperoxidase*

Atul K. Bhan

Immunopathology Unit, Department of Pathology, Massachusetts General Hospital,
Harvard Medical School, Boston, Massachusetts 02114

Immunoenzyme methods are designed to allow maximum sensitivity consistent with precise localization of antigens (68). A suitable substrate is needed for the marker enzyme to produce a visible, insoluble product at the place of antigen-antibody reaction. Horseradish peroxidase is the most widely used enzyme, and produces reaction products with colors that depend on the chromogen (19,20,22,23,29,34,68–70). Therefore, most of the description of the immunoenzyme methods will be primarily devoted to the techniques in which horseradish peroxidase is used as the marker enzyme (immunoperoxidase techniques). Glucose oxidase (66), a microbial enzyme not present in human tissues, has the disadvantage that the reaction product is not as stable or insoluble as that of peroxidase. Recently, alkaline phosphatase has become popular, especially in double staining techniques for the simultaneous demonstration of two antigens (39,42).

ANTIBODIES

The success of immunohistologic staining is primarily dependent on the specificity of the antibody (8). Most commercially available antisera also contain antibodies of different specificities which must be removed prior to the use of the antisera (Chapter 16).

Monoclonal antibodies are restricted in specificity to a single antigenic determinant (epitope) (36). Commercially available monoclonal antibodies are mostly of murine origin and are prepared by hybridizing lymphocytes from immunized mice with a murine myeloma cell line (78). Selected hybrids are re-cloned, propagated in tissue culture and injected intraperitoneally into pristane primed mice to obtain ascitic fluid as the source of monoclonal antibodies (78).

Although monoclonal antibodies have proved to be highly specific reagents in immunohistochemistry, a number of problems can be encountered with their use in tissue staining (8) and are listed below.

1. Since monoclonal antibodies, in contrast with polyclonal antibodies, recognize a limited number of epitopes, a higher level of sensitivity of detection is needed when antigens are sparsely distributed. This problem may be minimized by a mixture (cocktail) of monoclonal antibodies against different epitopes of a given antigen.
2. During tissue processing, a selective loss of epitopes on a multivalent antigen may lead to loss of binding with monoclonal antibodies but not with polyclonal antisera (48).

3. Weak staining may be due to intrinsically lower affinity of the monoclonal antibody. Monoclonals to different epitopes on the same molecule may behave better than others (e.g., anti-Leu 3a vs OKT4).
4. Sharing of antigenic determinants between two different molecules (38) can lead to reactivity of a monoclonal antibody with an unexpected antigen.
5. Monoclonal antibodies are generally more sensitive than polyclonal antisera to repeated freezing and thawing, and should be stored in small aliquots at $-70°C$ or at $4°C$.

IMMUNOENZYME TECHNIQUES

Methods Employing Antibodies Conjugated with Enzymes

Direct Method

In this technique tissue sections are reacted with antibodies conjugated with an enzyme (e.g., peroxidase), followed by incubation in a suitable substrate (1). Although this method is simple, it is rarely used because it is less sensitive than other methods, often requiring the use of a higher concentration of the antibody.

Indirect Method

The tissue sections are incubated first with a primary antibody followed by washing and incubation with a peroxidase labeled secondary antibody directed against the primary antibody. This technique is more sensitive than the direct method and allows the primary antibody to be used in higher dilutions. However, more controls are needed to confirm the specificity of staining. The controls commonly used are sections incubated with saline instead of the primary antibody or with an irrelevant antibody from the same species (or isotype matched monoclonal antibody). Other controls include preabsorption of the antibodies with the antigen under study (Chapter 16). The immunoperoxidase techniques described in the following sections are modifications of this indirect technique. In situations where the primary antibody is from the same species as the tissue to be stained, specific staining without cross-reactivity with tissue elements can be achieved by using a primary antibody labeled with a hapten (13) (such as arsenilic acid or biotin) and an anti-hapten antibody (or avidin) conjugated with peroxidase as the secondary antibody.

Methods Employing Nonlabeled Antibodies

Conjugation with enzymes may lead to denaturation of the antibody as well as inactivation of the enzyme; therefore, alternative techniques have been developed. One clever, but as yet not widely used, technique employs bispecific hybrid antibodies with anti-peroxidase activity as one of the two halves (63,68). The preparation of hybrid antibodies requires enzymatic cleavage of antibodies prior to conjugation. The technique also requires the availability of highly purified antibodies (68), and the generation of monoclonal antibodies can greatly help in this regard. Hybridization of antibodies with different specificities has also been accomplished by the fusion of two hybrid cloned cells, each capable of secreting an antibody of a different specificity (61). However, because of technical difficulties, hybrid antibodies have not been widely used for staining.

The introduction of the immunoglobulin enzyme bridge method by Mason et al. (43) and the peroxidase-antiperoxidase method by Sternberger (63,64) greatly increased the sensitivity of the immunoperoxidase methods. The immunoglobulin enzyme bridge method involves four sequential incubations: 1) a primary antibody; 2) secondary antibody against the primary antibody; 3) an anti-peroxidase antibody from the same species as the primary antibody. (An excess of secondary (bridging) antibody is needed so that the second valency of the antibody is free for binding with the anti-peroxidase antibody); 4) peroxidase.

By using pre-formed peroxidase-anti-peroxidase (PAP) complexes instead of anti-peroxidase antibody, Sternberger (64) also developed a highly sensitive technique (63) (Fig. 1). The antibodies in the PAP complexes have to be from the same species as the primary antibody. Recently, PAP complexes made with antibodies from different species, including mouse, have become available from commercial sources (41). A modification allows the method to be used for any type of PAP complexes. A secondary antibody directed against primary murine monoclonal antibody is added. The following bridging antibody is directed against immunoglobulin species of the secondary antibody and that in the PAP complexes (8–10). PAP complexes, as usually prepared, contain two molecules of antibody and three molecules of peroxidase. The complexes appear to remain stable in high dilutions (63). Jasani et al. (35) have used hapten labeled PAP complexes and anti-hapten antibodies to increase the sensitivity and specificity of the PAP method even further. Alkaline phosphatase and anti-alkaline phosphatase complexes can be used instead of PAP complexes where tissues are rich in endogenous peroxidase activity or in conjunction with immunoperoxidase techniques for double immunoenzymatic staining (17).

Peroxidase-Anti-Peroxidase (PAP) Method

As the PAP method is widely used, the staining technique will be described in detail. The steps in this method are as follows:

1. Frozen tissue sections, 4 to 5 μm thick, are placed on Histostick (Accurate Chemical, Westbury, N.Y.) coated slides and stored at $-20°$C. The sections are air dried for 20

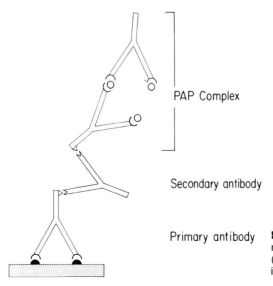

PAP Complex

Secondary antibody

Primary antibody

FIG. 1. PAP method. The basic steps in the method are: 1. primary antibody; 2. secondary (bridging) antibody; 3. peroxidase anti-peroxidase (PAP) complexes.

min on the day of staining and fixed with acetone for 10 min. In the case of formalin-fixed paraffin-embedded tissues, sections are placed on glue coated slides, deparaffinized with xylene and hydrated with graded alcohols. Fixatives used for frozen tissue sections can also be used for air dried cell smears, imprints and cytocentrifuge preparations (6,47,58).

Other fixatives can be used depending on the antigen. Optimal staining of most antigens, in formalin-fixed paraffin-embedded sections requires trypsin [(0.1% in phosphate buffered saline, pH 7.3 (PBS)] pre-treatment for 10–12 min at 37°C (after hydrating the sections). The enzyme is removed by washing the sections in water. In certain tissues such as liver and kidney, and tissues containing numerous granulocytes or erythrocytes (bone marrow), it is necessary to block endogenous peroxidase activity by treating sections with 0.3% hydrogen peroxide in PBS. This treatment may be performed before or after incubation with the primary antibody. Hydrogen peroxide in methanol can also be used to inhibit endogenous activity in situations where the antigen is not altered by treatment with methanol (68). There are other procedures for inhibiting endogenous peroxidase activity (29,68).

2. Wash the deparaffinized slides twice with PBS.
3. Incubate the sections for 10 min with 10% nonimmune serum from the same species from which the secondary antibody has been obtained. Drain off the excess serum. Do not rinse.
4. Incubate sections with an optimal dilution of primary antibody (50 to 100 μl are usually sufficient to cover the sections) for 60 min at room temperature in a moist chamber. With paraffin-embedded sections more intense staining may be obtained by overnight incubation at 4°C with the primary antibody.
5. Rinse the slides in PBS (three changes) for 5 min.
6. Incubate the sections with an optimal dilution of the secondary (bridging) antibody for 30 min at room temperature in a moist chamber.
7. Rinse the slides in PBS (three changes) for 5 min.
8. Incubate the sections with an optimal dilution of PAP soluble complexes for 45 min at room temperature in a moist chamber.
9. Rinse in PBS (three changes) for 5 min.
10. Incubate sections in a solution containing (a) 3,3′-diaminobenzidine or (b) 3-amino-9-ethyl carbazole, made as follows:

    (a) Dissolve 25 mg of diaminobenzidine in 50 ml of 0.05 M Tris saline buffer, pH 8.0 (Sigma Chemical Company, St. Louis, MO), add 25 μl of 30% hydrogen peroxide; filter the solution before use.

    (b) Dissolve 15 mg of amino-ethyl carbazole in 2.5 ml of N,N dimethylformamide, add 50 ml of 0.1 M acetate buffer, pH 5.0 (to prepare 0.1 M acetate buffer, mix seven volumes of 0.1 M sodium acetate with 3 volumes of 0.1 M acetic acid). Add 25 μl of 30% hydrogen peroxide; filter the solution before use.

    The staining should be monitored by frequent microscopic examinations of the sections. Incubation time is usually 2 to 5 min for frozen tissue sections or 4 to 10 min for paraffin-embedded sections. Since chromogens may be carcinogenic, chromogen solutions should be prepared under the hood and gloves should be worn while handling the solutions (58,72).
11. The reaction can be stopped by dipping the slides either in the staining buffer or in distilled water.
12. Counterstain as desired. In our laboratory, frozen tissue sections are stained with

amino-ethyl carbazole and counterstained with Gill's single strength hematoxylin (Lerner Lab., New Haven, CT) and coverslipped with Dako glycergel (Dako Corporation, Santa Barbara, CA). Paraffin-embedded sections are counterstained with Gill's triple strength hematoxylin. Frozen tissue sections are usually post fixed in 4% formaldehyde prior to being counterstained. Sections stained with diaminobenzidine can be counterstained either with Gill's hematoxylin, Harris Hematoxylin, periodic acid Schiff reagent (PAS) or methyl green, dehydrated in graded alcohols, cleared in xylene and coverslipped with Permount.

As the reaction product obtained with amino-ethyl carbazole is alcohol soluble, counterstains that require alcohol differentiation cannot be used with this substrate. By contrast, the reaction product obtained with diaminobenzidine is insoluble in alcohol and the brown color of the reaction product can be enhanced by treatment with nickel chloride (34) osmium tetroxide (10) or 2.0% copper sulfate in 1 N NaCl. Furthermore, the reaction product of diaminobenzidine is electron dense, allowing it be to used for immunoelectron microscopic studies (14,37,46).

Placement of sections on glue coated slides prevents the sections from floating off the slides, and is necessary when the sections are to be treated with enzymes (e.g., trypsin). Incubation of the sections with normal nonimmune serum in step 3, although not always necessary, is used to prevent nonspecific binding of primary or secondary antibodies to tissues; the immunoglobulins and other proteins in the normal serum occupy the nonspecific binding sites, including Fc receptors. It is important that the antibodies in the staining procedure do not react with any of the components of this normal serum. Optimal dilutions of primary and secondary antibodies and PAP complexes are determined by staining with serial dilutions (checkerboard titration) of the reagents. In practice, the commercially available staining kits either contain the reagents in ready to use diluted form or indicate the optimal dilutions. However, it may be necessary to vary the dilutions of the reagents to obtain the greatest intensity of specific staining with the least amount of background staining. In our experience, the red reaction product obtained from amino-ethyl carbazole is finer and more easily differentiated from the pigments present in tissues (melanin, hemosiderin), than is the brown reaction product obtained from diaminobenzidine. Other chromogens for peroxidase are 4-chloro-1-naphthol (blue reaction product) and p-phenylenediamine dihydrochloride/pyrocatechol (Hanker-Yates reagent) (dark-brown reaction product) (26). The reaction product of chloro-naphthol tends to diffuse from the reaction site and is alcohol soluble. The reaction product of Hanker-Yates reagent is insoluble in alcohol, and like the reaction product of diaminobenzidine, its intensity can be enhanced with nickel chloride (58).

Application of Protein A in Immunoperoxidase Techniques

The ability of Protein A (a 42 Kd protein derived from staphylococcus) to bind with the Fc portion of IgG from certain species has been utilized to develop sensitive and rapid immunoperoxidase techniques (23,50,56,68,71). Protein A conjugated with peroxidase can be used to bind directly with a primary or secondary antibody. It can also be used instead of a bridging antibody in the PAP method (22,68). However, the affinity of Protein A varies from species to species and also within IgG subclasses, thus restricting its widespread use. Protein A binds to human IgG in frozen tissue leading to unacceptable nonspecific staining. This background staining does not occur in paraffin-embedded sections as the Fc fragment of tissue IgG is apparently altered during tissue processing. Protein A-peroxidase complexes are considerably smaller than PAP complexes (or antibodies conjugated with peroxidase) and can better penetrate the tissue. Protein A conjugated gold particles have achieved great popularity in immunoelectron microscopy (55,56) and can be used by light microscopy (30,75). The electron dense gold particles are easily detectable and their small size allows identification of the underlying cellular structure. Simultaneous localization of two antigens can be achieved by the use of gold particles of different sizes conjugated with Protein A or immunoglobulins (55,56).

Avidin-Biotin Systems

A major advance in immunohistochemistry resulted from the application of the high affinity of avidin for biotin to link reactants in multistep staining procedures (25). Avidin, an egg white 68 Kd glycoprotein, has four binding sites for the vitamin biotin. Either avidin or biotin can be conjugated to antibodies or enzymes (as well as to other markers such as fluorescein or lectins) (31). Generally, biotin has been conjugated with antibodies and avidin has been conjugated to enzymes or used as a bridge between a biotin related antibody and a biotin related enzyme. In one technique (76), a high level of staining was achieved by incubating sections first with a primary antibody, then with sequential incubations of a biotin related secondary antibody and an avidin conjugated peroxidase. Hsu et al. (31–33) by using avidin-biotin-peroxidase complexes (ABC) instead of avidin conjugated with peroxidase, developed a very sensitive technique which allowed both primary and secondary antibodies to be used in high dilutions (Fig. 2). The ABC technique can be used as a two step method when biotinylated primary antibodies are used. The sensitivity of the technique may be due to the presence of several peroxidase molecules in the ABC complexes, and has been reported to be more sensitive than other immunoperoxidase techniques, including the PAP method. However, some investigators have not found a significant difference in the sensitivity between the ABC method and PAP method (65,68). In a recent study, the Sternbergers (65) found the PAP method more sensitive than the ABC method, which was unsuitable for distinguishing high from low concentrations of antigens. They speculated that binding of the large complex of avidin with biotin-labeled peroxidase to the antigen site may lead to steric hindrance when the antigens are densely distributed (65). This may result in a lack of increased staining with increased concentrations of the antigen. In our laboratory, the ABC method is routinely used to stain sections, and we find the method to be highly sensitive and reliable (8,14,15).

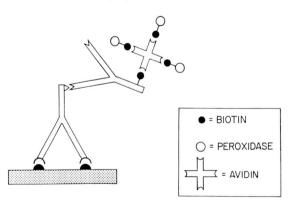

● = BIOTIN

○ = PEROXIDASE

= AVIDIN

FIG. 2. ABC Method. The basic steps in the method are: 1. primary antibody; 2. biotinylated secondary antibody; 3. avidin-biotin-peroxidase complexes.

Avidin-Biotin-Peroxidase Complex (ABC) Method

1. Prepare frozen or paraffin-embedded sections as described in the PAP method.

    (a) Deparaffinize paraffin-embedded sections and rinse in PBS for 5 min (2 changes)

    (b) Incubate the paraffin-embedded sections which need enzyme digestion in a 0.1% solution of porcine trypsin in PBS in a water bath at 37°C for 12 min. Stop the enzymatic reaction by rinsing in distilled water, then place the slides in PBS.

2. Incubate the sections (paraffin-embedded or frozen) with one or two drops of 1% normal serum (from the same species as the biotinylated secondary antibody) diluted in PBS, for 20 min in a moist chamber at room temperature. If the tissue is likely to contain endogenous biotin, add 2 drops of avidin (100 μg/ml in PBS) to the serum.

3. Drain the excess serum off the slides (do not rinse).

4. Cover the tissues with a sufficient quantity (about 50 to 100 μl) of optimally diluted primary antibody. Incubate frozen tissue sections for 60 min at room temperature. Incubate paraffin-embedded sections overnight in a moist chamber at 4°C.

5. Rinse in PBS (3 changes of 2 min each), and if necessary, proceed with blocking steps (a) or (b).

    (a) Place sections that have been incubated with avidin in a solution of biotin (1 mg/100 ml in PBS) with 0.3% hydrogen peroxide for 20 min at 37°C (add the hydrogen peroxide to the solution immediately before use).

    (b) Incubate sections of tissues which are likely to contain endogenous peroxidase activity in a 0.3% solution of hydrogen peroxide in PBS for 20 min at 37°C.

    (c) Following the above incubations (a or b) rinse the slides in PBS (3 changes of 2 min each).

6. Incubate the sections in a moist chamber with an optimal dilution of biotinylated secondary antibody (diluted in 1% bovine serum albumin in PBS) for 30 to 45 min at room temperature.

7. Rinse the sections in PBS (3 changes of 2 min each).

8. Incubate the sections in an optimal dilution of avidin-biotin-peroxidase complexes (diluted in PBS) for 60 min at room temperature.

9. Rinse the slides in PBS (3 changes of 2 min each).

10. Incubate the sections in a solution containing either (a) diaminobenzidine or (b) aminoethyl-carbazole as described in the PAP method.

11. Counterstain and mount as in the PAP method.

The presence of nonspecific staining in the ABC technique can be due to the presence of endogenous biotin in tissues (2,77) such as liver and kidney (77). Suppression of the avidin binding activity can be achieved by incubations of the sections with avidin and biotin as described in steps 2 and 5. Avidin binds with the biotin in the tissues and the extra binding sites of the avidin are then blocked by the incubation with free biotin in step 5. (As biotin has only one binding site for avidin, biotin which has interacted with tissue bound avidin cannot interact with avidin in avidin-biotin-peroxidase complexes.) Biotinylated peroxidase (5 μg/ml) and avidin (20 μg/ml) are mixed together to form complexes no more than 3 days before use, preferably on the day of staining. Recently, reagents have become available to prepare complexes of avidin and biotinylated alkaline phosphatase and ABC method staining kits are available from commercial sources (Vector Laboratories, Burlingame, CA).

Alkaline phosphatase is widely distributed in human tissues and is destroyed by routine fixation and paraffin-embedding procedures. Since the enzyme is preserved in frozen tissue sections and cell smears, endogenous alkaline phosphatase activity needs to be blocked by adding levamisole to the enzyme substrate during the staining procedure (11). Levamisole inhibits most endogenous alkaline phosphatase activity but has no effect on intestine alkaline phosphatase, which is usually used for preparation of alkaline phosphatase labeled reagents. The important causes of nonspecific staining in immunoperoxidase techniques are listed in Table 1.

DOUBLE STAINING TECHNIQUES

Studies carried out with monoclonal antibodies in the last few years have clearly established that for precise characterization of different cell types, such as functionally distinct

TABLE 1. *Common technical problems in immunoperoxidase staining*

PROBLEM A
High background staining
or
Nonspecific staining

Cause		Solution
1. Endogenous peroxidase activity	(1)	Blocking of endogenous peroxidase activity by pretreatment of sections with H_2O_2.
2. Endogenous biotin activity	(2)	Pretreatment of sections with avidin and biotin to block avidin binding sites.
3. Presence of antibodies of unwanted specificity in the antisera	(3)	(i) Absorption of antisera with unrelated antigens (tissue powders, serum proteins)
		(ii) High dilution of antisera (if nonspecific antibodies are at lower concentrations than the specific antibodies)
		(iii) Use of different batches of antisera if (i) or (ii) does not remove nonspecific reactivity.
4. Fc-receptor mediated or non-specific (charge) related binding of the specific antibody	(4)	(i) Preincubation of sections with serum from the species of the secondary (bridging) antibody
		(ii) Use of Fab or F(ab′)$_2$ fragments of the primary antibody to prevent Fc-mediated binding (usually not necessary when staining fixed tissue sections).
5. Presence of serum proteins in the stroma or in the cells due to ingestion	(5)	(i) Recognition of the problem by observing similar staining for serum protein (albumin) other than the antigen in question (immunoglobulins). Staining for IgG is often observed in the interstitium. Presence of kappa and lambda light chains in the same cells indicates either passive cellular uptake or absorption of IgG via Fc receptors.
		(ii) Sometimes the use of a less sensitive staining method (peroxidase labeled primary antibodies) may lead to decreased background staining, especially when the density of the antigen is greater in the cells than in the interstitium
6. Nonspecific binding to necrotic areas	(6)	Ignore necrotic areas while evaluating staining.
7. Nonspecific binding due to alterations of antigens during tissue processing or fixation.	(7)	(i) Select the appropriate fixative(s). (ii) Use frozen tissue sections.

PROBLEM B

Inadequate Staining

Cause	Solution
1. Alteration of the antigen by fixation	(1) (i) Pretreatment of paraffin-embedded sections with enzymes (e.g., trypsin) (caution: some antigens are destroyed by enzymatic reaction and prolonged incubation may alter most antigens).
	(ii) Prolonged (overnight) incubation with primary antibody.
	(iii) Selection of a fixative which does not cause a marked alteration of the antigen.
	(iv) Use of another source of antibody reactive with determinants not altered by fixation. If necessary use polyclonal antisera or a mixture of monoclonal antibodies rather than a single monoclonal antibody.
	(v) Use of frozen tissue sections rather than paraffin-embedded sections.
2. Low titer of primary antibody	(2) (i) Increase of primary antibody concentration.
	(ii) Use of a different batch or source of antibody.
	(iii) Application of the procedures listed above for alteration of antigens by fixatives.
3. Inadequate secondary antibody or other reagents (ABC and PAP complexes) used in staining.	3. Use of different batches or sources of the reagents (inclusion of adequate control sections can help determine this problem).
4. Diffusion of intracellular antigens	4. Prompt fixation of tissue samples or frozen tissue sections with appropriate fixatives.

lymphocyte subsets, it is essential that two or more different antigens be simultaneously demonstrated on the cells. Therefore, there is a great need to develop sensitive double immunoenzyme techniques to identify cell subsets in tissue sections.

In the past double staining has been performed primarily with immunofluorescence techniques using fluorochromes (such as fluorescein or rhodamine), to produce contrasting green and red fluorescence or more recently the phycobiliproteins (Chapter 16). The availability of different enzymes capable of producing reaction products of contrasting colors has made it possible to use immunoenzyme methods for double staining (22). For example, by using different chromogens, reaction products of brown (with 3-3-diaminobenzidine), red (with 3-amino-9-ethyl carbazole) or blue (with 4-chloro-1-naphthol) colors can be produced with horseradish peroxidase. Furthermore, by adding metallic ions ($NiCl_2$, $CoCl_2$, $CuSO_4$) to a solution containing diaminobenzidine, intensification and color modification of the reaction product can be accomplished (34). Similarly, several suitable substrates of alkaline phosphatase are available which allow development of reaction products of blue or red colors (21,39,42).

Double staining involves the incubation of a section with one set of reagents to stain for one antigen followed by incubation with a second set to stain for the other antigen (73,74).

One major problem associated with double staining is that cross-reactivity of the antibodies used for the second antigen with the first set of reagents can lead to nonspecific staining. This can be prevented either by using primary antibodies conjugated with different enzymes, haptens or biotin, or from different species. Elution of antibodies used in the first set of reactions by dissociation has not been widely used (68). The reaction product from first enzyme can lead to blocking of antigenic sites of the first set of antibodies as well as the reactive sites of the enzyme, allowing the use of the second set of reagents (16,74) without producing cross reactivity with the first set of reagents. Thus, we have been able to use murine monoclonal antibodies and ABC method to stain simultaneously two different antigens in tissue sections. This involves staining of the sections first with one monoclonal antibody employing avidin-biotin-alkaline phosphatase (Vector Laboratories) complexes to produce a blue reaction product, followed by staining with a second monoclonal antibody employing avidin-biotin-peroxidase complexes to produce a red or brown reaction product. Biotinylated horse anti-mouse antibodies (Vector) are used as secondary antibodies in both staining reactions.

A second major problem is the blocking of antibodies for the second antigen by the reaction product developed with the first enzyme (especially when the two antigens are in close proximity) (73). Double staining immunoenzyme methods have been successfully employed when the two antigens are either associated with different cell types or located in different parts of the same cell (21). However, when the two antigens are closely associated with each other, as on the cell membrane, simultaneous demonstration of the antigens by the immunoenzyme methods has been extremely difficult. This, as stated above, is due to covering of the second antigen with the reaction product obtained for staining of the first antigen. Thus, intense staining with one enzyme can obscure weak staining by the other enzyme. In situations where double staining has been successfully achieved for closely associated antigens, mixing of the two different colored reaction products has resulted in development of a new color (mixing of red and blue reaction products leads to development of a purple color) (16).

TISSUE FIXATION AND PROCESSING

Characterization of lymphoid cells by the use of monoclonal antibodies is best performed in frozen tissue sections and cell smears (6,8–10,14,27,40). Recently, a technique of tissue fixation in acetone followed by paraffin embedding has been described which allows for the detection of lymphocyte associated antigens with monoclonal antibodies (57). Monoclonal antibodies capable of reacting with T cells and B cells in routine paraffin-embedded tissue sections have become available (49,51,54). As only part of the cell membrane is available for staining in tissue sections, it is essential that highly sensitive techniques (PAP or ABC methods) be used to stain the cells. Fixation of frozen tissue sections with acetone or periodate-lysine-paraformaldehyde generally yields better results than frozen sections stained after no fixation (8). Frozen tissue sections should also be employed in situations where there is poor preservation of antigens in paraffin-embedded sections. Tissues to be transported for immunohistochemical studies can be frozen in O.C.T. compound (Ames, divison of Miles Laboratories, Inc., Elkhart, IN) and sent to the laboratory in dry ice. Tissues can be also sent without freezing in transport medium (24). However adequate preservation of the antigen may not always be obtained by placing the tissue in transport medium (58) and, therefore, it is not recommended for routine use.

The application of immunohistochemical techniques is greatly influenced by the fixatives routinely used for histopathologic diagnosis (52). Small antigens (peptide hormones) can be best immobilized by fixatives capable of forming cross-linkages (formaldehyde, glutaraldehyde, carbodiimide) (12). Extensive cross-linking of proteins in high concentrations can also lead to the masking or destruction of antigens. Buffered 10% formalin is the fixative commonly used for tissue samples in routine diagnostic pathology. Fortunately, a large number of antigens survive treatment with formalin (52, Chapter 8). Prolonged storage of tissue in formalin, however, may lead to a loss of antigenicity (4).

The loss of staining in formalin-fixed tissue can be restored to a certain extent by pretreatment of tissue sections with enzymes (trypsin, pepsin, pronase, papain) (28,59). The exact mechanism of this unmasking of antigens by enzymes is not clear but may be due to dissociation of cross linkages of proteins produced by fixation, leading to the revealing of the antigenic sites. In a study of the effect of protease digestion and fixation on the staining for keratin by Battifora and Kopinski (4), formalin fixed tissues showed weak or no staining for keratin unless tissue sections were treated with proteolytic enzymes. In contrast, there was excellent staining for keratin in ethanol-fixed tissues and pretreatment of tissue sections with enzymes did not lead to improvement of staining but caused rapid tissue disintegration (4).

The optimal duration of proteolysis in formalin-fixed tissues was found to be generally related to the degree of fixation with tissues fixed for weeks in formalin requiring prolonged treatment with enzymes (4). Tissues fixed for less than 24 hr in formalin, like alcohol fixed tissues, were more susceptible to overdigestion of enzymes than tissues fixed for a prolonged period. Different lots of the same enzyme (trypsin) can vary in their ability to increase staining for keratin (53). Recently Shintaku and Said (60) have demonstrated that pretreatment of formalin-fixed paraffin embedded sections with DNase can lead to exposure of antigen associated with estrogen receptors in routinely processed tissues. Since demonstration of some antigens may not be increased by enzymatic treatment of tissue sections, it is wise not to use enzymes indiscriminately for the detection of an antigen whose sensitivity to the enzymes has not been established. In fact some antigens may be susceptible to the enzymatic reaction, leading to the loss of antigenic determinants. In our experience trypsin treatment of formalin-fixed paraffin-embedded sections leads to the loss of reactivity with commercially available antibodies to vimentin and actin. Enzymatic treatment of sections can lead to the loss of sections from slides; this annoying problem can be prevented by placing the sections on glue coated slides.

The staining of cytoplasmic immunoglobulins in paraffin-embedded sections is optimal in tissue samples fixed in mercuric chloride fixatives such as B5 or Zenker's (formalin and mercuric chloride) (5). These fixatives preserve morphologic details better than formalin and often need shorter fixation time (less than four hr). Sections fixed in B5 do not need enzyme treatment prior to the immunoperoxidase staining (18). One problem associated with mercury containing fixatives is the development of black precipitates of mercury in the tissues. These can be removed by treating the sections with 0.5% iodine in 80% alcohol for 1 min, rinsing in distilled water, incubating in a 5% sodium thiosulphate bath for 1 min and rinsing again in distilled water. This procedure is performed in our laboratory following the deparaffinization of tissue sections. Carnoy's fixative (alcohol, formalin and acetic acid) has been reported to be the fixative of choice for certain antigens such as intermediate filament proteins and lactoferrin (68). Similarly, peptide hormones appear to be well preserved in picric acid containing fixatives (Bouin's and Zamboni's fixatives). Bouin's fixative has also been reported to allow better demonstration of intracellular immunoglobulins.

Fixatives such as paraformaldehyde and periodate-lysine-paraformaldehyde (45) have been used for immunoelectron microscopy, as these fixatives allow adequate preservation of ultrastructural features without substantial loss of reactivity of most antigens with antibodies (14,46). The embedding procedures employed in immunoelectron microscopy have also been used to obtain one micron thick sections for immunoenzyme staining (7). This permits better demonstration of morphologic details of stained cells than has been observed with frozen tissue or paraffin-embedded sections (7).

It is important to note that prolonged fixation in any fixative will lead to progressive denaturation of the antigen. Therefore, the tissues should be fixed for the minimal period necessary for adequate preservation of morphologic details. The size of the tissue sample can also influence the duration of the fixation time. In a large tissue sample, inadequate fixation can lead to the preservation of morphologic details and antigens at the periphery but loss of morphologic details and antigens at the center, whereas prolonged fixation may lead to the loss of antigens at the periphery but preservation of antigen reactivity at the center.

Although the effect of embedding media and other steps involved in tissue processing have not been clearly defined yet, studies so far indicate that the loss of antigenic reactivity in paraffin-embedded sections can be mostly attributed to tissue fixation and dehydration (68). By using freeze dried unfixed tissue, Stein et al. (62) were able to demonstrate reactivity with monoclonal antibodies to lymphocyte associated antigens in paraffin-embedded sections. Furthermore, the antigens in freeze dried paraffin-embedded sections were resistant to fixatives which would cause their rapid destruction in frozen tissue sections (62). Xylene, which is used routinely in the preparation of paraffin-embedded sections, may also have a deleterious effect on tissue antigens (44). High melting point embedding media should be avoided because high temperatures may lead to antigenic denaturation (58). Some decalcification procedures also severely affect the antigenicity of many molecules (68).

CONCLUSIONS

Immunoenzyme techniques have become essential tools in routine diagnostic pathology and have replaced many special stains used for the demonstration of specific cell products. However, it is unlikely that in the immediate future the methods used for tissue processing are going to be radically changed to allow optimal preservation of antigens for immunohistochemical studies. In fact, immunohistochemical studies are often performed on tissue samples which have been either over-fixed or fixed with fixatives which do not allow optimal preservation of the antigen. Therefore, it is essential that adequate controls be included during immunohistochemical staining. The most reliable control under these circumstances is the presence of positive reactivity with cells which contain the antigen in question and lack of reactivity with cells which do not express the antigen.

Recently, Battifora (3) has described a method of embedding 100 or more different tissue samples in a normal sized paraffin block. This allows simultaneous immunohistologic testing of numerous tissues with a broad range of antigen densities and tissues fixed with different fixatives (3). Although enzymatic treatment of sections, in particular formalin-fixed paraffin-embedded sections, allows for the restoration of antigenic reactivity in many instances, the results of proteolytic digestion may be variable, not only for different antigens but also for the same antigen.

Whenever possible, attempts should be made to freeze a sample of the speciman in case the antigen to be studied is not preserved by the tissue processing used in the laboratory. Traditionally, tissue samples from organs such as kidney and skin are routinely frozen, especially when immunohistochemical studies are expected to be performed. The recent application of monoclonal antibodies against lymphocyte associated antigens in the diagnosis of lymphoproliferative disorders has made it necessary to routinely freeze tissues for immunohistochemic ' studies in situations where staining for lymphoid markers needs to be performed (Chapter 11).

The selection of an immunoenzyme technique is largely dependent upon the amplification of staining necessary for the demonstration of the antigen in question and the experience of the laboratory in using various immunoenzyme techniques. The PAP method and the ABC method have become the most popular immunoenzyme methods in diagnostic pathology. The great sensitivity of these techniques allows the antisera to be used in high dilutions leading to the elimination of staining due to the presence of nonspecific antibodies that are present in low concentrations in the antiserum. Swanson et al. (67) have combined the PAP and ABC methods to develop a more sensitive method, which can help in the visualization of antigens when the ABC and PAP methods yield suboptimal results. However, augmentation of sensitivity may be associated with increased nonspecific background staining. We have found the commercially available staining kits for the ABC method to be highly reliable and easy to use for both diagnostic and research purposes. Recently, immunogold-silver techniques have been used for the detection of antigens in tissue sections by light microscopy without the use of enzyme conjugated reagents (30,75). These techniques along with immunoenzyme methods are likely to be useful in double staining for the simultaneous detection of more than one antigen.

ACKNOWLEDGMENT

The expert technical assistance of Mr. Bruce Kaynor and Ms. Kathleen Bain is gratefully acknowledged.

REFERENCES

1. Avrameas, S. (1969): Coupling of enzymes to proteins with glutaraldehyde. Use of conjugates for the detection of antigens and antibodies. *Immunochemistry*, 6:43–52.
2. Banerjee, D., and Pettit, S. (1984): Endogenous avidin-binding activity in human lymphoid tissue. *J. Clin. Pathol.*, 37:223–225.
3. Battifora, H. (1986): The multitumor (sausage) tissue block: Novel method for immunohistochemical antibody testing. *Lab. Invest.*, 55:244–248.
4. Battifora, H., and Kopinski, M. (1986): The influence of protease digestion and duration of fixation on the immunostaining of keratins. A comparison of formalin and ethanol fixation. *J. Histochem. Cytochem.*, 34:1095–1100.
5. Banks, P. M. (1979): Diagnostic applications of an immunoperoxidase method in hematopathology. *J. Histochem. Cytochem.*, 27:1192–1194.
6. Banks, P. M., Caron, B. L., and Morgan, T. W. (1983): Use of imprints for monoclonal antibody studies. Suitability of air dried preparations from lymphoid tissue with an immunochemical method. *Am. J. Clin. Pathol.*, 79:438–442.
7. Beckstead, J. H. (1985): Optimal antigen localization in human tissues using aldehyde-fixed plastic-embedded sections. *J. Histochem. Cytochem.*, 33:954–958.
8. Bhan, A. K. (1984): Application of monoclonal antibodies to tissue diagnosis. In: *Advances in Immunohistochemistry*, edited by R. A. DeLellis, pp. 1–29. Masson Publishing, New York.
9. Bhan, A. K., Reinherz, E. L., Poppema, S., McCluskey, R. T., and Schlossman, S. F. (1980): Location of T-cell and major histocompatibility complex antigens in the human thymus. *J. Exp. Med.*, 152:771–782.
10. Bhan, A. K., Nadler, L. M., Stashenko, P., McCluskey, R. T., and Schlossman, S. F. (1981): Stages of B-cell differentiation in human lymphoid tissues. *J. Exp. Med.*, 154:737–749.
11. Borges, M. (1973): The cytochemical application of new potent inhibitors of alkaline phosphatases. *J. Histochem. Cytochem.*, 21:812–824.

12. Brandtzaeg, P. (1982): Tissue preparation methods for immunocytochemistry. In: *Techniques in Immunochemistry*, Vol. I, edited by G. R. Bullock and P. Petrusz, pp. 1–76. Academic Press, Inc., New York.

13. Cammisuli, S. (1981): Hapten-modified antibodies specific for cell surface antigens as a tool in cellular immunology. In: *Immunological Methods*, Vol. 2, edited by I. Lefkovits and B. Permis, pp. 139–162. Academic Press, Inc., New York.

14. Cerf-Bensussan, N., Schneeberger, E. E., and Bhan, A. K. (1983): Immunohistologic and immunoelectron microscopic characterization of the mucosal lymphocytes of human small intestine by the use of monoclonal antibodies. *J. Immunol.*, 130:2615–2622.

15. Charpin, C., Bhan, A. K., Zurawski, V. R., Jr., and Scully, R. E. (1982): Carcinoembryonic antigen (CEA) and carbohydrate determinant 19-9 (CA 19-9) localization in 121 primary and metastatic ovarian tumors. An immunohistochemical study with the use of monoclonal antibodies. *Int. J. Gynecol. Pathol.*, 1:231–245.

16. Chen, K., Demetris, A. J., Van Thiel, D. H., and Whiteside, T. C. (1987): Double immunoenzyme staining method for analysis of tissue and blood lymphocyte subsets with monoclonal antibodies. *Lab. Invest.*, 56:114–119.

17. Cordell, J. L., Falini, B., Erber, W. N., Ghosh, A. K., Abdulaziz, Z., MacDonald, S., Pulford, K. A., Stein, H., and Mason, D. Y. (1984): Immunoenzymatic labeling of monoclonal antibodies using immune complexes of alkaline phosphatase and monoclonal anti-alkaline phosphatase (APAAP complexes). *J. Histochem. Cytochem.*, 32:219–229.

18. Curran, R. C., and Gregory, J. (1978): Effects of fixation and processing on immunohistochemical demonstration of immunoglobulin in paraffin sections of tonsil and bone marrow. *J. Clin. Pathol.*, 33:1047–1057.

19. DeLellis, R. A. (1981): Basic techniques in immunohistochemistry. In: *Diagnostic Immunohistochemistry*, edited by R. A. DeLellis, pp. 7–16. Masson Publishing Inc., New York.

20. DeLellis, R. A., Sternberger, L. A., Mann, R. B., Banks, P. M., and Nakane, P. K. (1979): Immunoperoxidase technics in diagnostic pathology. Report of a workshop sponsored by the National Cancer Institute. *Am. J. Clin. Pathol.*, 71:483–488.

21. Falini, B., De Solas, I., Halverson, C., Parker, J. W., and Taylor, C. R. (1982): Double labeled-antigen method for demonstration of intracellular antigens in paraffin-embedded tissues. *J. Histochem. Cytochem.*, 30:21–26.

22. Falini, B., and Taylor, C. R. (1983): New developments in immunoperoxidase techniques and their application. *Arch. Pathol. Lab. Med.*, 107:105–117.

23. Farr, A. G., and Nakane, P. K. (1981): Immunohistochemistry with enzyme labelled antibodies. A brief review. *J. Immunol. Method.*, 47:129–144.

24. Giorno, R. (1982): Evaluation of a tissue transport medium for immunological characterization of benign and malignant lymphoid tissues. *Am. J. Clin. Pathol.*, 78:8–13.

25. Guesdon, J. L., Ternynck, T., and Avrameas, S. (1979): The use of avidin-biotin interaction in immunoenzymatic techniques. *J. Histochem. Cytochem.*, 27:1131–1139.

26. Hanker, J. S., Yates, P. E., Metz, C. B., and Rushoni, A. (1977): A new specific sensitive and non-carcinogenic reagent for the demonstration of horseradish peroxidase. *Histochem. J.*, 9:789–792.

27. Harris, N. L., Poppema, S., and Data, R. E. (1982): Demonstration of immunoglobulin in malignant lymphomas: Use of an immunoperoxidase technique on frozen sections. *Am. J. Clin. Pathol.*, 78:14–21.

28. Hautzer, N. W., Wittkauhn, J. F., and McCaughey, W. T. (1980): Trypsin digestion in immunoperoxidase staining. *J. Histochem. Cytochem.*, 28:52–60.

29. Heyderman, E. (1979): Immunoperoxidase technique in histopathology: Applications, methods and controls. *J. Clin. Pathol.*, 32:971–978.

30. Holgate, C. S., Jackson, P., Cowen, P. N., and Bird, C. C. (1983): Immunogold-silver staining. A new method of immunostaining with enhanced sensitivity. *J. Histochem. Cytochem.*, 31:936–944.

31. Hsu, S. M., Raine, L. (1984): The use of avidin-biotin-peroxidase complex (ABC) in diagnostic and research pathology. In: *Advances in Immunohistochemistry*, edited by R. A. DeLellis, pp. 31–42. Masson Publishing Inc., New York.

32. Hsu, S. M., Raine, L., and Fanger, H. (1981): Use of avidin-biotin-peroxidase complex (ABC) in immunoperoxidase techniques: A comparison of ABC and unlabeled antibody (PAP) procedure. *J. Histochem. Cytochem.*, 29:577–584.

33. Hsu, S. M., Raine, L., and Fanger, H. (1981): A comparative study of the peroxidase-antiperoxidase method and an avidin-biotin complex method for studying polypeptide hormones with radioimmunoassay antibodies. *Am. J. Clin. Pathol.*, 75:734–738.

34. Hsu, S. M., and Soban, E. (1982): Color modification of diaminobenzidine (DAB) precipitation by metallic ions and its application for double immunohistochemistry. *J. Histochem. Cytochem.*, 30:1079–1082.

35. Jasani, B., Wynford, T. D., and Williams, E. D. (1981): Use of monoclonal antihapten antibodies for immunolocalization of tissue antigens. *J. Clin. Pathol.*, 34:1000–1002.

36. Kohler, G., and Milstein, C. (1975): Continuous cultures of fused cells secreting antibody of predefined specificity. *Nature*, 256:495–497.

37. Kuhlmann, W. D., and Peschke, P. (1982): Advances in ultrastructural postembedment localization of antigens in Epon sections with peroxidase-labelled antibodies. *Histochemistry*, 75:151–161.

38. Lafer, E. M., Rauch, L., Andrezejewski, C., Jr., Mudd, D., Furie, B., Furie, B., Schwartz, R. S., and

Stollar, B. D. (1981): Polyspecific monoclonal lupus autoantibodies reactive with both polynucleotides and phospholipids. *J. Exp. Med.*, 153:897–909.

39. Mason, D. Y., Abdulaziz, Z., and Falini, B. (1983): Single and double immunoenzymatic techniques for labeling tissue sections with monoclonal antibodies. *Ann. N.Y. Acad. Sci.*, 420:127–133.
40. Mason, D. Y., and Biberfeld, P. (1980): Technical aspects of lymphoma immunohistology. *J. Histochem. Cytochem.*, 28:731–745.
41. Mason, D. Y., Cordell, J. L., Abdulaziz, Z., Naiem, M., and Bordenave, G. (1982): Preparation of peroxidase antiperoxidase (PAP) complexes for immunohistological labeling of monoclonal antibodies. *J. Histochem. Cytochem.*, 30:1114–1122.
42. Mason, D. Y., and Woolston, R. E. (1982): Double immunoenzymatic labelling. In: *Techniques in Immunocytochemistry*, Vol. 1, edited by G. R. Bullock and P. Petruzz, pp. 135–153. Academic Press, New York.
43. Mason, T. E., Phifer, R. F., Spicer, S. S., Swallow, R. A., and Dreskin, R. B. (1969): An immunoglobulin-enzyme bridge method for localizing tissue antigens. *J. Histochem. Cytochem.*, 17:563–569.
44. Matthews, J. B. (1981): Influence of clearing agent on immunohistochemical staining of paraffin-embedded tissue. *J. Clin. Pathol.*, 34:103–105.
45. McLean, I. W., and Nakane, P. K. (1974): Periodate-lysine-paraformaldehyde fixative. A new fixative for immunoelectron microscopy. *J. Histochem. Cytochem.*, 22:1077–1083.
46. Murphy, G. F., Harrist, T. J., Bhan, A. K., and Mihm, M. C., Jr. (1983): Distribution of cell-surface antigens in histiocytosis X cells. Quantitative immunoelectron microscopy using monoclonal antibodies. *Lab. Invest.*, 48:90–97.
47. Nadji, M. (1980): The potential value of immunoperoxidase techniques in diagnostic cytology. *Acta Cytol.*, 24:442–447.
48. Naritoku, W. Y., and Taylor, C. R. (1982): A comparative study of the use of monoclonal antibodies using three different immunohistochemical methods: An evaluation of monoclonal and polyclonal antibodies against human prostatic acid phosphatase. *J. Histochem. Cytochem.*, 30:253–260.
49. Norton, A. J., Ramsay, A. D., Smith, S. H., Beverley, P. C., and Isaacson, P. G. (1986): Monoclonal antibody (UCHL1) that recognizes normal and neoplastic T cell in routinely fixed tissues. *J. Clin. Pathol.*, 39:399–405.
50. Notani, G. W., Parson, J. A., Erlandsen, S. L. (1979): Versatility of staphylococcus aureus Protein A in immunocytochemistry. Use of unlabeled antibody enzyme system and fluorescent methods. *J. Histochem. Cytochem.*, 27:1438–1444.
51. Okon, E., Felder, B., Epstein, A., Lukes, R. J., and Taylor, C. R. (1985): Monoclonal antibodies reactive with B-lymphocytes and histiocytes in paraffin sections. *Cancer*, 56:95–104.
52. Pinkus, G. S. (1982): Diagnostic immunocytochemistry of paraffin-embedded tissues. *Hum. Pathol.*, 13: 411–415.
53. Pinkus, S. P., O'Connor, E. M., Elheridge, L. L., and Corson, J. M. (1985): Optimal immunoreactivity of keratin proteins in formalin-fixed, paraffin-embedded tissue requires preliminary trypsinization. An immunoperoxidase study of various tumors using polyclonal and monoclonal antibodies. *J. Histochem. Cytochem.*, 33:465–473.
54. Poppema, S., Hollema, H., Visser, L., and Vos, H. (1987): Monoclonal antibodies (MT1, MT2, MB1, MB2, MB3) reactive with leukocyte subsets in paraffin embedded sections. *Am. J. Pathol.*, 127:418–429.
55. Roth, J. (1984): Light and electron-microscopic localization of antigens with the protein A-gold (pAg) technique. In: *Advances in Immunohistochemistry*, edited by R. A. DeLellis, pp. 43–65. Masson Publishing U.S.A., Inc., New York.
56. Roth, J. (1986): Post embedding cytochemistry with gold-labelled reagents: A review. *J. Microscopy*, 143: 125–137.
57. Sato, Y., Mukai, K., Watanabe, S., Goto, M., and Shimosato, Y. (1986): The AMEX method. A simplified technique of tissue processing and paraffin embedding with improved preservation of antigens for immunostaining. *Am. J. Pathol.*, 125:431–435.
58. Sheibani, K., and Tubbs, R. R. (1984): Enzymes immunohistochemistry. Technical aspects. *Sem. Diagnost. Pathol.*, 4:235–249.
59. Shinshi, J., Ghazizadeh, M., Ogura, T., Aihara, K., and Araki, T. (1986): Immunohistochemical localization of CA 125 antigen in formalin-fixed paraffin sections of ovarian tumors with use of Pronase. *Am. J. Clin. Pathol.*, 85:595–598.
60. Shintaku, I. P., and Said, J. W. (1987): Detection of estrogen receptor with monoclonal antibodies in routinely processed formalin-fixed paraffin sections of breast carcinoma. Use of DNase pretreatment to enhance sensitivity of the reaction. *Am. J. Clin. Pathol.*, 87:161–167.
61. Staerz, U. D., and Bevan, M. J. (1986): Hybrid hybridoma producing a bispecific monoclonal antibody that can focus effector T-cell activity. *Proc. Natl. Acad. Sci. U.S.A.*, 83:1453–1457.
62. Stein, H., Gatter, K., Asbahr, H., and Mason, D. Y. (1985): Use of freeze-dried paraffin-embedded sections for immunohistologic staining with monoclonal antibodies. *Lab. Invest.*, 52:676–683.
63. Sternberger, L. A. (1979): *Immunocytochemistry*, 2nd Ed. John Wiley & Sons, New York.
64. Sternberger, L. A., Hardy, P. H., Jr., Cuculis, J. J., and Meyer, H. G. (1970): The unlabeled antibody enzyme method of immunohistochemistry. Preparation and properties of soluble antigen-antibody

complex (horseradish peroxidase-antihorseradish peroxidase) and its use in the identification of spirochetes. *J. Histochem. Cytochem.*, 18:315–333.

65. Sternberger, N. H., and Sternberger, L. A. (1986): The unlabelled antibody method. Comparison of peroxidase-antiperoxidase with avidin-biotin complex by a new method of quantification. *J. Histochem. Cytochem.*, 34:599–605.

66. Suffin, S. C., Muck, K. B., Young, J. C., Klaus, L., and Porter, D. D. (1979): Improvement of the glucose oxidase immunoenzyme technic. Use of tetrazolium whose formazan is stable without heavy metal chelation. *Am. J. Clin. Pathol.*, 71:492–496.

67. Swanson, P. E., Hagen, K. A, and Wick, M. R. (1987): Avidin-biotin-peroxidase-antiperoxidase (ABPAP) complex. An immunocytochemical method with enhanced sensitivity. *Am. J. Clin. Pathol.*, 88:162–176.

68. Taylor, C. R. (1986): *Immunomicroscopy: A Diagnostic Tool for the Surgical Pathologist.* W.B. Saunders Company, Philadelphia.

69. Taylor, C. R. (1978): Immunoperoxidase techniques. Practical and theoretical aspects. *Arch. Pathol. Lab. Med.*, 102:113–121.

70. Trojanowski, J. Q., Obrocka, M. A., and Lee, V. M. (1983): A comparison of eight different chromogen protocols for the demonstration of immunoreactive neurofilaments or glial filaments in rat cerebellum using the peroxidase-antiperoxidase method and monoclonal antibodies. *J. Histochem. Cytochem.*, 31:1217–1223.

71. Trost, T. H., Steigleder, G. K., and Bodeux, E. (1980): Immuno-electron microscopical investigations with a new tracer: Peroxidase-labeled protein A. Application for detection of pemphigus and bullous pemphigoid antibodies. *J. Invest. Dermatol.*, 75:328–330.

72. Tubbs, R. R., and Sheibani, K. (1982): Chromogens for immunohistochemistry. *Arch. Pathol. Lab. Med.* (Letter), 106:205.

73. Valnes, K., and Brandtzaeg, P. (1982): Comparison of paired immunofluorescence and paired immunoenzyme staining methods based on primary antisera from the same species. *J. Histochem. Cytochem.*, 30:518–524.

74. Valnes, K., and Brandtzaeg, P. (1984): Paired indirect immunoenzyme staining with primary antibodies from the same species. Application of horseradish peroxidase and alkaline phosphatase as sequential labels. *Histochem. J.*, 16:477–487.

75. Waele, M. D., Mey, J. D., Reynaert, P., Dehou, M-F., Gepts, W., and Camp. B. V. (1986): Detection of cell surface antigens in cryostat sections with immunogold-silver staining. *Am. J. Clin. Pathol.*, 85:573–578.

76. Warnke, R., and Levy, R. (1980): Detection of T and B cell antigens hybridoma monoclonal antibodies: A biotin-avidin-horseradish peroxidase method. *J. Histochem. Cytochem.*, 28:771–776.

77. Wood, G. S., and Warnke, R. (1981): Suppression of endogenous avidin-binding activity in tissues and its relevance to biotin-avidin detection system. *J. Histochem. Cytochem.*, 29:1196–1204.

78. Zola, H., and Brooks, D. (1982): Techniques for the production and characterization of monoclonal hybridoma antibodies. In: *Monoclonal Hybridoma Antibodies: Techniques and Applications*, edited by J. G. R. Hurrell, pp. 1–58. CRC Press, Inc., Boca Raton, Florida.

Diagnostic Immunopathology,
edited by R.B. Colvin,
A.K. Bhan, and R.T. McCluskey.
Raven Press, New York © 1988.

18 / *Flow Cytometry*

Frederic I. Preffer

Department of Pathology, Massachusetts General Hospital, Harvard Medical School,
Boston, Massachusetts 02114

Flow cytometry has emerged from the research laboratory to play an increasingly important role in diagnostic pathology. Flow cytometry offers the ability to examine rapidly thousands of cells stained with monoclonal antibodies conjugated with fluorescent dyes. Each cell is individually assessed for a variety of characteristics such as size, shape and biochemical or antigenic composition. The limit of detectable fluorescence can be as little as 130 molecules of free fluorescein (117). High precision and sensitivity, combined with the large numbers of cells that can be examined, allow resolution of even minor subpopulations from complex mixtures with high levels of statistical validity. The ability to separate physically these populations by flow sorting allows further functional and morphologic correlations based on the detected markers. Material may be stained either when fresh, or after storage as frozen or paraffin embedded tissue (37).

Until recently, the initial cost and maintenance of flow cytometers limited their practical application. Fortunately, advances in computer, software and laser based technologies has permitted the introduction of multiparametric non-sorting analyzers from both Becton-Dickinson (FACScan) and Coulter (EPICS Profile) that specifically address the needs of modern clinical laboratories in their automation, high throughput, ease of operation, and initial "low" cost ($80,000) and upkeep. These instruments and their successors should have a major impact on the inclusion of flow cytometry in pathology laboratories in the detection of multiple lymphocyte markers, cell cycle analysis, reticulocyte counts and possibly the detection of oncoproteins.

The identification and enumeration of lymphocytes in peripheral blood has already proven useful in organ and bone marrow transplantation (17,18,21,106), and in detecting (88,94) and characterizing leukemias (Chapter 10), non-Hodgkin's lymphoma (Chapter 11), autoimmune and immunodeficiency diseases (Chapter 6) (8,31,64,102). Direct staining of cellular DNA and RNA is also possible, and has been shown to have prognostic significance in detecting and evaluating ploidy abnormalities in human neoplasms (6). Flow karyotyping (57,65), oncogene detection (2,115), nuclear antigen analysis (15) and the detection of genetic abnormalities (9) is now at the research stage.

In this chapter, a brief overview of the principles of cytometry is presented, along with practical information concerning multi-color surface and nucleic acid staining techniques. Selected new developments in flow cytometry that may aid diagnostic pathology in the future are also mentioned.

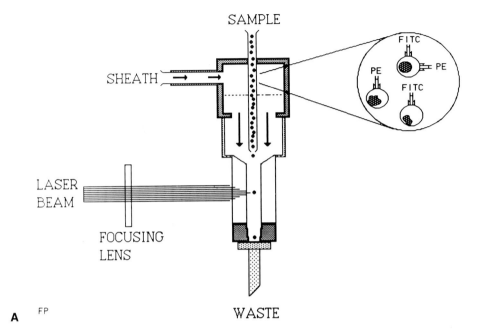

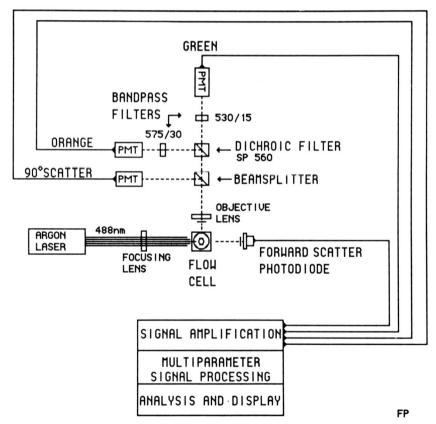

FIG. 1. General features of a flow cytometer.

PRINCIPLES AND INSTRUMENTATION OF FLOW CYTOMETRY

Signal Generation

The principles of flow cytometric analysis are illustrated in a model two-color system (Fig. 1A). A suspension of cells stained with two monoclonal antibodies conjugated with either a green or orange emitting fluorescent dye is coaxially introduced (1 mm/sec) into the laminar flow of a confining sheath fluid within the flow cell of a cytometer, a process referred to as hydrodynamic focusing. The rapidly moving sheath (10 m/sec) separates cells and ensures individual and uniform interrogation by the precisely focused laser light source (74).

The presence of a cell in the path of the laser scatters light in all directions and excites the fluorescent dyes conjugated to the monoclonal antibodies bound to the cell. Light scattered in the orthogonal, or forward direction ($2°$ to $13°$ relative to the path of the laser) is mostly due to diffraction, correlates with cell volume, and is useful in distinguishing a viable cell population from dead cells (77). Light scattered at right angles (side, or $90°$ scatter) is related more to refraction, and correlates with internal cellular structure. A correlated measurement of forward and side scatter can resolve red cells, lymphocytes, monocytes and granulocytes from whole blood (95,96).

Light is also blocked by a cell in the path of the laser beam ($0°$), a process referred to as axial light extinction. The measure of this light loss, in comparison to a standard particle, can give information about cellular cross-sectional area independent of light scatter measurements (103). A Coulter volume measurement (22) may also be taken instead of (or in addition to) a forward angle scatter or axial extinction measurement. Other measures include fluorescence polarization, which detects changes in macromolecular conformation of the plasma membrane in early stages of cell activation (92), and slit-scan or "time-of-flight" measurements, in which the times the cytoplasm and the nucleus of a cell take to pass in and out of the laser beam are measured. Time-of-flight measures have been used to determine cellular nuclear to cytoplasmic size ratios (118) and chromosomal centromeric indices (66).

Signal Detection, Processing and Representation

Light Scatter Detection

Forward light scatter is collected by a light sensitive diode and converted into electronic signals. These signals are commonly used to initiate, or "trigger", related right angle and fluorescence analysis. Alternatively, the cytometer can be set to trigger analysis on the basis of fluorescence. This is useful for multi-color (> 2) analysis, or the cell-cycle analysis of rare nucleated cells in hemorrhagic effusions.

A microscope objective mounted at right angles to both the moving stream and the laser collects right angle scatter and the fluorescent emissions of the dyes conjugated to the antibodies. These are directed to individual photomultiplier tubes (PMTs). PMTs are extremely sensitive light detectors that provide a current output proportional to incident light intensity. The electronic signals from the detectors are amplified and digitalized, and displayed or stored by computer.

Fluorescence Detection

Most applications rely on fluorescent dyes that bind to nuclear or cytoplasmic components, or that are conjugated to antibodies. These are excited by the incident laser beam and emit longer wavelength light. Dichroic reflectors and narrow band-pass filters selectively direct these signals to PMTs, allowing several fluorescent tags to be applied and distinguished (Fig. 1B). Dichroic reflectors, also referred to as beam-splitters, are placed at a 45° angle to the light path to reflect wavelengths longer than a designated value, and to transmit wavelengths less than that value (short-pass filter). Band-pass filters are described by the center wavelength of transmission and the bandwidth around this center. These are placed directly in front of PMTs, restricting their reception to the emission of a specific fluorochrome (e.g., a 530/30 filter for fluorescein isothiocyanate emission) (63).

Fluorescence Compensation

The spectral emissions of two dyes such as fluorescein isothiocyanate (FITC) and phycoerythrin (PE) excited by a single light source are often separated incompletely by dichroic and band-pass filtration. Compensation circuits perform a linear subtraction of the undesired emission out of each color channel by cross coupling one to the other via a differential amplifier system (62). Setting the compensation involves running singly stained cell preparations (or beads) until no overlap of color is present. This should be done at fixed PMT voltages, amplification and laser power, with a relatively "bright" marker (e.g., anti-CD8 on resting lymphocytes, anti-HLA-DR on lymphoblasts). New software is available (AutoCOMP from Becton-Dickinson) to fully automate this process. Compensation often is unnecessary between the widely separated emissions produced by two-laser excitation systems.

Signal Amplification

Linear amplification is useful for forward scatter measures, and when fluorescence can be related stoichiometrically to the target, such as in the DNA content of a cell. Logarithmic amplification of fluorescence (or side scatter) signals increases the dynamic range of display, allowing both weakly staining and very brightly staining cells to be compared on the same scale. Additionally, the shapes of the display are not affected by amplification or PMT voltage (75).

Data Representation

Data may be represented for single color fluorescence as a distribution histogram. A predefined threshold of "positivity" is selected as the level of fluorescence which only a minority of the control cells exceed. An unusual subpopulation may appear as a peak in a unique location. Consideration of the movement of the mean peak channel is useful when all cells are "positive" for the probe in question.

Dual color immunofluorescence may be shown as an X by Y dot plot, contour or isometric display (Figs. 2 to 4). Storage of each independent value per cell (list mode storage) permits recollection of any possible combination. As the number of parameters measured

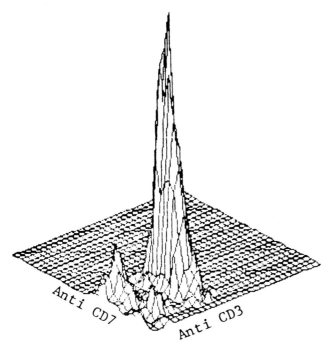

FIG. 2. Isometric (3-dimensional) representation of fresh peripheral blood lymphocyte population double stained with anti CD3 PE (x axis, 5 log decades), and anti CD7 FITC (y axis, 5 log decades). Out of the x versus y plane (z axis, scale = 700), the number of events are depicted, with hidden lines erased for clarity. The figure is displayed with a latitude 20° above the horizontal, and a longitude 40° "west" of the original y axis. Three distinct populations of interest are evident: 10% CD3−CD7+, 76% CD3+ CD7+, and 4% CD3−CD7−. The remaining cells are CD3+ with decreasing expression CD7. Data generated on a FACS 440 with a 5 watt Spectra Physics argon laser emitting 300 mw. Figure drawn on Consort 30/ Hewlett-Packard series 200 computer running FACSDRAW software (kindly provided by M. Conrad, Becton-Dickinson Immunocytometry Systems).

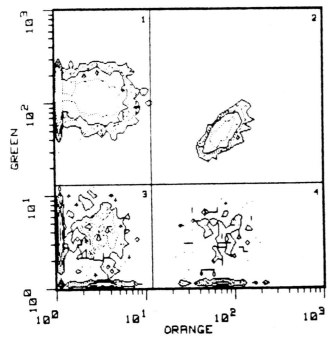

FIG. 3. Contour representation of peripheral blood lymphocytes and monocytes stained simultaneously with one reagent containing titrated amounts of anti CD3 FITC, anti HLA-DR PE, and anti CD14 FITC plus anti CD14 PE. This type of staining provides a rapid method for calculating the total percentage of T-cells, B-cells and monocytes, respectively. Electronic forward versus side scatter gating on the lymphocytes would exclude the staining in quadrant 2. Other possible combinations might substitute a combination of anti CD4 plus anti CD8 PE for anti CD3, and/or anti CD19 for anti HLA-DR. Data generated on a FACS Analyzer with "TBM" stain from an Immune Monitoring Kit (provided by Becton-Dickinson). Contours drawn to include 3, 6, 10 and 20 events.

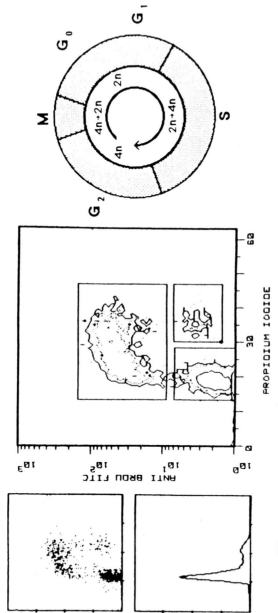

FIG. 4. Comparison of bivariate dot-plot (top left), single parameter histogram (bottom left), and bivariate contour plot (center) depicting the identical cell-cycle (right) data from an Epstein-Barr virus transformed lymphoblastoid cell line. On all three graphs, the x axis is measuring DNA content in linear units by propidium iodide (5 μg/ml) incorporation. The y axis, measured over 3 log decades on the bivariate distributions, indicates BrdU incorporation. The 2-parameter distributions, unlike the histogram, permit quantification of specific S-phase staining distinct from G_1 and G_2 staining; $G_0G_1 = 59\%$, $S = 34\%$, $G_2M = 4\%$ (center).

increases, efficiency of storage and display of data become major concerns. Visualization of multi-parametric data necessitates either three dimensional (50,104), reductive (69) or cluster (68,78) analysis techniques.

Light Sources

Lasers provide light sources that illuminate cells uniformly and intensely for a very short period of time. Argon lasers are popular due to their ideal excitation (488 nm) of FITC and PE. Helium-neon lasers (633 nm) can be used in conjunction with argon lasers for multi-color (> 2) analysis, by exciting allophycocyanin and C-phycocyanin. Helium-neon lasers excite the endogenous flavin and pyridine nucleotides less efficiently, allowing examination of cells too autofluorescent for study with argon lasers (7,60).

Mercury arc lamps are much less expensive and smaller than lasers, and offer a broad range of available wavelengths (200 to 600 nm), but are not as powerful or as stable (51,81). In non-sorting applications, when samples may be run more slowly (allowing each signal to be collected for a longer period of time) arc lamps have been useful, such as in the FACS Analyzer (Becton-Dickinson Immunocytometry Systems). The introduction of small air-cooled lasers into commercial flow cytometers results in small and relatively inexpensive instruments with all the advantages of a laser light source (FACScan by Becton-Dickinson; Profile by Coulter) and have currently superseded arc lamp based systems for multicolor cell-surface analyses (100).

Cell Sorting

Cell sorting permits the physical recovery of pure, viable populations for individual study. No other method separates cells as accurately by their quantitative expression of molecules or by their combination of predefined attributes (82). Sorting of cells by DNA content (108), tumor antigens (23), hormone receptors (70,109) or oncogene products (2) has the potential, as yet unrealized, for assisting in morphologic cytologic screening by providing an essential element of quality control.

In a fluorescence activated cell sorter (10), two individual cell populations may be physically separated from the bulk population by accurately trapping cells in positively or negatively charged droplets, formed by vibrating the flowcell at high frequencies (20–40 kHz). The charged droplets are directed through an electronic field and attracted to either the left or right of the residual population. Thus, relatively rare cells (1% to 5%) may be enriched to a high degree of purity (> 99%) for direct visual examination or placed into tissue culture (83).

While the analytic and sorting speed (≤ 5,000 cells/sec) of a flow sorter is useful for cloning, or sorting relatively small (depending upon rarity of cell) populations for subsequent growth in tissue culture, commercially available instruments are too slow for generating bulk cultures for direct functional, biochemical or molecular study. Unless sorting speeds can be greatly increased, clinical applications, such as sorting fetal from maternal bloods for prenatal diagnosis (40), remain unlikely. Alternative methods of cell separation, such as panning or complement mediated depletion, offer advantages of simplicity and higher yields. These techniques can be more cost and time effective than flow sorting when large numbers (> 10^7) of cells are needed and when purity is not critical.

IMMUNOFLUORESCENCE STAINING TECHNIQUES
FOR FLOW CYTOMETRY

The principle diagnostic application of flow cytometry is the immunophenotyping of circulating leukocytes and leukemia/lymphoma cells (1) (see Chapters 6, 7, 10, 11). A variety of reagents are available for T-cells (CD3, CD5), B-cells (CD19, CD20) and monocytes (CD14, CD15) though none specifically identify unique functional subsets (Table 1). However, by combining different monoclonal antibodies, each distinguished by a particular fluorochrome, it is possible to recognize distinct functional (73) or activated (87,111) T-cell subpopulations.

Cell Preparation

Lymphocytes obtained from peripheral blood for staining are generally enriched by density gradient centrifugation, or red cell lysis of whole blood or the buffy coat, with an ammonium chloride buffer (42). The latter two methods offer a more rapid approach, especially when combined with cell staining in 96 well microtiter plates and automated cell aspiration by the flow cytometer (e.g., FACS AutoMATE). Buffy coat preparations (versus whole blood) also offer the advantage of concentrating cells from lymphopenic patients. Density gradient centrifugation (e.g., Ficoll-Hypaque) efficiently removes red blood cells and granulocytes, but can selectively deplete $CD8^+$ cells, and should be avoided when the "helper-suppressor" (CD4/CD8) ratio is of significant clinical importance (89).

If collected whole blood cannot be stained immediately, it should be stored at 22°C diluted with tissue culture medium. Storage in this fashion permits staining to be delayed for 24 (38) to 72 (76) hr without spurious results. Cultured cell lines generally need only to be washed free of supportive culture medium prior to staining.

Direct and Indirect Staining Techniques

The relative advantages of direct or indirect staining for flow cytometry are similar to those for immunofluorescence or immunoperoxidase microscopy (49) (see Chapters 16, 17). However, most surface staining is done on viable cells which reduces the nonspecific binding of antibodies to dead cells.

Verification that only live cells are analyzed is possible by electronically gating out dead cells that stain with the nucleic acid specific stain propidium iodide (PI) which cannot pass through the surface membrane of a live cell (52). Electronic gating also permits analysis of selected cells. For example, lymphocytes may be distinguished by light scatter from monocytes which might stain nonspecifically due to Fc receptor binding. Flow cytometry also offers the ability to gauge precisely and relate the size of each individual cell with cell surface markers and/or the cell cycle.

For direct immunofluorescence, a cell suspension is incubated with antibody, and subsequently washed free of unbound reagent. Directly conjugated antibodies should be matched with irrelevant non-reactive isotype-matched controls with the same fluorescent tag. For controlling indirect staining, an irrelevant primary antibody should be isotypically matched to the test antibody, followed by the second antibody. In the absence of an irrelevant primary antibody, the second anti-primary immunoglobulin is added alone. Direct staining is quicker than indirect, but is not as sensitive, and requires all reagents to be conjugated with fluorochrome, which increases the cost. Direct staining is clearly the technique of choice for multi-color immunofluorescence, to avoid cross-reactivity of second antibodies. Alternatively, a biotinylated primary antibody can be detected with a strepavidin-fluorochrome combination, and be combined with direct reagents. Nonspecific binding of avidin can be a problem and should be monitored by the addition of the strepavidin-fluorochrome reagent alone. When working with dual and triple color stain combinations, it is essential to include singly stained preparations to set the compensation circuitry properly.

Our current protocol for two-color staining of lysed whole blood is as follows:

1. For each sample, 20 μl of Simultest (Becton-Dickinson) reagent, or an appropriate volume of single PE and FITC conjugate reagent, is added to a 12 mm × 75 mm tube, followed by a 100 μl of anticoagulated (acid citrate dextrose) whole blood. The tubes are vortexed gently and incubated at room temperature, and covered to prevent light exposure.
2. After 15 min, 2.0 ml of FACS Lysing Solution (Becton-Dickinson) is added to each tube. The tubes are vortexed, and incubated for 10 min in the dark.
3. The tubes are centrifuged at 200 × g for 5 min at room temperature.
4. Without disturbing the pellet, aspirate the supernatant leaving about 50 μl in the tube.
5. Add 3.0 ml of PBS containing 0.1% sodium azide to each tube, and vortex.
6. Centrifuge at 300 × g for 5 min at room temperature, and aspirate as in step 4.
7. Resuspend each pellet in 0.7 ml of 1% paraformaldehyde in PBS + 0.1% sodium azide (pH 7.3).
8. Samples may be stored in the dark at 4°C, or run directly on the flow cytometer.

Practical Staining and Operating Procedures

Optimal staining necessitates removal of aggregates from reagents by airfuge at 100,000 g for 10 min, and maintenance of the staining samples at 4°C in buffers containing 0.1% sodium azide to inhibit the modulation and capping of surface antigens. Irrelevant proteins, such as 5% human serum or 1% bovine serum albumin should be included in the staining buffer to saturate non-specific protein binding sites. Nonspecific binding of reagents to the Fc receptors commonly found on monocytes and macrophages may require the utilization of affinity purified F(ab′)$_2$ fragments. Nonspecific fluorescence may result from inadequate washing between steps, and the resulting presence of unbound reagent. Stained preparations should also be removed from exposure to light to maintain the integrity of the fluorescent dye (80).

Fixation

Preservation of surface antibody binding and fluorescent conjugation is ensured by fixing the samples in paraformaldehyde (1% w/v in phosphate buffered saline, PBS) for 10 min, followed by resuspension and maintenance in cold PBS (55). This technique also preserves the light scatter characteristics and Coulter volume of the cells for several weeks. Paraformaldehyde (0.5% to 1.0%) and gluteraldehyde (0.05% to 0.1%) may also preserve selective cell surface antigens, permitting monoclonal antibody staining after fixation (112).

Viable cells prepared for sorting should be maintained on ice (not azide) through the sorting procedure to prevent modulation or shedding of the antigen-antibody complexes.

TABLE 1. Cluster designation of leukocyte associated molecules[a,b]

CD	Common name(s)	MW(Kd)[c]	Monoclonal antibodies	Function/comment	Major normal distribution
1 a	T6/gp49	+ 49	Leu6, T6, OKT6, NA1/34	MHC Class I related	Thymocytes, Langerhans' cells, Histiocytosis X
1 b	T6/gp45	+ 45	WM25, 7C4, 4A76, NU-T2		Thymocytes, Langerhans' cells
1 c	T6/gp43	+ 43	L161, 10C3, M241		Thymocytes, Langerhans' cells, mantle zone in lymphoid organs
2	T11/SER/LFA-2	+ 50	Leu5t, T11, OKT11, RT11	LFA-3 R/Activation	T pan, thymocytes, NK cells
3	T3	+ γ26,δ20,ε20	Leu4, T3, OKT3, RT3.1, UCHT1	Signal transduction	*T pan, T specific, thymocytes
4	T4	+ 60	Leu3ε, T4, OKT4, RT4.1	MHC II R, HTLV R	T subset (MHC Class II restricted), monocytes, thymocytes
5	T1	67	Leu1, T1, OKT1, RT1, T101		T pan, some B cells, (B-CLL)
6	T12	120	T12, TU33		T pan, medullary thymocytes
7	3A1	+ 40	Leu9, 3A1, RT7.1, TU14		Prothymocytes, most circulating T cells, NK subset
8	T8	+ 32	Leu2a, T8, OKT8, RT8.1	MHC 1 R	T subset (MHC Class I restricted), NK subset, thymocytes,SCS
9	BA-2/p24	24	BA-2, J2	Platelet aggregation	Monocytes, pre-B, platelets, activated T cells
10	CALLA	100	Anti-CALLA, J5, OKB-cALLa		Bone marrow, pre-B, kidney, (ALL)
11 a	LFA-1 α chain	180(95)	LFA-1, 2H8.3, 8F2.7	Adhesion to ICAM	Leukocytes, thymocytes
11 b	MAC1/p160/CR3	160(95)	Leu15, Mo1, OKM1	iC3b R	Monocytes, granulocytes
11 c	p150/95	150(95)	LeuM5		Monocytes, activated granulocytes
w12			M67, MG14		Monocytes, granulocytes, platelets
13	gp150	150	MY7		Granulocyte pan, monocytes
14	gp55	55	LeuM3, Mo2, MY4		Monocytes, FDRC, (granulocytes)
15	X Hapten	180,110,68,50	LeuM', MY1	LNFP	Monocytes, activated T cells, granulocytes
16	IgG FcRIII	50–60	Leu11	IgG FcR (low affinity)	Neutrophils, NK pan, some macrophages
17	Lactosylceramide		T5A7, (G)035		Granulocyte pan, platelets
18	LFA β chain	95	60.3, MHM23	Adhesion, with CD11	Leukocytes
19	B4	+ 95	Leu12, B4, 1F1		*B pan, B pre, B activated
20	B1	35	Leu16, B1	Inhibits differentiation	B pan, FDRC
21	CR2	140	Anti-CR2, B2, OKB7	C3d R, EBV R	B pan, C3d red cells, FDRC
22	B3/p135	+ 135	Leu14, TO15, SHCL1, B3		*B pan
23	Blast-2	45	Leu20, B6, Blast-2	IgE FcR	B activation, FDRC
24	BA-1	45,55,65	OKB2, BA1, HB8, HB9		B pan, granulocytes, monocytes
25	IL2 R	55	Anti-IL2R, Tac, 7E11	IL-2 R (low affinity)	Activated T and B Cells, monocytes, thymocytes
w26		130	Ta1, TS145		Activated T culture cell lines
27		55,[120]	OKT18A, S152, VIT14	Lost with culture	T cells, plasma cells (cytoplasmic stain)
28	Tp44	+ 44	9.3, KOLT 2		T subset (cytotoxic precursors)

462

CD	Name	MW (kDa)[c]	Function	Antibodies	Cellular distribution
w29	4B4	135	Activation related	4B4, K20	T subset (helper cells), B cells, monocytes
30	Ki-1	110,95		BERH8, BERH6, BERH4, VIP1	Activated T and B cells, (Reed-Sternberg cells)
31	gp130-140	130–140	(?)gpIIa	SG134, TM3	Monocytes, granulocytes, platelets (T cells)
w32	IgG FcRII	+ 40	IgG FcR (low affinity)	2E1, CIKM5	Monocytes, granulocytes, platelets, B cells
33	gp67	67		MY9, L4F3, L1B2	Myeloid precursors, acute myelogenous leukemia
34	gp115	115		My10, BI-3C5	Myeloid precursors(early),(myeloid,lymphoblastic leukemias)
35	CR1	220	C3b R	Anti-CR1, c3bR	Monocytes, B cells, red cells, kidney prodocytes, FDRC
36	gpIV	85		OKM5, 5F1, CIMeg1	Monocytes, platelets
37	gp40-45	40–45		G28/1, BL14, HD28	B cells (mature), neutrophiles, monocytes
38	T10/gp45	45		Leu17, OKT10	Activated T cells, plasma cells, monocytes
39	p80	80		G28/8, G28/10	B cells, macrophages, endothelium
w40	p50	50	B cell proliferation	G28/5, S2C6	B cell, carcinoma, interdigitating reticulum cells
w41	gpIIb/IIIa	106,96	Fg/Fn R	J15, BC5-C4, P2, P256	*Platelets, megakaryocytes
42	gpIb	125,18	VHFR	HPL14, AN51	*Platelets, megakaryocytes
43	p95	95		84-3C1, G10-2, G19-1	T cells, granulocytes, red cells, brain
w44	p65-85	65–85		1-173, F10-44-2, 106-4D5	T cells, pre-B, brain, granulocytes
45	LCA/T200	220,200,180,160	IL2 R modulation	HLe-1, LCA	Leukocyte common antigen, all leukocytes except plasma cells
45R	LCA-R	220,205		Leu18, 2H4	Restricted T200, T suppressor-inducer and B cell subsets
45R1	LCA-R1	180		UCHL1	T helper cells, thymocytes, granulocytes, monocytes
Leu8	Leu8	80		Leu8, TQ1	T helper cells, B cells, neutrophils, monocytes
NKH-1	NKH-1	205		Leu19, NKH-1A	Pan NK, activated T cells, lung cancer cell lines
HNK-1	HNK-1			Leu7	T cell and NK cell subset, lung cancer cell lines
HLA-DR/Ia-like	HLA-DR/Ia-like	+ α34,β28	MHC Class II Antigen	HLA-DR, I2, OKIaI	B cells, mono/macrophages, active T, dendritic and endothelial
HLA-DQ/(DC)	HLA-DQ/(DC)	+ α32,β27	MHC Class II Antigen	Leu10, Genox 353	B cells, monocytes, activated T cells
HLA-DP/(SB)	HLA-DP/(SB)	+ α35,β25	MHC Class II Antigen	HLA-DP	B cells, monocytes
TdT	TdT		Stem cell marker	Anti-TdT	T and B cell precursors, cortical thymocytes
ATnfR	ATnfR	90[180]	Iron transport	Anti-Transferrin, OKT9	Lymphoblasts, tumor cell lines, monocytes
TCR/Ti, TCR2	TCR/Ti, TCR2	+ α43,β42	Antigen + MHC	BMA031, BMA032, WT-31, BF 1	*T cells, HPB-ALL, HUT 78, PEER negative
TCR1	TCR1	+ γ55λ40	MHC unrestricted cytotoxicity	δTCS1, anti-TCRδ1, Ti-γA	*T cells

[a] Adapted from Michael, A.J., ed. (1987). *Leukocyte Typing III — White Cell Differentiation Antigens.* Oxford University Press, Oxford, U.K.

[b] Abbreviations:

+ = Immunoglobulin gene superfamily member. * = Lineage specific. MHC = Major histocompatibility complex. R = Receptor. SER = Sheep erythrocyte receptor. SCS = Sinusoidal cells in spleen. CALLA = Common acute lymphoblastic leukemia antigen. LFA = Lymphocyte function-associated antigen. FDRC = Follicular dendritic reticulum cells. FcR = Fc receptor. EBV = Epstein Barr virus. LNFP = Lacto-N-fucose pentaosyl III. FgFn = Fibrinogen/fibronectin. VHFR = von Hillebrand factor receptor. LCA = Leucocyte common antigen. TdT = Terminal deoxynucleotidyl transferase. ATnfR = Anti-transferrin receptor. TCR = T cell receptor. ICAM = Intercellular adhesion molecule.

[c] Molecular Weight (kilodaltons) reduced, except [x] = unreduced form; Weak reactions in parentheses.

Antibody binding to cellular structures may perturb cell function, such as anti-CD3 binding to the T-cell receptor, and influence the properties of positively selected cells.

Clogging

Clogging of the nozzle tip or flow cell is best prevented by passing stained cell suspensions through nylon mesh filter material prior to analysis. This is available in a range of pore sizes; mesh ⅓ the inner diameter of the flow cell/nozzle tip is effective at preventing obstruction. For sterile sorting, the filter should be mounted in a small filter holder and sterilized in ethanol. The cell suspension, contained in a 1 ml syringe, is slowly passed through the filter, after rinsing out the alcohol with a large volume of sterile saline.

Fluorochromes for Surface Staining

Fluorescein

FITC is the most popular fluorescent dye due to its high quantum efficiency and its ease of conjugation to antibody. Additionally, it is relatively hydrophilic and easily excited by argon lasers and mercury arc lamps at 488 nm. It is generally the fluorochrome of choice for single color immunofluorescence. Table 2 lists fluorochromes useful for surface and nucleic acid staining.

TABLE 2. *Fluorochromes for surface and nucleic acid staining*

Fluorescent stain	Detect Reaction target	Peak excitation(nm)	Peak emission(nm)
Antibody conjugation			
Fluorescein isothiocyanate	Antigens	495	525
B-Phycoerythrin	Antigens	545/565	575
R-Phycoerythrin	Antigens	480/545/565	578
Texas Red	Antigens	596	615
Allophycocyanin	Antigens	650	660
C-Phycocyanin	Antigens	620	648
DNA/RNA			
Mithramycin	G-C Base Pairs	425	575
Chromomycin A3	G-C Base Pairs	425	575
7-amino actinomycin D	G-C Base Pairs	488	650
Hoechst 33258	A-T Base Pairs	352	465
Hoechst 33342	A-T Base Pairs	361	450
Propidium iodide	Intercalator	340/530	615
Ethidium bromide	Intercalator	345/530	605
Acridine orange	Intercalator	492	520
Pyronin Y	RNA	545	575
Thiazole orange	RNA	509	533

Phycoerythrin

The "R" and "B" phycoerythrins, auxiliary photosynthetic pigments derived from red algae and cyanobacteria, respectively, exhibit excellent labeling characteristics due to their high quantum yields (> 90%) over a broad pH range and a large Stokes shift. These proteins are highly soluble, stable and easily purified, and can be linked to antibodies, biotin or avidin with succinimide esters (79). As with FITC, PE is also excited by the 488 nm line of an argon laser or mercury arc lamp, while emitting further into the red at 575 nm. Thus, pairing these two fluorochromes results in an ideal two-color combination, as long as the spectral overlap of FITC is subtracted from the PE sensitive PMT by appropriately adjusted compensation circuitry. Increased sensitivity (5 to 10-fold) over similar fluorescein conjugates is possible utilizing the phycobiliproteins. Some problems may arise due to the large size of PE (240 Kd), which slows its diffusion in solution (increased staining time must be allowed) and increases the potential for steric hindrance, especially through permeabilized cell membranes (45).

Multi-color (> 2) Analysis

Three and four color surface analysis currently requires two lasers focused at different points of the flow stream and appropriate time delay electronics to coordinate emissions from a single cell. This requires stringent alignment and calibration of the instrument. Independent detection of the fluorophores and the possibility of energy transfer between fluorescent reagents are additional potential complications of multi-color analysis.

Utilization of a pumped-dye laser to excite Texas Red (sulfonyl-chloride rhodamine) conjugated antibodies (54,61), or a helium-neon laser to excite allophycocyanin (53,56), in addition to an argon laser, has demonstrated the potential of multi-color flow cytometric analysis to identify unique cell populations in the peripheral blood and thymus. A new and creative course to triple color analysis with only a single argon laser is also possible. This requires exciting FITC and PE as well as a third tandem-conjugate of two fluorochromes; one (PE) to be excited at 488 nm, which would then excite the second (allophycocyanin) by resonance energy transfer, and thus emit further (660 nm) than PE (578 nm) into the red spectrum. Texas Red, with a peak emission at 615 nm, could also serve in such a conjugate with PE. This technique would permit triple (and higher) -color cell surface analysis in a benchtop cytometer, as PE can also be conjugated with phycocyanin and allophycocyanin B which has shorter and longer emission wavelengths, respectively, than allophycocyanin (34). Utilization of the DNA specific 7-amino-actinomycin D in conjunction with FITC and PE makes simultaneous cell-cycle and two-color surface staining feasible with a single argon laser (85). This is due to the peak emission of 7-amino-actinomycin D occurring further into the red spectrum (650 nm) than PE (578 nm).

Scatter-gate Control

If the analysis of a mixed-cell population (e.g., whole human blood) is based upon an electronic scatter gate, it is necessary to prepare control stains to detect the presence of contaminating cells within the selected population. This may be accomplished by examination of an anti-CD3/CD14 or -CD45/CD14 two-color stain combination to assess the extent of monocytes within the lymphocyte forward versus side scatter gate. This is of particular importance in the study of activated peripheral blood lymphocytes, which due to their greater size tend to fall into a region usually occupied by small monocytes. "Backgating" from fluorescence to forward versus side scatter permits evaluation of the size of all cells positive (or negative) for a particular marker(s), and is especially useful in defining the proper borders of a scatter gate. Routine two-color analysis has been speeded by premixed monoclonal antibody "cocktails" and software that automatically sets the lymphocyte and monocyte gates based upon criteria similar to that described above (Simultest Reagents and Software from Becton Dickinson).

Aid in the analysis of multiparametric research data has recently been addressed by software ("Paint-A-Gate" from Becton Dickinson) that "follows" cell populations on a color monitor through all possible permutations of parameter versus parameter by "painting" subpopulations with a particular color. The Pyramid System (Coulter) aids in both the analysis and sorting of cell populations stained with three or four markers by reducing immunofluorescence data to a real-time eight or sixteen channel bar chart.

DNA ANALYSIS BY FLOW CYTOMETRY

Oncology

An important clinical application of flow cytometric analysis has been the evaluation of cellular DNA content in order to assess ploidy and the frequency of cells in various phases of the cell cycle (Fig. 4). The phenotypic and genetic features of malignant cells quantified by cytometry help in diagnosis, prognosis and choice of therapy. For example, abnormal DNA content in colon (5), ovarian (91), breast (20) and prostatic (67) malignancies has been correlated with a poor prognosis. Identical aneuploid DNA patterns present in separate colonic lesions most probably originated from the same clone, rather than multiple primary tumors, as suggested by histopathologic criteria (97). The relations between ploidy and prognosis depends upon the particular malignancy and treatment mode (radiation or chemotherapy) (5,6,19,105). Cells for analysis have been obtained by fine needle aspiration biopsies (4,93) and paraffin blocks (see below).

Examination of bladder epithelial cells for aneuploid populations by flow cytometry has achieved levels of accuracy comparable to conventional exfoliative cytology, especially with simultaneous examination of cellular RNA, using acridine orange (26,71,72). Simultaneous cytokeratin staining and DNA analysis can distinguish carcinoma cells from stromal and inflammatory cells (32,46). The extension of this approach to other markers should be useful in restricting the cell-cycle analysis provided by DNA specific stains to the malignant cells (12).

Archived Specimens, Oncoproteins and Nuclear Antigens

The discovery that whole nuclei can be recovered from paraffin embedded tissue blocks (36,37) led to routine and retrospective analysis of DNA content by flow techniques (20, 67,91). Comparison of DNA histograms between fresh and paraffin embedded samples has shown good agreement (13,48). Particular areas of a paraffin block can be sampled based upon conventional histological criteria for diploid control cells, or analysis of variations in pathologic grade (110).

Monoclonal antibodies raised against synthetic peptide sequences have recently yielded probes permitting analysis of oncogene expression in human cells (84). These have been valuable in the analysis of the c-myc oncoprotein found in nuclei obtained from deparaffinized testicular tumors. Greater expression of the oncoprotein was shown to correlate with increasing differentiation of the tumor, and an improved prognosis, whereas more aggressive tumors had lower levels of expression (116).

Examination of nuclear antigens in conjunction with the cell-cycle holds promise as a more precise indicator of cell proliferation status and tumor aggressiveness (15,39). These proteins (e.g., p53, p105) appear to serve as "competency factors" in regulating transcription (16). Increasingly sensitive levels of detection (117) may soon allow resolution of specific DNA hybridization probes (107).

Fluorochromes for Nucleic Acid Analysis

Intercalative and Nonintercalative Dyes

The phenanthridinium dyes propidium iodide (PI) and ethidium bromide (EB) intercalate stoichiometrically into double stranded nucleic acids, and measure the cellular DNA content as fluorescence. These stains do not enter intact cells, so that alcohol fixation (70% $-20°C$ ethanol) or detergent treatment (0.1% Triton-X) (14) is used to permeabilize the cell membrane. RNAase should be added to the cells, as PI or EB also bind to RNA (25). PI can also be used (5 to 10 $\mu g/ml$) to correlate DNA content with surface antigen expression, utilizing a fluorescein tagged antibody, and the 488 nm line of an argon laser (11). DNA can be measured after hypotonic lysis (52,113), but this disaggregates metaphase nuclei, and decreases the percentage of cells measured in G_2/M-phase (24).

Vital staining of DNA with nonintercalative dyes has been obtained with both Hoechst 33342 and 33258 (3,90). The principal liability of these dyes is that cells stained with sufficient concentrations for a good DNA histogram are not all capable of subsequent division (33,59), especially after passage through ultraviolet wavelengths (99). Vital staining of RNA has been achieved with the stain pyronin Y (98). RNA specific stains are also used to enumerate reticulocytes in peripheral blood. A recently available RNA stain excited with the 488 nm line of an argon laser is thiazole orange (58).

S-phase Specific Staining

The histograms produced by the intercalative dyes distinguish the DNA content of resting and dividing cell populations, but do not adequately discriminate cells entering or leaving S-phase (Fig. 4). Attempts to distinguish S-phase cells from G_0/G_1- and $G_2/$ M-phase cells have been made by various mathematical curve fitting models, all of which have shortcomings as the measured populations depart from the "ideal" (27,28). S-phase may be measured directly by pulsing (10 μM for 2–30 min) living populations of cells with the S-phase specific thymidine analog bromodeoxyuridine (BrdU) fixing in 70% $-20°C$ ethanol, and assaying for uptake with a fluoresceinated monoclonal anti-BrdU (Fig. 4) (35). Anti-BrdU has specificity only towards single-stranded DNA, and thus requires acid denaturation (3N HCl) of the nucleic acid (30). The combination of anti-BrdU FITC with G_0/G_1 and G_2/M-phase specific staining (e.g., EB) permits direct assessment of each particular cell cycle phase, and permits study of the rate of synthesis. When used in conjunction with a third fluorescent surface marker, such as Texas Red, complete cell cycle information can be correlated with the expression of surface antigen (45). Since BrdU is neither radioactive, nor toxic at low levels, intravenous administration of BrdU to patients with various brain tumors (44) or lymphoproliferative malignancies (86) permits study of the DNA synthesis rate *in situ*.

Controls for DNA Analysis

To determine the DNA content of a fresh or deparaffinized sample tumor tissue, normal cells from the same source serve as ideal control reference cells, as these have been through the same preparative conditions. In the absence of normal tissue cells, autologous peripheral blood cells should be used. An index of DNA abnormality should be calculated and reported as the mode (or mean) of the relative DNA content of the $G_0/1$ cells of the test population divided by the mode (or mean) of the $G_0/1$ reference population (41). Thus, cells with a normal diploid karyotype should have a DNA index of 1.0. Internal standards such as chicken and trout red blood cells, or fluorescent beads, should be intermixed with the test population before staining for instrument calibration (47,114). The discrimination of single cells from cell aggregates is best determined by pulse width measurement. This allows accurate resolution of doublets of G_0/G_1 cells from G_2/M-phase cells, and large clumps from single cells having abnormally high DNA contents (101). Standards for flow cytometry in clinical laboratories are currently being developed jointly by the American Society of Histocompatibility and Immunogenetics (ASHI), the Society of Analytical Cytology (SAC) and the College of American Pathologists (CAP).

CALIBRATION AND MAINTENANCE

The interdependence of each subsystem in a flow cytometer makes control over and calibration of each an absolute necessity. Standard calibration conditions are achieved by precise mechanical alignment of the fluid stream with the light beam and detection optics at standard flow rates, PMT voltages, amplification and laser power. For this, lasers must be operating in TEMoo mode, and peaked for efficient light output at the line of operation, after a suitable warm-up.

Uniform, cell-sized and stable fluorescent beads provide a useful tool to relate fluorescence measurements between experiments, and to indicate when all systems are properly aligned, by reproducibly falling into predetermined scatter and fluorescence channels. Highest accuracy is accomplished when the fluorochrome bound to the bead has the same emission spectrum as that conjugated to the antibody; both FITC and PE conjugated to cell-sized beads are available (Calibright Beads from Becton-Dickinson). Fluorescence and antigen density may be quantitated by using a series of standard beads of known size and fluorescence such as those available through Flow Cytometry Standards Corporation (Research Triangle Park, North Carolina).

Due to the complexity of the instrumentation, proper alignment and quality control is of utmost importance when interpreting flow data, which can be voluminous, due to multiparametric acquisition. Objective lenses, prisms and other optical surfaces must be free of dirt and films, and optical paths clear of obstruction. In stream-in-air sorters, the ninety degree objective lens may be splashed with saline, attenuating signals to the photomultipliers. The lens is best cleaned with filtered water, rather than organic solvents, which would tend to loosen the lens after repeated cleanings.

A fluid delivery system free of kinks and obstructions is also of obvious importance and these systems require stable pressurization. Fluidic lines, removable nozzle tips and nozzle holders should never be left to dry, as air drying causes the precipitation of salts on their surfaces. Many helpful tips regarding the maintenance and operation of flow cytometers have been published (29,43,82).

CONCLUSION

The major limitation of flow cytometry is the requirement for single cell suspensions. This does not limit analysis of blood or effusions, but is a major drawback for the study of surface markers on the cells of solid tissue. These must be enzymatically or mechanically disaggregated, which can modify cell surface antigens and yield unrepresentative populations. Immunofluorescence or immunoperoxidase based microscopy can better provide the information about the location of cells with respect to the surrounding tissue architecture, and the distribution of cellular staining. Thus, it is most appropriate to apply flow cytometric techniques when the sensitivity, multiparametric and quantitative capabilities it provides are critical.

ACKNOWLEDGMENTS

I would like to thank Dr. Robert Colvin for discussions related to flow cytometry, and Ms. JoAnne Phelan and Ms. Elizabeth Sabga for technical assistance and help in preparation of the manuscript. Supported in part by grants from the National Institutes of Health (HL-18646 and CA43244-02).

REFERENCES

1. Andreeff, M., editor (1986): Clinical cytometry. *Ann. N.Y. Acad. Sci.*, 468:1–408.
2. Andreeff, M., Slater, D. E., Bressler, J., and Furth, M. E. (1986): Cellular ras oncogene expression and cell cycle measured by flow cytometry in hematopoietic cell lines. *Blood*, 67:676–681.
3. Arndt-Jovin, D. J., and Jovin, T. M. (1977): Analysis and sorting of living cells according to deoxyribonucleic acid content. *J. Histochem. Cytochem.*, 25:585–589.
4. Azavedo, E., Tribukait, B., Konaka, C., and Auer, G. (1982): Reproducibility of the cellular DNA distribution patterns in multiple fine needle aspirates from human malignant tumors. *Acta Pathol. Microbiol. Immunol. Scand.*, 90:79–83.
5. Banner, B. F., Tomas-De La Vega, J. E., Roseman, D., and Coon, J. S. (1985): Should flow cytometric DNA analysis precede definitive surgery for colon carcinoma? *Ann. Surg.*, 202:74–78.
6. Barlogie, B., Raber, M. N., Schumann, J., Johnson, T. S., Drewinko, B., Swartzendruber, D. E., Gohde, W., Andreeff, M., and Freireich, E. J. (1983): Flow cytometry in clinical cancer research. *Cancer Res.*, 43:3982–3997.
7. Benson, R. C., Meyer, R. A., Zaruba, M. E., and McKhann, G. M. (1979): Cellular autofluorescence—Is it due to flavins? *J. Histochem. Cytochem.*, 27:44–48.
8. Berliner, N., Ault, K. A., Martin, P., and Weinberg, D. S. (1986): Detection of clonal excess in lymphoproliferative disease by kappa/lambda analysis: Correlation with immunoglobulin gene DNA rearrangement. *Blood*, 67:80–85.
9. Bianchi, D. W., Harris, P., Flint, A., and Latt, S. A. (1987): Direct hybridization to DNA from small numbers of flow-sorted nucleated newborn cells. *Cytometry*, 8:197–202.
10. Bonner, W. A., Hulett, H. R., Sweet, R. G., and Herzenberg, L. A. (1972): Fluorescence activated cell sorting. *Rev. Sci. Instrum.*, 41:404–409.
11. Braylan, R. C., Benson, N. A., Nourse, V., and Kruth, H. S. (1982): Correlated analysis of cellular DNA, membrane antigens and light scatter of human lymphoid cells. *Cytometry*, 2:337–343.
12. Braylan, R. C., Benson, N. A., and Nourse, V. A. (1984): Cellular DNA of human neoplastic B-cells measured by flow cytometry. *Cancer Res.*, 44:5010–5016.

13. Camplejohn, R. S., and Macartney, J. C. (1985): Comparison of DNA flow cytometry from fresh and paraffin-embedded samples of non-Hodgkin's lymphoma. *J. Clin. Pathol.*, 38:1096–1099.

14. Clevenger, C. V., Bauer, K. D., and Epstein, A. L. (1985): A method for simultaneous nuclear immuno-fluorescence and DNA quantitation using monoclonal antibodies and flow cytometry. *Cytometry*, 6:208–214.

15. Clevenger, C. V., Epstein, A. L., and Bauer, K. D. (1987): Quantitative analysis of a nuclear antigen in interphase and mitotic cells. *Cytometry*, 8:280–286.

16. Clevenger, C. V., Epstein, A. L., and Bauer, K. D. (1987): Modulation of the nuclear antigen p105 as a function of cell-cycle progression. *J. Cell. Physiol.*, 130:336–343.

17. Colvin, R. B. (1984): Flow cytometric analysis of T cells: diagnostic applications in transplantation. *Ann. N.Y. Acad. Sci.*, 428:5–13.

18. Colvin, R. B., and Preffer, F. I. (1987): New technologies in cell analysis by flow cytometry. *Arch. Pathol. Lab. Med.*, 111:628–632.

19. Coon, J. S., Landay, A. L., and Weinstein, R. S. (1986): Flow cytometric analysis of paraffin-embedded tumors: Implications for diagnostic pathology. *Hum. Pathol.*, 17:435–437.

20. Cornelisse, C. J., van de Velde, C. J. H., Caspers, R. J. C., Moolenaar, A. J., and Hermans, J. (1987): DNA ploidy and survival in breast cancer patients. *Cytometry*, 8:225–234.

21. Cosimi, A. B. (1983): Diagnostic and therapeutic applications of monoclonal antibodies to human T-cell subsets in renal transplant recipients. *Urol. Clin. N. Am.*, 10:289–299.

22. Coulter, W. H. (1953): Means for counting particles suspended in a fluid. U.S. Patent 2,656,508.

23. Czerniak, B., Papenhausen, P. R., Herz, F., and Koss, L. G. (1985): Flow cytometric identification of cancer cells in effusions with Ca1 monoclonal antibody. *Cancer*, 55:2783–2788.

24. Darzynkiewicz, Z. (1979): Acridine orange as a molecular probe in studies of nucleic acids in situ. In: *Flow Cytometry and Sorting*, edited by H. R. Melamed, P. F. Mullaney, and M. L. Mendelsohn, pp. 283–316. John Wiley, New York.

25. Darzynkiewicz, Z., Traganos, F., Kapuscinski, J., Staiano-Coico, L., and Melamed, M. R. (1984): Accessibility of DNA in situ to various fluorochromes: Relationship to chromatin changes during erythroid differentiation of friend leukemia cells. *Cytometry*, 5:355–363.

26. Darzynkiewicz, Z., Traganos, F., and Melamed, M. R. (1980): New cell cycle compartments identified by multiparameter flow cytometry. *Cytometry*, 1:98–108.

27. Dean, P. N. (1980): A simplified method of DNA distribution analysis. *Cell Tissue Kinet.*, 13:299–308.

28. Dean, P. N. (1985): Methods of data analysis in flow cytometry. In: *Flow Cytometry: Instrumentation and Data Analysis*, edited by M. A. Van Dilla, P. N. Dean, O. D. Laerum and M. R. Melamed, pp. 195–223. Academic Press, London.

29. Dean, P. N. (1985): Helpful hints in flow cytometry and sorting. *Cytometry*, 6:62–64.

30. Dolbeare, F., Gratzner, H., Pallavicini, M. G., and Grey, J. W. (1983): Flow cytometric measurement of total DNA content and incorporated bromodeoxyuridine. *Proc. Natl. Acad. Sci.*, 80:5573–5577.

31. Fahey, J. L., Prince, H., Weaver, M., Groopman, J., Visscher, B., Schwartz, K., and Detels, R. (1984): Quantitative changes in T helper or T suppressor/cytotoxic lymphocyte subsets that distinguish acquired immune deficiency syndrome from other immune subset disorders. *Am. J. Med.*, 76:95–100.

32. Feitz, W. F. J., Beck, H. L. M., Smeets, A. W. G. B., Debruyne, F. M. J., Vooijs, G. P., Herman, C. J., and Ramaekers, F. C. S. (1985): Tissue-specific markers in flow cytometry of urological cancers: Cytokeratins in bladder carcinoma. *Int. J. Cancer*, 36:349–356.

33. Fried, J., Doblin, J., Takamoto, S., Perez, A., Hansen, H., and Clarkson, B. (1982): Effects of Hoechst 33342 on survival and growth of two tumor cell lines and on hematopoietically normal bone marrow cells. *Cytometry*, 3:42–47.

34. Glazer, A. N., and Stryer, L. (1983): Fluorescent tandem phycobiliprotein conjugates. Emission wavelength shifting by energy transfer. *Biophys. J.*, 43:383–386.

35. Grey, J., Guest Editor (1985): Special Issue: Monoclonal antibodies against bromodeoxyuridine. *Cytometry*, 6:499–673.

36. Hedley, D. W., Friedlander, M. L., and Taylor, I. W. (1985): Application of DNA flow cytometry to paraffin-embedded archival material for the study of aneuploidy and its clinical significance. *Cytometry*, 6:327–333.

37. Hedley, D. W., Friedlander, M. L., Taylor, I. W., Rugg, C. A., and Musgrove, E. A. (1983): Method for analysis of cellular DNA content of paraffin-embedded pathological material using flow cytometry. *J. Histochem. Cytochem.*, 31:1333–1335.

38. Hensleigh, P. A., Waters, V. B., and Herzenberg, L. A. (1983): Human T lymphocyte differentiation antigens: Effects of blood sample storage on Leu antibody binding. *Cytometry*, 3:453–445.

39. Herman, C. J., McGraw, T. P., Marder, R. J., and Bauer, K. D. (1987): Recent progress in clinical quantitative cytology. *Arch. Pathol. Lab. Med.*, 111:505–512.

40. Herzenberg, L. A., Bianchi, D. W., Schröder, J., Cann, H. M., and Iverson, G. M. (1979): Fetal cells in the blood of pregnant women: Detection and enrichment by fluorescence-activated cell sorting. *Proc. Natl. Acad. Sci.*, 76:1453–1455.

41. Hiddemann, W., Schumann, J., Andreeff, M., Barlogie, B., Herman, C., Leif, R. C., Mayall, B. H., Murphy, R. F., and Sandberg, A. A. (1984): Convention on nomenclature for DNA cytometry. *Cytometry*, 5:445–446.

42. Hoffman, R. A., Kung, P. C., Hansen, W. P., and Goldstein, G. (1980): Simple and rapid measurement of human T lymphocytes and their subclasses in peripheral blood. *Proc. Natl. Acad. Sci.*, 77:4914–4917.

43. Horan, P. K., and Loken, M. R. (1985): A practical guide for the use of flow systems. In: *Flow Cytometry: Instrumentation and Data Analysis*, edited by M. A. Van Dilla, P. N. Dean, O. D. Laerum, and M. R. Melamed, pp. 260–280. Academic Press, London.

44. Hoshino, T., Nagashima, T., Murovic, J., Levin, E. M., Levin, V. A., and Rupp, S. M. (1985): Cell kinetic studies of in situ human brain tumors with bromodeoxyuridine. *Cytometry*, 6:627–632.

45. Houck, D. W., and Loken, M. R. (1985): Simultaneous analysis of cell surface antigens, bromodeoxyuridine incorporation and DNA content. *Cytometry*, 6:531–538.

46. Huffman, J. L., Garin-Chesa, P., Gay, H., Whitmore, Jr., W. F., and Melamed, M. R. (1986): Flow cytometric identification of human bladder cells using a cytokeratin monoclonal antibody. *Ann. N.Y. Acad. Sci.*, 468:302–315.

47. Iversen, O. E., and Laerum, O. D. (1987): Trout and salmon erythrocytes and human leukocytes as internal standards for ploidy control in flow cytometry. *Cytometry*, 8:190–196.

48. Johnson, T. S., Williamson, K. D., Cramer, M. M., and Peters, L. J. (1985): Flow cytometric analysis of head and neck carcinoma DNA index and S-fraction from paraffin-embedded sections: Comparison with malignancy grading. *Cytometry*, 6:461–470.

49. Kabawat, S. E., Preffer, F. I., and Bhan, A. K. (1985): Monoclonal antibodies in diagnostic pathology. In: *Handbook of Monoclonal Antibodies: Applications in Biology and Medicine*, edited by S. Ferrone and M. P. Dierich, pp. 293–328. Noyes, New Jersey.

50. Kachel, V., and Schneider, H. (1986): On-line three-parameter data uptake, analysis, and display device for flow cytometry and other applications. *Cytometry*, 7:25–40.

51. Koper, G. J. M., Bonnet, J., Christiaanse, J. G. M., and Ploem, J. S. (1982): An epiilluminator/detector unit permitting arc lamp illumination for fluorescence activated cell sorters. *Cytometry*, 3:10–14.

52. Krishan, A. (1975): Rapid flow cytofluorometric analysis of mammalian cell cycle by propidium iodide staining. *J. Cell. Biol.*, 66:188–193.

53. Lanier, L. L., Allison, J. P., and Phillips, J. H. (1986): Correlation of cell surface antigen expression on human thymocytes by multi-color flow cytometric analysis: Implications for differentiation. *J. Immunol.*, 137:2501–2507.

54. Lanier, L. L., and Loken, M. R. (1984): Human lymphocyte subpopulations identified by using three-color immunofluorescence and flow cytometric analysis: Correlation of Leu-2, Leu-3, Leu-7, Leu-8, and Leu-11 cell surface antigen expression. *J. Immunol.*, 132:151–156.

55. Lanier, L. L., and Warner, N. L. (1981): Paraformaldehyde fixation of hematopoietic cells for quantitative flow cytometry (FACS) analysis. *J. Immunol. Methods*, 47:25–30.

56. Lanier, L. L., and Weiss, A. (1986): Presence of Ti(WT-31) negative T lymphocytes in normal blood and thymus. *Nature*, 324:268–270.

57. Lebo, R. V., Kan, Y. W., Cheung, M. C., Carrano, A. V., Yu, L.-C., Chang, J. C., Cordell, B., and Goodman, H. (1982): Assigning the polymorphic human insulin gene to the short arm of chromosome 11 by chromosome sorting. *Hum. Genet.*, 60:10–15.

58. Lee, L. G., Chen, C. H., and Chiu, L. A. (1986): Thiazole orange: A new dye for reticulocyte analysis. *Cytometry*, 7:508–517.

59. Loken, M. R. (1980): Simultaneous quantitation of Hoechst 33342 and immunofluorescence on viable cells using a fluorescence activated cell sorter. *Cytometry*, 1:136–142.

60. Loken, M. R., Keij, J. F., and Kelley, K. A. (1987): Comparison of helium-neon and dye lasers for the excitation of allophycocyanin. *Cytometry*, 8:96–100.

61. Loken, M. R., and Lanier, L. L. (1984): Three color immunofluorescence analysis of Leu antigens of human peripheral blood using two lasers on a fluorescence-activated cell sorter. *Cytometry*, 5:151–158.

62. Loken, M. R., Parks, D. R., and Herzenberg, L. A. (1977): Two-color immunofluorescence using a fluorescence-activated cell sorter. *J. Histochem. Cytochem.*, 25:899–906.

63. Loken, M. R., and Stall, A. M. (1982): Flow cytometry as an analytical and preparative tool in immunology. *J. Immunol. Methods*, 50:R85–R112.

64. Lovett, E. J., III, Schnitzer, B., Keren, D. F., Flint, A., Hudson, J. L., and McClatchey, K. D. (1984): Application of flow cytometry to diagnostic pathology. *Lab. Invest.*, 50:115–140.

65. Lucas, J. N., and Grey, J. W. (1987): Centromeric index versus DNA content flow karyotypes of human chromosomes measured by means of slit-scan flow cytometry. *Cytometry*, 8:273–279.

66. Lucas, J. N., Grey, J. W., Peters, D. C., and Van Dilla, M. A. (1983): Centromeric index measurement by slit-scan flow cytometry. *Cytometry*, 4:109–116.

67. Lundberg, S., Carstensen, J., and Rundquist, I. (1987): DNA flow cytometry and histopathological grading of paraffin-embedded prostate biopsy specimens in a survival study. *Cancer Res.*, 47:1973–1977.

68. Mann, R. C. (1987): On multiparameter data analysis in flow cytometry. *Cytometry*, 8:184–189.

69. Mann, R. C., Popp, D. M., and Hand, Jr., R. E. (1984): The use of projections for dimensionality reduction of flow cytometric data. *Cytometry*, 5:304–307.

70. Maron, R., Taylor, S. I., Jackson, R., and Kahn, C. R. (1984): Analysis of insulin receptors on human lymphoblastoid cell lines by flow cytometry. *Diabetologia*, 27:118–120.

71. Melamed, M. R. (1984): Flow cytometry of the urinary bladder. *Urol. Clin. N. Amer.*, 11:599–608.

72. Melamed, M. R., and Klein, F. A. (1984): Flow cytometry of urinary bladder irrigation specimens. *Human Pathol.*, 15:302–305.

73. Morimoto, C., Hafler, D. A., Weiner, H. L., Letvin, N. L., Hagen, M., Daley, J., and Schlossman, S. (1987): Selective loss of the suppressor-inducer T-cell subset in progressive multiple sclerosis: Analysis with anti-2H4 monoclonal antibody. *N. Engl. J. Med.*, 316:67–72.

74. Muirhead, K. A., Horan, P. K., and Poste, G. (1985): Flow cytometry: Present and future. *Bio/Technology*, 3:337–356.

75. Muirhead, K. A., Schmitt, T. C., and Muirhead, A. R. (1983): Determination of linear fluorescence intensities from flow cytometric data accumulated with logarithmic amplifiers. *Cytometry*, 3:251–256.

76. Muirhead, K. A., Wallace, P. K., Schmitt, T. C., Frescatore, R. L., Franco, J. A., and Horan, P. K. (1986): Methodological considerations for implementation of lymphocyte subset analysis in a clinical reference laboratory. *Ann. N.Y. Acad. Sci.*, 468:113–127.

77. Mullaney, P. F., and Dean, P. N. (1970): The small light scattering of biological cells. *Biophys. J.*, 10:764–772.

78. Murphy, R. F. (1985): Automated identification of subpopulations in flow cytometric list mode data using cluster analysis. *Cytometry*, 6:302–309.

79. Oi, V. T., Glazer, A. N., and Stryer, L. (1982): Fluorescent phycobiliprotein conjugates for analyses of cells and molecules. *J. Cell Biol.*, 93:981–986.

80. Parks, D. R., Lanier, L. L., and Herzenberg, L. A. (1986): Flow cytometry and fluorescence activated cell sorting (FACS). In: *Handbook of Experimental Immunology*, edited by D. M. Weir, L. A. Herzenberg, C. Blackwell, and L. A. Herzenberg, Chapter 29. Blackwell Scientific Publishing, Edinburgh.

81. Peters, D. C. (1979): A comparison of mercury arc lamp and laser illumination for flow cytometers. *J. Histochem. Cytochem.*, 27:241–245.

82. Preffer, F. I., and Colvin, R. B. (1987): Analysis and sorting by flow cytometry: Applications to the study of human disease. In: *Cell Separation: Methods and Selected Applications*, edited by T. Pretlow and T. Pretlow, pp. 311–347. Academic Press, New York.

83. Preffer, F. I., Colvin, R. B., Leary, C. P., Boyle, L. A., Tuazon, T. V., Lazarovits, A. I., Cosimi, A. B., and Kurnick, J. T. (1986): Two color flow cytometry and functional analysis of lymphocytes cultured from human renal allografts: Identification of a Leu 2^+3^+ subpopulation. *J. Immunol.*, 137:2823–2830.

84. Rabbitts, P. H., Watson, J. V., Lamond, A., Forster, A., Stinson, M. A., Evan, G., Fischer, W., Atherton, E., Sheppard, R., and Rabbitts, T. H. (1985): Metabolism of c-myc gene products: c-myc mRNA and protein expression in the cell cycle. *Embo. J.*, 4:2009–2015.

85. Rabinovitch, P. S., Torres, R. M., and Engle, D. (1986): Simultaneous cell cycle analysis and two-color surface immunofluorescence using 7-amino-actinomycin D and single laser excitation: Application to study of cell activation and the cell cycle of murine Ly-1 B cells. *J. Immunol.*, 136:2769–2775.

86. Raza, A., Ucar, K., and Preisler, D. (1985): Double labeling and in vitro versus in vivo incorporation of bromodeoxyuridine in patients with acute nonlymphocytic leukemia. *Cytometry*, 6:633–640.

87. Redelman, D. (1987): Simultaneous increased expression of E-rosette receptor (CD2, T11) and T cell growth factor receptor on human T lymphocytes during activation. *Cytometry*, 8:170–183.

88. Redner, A., Andreeff, M., Miller, D. R., Steinherz, P., and Melamed, M. (1984): Recognition of central nervous system leukemia by flow cytometry. *Cytometry*, 5:614–618.

89. Renzi, P., and Ginns, L. C. (1987): Analysis of T cell subsets in normal adults. Comparison of whole blood technique to ficoll-hypaque separation by flow cytometry. *J. Immunol. Methods*, 98:53–56.

90. Rice, G. C., Dean, P. N., Gray, J. W., and Dewey, W. C. (1984): An ultra-pure in vitro phase synchrony method employing centrifugal elutriation and viable flow cytometric cell sorting. *Cytometry*, 5:289–298.

91. Rodenburg, C. J., Cornelisse, C. J., Heintz, P. A. M., Hermans, J., and Flueren, G. J. (1987): Tumor ploidy as a major prognostic factor in advanced ovarian cancer. *Cancer*, 59:317–323.

92. Rolland, J. M., Dimitropoulos, K., Bishop, A., Hocking, G. R., and Nairn, R. C. (1985): Fluorescence polarization assay by flow cytometry. *J. Immunol. Methods*, 76:1–10.

93. Ronstrom, L., Tribukait, B., and Esposti, P. L. (1981): RNA pattern and cytological findings in fine needle aspirates of untreated prostatic tumors. A flow cytofluorometric study. *Prostate*, 2:79–88.

94. Ryan, D. H., Mitchell, S. J., Hennessy, L. A., Bauer, K. D., Horan, P. K., and Cohen, H. J. (1984): Improved detection of rare calla-positive cells in peripheral blood using multiparameter flow cytometry. *J. Immunol. Methods*, 74:115–128.

95. Salzman, G. C., Crowell, J. M., Martin, J. C., Trujillo, B. S., Romero, A., Mullaney, P. F., and LaBauve, P. M. (1975): Cell classification by laser light scattering: identification and separation of unstained leukocytes. *Acta Cytologica*, 19:374–377.

96. Salzman, G. C., Mullaney, P. F., and Price, B. J. (1979): Light-scattering approaches to cell characteriza-

tion. In: *Flow Cytometry and Sorting*, edited by H. R. Melamed, P. F. Mullaney, and M. L. Mendelsohn, pp. 105–124. John Wiley, New York.

97. Schwartz, D., Banner, B. F., Roseman, D. L., and Coon, J. S. (1986): Origin of multiple "primary" colon carcinomas. A retrospective flow cytometric study. *Cancer*, 58:2082–2088.

98. Shapiro, H. M. (1981): Flow cytometric estimation of DNA and RNA content in intact cells stained with Hoechst 33342 and Pyronin Y. *Cytometry*, 2:143–150.

99. Shapiro, H. M. (1985): *Flow Cytometry*. Alan R. Liss, Inc., New York.

100. Shapiro, H. M. (1986): The little laser that could: applications of low power lasers in clinical flow cytometry. *Ann. N.Y. Acad. Sci.*, 468:18–27.

101. Sharpless, T., Traganos, F., Darzynkiewicz, Z., and Melamed, M. R. (1975): Flow cytofluorimetry: discrimination between single cells and cell aggregates by direct size measurements. *Acta Cytolog.*, 19:577–581.

102. Smith, B. R., Weinberg, D. S., Robert, N. J., Towle, M., Luther, E., Pinkus, G. S., and Ault, K. A. (1984): Circulating monoclonal B lymphocytes in non-Hodgkin's lymphoma. *N. Engl. J. Med.*, 311:1476–1481.

103. Steinkamp, J. A. (1984): Flow cytometry. *Rev. Sci. Instrum.*, 55:1375–1400.

104. Stewart, S. S., and Price, G. B. (1986): Realtime acquisition, storage, and display of correlated three-parameter flow cytometric data. *Cytometry*, 7:82–88.

105. Teodori, L., Tirindelli-Danesi, D., Cordelli, E., Uccelli, R., DeVita, R., Spano, M., Mauro, F., Schillaci, A., Moraldi, A., Capurso, L., and Stipa, S. (1986): Potential prognostic significance of cytometrically determined DNA abnormality in GI tract human tumors. *Ann. N.Y. Acad. Sci.*, 468:291–301.

106. Thistlewaite, J. R., Buckingham, M. R., Stuart, J. K., and Stuart, F. P. (1986): Detection of presensitization in renal allograft recipients using a flow cytometric immunofluorescence crossmatch. *Transplant. Proc.*, 18:676–679.

107. Trask, B., Van Den Engh, G., Landegent, J., In De Wal, N. J., and Van Der Ploeg, M. (1985): Detection of DNA sequences in nuclei in suspension by in situ hybridization and dual beam flow cytometry. *Science*, 230:1401–1403.

108. Tyrer, H. W., Pressman, N. J., Albright, C. D., and Frost, J. K. (1985): Automatic cell identification and enrichment in lung cancer: V. Adenocarcinoma and large cell undifferentiated carcinoma. *Cytometry*, 6:37–46.

109. Van, N. T., Raber, M., Barrows, G. H., and Barlogie, B. (1984): Estrogen receptor analysis by flow cytometry. *Science*, 224:876–879.

110. Van Driel-Kulker, A. M. J., Eysackers, M. J., Dessing, M. T. M., and Ploem, J. S. (1986): A simple method to select specific tumor areas in paraffin blocks for cytometry using incident fluorescence microscopy. *Cytometry*, 7:601–604.

111. Van Es, A., Meyer, C. J., Oljans, P. J., Tanke, H. J., and Van Es, L. A. (1984): Mononuclear cells in renal allografts. Correlation with peripheral blood T lymphocyte subpopulations and graft prognosis. *Transplantation*, 37:134–139.

112. Van Ewijk, W., Van Soest, P. L., Verkerk, A., and Jongkind, J. F. (1984): Loss of antibody binding to prefixed cells: Fixation parameters for immunocytochemistry. *Histochem. J.*, 16:179–193.

113. Vindeløv, L. L., Christensen, I. J., and Nissen, N. I. (1983): A detergent-trypsin method for the preparation of nuclei for flow cytometric DNA analysis. *Cytometry*, 3:323–327.

114. Vindeløv, L. L., Christensen, I. J., and Nissen, N. I. (1983): Standardization of high-resolution flow cytometric DNA analysis by the simultaneous use of chicken and trout red blood cells as internal reference standards. *Cytometry*, 3:328–331.

115. Watson, J. V., Sikora, K., and Evan, G. I. (1985): A simultaneous flow cytometric assay for c-myc oncoprotein and DNA in nuclei from paraffin embedded material. *J. Immunol. Methods*, 83:179–192.

116. Watson, J. V., Stewart, J., Evan, G. I., Ritson, A., and Sikora, K. (1986): The clinical significance of flow cytometric c-myc oncoprotein quantitation in testicular tumor. *Br. J. Cancer*, 53:331–337.

117. Watson, J. V., and Walport, M. J. (1986): Molecular calibration in flow cytometry with sub-attogram detection limits. *J. Immunol. Methods*, 93:171–175.

118. Wheeless, L. L. (1979): Slit-scanning and pulse width analysis. In: *Flow Cytometry and Sorting*, edited by H. R. Melamed, P. F. Mullaney, and M. L. Mendelsohn, pp. 125–136. John Wiley, New York.

Diagnostic Immunopathology,
edited by R.B. Colvin,
A.K. Bhan, and R.T. McCluskey.
Raven Press, New York © 1988.

19 / *In Situ* Hybridization

David Myerson

*Division of Clinical Research, Fred Hutchinson Cancer Research Center, and
Department of Pathology, University of Washington, Seattle, Washington 98104*

In situ hybridization is a procedure which utilizes a labeled nucleic acid probe to detect the complimentary nucleic acid sequences within a tissue. Nucleic acid probes may be constructed to detect virtually any foreign DNA in a cell, such as bacteria or viruses, or establish the chromosomal location of genes. In addition intracellular RNA may be detected, including foreign RNA virus genomes, or viral or cell messenger RNA. The specific procedure for performing *in situ* hybridization differs, depending largely on how the tissue has been fixed and whether DNA or RNA is to be detected. Viral disease has been studied by *in situ* hybridization using both radioactive (2,10,16,17,21,25,28,35, 36,38,39,41,45,58,61,69,74,78,81,88,89,92,93,103,104) and nonradioactive probes, (1,4,12,13,19,23,29,32,64–66,68,76,85,86,95) sometimes combined with immunohistochemistry (8,11,17,27,36). Tissue embedded in paraffin has resulted in good tissue morphology as well as hybridization (4,9,12,18,28,34,35,50,62,65,68,74,91,102). Plastic embedded tissue has also been used (6,21,44). Different protocols may vary in their reproducibility and in their sensitivity (13,18,37,40,70,83,101).

This chapter is restricted to providing practical procedures and commentary for the clinical use of *in situ* hybridization for the detection of DNA viruses in routinely formalin-fixed tissue sections. Because the intent is for general clinical use, only a nonradioactive probe is considered. Examples including cytomegalovirus (CMV), herpes simplex virus (HSV), varicella-zoster virus (VZV), and human papilloma virus (HPV) are presented. These techniques are applicable to other viruses (e.g., HIV) and normal cytoplasmic mRNA. Radioactive probes (e.g., ^{35}S) provide increased sensitivity at the price of some inconvenience and delay.

DNA HYBRIDIZATION

DNA consists of two intertwined strands in the form of a double helix. Each strand is composed of a sequence of nucleotides. Each nucleotide contains one of four bases, adenine (A), thymine (T), guanine (G), or cytosine (C). They are expressed as their sequence order (e.g., TGCCA). Pairing of the two strands comprising the double stranded DNA molecule is specific—A with T, and G with C, (e.g., TGCCA, ACGGT). This specific base pairing of "complementary" strands is the basis of the specificity of the hybridization reaction. To hybridize a "probe" DNA to a "target" DNA both (double stranded) DNA's

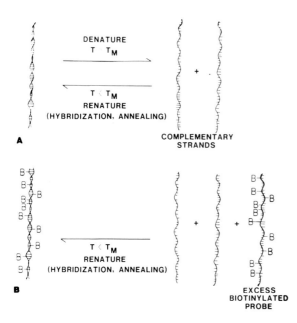

FIG. 1. The DNA denaturation and hybridization reactions. **(A)** The denaturation of double stranded DNA is reversed at temperatures below the T_m. **(B)** Excess biotinylated probe has been added to the denatured target DNA. Renaturation or "hybridization" results in a labeled target.

are heated to separate or "denature" the strands (Fig. 1A). The resulting single stranded probe DNA and single stranded target DNA will "anneal" or "hybridize" if and only if the probe DNA is complementary to the target DNA. They form a stable double-stranded DNA molecule, one strand being composed of probe DNA and the other strand of target DNA (Fig. 1B). In a tissue section the target DNA is immobile and a specially labeled probe can therefore localize the target DNA for microscopic inspection.

The reaction is characterized by a specific melting temperature (the T_m) below which hybridization takes place. The approximate T_m of two sufficiently long complementary strands of DNA can be determined from the following formula: (see 52,59).

$$T_m = 81.5 + 16.6(\log[Na^+]) + 0.41(\%GC) - 0.72(\%\text{formamide})$$

The T_m is affected by the ionic strength of the solution, increasing about 4.6°C for each doubling of $[Na^+]$ (79); by the relative amount of G and C versus A and T in the product increasing about 0.4°C for each percent of G + C over 50% (53); and by the amount of formamide in the solution, decreasing about 0.7° for each 1% of formamide (57). For any given probe and target which are perfectly complementary, the T_m may therefore be calculated.

The specificity of hybridization is dependent on the nucleotide sequence. For each 1 out of 100 mismatched bases, the T_m decreases about 1.2°C (94). Hybridization may be performed at temperatures considerably below the calculated T_m, resulting in the detection of related but nonidentical viruses. (See Hybridization Stringency.)

NONRADIOACTIVE PROBES

The DNA of interest may be isolated from the organism or virus, or may be molecularly cloned in a vector and grown in bacteria. Generally, the DNA plasmid with the viral insert of interest can be mailed at room temperature either in solution or precipitated in alcohol.

Upon receipt, the plasmid is transfected into a suitable bacteria culture and the resulting large quantity of plasmid DNA (with viral insert) chemically isolated from bacterial DNA. These procedures are standard molecular biology laboratory procedures and are well explained in the manuals by Maniatis et al. (52) and Glover (30).

For *in situ* hybridization the whole plasmid including the viral insert is usually labeled. There are regions in the plasmid which may cross react with bacteria, but these have not caused problems in diagnostic pathology because bacteria are readily identifiable as such. There may also be regions in the viral insert which cross hybridize to portions of the human genome at insufficiently high stringency (e.g., CMV, HSV) (77). These are not usually a problem because single copy sequences in nuclei are not detected sensitively enough to be a cause of background. Any offending DNA sequences which cause problems must be cut out enzymatically either prior to cloning or after DNA extraction.

The general clinical utility of DNA hybridization has depended on the development of a nonradioactive label. In 1981 Dr. David Ward and coworkers reported the synthesis of a biotin labeled analogue of thymidine triphosphate, 5-[N-(N-biotinyl-ε-aminocaproyl)-3-aminoallyl] deoxyuridine triphosphate. "Bio-11-dUTP" or "B11-dUTP" for short (13,46, Enzo Biochem, New York, NY; BRL, Bethesda, MD) (Fig. 2). The biotinylated uracil base has a biotin "reporter" molecule attached to it in a position not involved with base pairing. When incorporated into DNA the modified deoxynucleotide can therefore bond normally to the adenine base in the complementary strand with little affect on the T_m.

Other systems of nonradioactive labeling have been used for labeling long nucleic acid molecules. Other biotinylated uracil bases and biotinylated adenine and cystosine bases have been synthesized and are available as deoxynucleotide triphosphates. (BRL, Enzo, Calbiochem-Behring, San Diego, CA). Direct chemical (96,98), photochemical (24) or biochemical (18,90) biotinylation of nucleic acid has been described. Nonradioactive probes with other reporter molecules (3,33,42,73,92,97; Orgenics/FMC Colloids, Philadelphia, PA; Dupont/NEN, Boston, MA) have been synthesized.

Nick Translation (Table 1)

Like thymidine triphosphate (dTTP), B11-dUTP can readily be incorporated into DNA by the "nick translation" enzymatic reaction (52). A test tube containing the isolated or cloned double stranded DNA of interest is treated with a nuclease which introduces random single stranded breaks or "nicks." These nicks are utilized by DNA polymerase to start

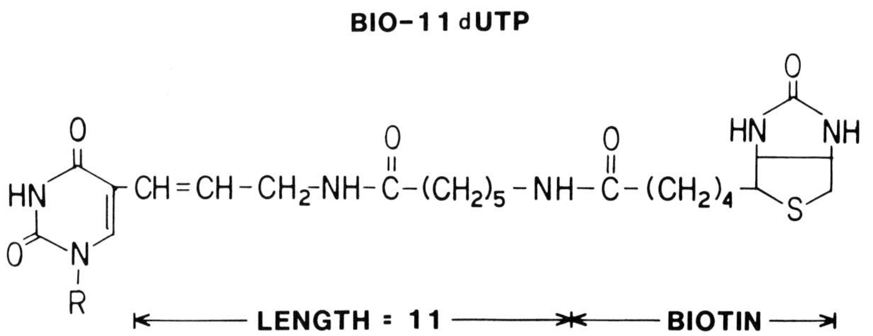

BIO-11 dUTP

FIG. 2. A biotinylated thymidine homologue. The B-11 dUTP extends a linker arm (length 11) to a biotin reporter molecule using a carbon not involved in base pairing.

TABLE 1. *Nick translation protocol*

A.   Nick Translation

Hands should be gloved and washed to remove powder. Do in pairs for each probe, one with a B11-dUTP label and one with dTTP as a nick translation control. All reagents and reactions at 0°C (on ice) unless noted. Put 10ml of distilled water on ice in preparation for step #8. Avoid frost free freezers for storage at −20°C (see 30,52).

1.   Dry tracer 5μCi(=5μl) ^{3}H-=dATP in 1.5 ml microfuge tube. The tracer comes in 50% ethanol. Cool aliquot to −60°C and put in dessicator with drying agent (NaOH pellets or other agent) and draw vacuum. This should take 45 min or less.

2.   Add 10 μl 10XNTB.

3.   Add distilled water as required for final 100 μl volume.

4.   Add 4,000 pmole each dATP, dCTP, dGTP.
     2 μl each of a 2 mM stock, for example. The stocks may be combined and added in one step.

5.   Add 4,000 pmole B11-dUTP *or* dTTP(control).
     Calculate amount depending on stock concentration.

6.   Add 2 μg DNA.
     Calculate proper volume. DNA concentration of stock must be accurately determined. A fluorimeter is best for this. Comparison of staining intensity with controls on an ethidium stained gel is satisfactory.

7.   Mix, and spin a few seconds in microfuge to consolidate on bottom of tube.

8.   Add 2 μl DNase I from diluted stock.
     To make diluted stock pipet 1 μl of stock into 10 ml of water precooled to 0°C in a capped plastic tube (50 ml disposable centrifuge tube). Mix by tilting tube very gingerly.
     Do not swirl as the enzyme will denature. Titrate DNase to determine proper dilution for each new lot.

9.   Add 2 μl DNA polymerase I, (15–20 units).

10. Mix gently and spin a few seconds in microfuge.
     Mix by hand with gentle rapping of tube. The glycerinated pol I should be seen swirling up and mixing.

11. Place into 14°C water bath, 2 hr.
     A "boat" may be constructed of a bit of styrofoam sheet by poking holes to fit the microfuge tubes. The bath may be in an ice bucket or styrofoam box with ice cooled water. Cover and adjust temperature with additional ice as necessary. The bath may also be a regulated water bath in a cold room.

12. Stop by adding 10 μl 0.3 M EDTA and heating at 60° to 68°C for 5 min.

B.   Separate unreacted nucleotides and quantitate incorporation.

13. Sample 2 μl for total counts and put into scintillation vial.
     Fill vial with scintillation fluid first for ease.

14. Make spin-column.
     Construct spin-column of 1 ml syringe, remove plunger and needle, put in glass fiber filter cutout on bottom with plunger, fill to brim with Sephadex slurry. Place the syringe into a 15ml plastic centrifuge tube with hole cut in the cap or 15 ml plastic test tube (Falcon 2017). The wings of the syringe should hold it from falling in. The tip should be well off the bottom. (modification of Maniatis et al. (52).

15. Prespin 700 × g in tabletop centrifuge, room temperature (RT), 2 min.
     Leave liquid in test tube. If slurry is at proper concentration .7–.8 ml bed volume should remain.

16. Place receiving tube.
     Place first a microfuge tube with a lid cut off and then the syringe into the test tube. The wings of the syringe should hold it from falling in and the tip should reside inside but not touching the bottom of the microfuge tube.

17. Pipet the nick translation mixture onto top of bed.
     Start by very slow drops so the bed on top swells and nothing runs down the side.

18. Spin 700 × g, RT, 2 min.

19. Remove syringe and discard in radioactive waste.

20. Remove microfuge tube with fine forceps.

21. Mix vigorously by hand after capping.

22. Sample 2 μl for incorporated counts into scintillation vial.

23. Store probe in microfuge tube at −20°C.

C.   Determine thymidine replacement. [example given]

24. Count ^{3}H in scintillation counter for total [50,940 cpm] and incorporated [8,487 cpm] counts.

25. Calculate % incorporation of ^{3}HdATP [16.7%=8,487/50,940].

26. Determine the theoretical maximum incorporation for the reaction conditions and the GC content.
   Total A in DNA [1,805 pmole] = [2 μg] DNA $\times$ 765 pmole/μg $\times$ [59/50]
   (765 pmole of each base/μg DNA is a constant; 59/50 is the correction factor for a known GC content of 41%, amounting to 59% AT (100% to 41%)) Amount dATP [4,185 pmole] = cold dATP [4,000 pmole] + [3]HdATP [185 pmole]
   (Use specific activity of [3]HdATP [l mmole/27Ci $\times$ 5 μCi = 185 pmole])
   Theoretical maximum incorporation [43%] = Total A in DNA / Amount dATP [= 1,805/4,185]
27. Calculate % replacement [39%] = % incorporation / Maximum theoretical incorporation [16.7/43]

D. Reagents

[3]H-dATP: Purchase (ICN 24012,Irvine,CA, or other).
10XNTB: 0.5M Tris HCl pH 7.8, 0.05M $MgCl_2$, 0.1 M
   2-mercaptoethanol, 0.5 mg/ml nuclease free BSA
Distilled water: Always use glass distilled water.
dXTPs: Prepare according to Maniatis et al. (53) or purchase in solution (Pharmacia,Piscataway,NJ).
   10 mM and 2 mM are typical concentrated and moderately dilute stocks.
BII-dUTP: Purchase (BRL 9507SA or Enzo EBP-806-15), or other dUTP or dXTP (BRL,Calbiochem,Enzo).
DNase I: Make up DNase I (Cooper Biomedical 6330 or other) stock at 5mg/ml in 1 part NTB: 1 part
   glycerol and store at $-20°C$.
DNA pol I: Purchase (BRL 80105A or other).
EDTA: 0.3 Na_2EDTA pH 8.0
TE: 0.01M Tris HCl pH 7.6, 0.001M EDTA pH 8.
Sephadex slurry: G-50 Fine Sephadex(Pharmacia) in 20 fold excess TE. Autoclave. Pour off TE after
   settling to produce 0.7ml bed in spin column. Store at 4°C. Warm a little towards RT
   before use.
Glass fiber filter for spin-column: Cut out the filters (Whatman GF/C) using a #2 cork borer (American
   Scientific Products C8270-1 or other; must produce disks large enough not to fall through the
   syringe opening upon centrifugation).
Scintillation fluid: Type not critical.

---

synthesizing new DNA from fresh nucleotide triphosphates. The new DNA is complementary to the opposite strand, but contains biotinylated uridine in place of thymidine. The result is a biotin labeled DNA probe.

Although nick translation is a standard procedure in molecular biology, there may be a slight difference in its application with a nonisotopic probe and the detailed procedures are therefore presented in Table 1. For the nick translation of small amounts of DNA (1 or 2 μg), 5 μC$_i$ of ^{3}H-dATP or another tritiated deoxynucleotide triphosphate is utilized as a tracer to determine the success of the nick translation. The nick translation reaction should be carried out with equal quantities of B11-dUTP and each of the remaining three unlabeled triphosphates. Good incorporation is obtained with a 2–4 : 1 molar excess of triphosphates to DNA bases. With greater amounts of DNA, the volume and enzymes should be increased proportionately but the lower triphosphate molar excess may be used. The labeled DNA is readily separated from the unreacted nucleotides in a spin-column. The fraction of thymidines replaced can be determined from the fraction of ^{3}H-dATP tracer incorporated into the labeled DNA. A good nick translation reaction replaces 25% to 50% of the thymidines.

A completely nonradioactive probe can be easily synthesized. This is most convenient when biotinylating larger amounts of DNA. The nick translation reaction is made up without tritiated tracer. A small aliquot from this microfuge tube is then placed into another tube with the dried down tritiated dATP. Both nick translation reactions are then conducted simultaneously. The success of incorporation can be assessed from the tritiated tube, while most of the probe remains completely free of radioactivity.

The biotinylated probe is chemically stable and is normally stored frozen at $-20°C$.

It readily withstands repeated freezing and thawing, and withstands room and greater temperatures.

Compounding the Probe (Table 2)

The formamide wets plastic and is difficult to pipet in small quantities. A micropipet with a tip marked for the proper volume of water or a positive displacement syringe should be used to ensure accuracy. The hybridization mixture contains dextran sulfate to enhance hybridization kinetics (100). Since the stock dextran solution is quite viscous it too must be similarly pipetted with care. Accurate concentrations are important in promoting the kinetics and ensuring the stringency of the reaction. The hybridization probe mixture is compounded with the concentration of probe DNA a nominal 1 μg/ml but may vary. (See Complexity.) The hybridization probe mixture may be stored at $-20°C$ and is stable for at least six months.

In order to reduce background, other probe mixtures have included bovine serum albumin (BSA), sodium dodecyl sulfate (SDS), Denhardt's solution (Ficoll, polyvinyl pyrrolidone, BSA) (11), or heparin (84). They are not generally needed in the protocol presented here.

IN SITU HYBRIDIZATION

In 1983 Brigati et al. (13) reported *in situ* hybridization in standard formalin-fixed paraffin-embedded tissue sections with a nonradioactive probe. *In situ* hybridization involves

TABLE 2. *Compounding the hybridization probe mixture*

A. 100 μl of hybridization mixture is made in the example. May be scaled up or down. May prepare at RT. Hands should be gloved and washed.
1. Add 50 μl deionized formamide.
    Pipet by marking tip, as formamide will wet plastic and excess may be drawn up.
2. Add 20 μl dextran sulfate (DS) stock.
    Widen the bore by cutting off the pipet tip. Then mark the micropipet tip using proper volume of water, as the DS is very viscous and may not pipet accurately.
3. Add 10 μl 20 X SSC to microfuge tube.
4. Add 11 μl distilled water.
5. Add 4 μl salmon sperm DNA stock as carrier.
6. Mix well.
7. Add 5 μl BII-labeled probe DNA [nominal 20 μg/ml].
    Amount may vary. Adjust distilled water as necessary. See text.
8. Mix and spin a few sec in microfuge.
9. Store at $-20°C$ (months to years).

20 X SSC: 3M NaCl, 0.3M Na_3citrate, pH to 7.2.
Formamide: Purchase reagent grade. Deionize with mixed bed resin (AG501-X8 Biorad) 4 g/100 ml by stirring 30 min and filtering twice (Whatman #1). Store at 4°C medium term and aliquot and store at $-20°C$ long term.
Dextran Sulfate: Purchase (Pharmacia 17-0340 or other). Different lots of DS may produce differing background intensities. Find a good lot. Prepare stock of 1 part DS: 2 parts water (w/w) with vigorous mixing to wet, and warming 65–99°C until dissolved (e.g., 50 mg DS + 100 μl water). The stock solution has been stored at $-20°C$, probably without deleterious effect.
Salmon sperm DNA: Make stock 10 mg/ml using purified DNA (Sigma 1626, St.Louis,MO; or better quality DNA). Sonicate, or shear by forcing through syringe and needle, to put easily into solution.

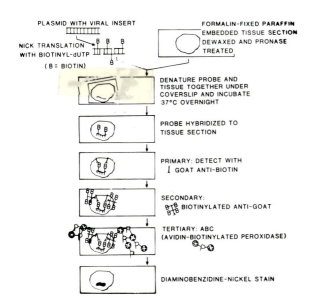

PLASMID WITH VIRAL INSERT

NICK TRANSLATION
WITH BIOTINYL-dUTP
(B = BIOTIN)

FORMALIN-FIXED PARAFFIN
EMBEDDED TISSUE SECTION
DEWAXED AND PRONASE
TREATED

DENATURE PROBE AND
TISSUE TOGETHER UNDER
COVERSLIP AND INCUBATE
37°C OVERNIGHT

PROBE HYBRIDIZED TO
TISSUE SECTION

PRIMARY: DETECT WITH
I GOAT ANTI-BIOTIN

SECONDARY:
BIOTINYLATED ANTI-GOAT

TERTIARY: ABC
(AVIDIN–BIOTINYLATED PEROXIDASE)

DIAMINOBENZIDINE-NICKEL STAIN

FIG. 3. Schematic of the *in situ* hybridization protocol.

three steps: 1) preparation and prehybridization treatment of the slides, 2) hybridization, and 3) detection (Fig. 3, Table 3). No specialized molecular biology equipment is necessary to perform the *in situ* hybridization procedure.

Preparation and Pretreatment (Table 3A,B,C)

One important technical detail of slide preparation is the secure attachment of the section to the glass slides (Table 3A). Good adhesion can be obtained by applying poly-D-lysine to acid cleaned slides. Poly-L-lysine has also been extensively used (54). Others have cleaned slides with alcohol (51). Use of a covalent crosslinking agent has also been reported (5).

When sectioning the paraffin blocks it is important that there be no gelatin whatever in the section flotation bath (Table 3B). After application to the glass slide the sections should be baked in a 56°C oven (just above the paraffin melting temperature) for 2 to 72 hr. Longer baking does not seem to significantly affect hybridization and does help affix the sections better.

There are a few important points of pretreatment (Table 3C). Glass distilled water, not just deionized water, must be used in all reagents and washes to obtain reproducible results. Care must be taken to completely dewax, using fresh xylene in the final bath. Pretreatment with acetic anhydride to reduce background (18,83) has not been found necessary with the procedure presented here, possibly as a result of the greater sensitivity of the procedures with radioactive probes.

The pretreatment of the slides is the most disparate step among the various *in situ* hybridization protocols for tissue sections, as well as tissue culture cells, cytospin preparations, and chromosome spreads. A pretreatment procedure which works well for one type of fixation and preparation may very well be completely unsatisfactory for another (5–7, 18,27,31,34,37,40,51,55,56,62,67,70,72,82,83,86,101). In addition, procedures for the detection of DNA in tissue sections may differ markedly from those designed to detect

TABLE 3. *Hybridization protocol*

A. Slide preparation
  1. Wash slides in 100°C 1N Hcl 30 min.
  2. Rinse in tap water 4 hr.
  3. Rinse in deionized water.
  4. Transfer to 0.01% poly-D-lysine 30 min (a few minutes are probably sufficient).
     Store poly-lysine in freezer in plastic bottle to prevent breakage upon thawing. 1 liter is good for reuse to 1,000 slides.
  5. Rinse in distilled water twice.
  6. Air or oven dry.

B. Tissue sectioning
  1. Section paraffin block 4–6 μm
     The embedding material is Peraplast X-tra (Monoject, St. Louis, MO) or other.
  2. Float on water bath with *no added gelatin*.
     Alcohol may be used to spread sections.
  3. Take up section on treated glass slide.
  4. Heat in paraffin over 56°C overnight.
     Longer heating (3 days) may affix section better and does not seem deleterious to hybridization.
  5. Store slides in box RT.

C. Pretreatment
  Hands should be gloved and washed.
  1. Dewax in xylene 3 changes, 10 min each.
     If there is visible residual wax dissolved after first xylene, leave in xylene until it dissolves. Final xylene should be fresh.
  2. Rinse in absolute ethanol for 3 min.
  3. Quench endogenous peroxidase in freshly made 1% H202 in methanol, 30 min RT.
     Use 97 parts absolute methanol: 3 parts 30% hydrogen perioxide.
  4. Hydrate in absolute, 95%, 70% ethanol, water, water 1 min each.
  5. Apply pronase (nominal 5 mg/ml, must be titrated) 5 min (nominal, may need optimization), RT.
     Time with care. See text.
  6. Stop pronase and postfix by draining slide and applying freshly made 4% paraformaldehyde in PBS, 5 min, RT.
     Use 4 parts PBS: 1 part 20% paraformaldehyde.
  7. Rinse with 0.2% glycine in PBS, 3 changes, 3 min each.
  8. Rinse with 2 X SSC 3 min.
  9. Treat in 2 X SSC/50% formamide ≥3 min.
     Leave in until ready to apply probe.
     Make from 1 part 20 X SSC: 4 parts distilled water: 5 parts deionized formamide

D. Hybridization
  10. Drain slide and wipe around section with tissue wiper so section is still moist.
      Kimwipes wipers (Kimberly-Clark Co.) are used.
  11. Apply 4 to 30 μl of probe with micropipet.
      Use enough probe so it spreads completely after coverslip application. For a 20 × 20 mm coverslip, 15 μl is about right.
  12. Apply silanized coverslip immediately with a very fine forceps.
      Drop it a little so it spreads probe mixture evenly. Coverslips may be cut with a diamond pencil to reduce size and conserve probe.
  13. Seal with rubber cement (Carter's) and let dry well.
      Apply liberally with syringe and 18 gauge needle on both coverslip and slide to seal junction.
  14. Place in moist chamber.
      The chamber is a polyethylene freezer box (Freezette, Safeway). The slides are placed on a rack (old pipet tip holders, or other), which are on very wet paper towels, and the box is lidded.
  15. Denature in 95°C water bath, 15 min.
      Put box in bath. After denaturation, crack the lid for several seconds to dissipate water vapor, and reseal.
  16. Hybridize at 37°C overnight (≥4 hr).
      Put box in water bath or incubator.

E. Detection
  17. Take off cover glass gently with very fine forceps.
      Discard as radioactive if tritium tracer is present.

18. Wash in 2 X SSC, 4 changes, 10 min each, RT.
19. Suppress nonspecific binding by applying 5% rabbit serum-2% BSA in PBS, 10 min RT.
20. Drain, wipe, and apply goat anti-biotin freshly diluted 1:600 (Vector) in PBS-0.1%BSA.
21. Place slides in moist chamber, incubate 37°C, 1 hr.
    A slight increase in intensity is attainable with longer times.
22. Wash in PBS, 3 changes, 3 min each, RT.
23. Apply biotinylated rabbit anti-goat freshly diluted 1:250 (Vector) in PBS-0.1% BSA, 30 min, 37°C in moist chamber.
24. Wash in PBS, 3 changes, 3 min each, RT.
25. Apply ABC made up in PBS, 30 min, 37°C in moist chamber.
    Prepare according to supplier's directions.
26. Wash in PBS, 4 changes, 3 min each, RT.
27. Apply Ni-DAB without peroxide, 5 min, RT.
    Thaw DAB just before use. Add 400 µl 1% $NiCl_2$ to 5 ml DAB slowly while mixing. Filter (Whatman #1), the filter prewetted with PBS. Different lots and different sources of DAB vary in quality. See text. Note: possible carcinogen; inactivate with hypochlorite bleach (Chlorox or other).
28. Drain slide and apply Ni-DAB with peroxide, 4 to 10 min, RT.
    Prepare by adding 7 µl of 3% H_2O_2 to 2 ml of the previously prepared Ni-DAB. The color change may be monitored in a control slide under the microscope. Five minutes is usually ideal. Incubating for more than 10 minutes produces little increase in signal while producing diffuse background duskiness.
29. Terminate peroxidase reaction in water, 3 changes, RT.
30. Air dry (optional).
    Sections tend to stick better if dried at this point.
31. Counterstain with Gill's hematoxylin, or other stain.
    Gill's hematoxylin 10 sec, wash well in tap water, blue in lithium carbonate (saturated, 6 g/500 ml) 2 dips, wash very well (5 to 10 min), dehydrate in alcohol clear in xylene, and coverslip with mounting media (Permount,Fisher). Most any standard staining procedure may be used, including Hematoxylin & Eosin. Avoid acid alcohol.

F. Reagents
10 X PBS: 80 g NaCl, 11.5g Na_2HPO_4 (anhydrous), 2g KCl, 2g KH_2PO_4 to 1 liter. Final pH should be 7.0.
Poly-D-lysine: Purchase (Sigma P7886).
Hydrogen peroxide: 30% (Fisher H-325); 3% (Fisher H-324 or other reagent grade).
Absolute methanol: Reagent grade.
Pronase: Purchase nuclease free pronase. (Calbiochem 537088). Dissolve in 50 mM Tris pH 7.4, prepared from 1 M Tris stock pH 7.4. Aliquot in 1-5 ml and store at −60°C.
20% paraformaldehyde: Make 20% stock in water (in fume hood) by heating, then adding 1 drop of 10 N NaOH while stirring. Filter through .22 or .45 µm membrane filter. Store at 4°C. Has been used for months-year but lifetime is uncertain. See Singer et al. (82)
Silanized coverslips: Acid wash in holders; (in fume hood) 5% dimethyldichlorosilane [HIGHLY TOXIC!] in methylene chloride, 10 sec, wash well with 95% ethanol. Or use other procedures (52).
Glycine: Reagent grade.
Normal rabbit serum: Purchase (DAKO X9020)
Bovine serum albumen (BSA): Purchase, Fraction V. (Calbiochem-Behring 12659).
Goat anti-biotin: Purchase (Vector SP3000).
Biotinylated rabbit anti-goat: Purchase (Vector BA5000 or other)
DAB: Add 100 ml of PBS to a bottle containing 50 mg 3,3′-Diaminobenzidine Tetrahydrochloride (DAB) (Polysciences 4001, Warrington, PA). Filter (Whatman #1). Aliquot 5−10 ml and freeze at −60°C.

RNA. The application of cross linking fixatives such as formalin renders DNA and RNA unhybridizable in a time dependent fashion (82). However DNA is able to recover a large portion of its hybridizing ability after treatment with protease. RNA is less stable in part due to ubiquitous RNases. Pretreatment with detergent (e.g., 0.01% Triton X-100) is used in some procedures with less severe fixation, or in addition to protease. Protease treatment, therefore, enables the use of routinely formalin-fixed (i.e., fixed for 12 or more hr) paraffin-embedded sections for *in situ* hybridization of DNA. Hybridization for high copy number RNA in routinely formalin-fixed paraffin-embedded tissue has been reported (63, 88).

The procedure presented in this chapter works well for neutral buffered formalin, Millonig's formalin, paraformaldehyde, and B5 fixatives. (B5 fixed sections must be treated to remove the mercury pigment: After dewaxing and washing in absolute ethanol, treat with 0.5% iodine in 80% ethanol 5 min, water rinse, 5% sodium thiosulfate 2 min, water rinse.) Pretreatment with pronase (Streptomyces griseus protease, nuclease free; Calbiochem 537088) is used successfully with these fixatives (13,14,65,68). The proper amount of pronase must be experimentally determined with care, in order that sufficient peptide bonds are cleaved in the formalin cross linked proteins, yet the mechanical integrity of tissue section is preserved. Each preparation must be individually tested and titered with two-fold or closer dilutions. The results of the titration often indicate an optimum concentration of up to 5,000 μg/ml in a digestion at room temperature (20°C) for 5 min. Pronase solutions should be aliquoted, and must be stored at or below -60°C.

The pronase reaction is carried out by draining the slide, and applying the pronase solution to the tissue section on the lab bench at room temperature. The reaction is carried out for *exactly* the experimentally determined optimal time, and the slide is tilted on a paper towel to drain the pronase off and the paraformaldehyde solution directly and immediately applied to the tissue section.

The single most important cause of variation and lack of sensitivity in the in situ hybridization procedure is insufficient pronase activity. This results in a marked decrease in hybridization sensitivity. It can often be diagnosed by the failure of hybridization in the portion of the tissue section adjacent to the glass slide. This can be identified by using the high power oil objective to resolve different tissue planes. Poor pronase performance is usually due to poor storage conditions, age, or insufficient concentration, and may be due to excess salt in the buffer, excessive time between thawing of the pronase and its use, or factors unknown. Extension of the digestion time to 10 min or more has proven useful at lower room temperatures or with insufficiently active pronase solutions. If in any doubt, a new lot of pronase should be procured and compounded. Excessive pronase treatment causes severe mechanical destruction with loss of resolution as well as a reduction in hybridization, and should be remedied by diluting the pronase or shortening the time.

Hybridization (Table 3D)

The probe should be applied to the tissue section without dehydrating the section (82). The final 50% formamide/2XSSC wash is drained, the slide wiped around the section, and about 15 μl probe mixture applied (4 to 30 μl depending on the size of the coverslip). Apply enough probe mixture to cover the entire section without bubbles upon applying the coverslip. Apply with enough of a drop so the probe mixture spreads. The silanization helps keep the coverslip from sticking to the tissue. Rubber cement is applied liberally with a syringe to seal the edges of the coverslip and allowed to dry completely.

Some procedures utilize a more rigorous prehybridization procedure, with the addition of Denhardt's solution or other blocking agent and a few hours of "prehybridization" incubation to reduce background. This is not necessary with the procedure presented.

Although the section and probe DNAs may be denatured separately it is of no major benefit. The target and probe DNA on the slides are denatured together under the sealed coverlip on a rack in a tightly covered humidified plastic box. Unger et al. (95) found that a high temperature of denaturation of 105°C (in an oven) yielded optimal sensitivity, and theorized that it may favor penetrance of the probe into the tissue in air dried slides. Probe applied to moist sections may be used with a lower temperature of denaturation (95° to 99°C for 15 min) and produce similar results (71). A water bath is adequate to perform this procedure.

There are a few rules of thumb which have proven useful in the practical use of *in situ* hybridization. The hybridization reaction is generally carried out at 37°C. This is about 25°C below the calculated melting temperature ($T_m - 25°C$) (see Hybridization Stringency). A quite useable signal is detected at 2 hr and the hybridization is essentially complete at 4 hr (71,82,95). Note, however, the kinetics are dependent on the molar concentration of the probe (see Complexity). There is some suggestion that increasing the probe concentration may increase sensitivity (50), possibly in circumstances where network formation may take place (see Probe Size).

Detection (Table 3E)

Although detection can be carried out by a direct application of avidin or streptavidin coupled enzymes or complexes (13,71,82,95), the most sensitive procedures rely on an amplification step. One effective procedure is the use of a primary anti-biotin antibody (Vector Laboratories, Burlingame, CA; Enzo; Calbiochem), amplified by a secondary biotinylated anti-goat, and detected by a tertiary ABC (Vector). The chromogen nickel-DAB (43) has given the most reproducibly sensitive results and the black color is more readily distinguishable from brown tissue components than DAB without nickel. The amount of nickel may be varied and the stock concentration increased if necessary. Too little gives a brown color, too much gives a blue color hard to distinguish from hematoxylin.

An alternative which perhaps is slightly more sensitive but with a slightly higher background (especially on certain tissues such as liver) is a primary avidin reagent (Avidin DH diluted 1:100 [or Avidin DN], Vector) with a secondary biotinylated anti-avidin (1:250, Vector), detected by tertiary ABC.

The DAB signal from the peroxidase can be increased by silver enhancing procedures (15,26,71), at the potential risk of enhancing background. A streptavidin-gold primary may also be enhanced with silver (49,96), as may an antibody-protein A-gold amplification scheme (6,48).

There are commercially available procedures marketed for the detection of biotinylated DNA (Enzo, BRL). In general, the detection of the biotinylated DNA probe depends on detection of the biotin, and the reagents for doing so are commercially available from scores of immunochemical companies. The primary detection must depend on reactivity with anti-biotin, avidin, or streptavidin. One step detection is possible with antibodies, avidin, or streptavidin complexed to fluorescent, enzymatic, or gold bead labels. A modified avidin-biotinylated alkaline phosphatase complex has proven useful for direct detection *in situ* (47,95). Amplification may be obtained with multistep procedures. A primary streptavidin used as a bridge for biotinylated alkaline phosphatase has proven extremely sensitive. Unlike peroxidase, the chromogenic reaction may be run for hours (47,50,82, 95). A primary avidin bridge has not been successful in my hands. I have not performed a comparison of the sensitivities of the various procedures or reagents and can only offer assurance that either of the two procedures detailed will be successful. Other, possibly superior, detection procedures and modifications may be devised according to suggestions in this volume and elsewhere.

Interpretation

Like any pathologic interpretation, definite criteria must be developed to evaluate the hybridization result. In the case of CMV either a hybridizing nucleus or multiple clearly hybridizing cytoplasmic inclusions, are required to define a positive result (Fig. 4). With HSV, VZV, or HPV a clearly hybridizing nucleus is required for definitive DNA hybridization (Figs. 5–7).

In general the *in situ* hybridization procedure is remarkably free of background staining. However the cytoplasm of some cells may contain pigmented material—anthracotic pigment, melanin, hemosiderin, lipofuscin or melanosis. Therefore nuclear hybridization is the preferable criteria where appropriate for the virus. In any case these pigments can usually be readily distinguished from nickel-DAB using high power microscopy. If uncertainty exists the slide may be compared with a similarly stained unhybridized slide.

Scattered blobs may occasionally be present on the slide and may be mistaken for nuclei. They may be distinguished from bona-fide nuclei by the observation of an abrupt and often irregular edge upon high power microscopy. These blobs may sometimes be caused by a poor lot of dextran sulfate, too high a concentration of dextran sulfate, leaving the probe mixture on the slide too long before placing the coverslip, or poor quality carrier DNA.

By far the most difficult problem of interpretation arises when there is nonspecific binding of the biotinylated probe to various tissue components. This does not seem due to endogenous avidin-like activity, since inclusion of biotin monomer into the hybridization mixture is not generally inhibitory. Nor has endogenous biotin been a documented problem, as this would be detectable in a control without a biotinylated probe. If endogenous

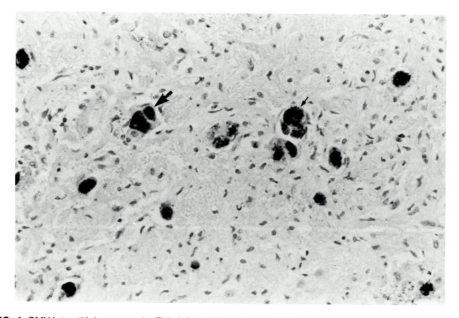

FIG. 4. CMV interstitial pneumonia. This infected lung shows CMV containing cells hybridizing to both the nuclear (large arrow) and cytoplasmic (small arrow) viral inclusions. Sometimes cells hybridize only in the nucleus and may appear morphologically normal (64,65,102). The probe comprises 18% of the genome, purchased prelabeled from Enzo (× 650) final magnification.

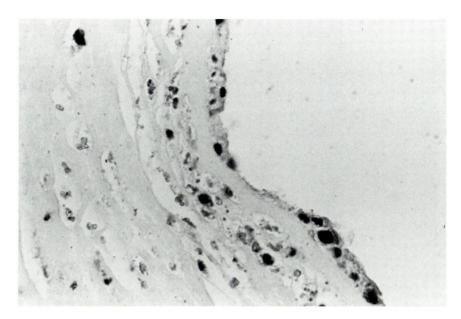

FIG. 5. Transplacental transmission of HSV. HSV-2 infected cells hybridize in the nucleus. A string of adjacent infected cells is seen in the amnion, with scattered infected cells present in the subamnionic chorion. The chorion contains inflamed lesions typical of late HSV lesions at any site. Transplacental transmission of HSV-2 is demonstrated in this case which resulted in a stillbirth. This finding is in collaboration with Dr. J.A. Robb (Scripps Clinic, La Jolla, CA) (75). The probe comprises 82% of the viral genome, a gift from Drs. J.A. Nelson and D.A. Galloway ($\times$ 1600).

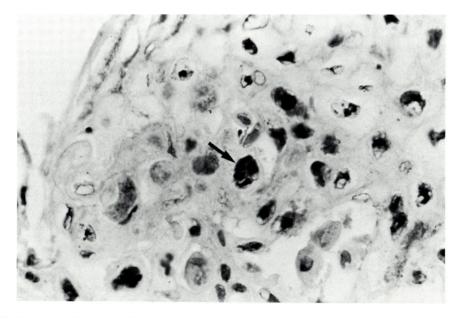

FIG. 6. Varicella-Zoster virus lesion in esophagus. The epithelium contains swollen and acantholytic cells with intranuclear inclusions. Each of 5 nuclei hybridize in a multinucleated cell (arrow). An occasional swollen cell hybridizes only weakly. The probe comprises a high proportion of the genome, a gift from Dr. S. E. Straus ($\times$ 1600).

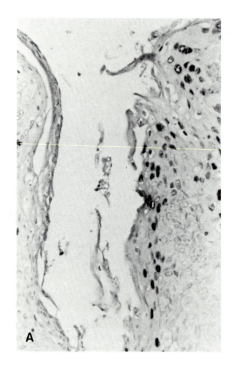

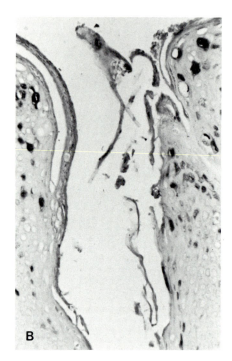

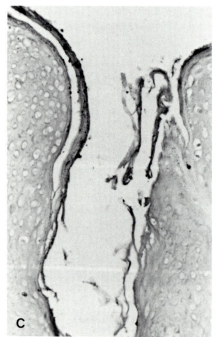

FIG. 7. Human papilloma virus in a dysplastic lesion of the vulva. (**A**) A probe constituted from a mixture of HPV-6, HPV-11, HPV-16, and HPV-18 detects HPV in this lesion in the more differentiated, often "koilocytotic," cells. (**B**) The HPV is typed by an unmixed HPV-16 probe at high stringency conditions. (**C**) Other probes, HPV-18 in this example, show no hybridization at high stringency conditions. There is a correlation between the HPV type, anatomic location, histologic appearance, and malignant potential in dysplastic squamous lesions (80). The probe comprises the entire viral genome, a gift from Drs. L. Gissmann and H. zurHausen ($\times$ 500).

avidin-like activity or endogenous biotin is a problem the slide may be pretreated with the usual avidin and biotin monomer reagents to block these sites (Vector).

With regard to nonspecific binding of biotinylated probe a few specific known problems should be noted. On occasion there is staining of argentaffin cell cytoplasm in gut sections. These cells are usually recognizable because of their location towards the base of the crypt with the cell cytoplasm staining near the basal lamina. Mucin may sometimes stain diffusely. The latter problem may be alleviated by increasing the hybridization stringency or including a high stringency wash. Another, and particularly nasty, nonspecificity is corpora amylacia in the brain. Some procedures use a detergent wash (e.g., 0.1% Triton X-100 in buffer) to reduce background (27).

All sources of nonspecific binding should be revealed by the proper control. *The most important control to rule out nonspecific binding is an unrelated biotinylated probe.* Unlike antibody procedures, in which a single antibody alone may have unique properties of nonspecificity, DNA molecules differ only in their base order and should all have the same properties of *nonspecific* binding (i.e., that binding which is not dependent on the order of the bases). The use of an unrelated biotinylated probe in the same vector followed by the complete detection system will test for nonspecific binding of the probe, and unwanted specific or nonspecific binding of the vector. Nonspecific staining in the detection step and staining due to tissue pigment is also assessed. A nonbiotinylated probe is not adequate to assess nonspecific binding. The confirmation of specific hybridization may be obtained by including excess unlabeled probe in the hybridization mixture to compete out the labeled probe.

The ABC detection procedure is generally free of background, except for the well known moderate disk-like staining of occasional mast cell granules. This background is not severe in formalin-fixed tissue. If problematic, another detection system such as PAP may be substituted. There are extremely rare cases in which endometrial gland nuclei nonspecifically bind to ABC (75). The primary avidin procedure presented gives a very slight diffuse duskiness. This is probably due to nonspecific avidin binding which is amplified to the point of slight visibility, and is worse in some tissues than others. For those who devise other detection procedures other sources of background may of course arise.

OPTIMIZATION AND PITFALLS

Probe Size

The diffusibility of the probe into the tissue section which is cross-linked by fixative is dependent on the fragment size resulting after nick translation (62). The probe size is mainly determined by the concentration of DNase in the nick translation reaction. Singer et al. (82) found that paraformaldehyde-fixed cells tolerate a broad range of probe sizes (50 to 1,000 bases). A longer radioactive probe which included plasmid sequences unrelated to the target sequences provided for network formation and increased the signal. However, signal was variable and backgrounds were often high. A very long probe is therefore not suitable for diagnostic use. In addition, a very long *biotinylated* probe failed to produce increased signal. It seems likely however, that Lo (50) has increased the signal of a biotinylated probe through network formation. No problems attributable to probe size should be expected provided the nick translation resulted in adequate thymidine replacement. If in doubt the probe length may be checked on a denaturing agarose gel (52).

Probe Complexity

For sensitive hybridization, the probe should incorporate as much of the virus genome as possible. The *complexity* of the probe is the length of the viral insert in a given probe mixture, assuming repeated sequences are not significant. This is distinct from probe size which is the length of the denatured DNA after nick translation.

The relationship of the complexity of the probe to the intensity of staining was investigated. A variety of cloned segments of HSV-2 (a gift from Drs. J.A. Nelson and D.A. Galloway) were nick translated with B11-dUTP and hybridized to a control tissue containing a herpes lesion. The staining intensity was assessed as 0 to 4 + . The intensity was closely correlated to the complexity of the probe (Fig. 8). It was not correlated to differences in the fraction of thymidines replaced by the biotinylated base (data not shown). A 1 + increase in intensity corresponded to a lengthening of the probe about threefold. Therefore, for maximum sensitivity of *in situ* hybridization, the use of the most complex available probe is indicated (assuming repeat sequences are not significant). For viral diagnosis, this indicates that a viral probe or a combination of probes should encompass the entire virus genome.

For a virus such as CMV, with a 230 kb genome, several plasmid clones are necessary to encompass clones of the entire genome (22). They may be nick translated separately and then mixed or they may be mixed first and then nick translated as a whole. Although

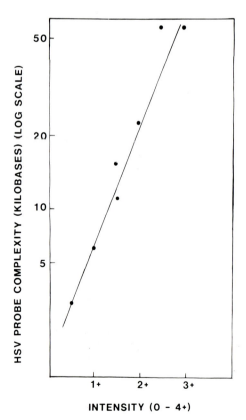

FIG. 8. Intensity of hybridization histochemistry versus probe complexity. A series of probes representing different lengths of the HSV genome (corrected for repeated sequences) were hybridized to a slide with a HSV lesion. The intensity was assessed blindly on a 0 to 4+ scale in ½+ increments. Plotting the intensity on a log scale, the intensity increased 1+ for each threefold increase in probe complexity.

separate nick translation is more accurate since the failure of one probe to a nick translate would be detectable, it is more laborious.

For a virus of high complexity such as CMV, sensitivity can be enhanced slightly by doubling the probe concentration in the hybridization mixture. For a virus of lower complexity such as HPV (8 kb), the concentration of the probe DNA can be lowered substantially and still retain the same sensitivity.

Sensitivity

The minimum sensitivity of *in situ* hybridization in formalin-fixed, paraffin-embedded tissues was directly determined in collaboration with Dr. Anne M. Beckmann (Fred Hutchinson Cancer Center, Seattle, WA). (The HPV probes were gifts from Drs. L. Gissmann and H. zurHausen.) A portion of a vulvar condyloma was divided in half. One-half was analyzed by Southern blotting and determined to contain 13 copies of the HPV-6 genome per cell. The other half was fixed in formalin and analyzed by *in situ* hybridization. The percentage of cells which hybridized was determined, using computer generated microscopic fields to ensure randomness. The intensities of the positive cells were also recorded according to a 1+ to 4+ scale. 1.7% of the cells were found to hybridize. In order to calculate the minimum sensitivity the most uneven distribution of DNA must be assumed to exist—all of the DNA being in the hybridizing cells and none of the DNA being in the cells which fail to hybridize. The minimum sensitivity is therefore 13/.017 or 760 genome copies per cell. If the demonstrated relationship between probe complexity and probe length is valid in this case (see Probe Complexity), a correction of threefold more DNA may be applied to each cell for each 1+ increase in signal greater than 1+. Taking this into account the minimum sensitivity was determined to be 370 copies per cell (data not shown). Since HPV is 8 kb long, these findings imply that 3000 kb or less can be detected with a biotinylated probe in a routinely fixed tissue section.

Much greater sensitivities have been obtained in cell, cytospin, tissue culture, or tissue section preparations in which the background is low and the fixation optimized.

The sensitivity of DNA hybridization for *in situ* procedures can only be obliquely compared with blot procedures such as "Southern" or "dot" blots. Blotting procedures employ disaggregation of the tissue or extraction of DNA rather than examination *in situ*. The maximum sensitivity of a DNA dot blotting procedure with disaggregation of tissue but intact cells (with a radioactive probe) has been estimated at 10,000 papilloma virus molecules, out of up to 10^6 cells per sample (99). The comparative *in situ* sensitivity depends on the distribution of virus DNA in the cells. A small amount of DNA which is evenly distributed might be detectable only by the blot procedure. An uneven distribution among the cells might be detected only by *in situ* hybridization.

When directly compared, the sensitivity of nonradioactive probes has been found lower than radioactive probes, but with a greater spatial resolution (18,60,66,82). Very high sensitivities have however been reported for nonradioactive probes (50,87). The useful sensitivity in routine tissue sections is determined by the balance between sensitivity, resolution, and background. The interpretation criteria must be stringent enough with either nonradioactive or radioactive probes to diagnose a single positive cell with relative certainty while disregarding a random cell with a high background out of a total of 10^6 cells.

Another measure of the sensitivity is the ability to make a diagnosis compared to other means. The following findings pertain to biotinylated probes for *in situ* hybridization and radioactive probes for blotting procedures. The sensitivity of detecting HPV in cervical neoplasia generally but not always has favored the blot procedures (19). *In situ* hybridization for CMV is about as effective as culture for the diagnosis of lung biopsy tissue, and far more effective than routine histology as many CMV infected cells are morphologically normal (58,102). The sensitivity increases slightly as more sections are examined. For the detection of hepatitis B virus (HBV) in liver tissue, *in situ* hybridization has proven generally less sensitive than blotting procedures, but sometimes has been more sensitive than antigen detection procedures, identifying a group antigen negative HBV cases (68,74). *In situ* hybridization was almost as sensitive as culture in a retrospective study of herpes encephalitis (23) and was effective in diagnosing adenovirus in nasopharyngeal secretions (32). Epstein-Barr virus (EBV) in oropharyngeal cells was as readily detected by hybridization as immunofluorescence (78), and more sensitively detected than by culture (86). JC virus has been more sensitively detected by hybridization than immunoperoxidase in brain sections with progressive multifocal leukoencephalopathy (1).

Mixtures of Probes

Since DNA of unrelated sequence exhibits no cross reactivity, biotinylated probes may be mixed with relative impunity. Probes for HPV types 6, 11, 16, and 18 were mixed together to create a combined probe which would detect any of them (Fig. 7). Such a combined probe was used for a papilloma virus screen. If a positive result was obtained, the probes were separately applied to determine the HPV type. The possible correlations between HPV type and oncogenicity and the possibility of diagnosis on Pap smears make this virus of prime interest for detection and typing by hybridization. Unrelated virus probes may also be combined to create a probe detecting any of the component viruses. In the case of a virus genome which is too long to be encompassed by a single plasmid (e.g., Herpesviridae), a combination of probes may be used to increase complexity and thereby sensitivity (see Probe Complexity).

Hybridization Stringency

Viruses which are related to but not identical with the probe may be detected by hybridization. At temperatures well below the T_m ($T_m - 42°C$), two DNA strands with only approximate complementarity of their sequences will successfully hybridize (see DNA Background). Under these "low stringency" conditions, for example, HPV 16 and 18 "cross hybridize". A probe made from one of these viruses can detect the other virus in a tissue section, with acceptably low background. These less stringent conditions are best attained by lowering the amount of formamide in the hybridization buffer rather than markedly lowering the hybridizing temperature. Under excessively nonstringent conditions, the viral probe will cross react with human genomic DNA and all the nuclei in the tissue sections will be stained. Nonstringent conditions are limited as screening procedures because of their potential for high background and false positivity.

Alternatively, the hybridization may be made more stringent. The stringency of CMV or HPV hybridization has been raised to at least $T_m - 12°C$ without significant loss of signal. This is usually done by increasing the temperature. The typing of HPV by high stringency *in situ* hybridization gives similar results to typing by blot hybridization (4,35) (Fig. 7).

General Comparison with Antibody and Culture

In situ hybridization may be more generally applied than antibody procedures because the protocol is invariant to the specific probe involved. Antibodies must be individually characterized and the satisfactory fixatives and pretreatment determined for each one. DNA hybridization has the advantage of a very well defined probe, predictable reactions, predictable cross reactions, relatively easy production in large quantity, stability, and the ability to engineer the probe and/or conditions to detect or not detect related viruses. DNA hybridization techniques utilize reagents which are readily produced in unlimited quantities in bioengineered bacteria, or alternatively can be directly isolated from the organism of interest. The reagents may be characterized by nucleotide sequencing, thereby making their hybridization properties predictable.

In general, antibody techniques are faster and somewhat simpler than *in situ* hybridization. Antibody techniques can yield a diagnosis ½ to 8 hr after biopsy, depending on the exact procedure, and in 24 hr with paraffin-embedded tissue. *In situ* hybridization using frozen sections can yield a diagnosis in 6 to 8 hr after biopsy (use a 15 min or less fixation in 4% paraformaldehyde and reduce or eliminate the pronase). For this the hybridization time is restricted to 2 hr and the hybridizing DNA is detected with a direct ABC with silver enhancement (71), modified alkaline phosphatase complex (95;BRL), or other rapid procedure (82;Enzo). The protocol presented in this chapter involves fixation and embedding of the specimen, usually taking overnight, and a subsequent 12 to 16 hr hybridization, making the total time to diagnosis 48 hr.

The *in situ* hybridization and antibody procedures are faster than viral culture, as viral culture may take several weeks with some viruses (e.g., CMV), or is not available (e.g., HPV, HBV). Tissue obtained under nonsterile conditions and contaminated tissue can be analyzed. Retrospective analyses can be realized using stored paraffin tissue blocks.

Commercial Availability of Viral Reagents

There are some commercially available biotinylated viral probes from Enzo for HSV-1/2, CMV, HBV, HPV-1, EBV, Hepatitis A Virus, Adenovirus type-5, JC, BK, and SV-40. Oligonucleotide probes directly labeled with alkaline phosphatase are available from DuPont (Boston, MA) for HSV-1, HSV-2, HSV-1/2, HBV surface antigen, and HBV core antigen. Of course the differentiation of HBV antigens could only be made by performing hybridization to RNA. Unlabeled adenovirus type-2 and SV-40 DNA is available (Sigma, Calbiochem). Virtually all the important DNA and RNA viruses have been cloned and are usually available from the researcher. Viral probes of high complexity for large viruses, either labeled or unlabeled, are not generally available commercially at the present time.

Unfortunately, as Edberg (20) points out, "the majority of work in the nucleic acid hybridization field is proprietary and is not being published. It may be that many [problems] have been solved, perhaps solved several times in different places, but [are] not available to the independent scientist. Progress will be hindered by this lack of public information. The intermediate steps necessary before a final product is generated will have to be discovered, analyzed, and overcome in multiple individual settings. This massive redundancy of scientific investigation is unprecedented, and the scientific community must find a way to obviate this recently developed situation." By providing a reliable annotated protocol together with some observations about intermediate steps, I hope that this chapter will lessen the effort required by the clinical community to implement this powerful diagnostic technique.

ACKNOWLEDGMENTS

Charles T. Mahan skillfully performed the hybridizations pertaining to procedural optimization. I thank Dr. Jim McDougall for his support and review of the manuscript. This work was supported by Institutional Cancer Grant IN-26Y from the American Cancer Society and NIH Grants CA-15704 and CA-18029.

REFERENCES

1. Aksamit, A. J., Sever, J. L., and Major, E. O. (1986): Progressive multifocal leukoencephalopathy: JC virus detection by in situ hybridization compared with immunohistochemistry. *Neurology*, 36:499–504.
2. Basle, M. F., Fournier, J. G., Rozenblatt, S., Rebel, A., and Bouteille, M. (1986): Measles virus RNA detected in Paget's disease bone tissue by in situ hybridization. *J. Gen. Virol.*, 67:907–913.
3. Bauman, J. G. (1985): Fluorescence microscopical hybridocytochemistry. *Acta Histochem*. Suppl., 31:9–18.
4. Beckmann, A. M., Myerson, D., Daling, J. R., Kiviat, N. B., and McDougall, J. K. (1983): Detection and localization of human papillomavirus DNA in human genital condylomas by in situ hybridization with biotinylated probes. *J. Med. Virol.*, 16:265–273.
5. Berger, C. N. (1986): In situ hybridization of immunoglobulin-specific RNA in single cells of the B lymphocyte lineage with radiolabelled DNA probes. *EMBO J.*, 5:85–93.
6. Binder, M., Tourmente, S., Roth, J., Renaud, M., and Gehring, W. J. (1986): In situ hybridization at the electron microscope level: localization of transcripts on ultrathin sections of Lowicryl K4M-embedded tissue using biotinylated probes and protein A-gold complexes. *J. Cell Biol.*, 102:1646–1653.
7. Bloch, B., Milner, R. J., Baird, A., Gubler, U., Reymond, C., Bohlen, P., le Guellec, D., and Bloom, F. E. (1984): Detection of the messenger RNA coding for preproenkephalin A in bovine adrenal by in situ hybridization. *Regul. Pept.*, 8:345–354.
8. Blum, H. E., Figus, A., Haase, A. T., and Vyas, G. N. (1985): Laboratory diagnosis of hepatitis B virus infection by nucleic acid hybridization analyses and immunohistologic detection of gene products. *Dev. Biol. Stand.*, 59:125–139.
9. Blum, H. E., Haase, A. T., and Vyas, G. N. (1984): Molecular pathogenesis of hepatitis B virus infection: simultaneous detection of viral DNA and antigens in paraffin-embedded liver sections. *Lancet*, 2:771–775.
10. Brahic, M., and Haase, A. T. (1978): Detection of viral sequences of low reiteration frequency by in situ hybridization. *Proc. Natl. Acad. Sci. USA*, 75:6125–6129.
11. Brahic, M., Haase, A. T., and Cash, E. (1984): Simultaneous in situ detection of viral RNA and antigens. *Proc. Natl. Acad. Sci. USA*, 81:5445–5448.
12. Brambilla, C., Tackney, C., Hirschman, S. Z., Columbo, M., Dioguardi, M. L., Donati, M., Paronetto, F. (1986): Varying nuclear staining intensity of hepatitis B virus DNA in human hepatocellular carcinoma. *Lab. Invest.*, 55:475–480.
13. Brigati, D. J., Myerson, D., Leary, J. J., Spalholz, B., Travis, S. Z., Fong, C. K. Y., Hsiung, G. D., and Ward, D. C. (1983): Detection of viral genomes in cultured cells and paraffin-embedded tissue sections using biotin-labeled hyridization probes. *Virology*, 126:32–50.
14. Brutlag, D., Schlehuber, C., and Bonner, J. (1969): Properties of formaldehyde-treated nucleohistone. *Biochemistry*, 8:3214–3218.
15. Burns, J., Chan, V. T. W., Jonasson, J. A., Fleming, K. A., and McGee, J. O'D. (1985): Sensitive system for visualising biotinylated DNA probes hybridised in situ: rapid sex determination of intact cells. *J. Clin. Pathol.*, 38:1085–1092.
16. Burrell, C. J., Gowans, E. J., Rowland, R., Hall, P., Jilbert, A. R., and Marion, B. P. (1984): Correlation between liver histology and markers of hepatitis B virus replication in infected patients: a study by in situ hybridization. *Hepatology*, 4:20–24.
17. Cash, E., Chamorro, M., and Brahic, M. (1985): Theiler's virus RNA and protein synthesis in the central nervous system of demyelinating mice. *Virology*, 15:290–294.
18. Cox, K. H., DeLeon, D. V., Angerer, L. M., and Angerer, R. C. (1984): Detection of mRNAs in sea urchin embryos by in situ hybridization using asymmetric RNA probes. *Develop. Biol.*, 101:485–502.
19. Crum, C. P., Nagai, N., Levine, R. U., and Silverstein, S. (1986): In-situ hybridization analysis of HPV-16 DNA sequences in early cervical neoplasia. *Am. J. Pathol.*, 123:174–182.

20. Edberg, S. C. (1986): Nucleic acid hybridization analysis to elucidate microbial pathogens. *Lab. Med.*, 17:735–738.

21. Falser, N., Bandtlow, I., Haus, M., and Wolf, H. (1986): Demonstration of pseudorabies virus DNA in the mouse inner ear by an in situ nucleic acid hybridization technique in plastic embedded bony material. *J. Microsc.*, 141:55–67.

22. Fleckenstein, B., Muller, I., and Collins, J. (1982): Cloning of the complete human cytomegalovirus genome in cosmids. *Gene*, 18:39–46.

23. Forghani, B., Dupuis, K. W., and Schmidt, N. J. (1985): Rapid detection of herpes simplex virus DNA in human brain tissue by in situ hybridization. *J. Clin. Micro.*, 22:656–658.

24. Forster, A. C., McInnes, J. L., Skingle, D. C., and Symons, R. H. (1985): Non-radioactive hybridization probes prepared by the chemical labelling of DNA and DNA with a novel reagent, photobiotin. *Nucleic Acids Res.*, 15:745–761.

25. Gallaway, D. A., Fenoglio, C., Shevchuk, M., and McDougall, J. K. (1979): Detection of herpes simplex RNA in human sensory ganglia. *Virology*, 95:205–208.

26. Gallyas, F., Gorcs, T., and Merchenthaler, I. (1982): High-grade intensification of the end-product of the diaminobenzidine reaction for peroxidase histochemistry. *J. Histochem. Cytochem.*, 30:183–184.

27. Gendelman, H. E., Moench, T. R., Narayan, O., Griffin, D. E., and Clements, J. E. (1985): A double labeling technique for performing immunocytochemistry and in situ hybridization in virus infected cell cultures and tissues. *J. Virol. Methods*, 11:93–103.

28. Gendelman, H. E., Narayan, O., Molineaux, S., Clements, J. E., and Ghotbi, Z. (1985): Slow, persistent replication of lentiviruses: role of tissue macrophages and macrophage precursors in bone marrow. *Proc. Natl. Acad. Sci. USA*, 82:7086–7090.

29. Gibson, P. E., Gardner, S. D., and Field, A. M. (1986): Use of a molecular probe for detecting JCV DNA directly in human brain material. *J. Med. Virol.*, 18:87–95.

30. Glover, D. M. (1985): *DNA Cloning. A Practical Approach*, Vol. I and II. IRL Press, Oxford, England.

31. Godard, C., and Jones, K. W. (1979): Detection of AKR MuLV-specific RNA in AKR mouse cells by in situ hybridization. *Nuc. Acids Res.*, 6:2849–2861.

32. Gomes, S. A., Nascimento, J. P., Siqueira, M. M., Krawczuk, M. M., Pereira, H. G., and Russell, W. C. (1985): In situ hybridization with biotinylated DNA probes: a rapid diagnostic test for adenovirus upper respiratory infections. *J. Virol. Methods*, 12:105–110.

33. Gratzner, H. G. (1982): Monoclonal antibody to 5-Bromo- and 5-Iododeoxyuridine: a new reagent for detection of DNA replication. *Science*, 218:474–475.

34. Guelin, M., Kejzlarova-Lepesant, J., and Lepesant, J. A. (1985): In situ hybridization: a routine method for parallel localization of DNA sequences and of their transcripts in consecutive paraffin sections with the use of 3H-labelled nick translated cloned DNA probes. *Biol. Cell*, 53:1–12.

35. Gupta, J., Gendelman, H. E., Naghashfar, Z., Gupta, P., Rosenshein, N., Sawada, E., Woodruff, J. D., and Shah, K. (1985): Specific identification of human papillomavirus type in cervical smears and paraffin sections by in situ hybridization with radioactive probes: a preliminary communication. *Int. J. Gynecol. Pathol.*, 4:211–218.

36. Haase, A. T. (1986): Analysis of viral infections by in situ hybridization. *J. Histochem. Cytochem.*, 34: 27–32.

37. Haase, A. T., Brahic, M., Stowring, L., and Blum, H. (1984): Detection of viral nucleic acids by in situ hybridization. In: *Methods in Virology*, Vol. 7, edited by K. Maramorosch and H. Koprowski, pp. 189–226. Academic Press, New York.

38. Haase, A. T., Gantz, D., Eble, B., Walker, D., Stowring, L., Ventura, P., Blum, H., Wietgrefe, S., Zupancic, M., Tourtellote, W., Gibbs, C. J., Jr., Norrby, E., and Rozenblatt, S. (1985): Natural history of restricted synthesis and expression of measles virus genes in subacute sclerosing panencephalitis. *Proc. Natl. Acad. Sci. USA*, 82:3020–3024.

39. Haase, A. T., Walker, D., Stowring, L., Ventura, P., Geballe, A., Blum, H., Brahic, M., Goldberg, R., and O'Brien, K. (1985): Detection of two viral genomes in single cells by double-label hybridization in situ and color microradioautography. *Science*, 227:189–192.

40. Harper, M. E., and Marselle, L. M. (1986): In situ hybridization—application to gene localization and RNA detection. *Cancer Genet. Cytogenet.*, 19:73–80.

41. Harper, M. E., Marselle, L. M., Gallo, R. C., and Wong-Staal, F. (1986): Detection of lymphocytes expressing human T-lymphotropic virus type III in lymph nodes and peripheral blood from infected individuals by in situ hybridization. *Proc. Natl. Acad. Sci. USA*, 83:772–776.

42. Hopman, A. H., Wiegant, J., and van Duijn, P. (1986): A new hybridocytochemical method based on mercurated nucleic acid probes and sulfhydryl-hapten ligands. II. Effects of variations in ligand structure on the in situ detection of mercurated probes. *Histochemistry*, 84:179–185.

43. Hsu, S. M., and Soban, E. (1982): Color modification of diaminobenzidine (DAB) precipitation by metallic ions and its application for double immunohistochemistry. *J. Histochem. Cytochem.*, 30:1079–1082.

44. Jamrich, M., Mahon, K. A., Gavis, E. R., and Gall, J. C. (1984): Histone RNA in amphibian oocytes visualized by in situ hybridization to methacrylate-embedded tissue sections. *EMBO J.*, 3:1939–1943.

45. Koenig, S., Gendelman, H. E., Orenstein, J. M., Dal Canto, M. C., Pezeshkpour, G. H., Yungbluth, M.,

Janotta, F., Aksamit, A., Martin, M. A., and Fauci, A. S. (1986): Detection of AIDS virus in macrophages in brain tissue from AIDS patients with encephalopathy. *Science*, 233:1089–1093.

46. Langer, P. R., Waldrop, A. A., and Ward, D. C. (1981): Enzymatic synthesis of biotin-labelled polynucleotides: Novel nucleic acid affinity probes. *Proc. Nat. Acad. Sci. USA*, 78:6633–6637.

47. Leary, J. J., Brigati, D. J., and Ward, D. C. (1983): Rapid and sensitive colorimetric method for visualizing biotin-labeled DNA probes hybridized to DNA or RNA immobilized on nitrocellulose: Bio-blots. *Proc. Natl. Acad. Sci. USA*, 80:4045–4049.

48. Lee, A. K., and Dellis, R. A. (1987): Immunohistochemical techniques and their applications to tissue diagnosis. In: *Histochemistry in Pathologic Diagnosis*, edited by S. S. Spicer, pp. 31–76.

49. Liesi, P., Julien, J. P., Vilja, P., Grosveld, F., and Rechardt, L. (1986): Specific detection of neuronal cell bodies: in situ hybridization with a biotin-labeled neurofilament cDNA probe. *J. Histochem. Cytochem.*, 34:923–926.

50. Lo, C. W. (1986): Localization of low abundance DNA sequences in tissue sections by in situ hybridization. *J. Cell Sci.*, 81:143–162.

51. Lum, J. B. (1986): Visualization of mRNA transcription of specific genes in human cells and tissues using in situ hybridization. *Biotechniques*, 4:32–40.

52. Maniatis, T., Fritsch, E. F., and Sambrook, J. (1982): *Molecular Cloning*, Cold Spring Harbor Laboratory, NY.

53. Marmur, J., and Doty, P. (1962): Determination of the base composition of DNA from its thermal denaturation temperature. *J. Mol. Biol.*, 5:109–118.

54. Mazia, D., Schatten, G., and Sale, W. (1975): Adhesion of cells to surfaces coated with polylysine. *J. Cell Biol.*, 66:198–200.

55. McAllistar, H. A., and Rock. D. L. (1985): Comparative usefulness of tissue fixatives for in situ viral nucleic acid hybridization. *J. Histochem. Cytochem.*, 33:1026–1032.

56. McCabe, J. T., Morrell, J. I., Ivell, R., Schmale, H. Richter, D., and Pfaff, D. W. (1986): In situ hybridization technique to localize rRNA and mRNA in mammalian neurons. *J. Histochem. Cytochem.*, 34:45–50.

57. McConaughy, B. L., Laird, C. D., and McCarthy, B. J. (1969): Nucleic acid reassociation in formamide. *Biochemistry*, 8:3289–95.

58. Minnigan, H., and Moyer, R. W. (1985): Intracellular location of rabbit poxvirus nucleic acid within infected cells as determined by in situ hybridization. *J. Virol.*, 55:634–643.

59. Minson, A. C., and Darby, G. (1982): Hybridization techniques. In: *New Developments in Practical Virology*, edited by C. Howard. Alan R. Liss, New York.

60. Mitchell, A. R., Ambros, P., Gosden, J. R., Morten, J. E., and Porteous, D. J. (1986): Gene mapping and physical arrangements of human chromatin in transformed, hybrid cells: fluorescent and autoradiographic in situ hybridization compared. *Somatic Cell Mol. Genet.*, 12:313–324.

61. Moar, M. H., and Klein, G. (1978): Detection of Epstein-Barr virus (EBV) DNA sequences using in situ hybridization. *Biochim. Biophys. Acta*, 519:49–64.

62. Moench, T. R., Gendelman, H. E., Clements, J. E., Narayan, O., and Griffen, D. E. (1985): Efficiency of in situ hybridization as a function of probe size and fixation technique. *J. Virol. Methods*, 11:119–130.

63. Morley, D. J., and Hodes, M. E. (1987): In situ localization of amylase in RN and protein. An investigation of amylase gene activity in normal human parotid gland. *J. Histochem. Cytochem.*, 35:9–14.

64. Myerson, D., Hackman, R. C., and Meyers, J. D. (1984): Diagnosis of cytomegaloviral pneumonia by in situ hybridization. *J. Infect. Dis.*, 150:272–277.

65. Myerson, D., Hackman, R. C., Nelson, J. A., Ward, D. C., and McDougall, J. K. (1984): Widespread presence of histologically occult cytomegalovirus. *Hum. Pathol.*, 15:430–439.

66. Nakamura, S., Tourtellotte, W. W., Shapshak, P., and Darvish, M. (1985): Patient with progressive multifocal leukoencephalopathy by in situ hybridization: comparison of in situ hybridization using isotopic and biotinylated probes. *No To Skinkei*, 37:359–364.

67. Nakane, P. K., Moriuchi, T., and Koji, T. (1986): Enzyme-immuno-histo in situ hybridization. *Gan To Kagaku Ryoho*, 13:740–746.

68. Negro, F., Berninger, M., Chiaberge, E., Gugliotta, P., Bassolati, G., Actis, G. C., Rizzetto, M., and Bonino, F. (1985): Detection of HBV-DNA by in situ hybridization using a biotin labeled probe. *J. Med. Virol.*, 15:373–382.

69. Orth, G., Jeanteur, P., and Croissant, O. (1971): Evidence for and localization of vegetative viral DNA replication by autoradiographic detection of RNA-DNA hybrids in sections of tumors induced by Shope papilloma virus. *Proc. Natl. Acad. Sci. USA*, 68:1876–1880.

70. Penschow, J. D., Haralambidis, J., Aldred, P., Tregear, G. W., and Coglan, J. P. (1986): Location of gene expression in CNS using hybridization histochemistry. *Methods Enzymol.*, 124:534–548.

71. Przepiorka, D., and Myerson, D. (1986): A single-step silver enhancement method permitting rapid diagnosis of cytomegalovirus infection in formalin-fixed, paraffin-embedded tissue sections by in situ hybridization and immunoperoxidase detection. *J. Histochem. Cytochem.*, 34:1731–1734.

72. Raap, A. K., Marijnen, J. G., Vrolijk, J., and van der Ploeg, M. (1986): Denaturation, renaturation, and loss of DNA during in situ hybridization procedures. *Cytometry*, 7:235–242.

73. Renz, M., and Kurz, C. (1984): A colorimetric method for DNA hybridization. *Nuc. Acids Res.*, 12:3435–3444.
74. Rijntijes, P. J. M., Van Ditzhuijsen, J. M., Van Loon, A. M., Van Haelst, U. J. G. M., Bronkhorst, F. B., and Yap, S. H. (1985): Hepatitis B virus DNA detected in formalin-fixed liver specimens and its relation to serologic markers and histopathologic features in chronic liver disease. *Am. J. Pathol.*, 120:411–418.
75. Robb, J. A., Benirschke, K., and Barmeyer, R. (1986): Intrauterine latent herpes simplex virus infection: I. Spontaneous abortion. *Hum. Pathol.*, 17:1196–1209.
76. Roy, P., Ritter, G. D., Jr., Akashi, H., Collisson, E., and Inaba, Y. (1985): A genetic probe for identifying bluetongue virus infections in vivo and in vitro. *J. Gen. Virol.*, 66:1613–1619.
77. Ruger, R., Bornkamm, G. W., and Fleckenstein, B. (1984): Human cytomegalovirus DNA sequences with homologies to the cellular genome. *J. Gen. Virol.*, 65:1351–1364.
78. Sauerbrei, A., Wutzler, P., Farber, I., Brichacek, B., Swoboda, R., and Macheleidt, S. (1986): Comparative detection of herpes viruses in tissue specimens by in situ hybridization and immunofluorescence. *Acta Virol. (Praha)*, 30:213–219.
79. Schildkraut, C. L., and Lifson, S. (1965): Dependence of the melting temperature of DNA on salt concentration. *Biopolymers*, 3:195–208.
80. Schneider, A., Kraus, H., Schuhmann, R., and Gissmann, L. (1985): Papillomavirus infection of the lower genital tract: detection of viral DNA in gynecological swabs. *Int. J. Cancer*, 35:443–448.
81. Simon, I., Lohler, J., and Jaenisch, R. (1982): Virus-specific transcription and translation in organs of BALB/Mo mice: comparative study using quantitative hybridization, in situ hybridization, and immunocytochemistry. *Virology*, 120:106–121.
82. Singer, R. H., Lawrence, J. B., and Villnave, C. (1986): Optimization of in situ hybridization using isotopic and non-isotopic detection methods. *Biotechniques*, 4:230–250.
83. Singer, R. H., Lawrence, J. B., and Rashtchian, R. N. (1986): Toward a rapid and sensitive in situ hybridization methodology using isotopic and non-isotopic probes. In: *In situ Hybridization: Application to Neurobiology*, edited by K. Valentino, J. Eberwine, and J. Barchas. Oxford University Press, New York.
84. Singh, L., and Jones, K. W. (1984): The use of heparin as a simple cost-effective means of controlling background in nucleic acid hybridization procedures. *Nucleic Acids Res.*, 12:5627–5638.
85. Sixbey, J. W., and Pagano, J. S. (1985): Biotin-labeled DNA probes for detection of Epstein-Barr virus by in-situ cytohybridization. *Clin. Lab. Med.*, 5:503–512.
86. Sixbey, J. W., Nedrud, J. G., Raab-Traub, N., Hanes, R. A., and Pagano, J. S. (1984): Epstein-Barr virus replication in oropharyngeal epithelial cells. *N. Engl. J. Med.*, 310:1225–1230.
87. Smith, G. H., Doherty, P. J., Stead, R. B., Gorman, C. M., Graham, D. E., and Howard, B. H. (1986): Detection of transcription and translation in situ with biotinylated molecular probes in cells transfected with recombinant DNA plasmids. *Anal. Biochem.*, 156:17–24.
88. Stoler, M. H., and Broker, T. R. (1986): In situ hybridization detection of human papillomavirus DNAs and messenger RNAs in genital condylomas and a cervical carcinoma. *Hum. Pathol.*, 17:1250–1258.
89. Stroop, W. G, Rock, D. L, and Fraser, N. W. (1984): Localization of herpes simplex virus in the trigeminal and olfactory systems of the mouse central nervous system during acute and latent infections by in situ hybridization. *Lab. Invest.*, 51:27–38.
90. Sybanen, A. C., Alanen, M., and Soderland, H. (1985): A complex of single-strand binding protein and M13 DNA as hybridization probe. *Nuc. Acids Res.*, 13:2789–2802.
91. Syrjanen, S., Syrjanen, K., Mantyjarvi, R., Parkkinen, S., Vayrynen, M., Saarikoski, S., and Castren, O. (1986): Human papillomavirus (HPV) DNA sequences demonstrated by in situ DNA hybridization in serial paraffin-embedded cervical biopsies. *Arch. Gynecol.*, 239:39–48.
92. Tchen, P., Fuchs, R. P. P., Sage, E., and Leng, M. (1984): Chemically modified nucleic acids as immunodetectable probes in hybridization experiments. *Proc. Natl. Acad. Sci. USA*, 81:3466–3470.
93. Tenser, R. B., Dawson, M., Ressel, S. J., and Dunstan, M. E. (1982): Detection of herpes simplex virus mRNA in latently infected trigeminal ganglion neurons by in situ hybridization. *Ann. Neurol.*, 11:285–291.
94. Ts'o, P. O. P. (1974): In the beginning. In: *Basic Principles in Nucleic Acid Chemistry*, edited by P. O. P. Ts'o, p. 42. Academic Press, London.
95. Unger, E. R, Budgeon, L. R., Myerson, D, and Brigati, D. J. (1986): Viral diagnosis by in-situ hybridization: Description of a rapid simplified colorimetric method. *Am. J. Surg. Path.*, 10:1–8.
96. Varndell, I. M., Polak, J. M., Sikri, K. L., Minth, C. D., Bloom, S. R., and Dixon, J. E. (1984): Visualization of messenger RNA directing peptide synthesis by in situ hybridization using a novel single-stranded cDNA probe. Potential for the investigation of gene expression and endocrine cell activity. *Histochemistry*, 81:597–601.
97. Viegas-Pequignot, E., Malfoy, B., Leng, M., Dutrillaux, B., and Tchen, P. (1986): In situ hybridization of an acetylaminofluorene-modified probe recognized by Z-DNA antibodies in vitro. *Cytogenet. Cell Genet.*, 42:105–109.
98. Viscidi, R. P., Connelly, C. J., and Yolken, R. H. (1986): Novel method for the preparation of nucleic acids for nonisotopic hybridization. *J. Clin. Micro.*, 23:311–317.
99. Wagner, D., Ikenberg, H., Boehm, N., and Gissmann, L. (1984): Identification of human papillomavirus in cervical swabs by deoxynucleic acid in situ hybridization. *Obstet. Gynecol.*, 64:767–672.

100. Wahl, G. M., Stern, M., and Stark, G. R. (1979): Efficient transfer of large DNA fragments from agarose gels to diazobenzyloxymethyl paper and rapid hybridization by using dextran sulfate. *Proc. Natl. Acad. Sci. USA*, 76:3683–3687.

101. Wilcox, J. N., Gee, C. E., and Roberts, J. L. (1986): In situ cDNA:mRNA hybridization: development of a technique to measure mRNA levels in individual cells. *Methods Enzymol.*, 124:510–533.

102. Wiley, C. A., Schrier, R. D., Denaro, F. J., Nelson, J. A., Lampert, P. W., and Oldstone, M. B. A. (1986): Localization of cytomegalovirus proteins and genome during fulminant central nervous system infection in an AIDS patient. *J. Neurol. Exp. Pathol.*, 45:127–139.

103. Wiley, C. A., Shrier, R. D., Nelson, J. A., Lampert, P. W., and Oldstone, M. B. (1986): Cellular localization of human immunodeficiency virus infection within the brains of acquired immune deficiency syndrome patients. *Proc. Natl. Acad. Sci. USA*, 83:7089–7093.

104. Wolf, H., Haus, M., and Wilmes, E. (1984): Persistence of Epstein-Barr virus in the parotid gland. *J. Virol.*, 51:795–798.

Subject Index